a LANGE medical book

UNDERSTANDING GLOBAL HEALTH

Second Edition

Edited by

William H. Markle, MD, FAAFP, DTM&H
Clinical Associate Professor Family Medicine
University of Pittsburgh School of Medicine
Senior Associate Director Family Medicine Residency
UPMC McKeesport

Melanie A. Fisher, MD, MSc
Professor of Medicine, Section of Infectious Diseases
Director of the International Health Program
Robert C. Byrd Health Sciences Center
West Virginia University

Raymond A. Smego, Jr., MD, MPH, FACP, FRCP, DTM&H, Deceased
Former Professor and Head, School of Medicine
University of the Free State
SOUTH AFRICA

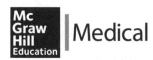 | Medical

New York   Chicago   San Francisco   Athens   London   Madrid   Mexico City
Milan   New Delhi   Singapore   Sydney   Toronto

Understanding Global Health, Second Edition

Copyright © 2014 by McGraw-Hill Education. All rights reserved. Printed in the United States of America. Except as permitted under the United States Copyright Act of 1976, no part of this publication may be reproduced or distributed in any form or by any means, or stored in a data base or retrieval system, without the prior written permission of the publisher.

1 2 3 4 5 6 7 8 9 0 DOC/DOC 18 17 16 15 14 13

ISBN-978-0-07-179100-7
MHID-0-07-179100-0

Notice

Medicine is an ever-changing science. As new research and clinical experience broaden our knowledge, changes in treatment and drug therapy are required. The authors and the publisher of this work have checked with sources believed to be reliable in their efforts to provide information that is complete and generally in accord with the standards accepted at the time of publication. However, in view of the possibility of human error or changes in medical sciences, neither the authors nor the publisher nor any other party who has been involved in the preparation or publication of this work warrants that the information contained herein is in every respect accurate or complete, and they disclaim all responsibility for any errors or omissions or for the results obtained from use of the information contained in this work. Readers are encouraged to confirm the information contained herein with other sources. For example and in particular, readers are advised to check the product information sheet included in the package of each drug they plan to administer to be certain that the information contained in this work is accurate and that changes have not been made in the recommended dose or in the contraindications for administration. This recommendation is of particular importance in connection with new or infrequently used drugs.

This book was set in Adobe Garamond by Cenveo® Publisher Services.
The editors were Jim Shanahan and Cindy Yoo.
The production supervisor was Richard Ruzycka.
Project management was provided by Raghavi Khullar, Cenveo Publisher Services.
The cover designer was Thomas De Pierro.
RR Donnelley/Crawfordsville was printer and binder.

This book is printed on acid-free paper.

Library of Congress Cataloging-in-Publication Data

Understanding global health / [edited] by William Markle, Melanie Fisher.—Second edition.
   p. ; cm.
Includes bibliographical references and index.
ISBN 978-0-07-179100-7—ISBN 0-07-179100-0
  I. Markle, William H., editor of compilation.   II. Fisher, Melanie A.,
editor of compilation.
   [DNLM: 1. World Health. 2. Public Health.   WA 530.1]
RA441
362.1—dc23   2013010281

Contents

Authors

Lisa V. Adams, MD (*Chapter 10*)
Associate Dean for Global Health
Assistant Professor, Section of Infectious Disease and
    International Health, Department of Medicine,
    and Coordinator, Global Health Initiative,
    Geisel School of Medicine at Dartmouth
Hanover, New Hampshire
Lisa.V.Adams@Dartmouth.edu

Jordi Alonso, MD, PhD (*Chapter 17*)
IMIM- Institut Hospital del Mar d'Investigacions
    Mèdiques,
Pompeu Fabra University (UPF),
CIBER en Epidemiología y Salud Pública, Barcelona,
    Spain.
jalonso@imim.es

Onil Bhattacharyya, MD, PhD (*Chapter 20*)
Assistant Professor, Department of Family and
    Community Medicine
Clinical Scientist, Li Ka Shing Knowledge Institute
St. Michael's Hospital, University of Toronto
Toronto, Ontario, Canada
BhattacharyyaO@smh.ca

John H. Bryant, MD (*Chapter 21*)
Adjunct Associate Professor
Department of Public Health Sciences
Senior Faculty Associate, Department
    of International Health
University of Virginia School of Medicine
Charlottesville, Virginia
Johns Hopkins University School of Public Health
Baltimore, Maryland
jbryantwcbr@gmail.com

Thuy D. Bui, MD (*Chapter 2*)
University of Pittsburgh School of Medicine
Director of the Global Health and Underserved
    Populations Track
Internal Medicine Residency Program
University of Pittsburgh Medical Center
Pittsburgh, Pennsylvania
buit@upmc.edu

John R. Butterly, M.D., FACP, FACC (*Chapter 7*)
Executive Medical Director, External Affairs,
    Dartmouth-Hitchcock Medical Center
Associate Professor, Dartmouth Medical School and
    The Dartmouth Institute of Healthcare Policy and
    Clinical Practice
Lebanon, New Hampshire
john.r.butterly@hitchcock.org

Kathleen Casey, MD (*Chapter 14*)
Director, Operation Giving Back
American College of Surgeons
Chicago, Illinois
kcasey@facs.org

Somnath Chatterji, MD (*Chapter 17*)
World Health Organization
Geneva, Switzerland
chatterjis@who.int

Kevin Chan, MD, MPH, FAAP, FRCPC
    (*Chapter 19*)
Assistant Professor, Department of Pediatrics
Faculty of Medicine, Hospital for Sick Children, and
University of Toronto
Toronto, Ontario, Canada
kevinjchan@aol.com

Kathryn Chu, MD, MPH, FACS (*Chapter 14*)
Assistant Professor of Surgery
Johns Hopkins Medical Institutions
Baltimore, Maryland
Honorary Assistant Professor of Surgery, National
    University of Rwanda
Adjunct Faculty, Brigham and Women's Hospital
    Center for Surgery and Public Health
Instructor in Surgery, Harvard Medical School
kathryn.chu@joburg.msf.org

Deyanira Gonzalez de Leon, MD, MPH (*Chapter 4*)
Professor, Department of Health Care
Universidad Autónoma Metropolitana Xochimilco
Mexico DF, Mexico
dgonzal@correo.xoc.uam.mx

Monika Doshi, MPH (*Chapter 4*)
Principal, Saath
West Hartford, Connecticut
mdoshi@saath.co

Emmanuel Elobu, MBBS, MMED (Surgery)
(*Chapter 14*)
Senior Scholar
Global Partners in Anesthesia and Surgery
Mulago National Referral Hospital
Kampala, Uganda
elobuemmy@yahoo.co.uk

Jessica Evert, MD (*Chapter 22*)
Clinical Faculty, UCSF Department of Family and
Community Medicine
Medical Director, Child Family Health International
San Francisco, California
jevert@fcm.ucsf.edu

Sheri Fink, MD, PhD (*Chapter 15*)
Senior Fellow, Harvard Humanitarian Initiative and
New America Foundation
New York, New York
sherifink@gmail.com

Jeffrey K. Griffiths, MD, MPH&TM (*Chapter 6*)
Director, Global Health
Associate Professor of Public Health, and of Medicine
Department of Public Health and Family Medicine
Tufts University School of Medicine
Boston, Massachusetts
Jeffrey.Griffiths@tufts.edu

Wayne A. Hale, MD, MS, FABFP, CAQ Geriatrics
(*Chapter 16*)
Associate Professor, Department of Family Medicine
University of North Carolina at Chapel Hill
Cone Health System Family Medicine
Residency Program
Area Health Education Centers
Greensboro, North Carolina
wayne.hale@conehealth.com

Yanling He, MD (*Chapter 17*)
Director, Department of Epidemiology
Shanghai Mental Health Center
Shanghai, People's Republic of China
heyl2001@yahoo.cn

Rooney Jagilly MBBS, MMED(Surgery) (*Chapter 14*)
General Surgeon
National Referral Hospital
Honiara, Solomon Islands
rjagilly@gmail.com

Jané D. Joubert, MA (*Chapter 16*)
Specialist Scientist
Burden of Disease Research Unit
South African Medical Research Council
PhD scholar, School of Population Health
The University of Queensland
jane.joubert@uqconnect.edu.au

Gregory Juckett, MD, MPH (*Chapter 11*)
Professor of Family Medicine
West Virginia University School of Medicine
Director, WVU International Travel Clinic
Morgantown, West Virginia
gjuckett@hsc.wvu.edu

Sebastiana Kalula, MBChB, MRCP, MMed, MPhil
(*Chapter 16*)
Clinical Head of Division of Geriatric Medicine
Department of Medicine
Institute of Aging in Africa
University of Cape Town, South Africa
Kalula@uctgsh1.uct.ac.za

Ronald Kessler, PhD (*Chapter 17*)
McNeil Family Professor of Health Care Policy
Department of Health Care Policy
Harvard Medical School
Boston, Massachusetts
kessler@hcp.med.harvard.edu

Rashida A. Khakoo, MD, MACP (*Chapter 12*)
Professor and Section Chief
West Virginia University
Robert C. Byrd Health Sciences Center
Morgantown, West Virginia
rkhakoo@hsc.wvu.edu

Amir A. Khaliq, MBBS, MSHS, MSc, PhD (*Chapter 1*)
Associate Professor of Public Health
Health Administration & Policy
College of Public Health
University of Oklahoma Health Sciences Center
Oklahoma City, Oklahoma
amir-khaliq@ouhsc.edu

Judy Lewis, MPhil (*Chapter 4*)
Director Global Health Education
Professor, Departments of Community Medicine and
    Pediatrics
University of Connecticut School of Medicine
Farmington, Connecticut
LewisJ@nso.uchc.edu

Paul R. Larson MD, MS, DTMH (*Chapter 9*)
UPMC St. Margaret Family Medicine Residency
    Program
Director, Global Health Education
UPMC St. Margaret
New Kensington, Pennsylvania
larsonpr@upmc.edu

Scott Loeliger, MD, MS (*Chapter 22*)
Faculty, Contra Costa Family Medicine Residency
Martinez, California
sloeliger@ccfamilymed.com

William H. Markle, MD, FAAFP, DTM&H
    (*Chapter 2*)
Clinical Associate Professor Family Medicine
University of Pittsburgh School of Medicine
Senior Associate Director Family Medicine Residency
University of Pittsburgh Medical Center
McKeesport, Pennsylvania
marklew@upmc.edu

Jeffrey F. Markuns, MD, EdM, FAAFP (*Chapter 8*)
Assistant Professor
Boston University
Executive Director, Boston University Family
    Medicine Global Health Collaborative
Boston, Massachusetts
Jeffrey.Markuns@bmc.org

Christopher Martin, MD, MSc (*Chapter 3*)
Professor and Director, International Programs
Robert C. Byrd Health Sciences Center
West Virginia University School of Medicine
Morgantown, West Virginia
cmartin@hsc.wvu.edu

Jeffry P. McKinzie, MD, FACEP (*Chapter 13*)
Assistant Professor of Emergency Medicine &
    Pediatrics
Vanderbilt University
Nashville, Tennessee
jeff.mckinzie@vanderbilt.edu

Mark W Meyer MD (*Chapter 9*)
UPMC Shadyside Family Medicine Residency
    Program
Director, UPMC Family Medicine Global Health
    Tracts
Shadyside, PA
meyermw@upmc.edu

Alain J. Montegut, MD (*Chapter 8*)
Associate Professor Family Medicine
Boston University
Vice President, Primary Care Development,
    Martins Point Health Care
Portland, Maine
alain.montegut@martinspoint.org

Eileen S. Natuzzi, MD, MS, FACS (*Chapter 14*)
San Diego State University, School of Public Health
Surgical Education Coordinator
San Diego, California
esnmd@mac.com

Thomas E. Novotny, MD, MPH (*Chapter 14*)
Professor and Associate Director for Border and
    Global Health
Graduate School of Public Health
Co-Director, Joint Global Health PhD Program
San Diego State University
San Diego, California
tnovotny@mail.sdsu.edu

Georges Ntakiyiruta, MMed, FCSECSA (*Chapter 14*)
Academic Head of the Department of Surgery,
National University of Rwanda
Kigali, Rwanda
georgentakiyiruta@yahoo.co.uk

Doruk Ozgediz, MD, MSc (*Chapter 14*)
Assistant Professor of Surgery
Yale University School of Medicine
Co-Founder of Global Partners in Anesthesia and
    Surgery (GPAS)
New Haven, Connecticut
doruk.ozgediz@yale.edu

Robin Petroze, MD (*Chapter 14*)
Resident in General Surgery
Research Fellow, National University of Rwanda
University of Virginia
Charlottesville, Virginia
rtp3z@virginia.edu

Clydette Powell, MD, MPH, FAAP (*Chapters 5, 7 & 15*)
Associate Professor
Department of Pediatrics
George Washington University School of Medicine and Health Sciences
Washington, DC
CPowell@USAID.gov

Amany Refaat, MD, MSc, MHPE, PhD (*Chapter 4*)
Public Health Faculty,
College of Health Sciences
Walden University
Minneapolis, MN
Amany.Refaat@walden.edu

Arif R. Sarwari, MD, MSc, MBA (*Chapter 12*)
Associate Professor
West Virginia University
Robert C. Byrd Health Sciences Center
Morgantown, West Virginia
asarwari@hsc.wvu.edu

Vera Sistenich, MD (*Chapter 15*)
Program on Humanitarian Policy and Conflict Research, Harvard University
Emergency Physician, Research Associate
Cambridge, Massachusetts
vsisteni@hsph.harvard.edu

Raymond A. Smego, Jr., MD, MPH, FACP, FRCP, DTM&H (*Chapter 1*)
Professor and Head, School of Medicine
University of the Free State
Bloemfontein, SOUTH AFRICA
Deceased

Gary Snyder, MS (*Chapter 18*)
Assistant Dean, Health Affairs Communications and Marketing
Geisel School of Medicine at Dartmouth
Hanover, New Hampshire
Adjunct Faculty Member
Ohio University Tropical Disease Institute
Gary.Snyder@dartmouth.edu

Anvar Velji, MD, FRCP(c), FACP, FIDSA (*Chapter 21*)
Associate Dean, Global Health Sciences
California Northstate University School of Medicine, Elk Grove, California
Chief Infectious Disease
Kaiser Permanente, South Sacramento
Clinical Professor of Medicine
University of California, Davis
Sacramento, California
anvarali.velji@kp.org

Philip S. Wang, MD (*Chapter 17*)
Division of Services and Intervention Research, National Institute of Mental Health
Bethesda, Maryland

Xiaolin Wei, MBBS, MPH, PhD, FFPH(UK) (*Chapter 20*)
Assistant Professor, Jockey Club School of Public Health and Primary Care, Chinese University of Hong Kong
Hong Kong, China
E-mail: xiaolinwei@cuhk.edu.hk

Edward Winant, PE, PhD (*Chapter 6*)
US Department of State, Vice-Consul
US Consulate General
Almaty, Kazakhstan
Winanteh@state.gov

Godfrey Woelk, BSc (Soc), MCOMMH, PhD (*Chapter 10*)
Former Professor of Epidemiology
Department of Community Medicine
University of Zimbabwe
Harare, Zimbabwe
Adjunct Associate Professor
The University of North Carolina at Chapel Hill
Gillings School of Global Public Health
Department of Health Behavior and Health Education
Chapel Hill, North Carolina
gwoelk@gmail.com

David Zakus, BSc, MES, MSc, PhD (*Chapter 20*)
Professor of Preventive Medicine and Director, Office of Global Health
Faculty of Medicine and Dentistry,
University of Alberta
Edmonton, Alberta, Canada
davidzakus@med.ualberta.ca

Preface

The first edition of this text has been well received and used throughout the world. After six years we feel a new edition is needed to reflect the changes in global health. As we write this preface with most of the book completed, the new Global Burden of Disease 2010 study has just been published.[1] In many ways the health of the world has improved. We see advancement in life expectancy, especially in the developing world, a continued reduction in infectious diseases and malnutrition, and a greater interest among funding agencies and governments in global health. Deaths in children are now much less and 43% of deaths in the world now occur at age 70 or older (compared to 33% in 1990). The HIV/AIDS epidemic has not grown as rapidly as originally predicted, although it remains a major problem in many of the lowest resource areas of the world. Although tuberculosis and malaria still caused 1-2 million deaths each in 2010 and HIV/AIDS caused about 1.5 million deaths, these figures are much less than the burden of the chronic noncommunicable diseases. Two of every three deaths were due to chronic illnesses in 2010. One in four deaths is due to heart disease or stroke (over 13 million). Eight million people died of cancer (38% more than in 1990) and the deaths from diabetes doubled since 1990 to claim 1.3 million lives. Road traffic deaths have increased by almost half.

There are still many areas of concern in global health. Many countries are now caught in the epidemiologic transition. They must continue to direct resources to fighting the old infectious and perinatal causes of morbidity and mortality, while trying to stem the growth of chronic and noncommunicable diseases. The main risk factors continue to be high blood pressure, tobacco, alcohol, and poor diet. Reduction of these risk factors requires much time and effort by public health professionals around the world.

Therefore we are pleased to present this new edition of *Understanding Global Health*. It is intended for anyone with an interest in this topic and is written especially with students in mind. We have continued to list learning objectives for each chapter with study questions at the end to stimulate thought and discussion. The original chapters have been updated, most of them by the original authors. We are indebted to every author, who has given time and expertise in producing an authoritative and useful text. Each author has done significant work to include the most current information. New chapters have been added to this edition on malaria and neglected tropical diseases; problems that continue to affect millions worldwide. Surgical issues are often at the forefront of needed services and a new chapter on surgery is included from the public health perspective. Mental health issues, especially depression, are major sources of disability-adjusted life years (DALYs) and a new chapter helps us understand this area. There is great interest currently in the problem of human trafficking. This is a global health issue and is addressed expertly in a new chapter. Finally new authors have been added to several chapters and have brought added expertise to the book.

It is with a sad heart that we must report the death of one of the editors, Dr. Ray Smego. He passed away suddenly December 15, 2012 in South Africa. Ray was serving as Dean of the School of Medicine, Faculty of Health Sciences at the University of the Free State in Bloemfontein at the time of his death. He had a long career in international medical education and had taught at schools in many countries around the world. He had served as a Fulbright scholar to Pakistan in the field of tropical medicine and public health and was the founding director of the international health program at West Virginia University. Ray had a true heart to improve health care for all peoples around the world and especially underserved peoples wherever they may be. The other editors have missed his expertise in the final stages of this book and wish to dedicate this book to him. He will be greatly missed by all who knew him.

We appreciate the help from the staff at McGraw-Hill, especially Jim Shanahan, Cindy Yoo, and Laura Libretti for their help and assistance. We hope this book will continue to contribute to better understanding of people around the world and better health for all.

William H. Markle, MD
Melanie Fisher, MD
Ray Smego, MD[†]

---

†Deceased.

Dedication

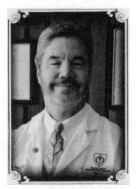

Raymond A. Smego, MD, MPH, FACP, FRCP, DTM&H (1952-2012)

We would like to dedicate this edition to Raymond Smego Jr., MD, MPH, DTM&H who was a co-editor of this book. Dr. Smego was passionately committed to global health for his entire medical career. He cared deeply for people everywhere. He dedicated his life to improving the health of people around the world through education, service, and scholarship. We honor his legacy through the writing of this book.

Melanie Fisher, MD, MSc
William Markle, MD, FAAFP, DTM&H

Global Health: Past, Present, and Future

1

Amir A. Khaliq and Raymond A. Smego, Jr.

LEARNING OBJECTIVES

- *Understand the history of global health and the role of forces and interventions that have helped shape the current state of health in the world*
- *Identify and discuss the major health problems and challenges facing the world today*
- *Propose and discuss suitable and promising solutions for these challenges to be considered by policymakers, planners, and health workers around the world*

DEFINING GLOBAL HEALTH

There are many different views on the definitions of "global health." To emphasize the need for collaborative actions across nations and geographic boundaries, Beaglehole and Bonita[1] proposed that Global Health is "collaborative trans-national research and action for promoting health for all." Other authors[2] have defined it as "health issues that transcend national boundaries and governments and call for actions on the global forces that determine the health of people." Still others[3] consider it to be the "worldwide improvement of health, reduction of disparities, and protection against global threats that disregard national borders." Koplan and colleagues[4] suggest that "The Global in global health refers to the scope of problems, not their location. Thus . . . global health can focus on domestic health disparities as well as cross-border issues." They propose that "global health is an area for study, research, and practice that places a priority on improving health and achieving equity in health for all people worldwide."

Although there is considerable overlap in the framework for action provided by several of the definitions, some experts make a distinction of terms with the assertion that international health primarily focuses on health issues in low-income countries, whereas public health focuses on the health of the population of a specific country or community. Others,[5] however, challenge such distinctions and contend that global, international, and public health all attempt to address the same underlying social, economic, and environmental factors that affect the health of populations whether locally, nationally, or globally.

HISTORICAL PERSPECTIVE

Throughout human history, numerous advances have improved the quality and longevity of life around the globe. Dating back to ancient civilizations, there is evidence of societies working to improve the health of the general public. The Babylonian sewage systems were among the first designed to protect the water supply from contamination and disease. The discovery of pasteurization by Louis Pasteur in the 1860s helped to ensure the safety of food supplies throughout the world. With the implementation of the constitution of the World Health Organization (WHO) in 1948, the mass tuberculosis (TB) immunization campaign with bacillus Calmette-Guérin vaccine in 1950, and the onset of the Malaria Eradication Program in 1955, many of the important developments related to global health in modern times occurred in the post–World War II period of the 1940s and 1950s. In 1980, smallpox was officially eradicated from the planet, and although polio and measles have not yet been eradicated, rapid progress is being made globally toward the goal of entirely protecting children and communities from these once debilitating diseases.

Table 1-1. Selected public health milestones during the 20th century.

Immunizations
Control of infectious diseases
Pasteurization
Fluoridation of drinking water
Maternal-child interventions
Family planning
Wastewater systems
Prevention and treatment of heart
  disease and stroke
Motor vehicle safety
Workplace safety
Safer and healthier foods
Tobacco control
Reducing firearm-related injuries
Preventing birth defects

Prior to these developments of the second half of the 20th century, improvements in living conditions and the availability of new technologies had already had a remarkable effect on the quality of life and health indicators in the industrialized countries of Europe, North America, and the Oceania. Public health is credited with adding almost 30 years to the life expectancy of people in the United States in the last century and more than 22 years elsewhere in the world. As a testament to the remarkable contributions of the field of public health for all peoples around the world, in 1999 the Centers for Disease Control and Prevention (CDC) formulated its list of 10 great public health achievements in the 20th century.[6] An expanded list of public health milestones is shown in Table 1-1.

Compared with the collective impact of improved living conditions including nutrition, sanitation, housing, education, and income, the impact of disease-oriented medical care on the overall health status of a country has been relatively small. There is now widespread recognition of the inextricable link between health, development, and sociopolitical stability. Technological, socioeconomic, and political factors all contribute to the overall well-being of a community. Internal strife and protracted political conflicts in a country, in contrast, lead to socioeconomic instability that negatively affects the health and welfare of its citizens. Unfortunately, developing countries around the globe have track records of long-standing conflicts and widespread corruption. Every year billions of dollars are siphoned from developing countries to banks in developed countries. Some have suggested that improvement in the health status of populations, particularly those in developing countries, can occur only through sociopolitical change, a global outlook, and local empowerment.

International aid agencies and voluntary groups are important partners in this effort. However, a lack of political will and geopolitical instability are major barriers in bringing about a positive change.

At the beginning of the 20th century, the most important public health problems throughout the world were largely infectious in nature. The life expectancy for a citizen living in the United States was 45.2 years, and the five leading causes of death were influenza and pneumonia, tuberculosis, diarrhea and enteritis, heart disease, and stroke (Figure 1-1). Life expectancy and median survival for persons residing in less developed countries was even less. However, 100 years later, life expectancy and health status of people all over the world had dramatically improved. In 2009, the average Japanese was living 83 years, the average American 79 years, the average Norwegian 81 years, and the average Malaysian 73 years. Many of the impoverished countries in Africa, Asia, and Latin America also made impressive public health gains in the last 100 years.[7]

Unfortunately, these gains have not been uniformly distributed across continents or among countries on the same continent. In some developing countries marred by poverty and political strife, the achievements in socioeconomic conditions and health indicators have been less than dramatic. In 2009, the average life expectancy of a person in Afghanistan was 48 years, in Bangladesh 65 years, in Chad 48 years, and in Guatemala 69 years (Figure 1-2). Sadly, the human immunodeficiency virus/acquired immunodeficiency syndrome (HIV/AIDS) pandemic, with its epicenter in Africa during the 1980s and 1990s, has contributed to huge setbacks in longevity in much of the African continent and elsewhere in the 30 years since its recognition. For example, the life expectancy of a Ugandan man was approximately 47.4 years in 1980–1985, 39.7 years in 1985–1990, and 38.9 years in 1995–2000. In 2009, the life expectancy of a Ugandan man had climbed back to only 48 years.[7]

In the transition to modernity, global populations are trading one set of diseases for another. In many countries, improved socioeconomic conditions that led to a reduction in the prevalence of infectious diseases and associated reductions in morbidity and mortality have led to a tremendous increase in lifestyle-related diseases such as obesity, coronary artery disease, hypertension, and diabetes. In most middle-income and lower-income countries in Asia, Africa, and Latin America, both communicable (e.g., pneumonia, diarrheal diseases, HIV/AIDS, tuberculosis, and malaria) and noncommunicable diseases (heart disease, cancer, diabetes) concurrently present major public health challenges as these countries continue their developmental, demographic, and epidemiologic transitions.

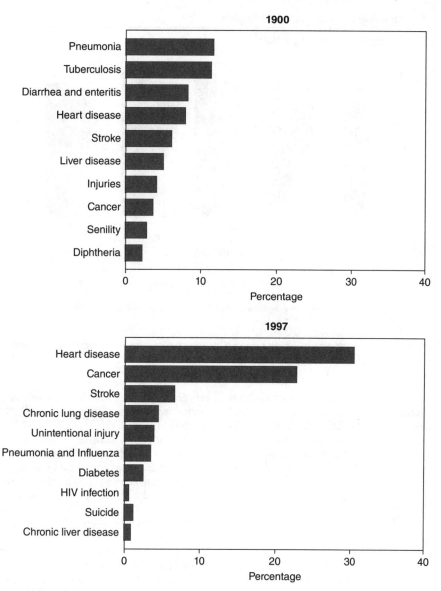

Figure 1-1. The 10 leading causes of death as a percentage of all deaths: United States, 1900 and 1997. From the Centers for Disease Control and Prevention. Achievements in Public Health, 1900–1999: Control of Infectious diseases. *MMWR* 48;621–629: 1999. (*Reproduced with permission.*)

The leading causes of mortality in most developed countries today are heart disease, cancer, stroke, chronic lung disease, and unintentional injury. In 2009, these diseases collectively accounted for 64% of all deaths in the United States, whereas pneumonia, influenza, and HIV/AIDS account for only 4.5% of annual deaths. However, the UN Population Division estimates that "group 1 diseases," which include maternal, perinatal, nutritional, and communicable diseases, are largely responsible for a reduction of more than 15 years of life expectancy in African countries. If developed countries' levels of group 1 diseases could be achieved in African countries, their life expectancy at birth would rise to about 72 years.[8-10] In all parts of the globe there is a transition taking place from first-generation or "group 1," diseases (e.g., common childhood infections, malnutrition, and reproductive risks) to second- (e.g., cardiovascular and cerebrovascular

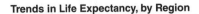

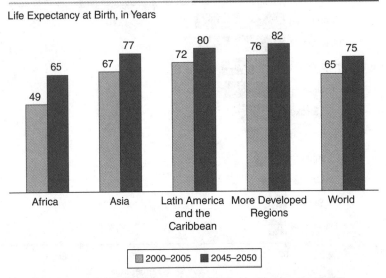

Trends in Life Expectancy, by Region

Life Expectancy at Birth, in Years

Source: United Nations, *World Population Prospects*: The 2004 *Revision* (medium scenario), 2005.
© 2006 Population Reference Bureau

Figure 1-2. Trends in life expectancy, by world region. From the Population Reference Bureau, 2006. *http://www. prb.org/presentations/g-trends-in-life-expect.ppt. (Reproduced with permission.)*

diseases, cancers, and degenerative diseases) and third-generation diseases (e.g., violence, drug abuse, and mental and psychosocial illness).[11] With this background, in the following sections we discuss some of the notable public health achievements and global health challenges.

GLOBAL HEALTH ACHIEVEMENTS AND CHALLENGES

Infectious Diseases

The 19th-century shift in population that accompanied industrialization and migration from countryside to cities led to overcrowding in poor housing served by inadequate or nonexistent public water supplies and waste-disposal systems. These conditions resulted in repeated outbreaks of cholera, dysentery, TB, typhoid fever, influenza, yellow fever, and malaria. Global urbanization accelerated dramatically during the last 4 decades of the 20th century, putting more and more people at risk for large-scale disease outbreaks. In 1960, an estimated 70% of the world's population lived in rural areas. Today, almost the same percentage lives in cities and large metropolitan areas. In 1994, the city of Shanghai, China, experienced an outbreak of viral hepatitis A involving more than 400,000 cases. Throughout the Indian subcontinent, virtually every major city has experienced outbreaks

of viral hepatitis E linked to contaminated municipal water systems, involving up to 200,000 persons per outbreak.

Public health control of infectious diseases after 1900 was based on the 19th-century discovery of microorganisms as the cause of many serious diseases such as cholera and tuberculosis.[12,13] Successes in disease control resulted largely from improvements in sanitation and hygiene, the discovery of antibiotics, and the implementation of universal childhood vaccination programs. Scientific and technologic advances played a major role in each of these areas and are the foundation for today's disease surveillance and control systems. In Western countries, the incidence of many infectious diseases began to markedly decline by 1900 because of public health improvements, implementation of which continued into the 20th century.

In Western countries, deaths from infectious diseases continued to decline at a steady pace during the 20th century. In particular, there has been a remarkable drop in infant and child mortality and a 29.2-year increase in life expectancy. For example, in the United States in 1900, 30.4% of all deaths occurred among children younger than 5 years; in 1997, that percentage was only 1.4%. In 1900, the three leading causes of death were pneumonia, tuberculosis, and diarrhea and enteritis, which (together with diphtheria) caused a third of all deaths. Of these deaths, 40% were among children younger than 5 years. In 1997, heart disease and cancers accounted for 54.7% of all deaths, with less than 5% attributable to pneumonia, influenza, and HIV infection.[6]

Despite this remarkable progress, infectious diseases remain among the greatest threats to persons living in developing countries of the world. More than 60% of children who die under the age of 5 die because of pneumonia, diarrhea, or measles. Together, pneumonia and diarrhea are still responsible for 40% of childhood deaths in the world, and only 39% of children with diarrhea receive oral rehydration therapy.[14] Even as the number of TB cases is at an all-time low in the United States, the global prevalence of tuberculosis is at an all-time high, with about 8 million new cases and 3 million deaths annually.[7] HIV/AIDS has become the most devastating epidemic in human history, supplanting the 1918 influenza pandemic that resulted in 20 million deaths. Since 1981, an estimated 33 million lives have been lost to HIV/AIDS, and almost 35 million more persons are believed to be infected worldwide, especially in sub-Saharan Africa, India, and Southeast Asia.[15-17] This pandemic is still in progress. In addition, more than 30 new diseases were discovered in the last 30 years (Table 1-2), demonstrating the

Table 1-2. Newly recognized pathogens or diseases since 1981.

Avian influenza
Acanthamebiasis
Australian bat Lyssavirus
Babesiosis
Bartonella henselae
Coronaviruses/Severe acute respiratory syndrome
  (SARS)
Ehrlichiosis
Hantavirus pulmonary syndrome
Helicobacter pylori
Hendra or equine morbilli virus
Hepatitis C virus
Hepatitis E virus
HIV/AIDS
Human herpesvirus 8
Human herpesvirus 6
Human T-cell lymphotropic virus I
Human T-cell lymphotropic virus II
Borrelia burgdorferi
Microsporidia
  Encephalitozoon cuniculi
  Encephalitozoon hellem
  Enterocytozoon bieneusi
Nipah virus disease
Parvovirus B19
Variant Creutzfeldt-Jakob disease

volatility of infectious diseases and the unpredictability of disease emergence. Many of the emerging infectious diseases, such as avian flu, severe acute respiratory syndrome (SARS), and hemolytic uremic syndrome, are zoonotic.

In many urban and rural areas of Asia, Africa, and Latin America, basic public health services such as provision of clean drinking water, sewage and solid waste disposal, food safety, and public education about hygienic practices (e.g., food handling and hand washing) are still lacking or inadequate. These deficiencies contribute to a continued global burden of major waterborne and foodborne diseases such as acute diarrheal illness (responsible for approximately 1.9 million deaths every year), viral hepatitis, enteric fever, and brucellosis. A third of the world's population suffers from diseases caused by unsafe food, and many of these people experience long-term complications or death. Furthermore, animal and pest control programs are inadequate worldwide and contribute to the persistence of diseases such as malaria, rabies, viral encephalitis, trypanosomiasis, plague, and anthrax.[7,9,10]

Antimicrobial Agents and Drug Resistance

Antibacterial drugs have been in civilian use for more than 60 years and have saved the lives of millions of individuals with streptococcal and staphylococcal infections, gonorrhea, syphilis, and other infections. Drugs have also been developed to treat viral diseases (e.g., herpes and HIV infection), fungal diseases (e.g., candidiasis and aspergillosis), and parasitic diseases (e.g., malaria). Penicillin, discovered fortuitously by Sir Alexander Fleming in 1928, was not developed for medical use until the 1940s, but it soon changed the face of medicine. The drug quickly became a widely available medical product that provided effective treatment for previously incurable bacterial illnesses, with a broader spectrum and fewer side effects than sulfa drugs.

Successes in reducing morbidity and mortality from infectious diseases during the first three quarters of the 20th century led to complacency about the need for continued research into the treatment and control of infectious microbes. However, the global appearance of AIDS, the emergence of multidrug-resistant (MDR) TB and extensively drug-resistant (XDR) TB, and an overall increase in infectious disease mortality during the 1980s and 1990s have provided additional evidence that as long as microbes can evolve, new diseases will appear.

Molecular genetics has provided valuable insights into the remarkable ability of microorganisms to evolve, adapt, and develop drug resistance in an unpredictable and dynamic fashion. Resistance genes are transmitted from one bacterium to another on plasmids, and viruses evolve through replication errors, reassortment of gene segments, and by crossing species barriers. Recent examples of microbial evolution include the development of a virulent strain of avian influenza in Hong Kong (1997–1998)[18] and the MDR W strain of *Mycobacterium tuberculosis* in the United States in 1991. The emergence of vancomycin-intermediate *Staphylococcus aureus* (VISA), vancomycin-resistant *S. aureus* (VRSA), and extensively drug-resistant gram-negative bacterial infections have become major causes of global concern among clinicians and microbiologists.

The increased development and use of antimicrobial agents has hastened the development of drug resistance. The emergence of drug resistance in many microorganisms is reversing some of the therapeutic miracles of the last 50 years and underscores the importance of disease prevention. Antimicrobial multidrug resistance is a serious and growing problem worldwide for community-based infections caused by *Plasmodium* species, *M. tuberculosis*, *Streptococcus pneumoniae*, *Salmonella*, and *Campylobacter* species, *Neisseria gonorrhoeae*, *Helicobacter pylori*, and HIV, as well as for nosocomial infections due to staphylococci, enterococci, Enterobacteriaceae, *Clostridium difficile*, and systemic fungi. (See Chapter 12 for more information on antimicrobial resistance.)

For continued success in controlling infectious diseases, the global public health system must prepare to address diverse challenges including the emergence of new infectious diseases, the reemergence of old diseases (sometimes in drug-resistant forms), large foodborne outbreaks, and acts of bioterrorism. Continued protection of health requires improved capacity for disease surveillance and outbreak response at the local, state, national, and global levels; the development and dissemination of new laboratory and epidemiologic methods; continued development of antimicrobial agents and vaccines; and ongoing research into environmental factors that facilitate disease emergence.[19] The global public health response to the SARS outbreak in 2004 and avian flu in 2010 demonstrated unprecedented cooperation in surveillance and dissemination of information. Ongoing research into the possible role of infectious agents (e.g., *Chlamydia trachomatis*, viruses) in causing or intensifying certain chronic diseases such as type 1 diabetes mellitus, some cancers, and atherosclerotic heart disease is also imperative.

Immunizations

Vaccine development to prevent the spread of communicable diseases is probably the single most important achievement in biomedical science and the most effective public health intervention in the history of humankind. At the beginning of the 20th century, infectious diseases exacted an enormous toll on the global population. It has only been since the middle of the 20th century that unprecedented achievements in the control of many vaccine-preventable diseases have been made.[20] The eradication of smallpox and the 95% or greater decline in morbidity and complications resulting from vaccine-preventable diseases included in the Expanded Program on Immunizations (EPI), initiated by WHO in 1974, attest to the remarkable efficacy of vaccines.

Although the first vaccine against smallpox was developed by Edward Jenner in 1796, more than 100 years later its use was still not widespread as evidenced by an outbreak in the United States between 1900 and 1904 that resulted in more than 48,000 cases in each of the 4 years. Four other vaccines—against rabies, typhoid, cholera, and plague—were developed late in the 19th century but were also not used widely by 1900. Since 1900, vaccines have been developed or licensed against 22 other diseases (Table 1-3). In 2012, an American child required 27 doses of vaccines by age 15 months to be protected against 14 childhood diseases.[21]

In 1974, when EPI was launched by the WHO, less than 5% of the world's children were immunized against the six initial target diseases—diphtheria, tetanus, pertussis (whooping cough), polio, measles, and tuberculosis—during their first year of life. Until then, immunization programs had been largely restricted to industrialized countries, and even there they were only partially implemented. By 1990, and, after a slight interim drop in coverage rates, again in recent years, almost 80% of the 130 million children born each year were immunized before their first birthday. In 2010 alone, 109 million children under the age of 1 year were inoculated with the three doses of the diphtheria-tetanus-pertussis (DTP3) vaccine.[22]

As coverage for each of the childhood vaccines has increased, now involving over 500 million immunization contacts with children every year, there has been a corresponding drop in the incidence of the targeted infectious diseases. The EPI (which today includes yellow fever and hepatitis B vaccines) now prevents the deaths of at least 3 million children a year. In addition, at least 750,000 fewer children are blinded, physically disabled, or mentally retarded as a result of vaccine-preventable diseases. Indeed, WHO's Millennium Development Goal # 4 (MDG4) essentially depends on widespread successful immunization of children to reduce by two thirds the global burden of under-5 mortality by the year 2015.[22,23]

The success of vaccination programs in the United States and Europe inspired the 20th-century concept of disease eradication, the idea that a carefully

Table 1-3. Vaccine-preventable diseases by year of vaccine development or U.S. licensure.

Disease	Year
Smallpox[a]	1798[b]
Rabies	1885[b]
Typhoid	1896[b]
Cholera	1896[b]
Plague	1897[b]
Diphtheria[a]	1923[b]
Pertussis[a]	1926[b]
Tetanus[a]	1927[b]
Tuberculosis	1927[b]
Influenza[a]	1945[c]
Yellow Fever	1953[c]
Poliomyelitis[a]	1955[c]
Measles[a]	1963[c]
Mumps[a]	1967[c]
Rubella[a]	1969[c]
Anthrax	1970[c]
Meningococcal Meningitis	1975[c]
Pneumococcal[a]	1977[c]
Adenovirus	1980[c]
Hepatitis B[a]	1981[c]
Haemophilus Influenza Type B[a]	1985[c]
Japanese B Encephalitis	1992[c]
Hepatitis A[a]	1995[c]
Varicella[a]	1995[c]
Lyme Disease	1998[c]
Rotavirus[a]	1998[c], 2006[c,d]
Human Papilloma Virus	2005[c]
Herpes Zoster	2006[c]

[a]Vaccine recommended for universal use in U.S. children. Routine smallpox vaccination ended in 1971.
[b]Vaccine developed (i.e., first published results of vaccine usage).
[c]Vaccine licensed for use in the United States. The first rotavirus vaccine was withdrawn from the market in 1999. Lyme Disease vaccine was withdrawn from the market in 2001.
[d]Live oral pentavalent vaccine.
Adapted from the Centers for Disease Control and Prevention. Achievements in Public Health, 1900–1999: Impact of vaccines universally recommended for children—United States, 1990–1998. *MMWR* 1999;48:243–248.

targeted disease could be eliminated from all human populations through global cooperation. In 1980, approximately a decade after it had been eliminated from the United States and the rest of the Western Hemisphere, smallpox was eradicated worldwide after a decade-long campaign involving 33 nations. International partnerships involving affluent industrialized nations, the WHO, and Rotary International are now seeking to eradicate polio. In fact, poliomyelitis caused by wild-type viruses has been nearly eliminated from all countries with the exception of Afghanistan, Nigeria, and Pakistan. Cases of measles and *Haemophilus influenzae* type b (Hib) among children younger than 5 years have been reduced to record low numbers. The disfiguring and debilitating disease known as dracunculiasis also shows the promise of being eradicated in the foreseeable future.[23,24]

Additional targets for disease control and eradication are presented by the relatively recent licensure of vaccines such as the seven-valent conjugated pneumococcal vaccine, tetravalent meningococcal vaccines, and the human papilloma virus vaccine. Anticipated new vaccines include those for influenza, parainfluenza, and chronic diseases (e.g., gastric ulcers and cancer caused by *Helicobacter pylori*, and rheumatic heart disease that occurs as a sequel to group A streptococcal infection). Given the constrained national health care resources in the 1990s, many developing countries were forced to re-examine epidemiologic data to set their infectious diseases priorities and choose between adding Hib or hepatitis B vaccine to their national EPI programs.[24]

Clinical trials are already Change to underway for a vaccine to prevent and/or treat HIV infection. The global immunization challenge of this century will be finding a way to finance the provision of an effective HIV vaccine for some of the poorest countries in the world where it is needed the most. Creative and innovative strategies to fund the worldwide distribution of an effective HIV vaccine, when it becomes available, are being aggressively discussed with potential funders such as the World Bank, the International Monetary Fund, and the Gates Foundation. The number of persons who will be candidates for a HIV vaccine will depend on whether the immunobiologic response is strictly preventive or therapeutic.

Additionally, efforts to control measles, which causes approximately 1 million deaths each year, and to expand rubella vaccination programs are also underway around the world. The use of existing vaccines in routine childhood vaccination programs worldwide must be expanded, and successful introduction of new vaccines must occur as they are developed. Such efforts regarding infectious diseases control and prevention can benefit both rich and poor countries by decreasing disease importations from developing countries. In the West, millions of cases of potentially preventable influenza, pneumococcal disease, and hepatitis B occur each year in adolescent and adult populations. New vaccines will be targeted at these age groups.

Despite the 3 million or so lives saved by DTP3 and measles vaccines every year and the high rates of immunizations reported in most countries,[23] there are serious challenges in terms of disparities within and across countries. In particular, countries in South Asia and Africa face challenges that at times are referred to as the "fallacy of coverage."[25] Namely the challenges have to do with suboptimal age-appropriate immunizations, social and gender inequity in immunizations, poor access, women's as well as both parents' education, and low vaccine efficacy rates that in some areas were found to be as low as 41.5%. To deal with these and other challenges, in 2006 WHO and the United Nations Children's Fund (UNICEF) launched a new initiative titled the Global Immunization Vision Strategy.[22] Other challenges include strategies for hard-to-reach populations, evidence-based prioritization of global initiatives to introduce new vaccines, and strengthening and expansion of the global immunization and surveillance infrastructure.[26]

National treasuries and vaccine delivery systems must be capable of successfully implementing an increasingly complex vaccination schedule. As is true for other public health interventions, national and international efforts to promote vaccine use largely depend on public health infrastructure, economic development, and political stability. With the proper mind-set and establishment of priorities, even low-income countries can achieve remarkable rates of vaccination coverage for their populations.

Coronary Heart Disease and Stroke

An estimated 17.3 million deaths—or 30% of total global deaths in 2008—resulted from various forms of cardiovascular disease (CVD): ischemic or coronary heart disease, cerebrovascular disease or stroke, hypertension, heart failure, and rheumatic heart disease. Of these, 7.3 million deaths were due to ischemic heart disease, 6.2 million to cerebrovascular disease, and an additional 3.9 million to hypertensive and other heart conditions.[27,28] At least 20 million people survive heart attacks and strokes every year, with a significant proportion of them requiring costly clinical care, which puts a huge burden on long-term care resources. CVD affects people in their midlife years, undermining the socioeconomic development not only of affected individuals but also of families and nations. Lower socioeconomic groups generally have a greater prevalence of risk factors, diseases, and mortality in developed countries. A similar pattern is emerging as the CVD epidemic matures in developing countries as well.

CVDs are no longer only a problem of the developed world. In 2005, some 80% of all CVD deaths worldwide took place in developing low- and middle-income countries, and these countries accounted for 86% of the global CVD disease burden. More than 60% of all coronary heart disease occurs in developing countries, partly as a result of increasing longevity, urbanization, and lifestyle changes. Furthermore, CVD is responsible for 10% of disability-adjusted life years (DALYs) lost in low- and middle-income countries and 18% in high-income countries. DALYs represent healthy years lost and indicate the total burden of a disease as opposed to simply the resulting death. The global burden of coronary heart disease is projected to rise from 46 million DALYs in 1990 to 82 million in 2020. The rise in the prevalence of CVD reflects a significant combination of unhealthy dietary habits, increased tobacco consumption worldwide, and reduced physical activity levels as a result of industrialization, urbanization, economic development, and food market globalization.[7,28]

More than half of the deaths and disability from heart disease and strokes each year can be reduced by a combination of simple cost-effective national efforts and individual actions to reduce major risk factors such as high blood pressure, diabetes mellitus, high cholesterol, obesity, and smoking. Obesity is one of the newest global epidemics, especially in developed and transitional countries. Because of obesity's association with CVD and diabetes, obesity control and weight loss must be considered an important global strategy to improve the health and well-being of people all over the world.

The WHO, in collaboration with the CDC, is presently working to provide actionable information to develop and implement appropriate national and international policies related to the global epidemic of heart attack and stroke. As part of such efforts, the WHO has produced *The Atlas of Heart Disease and Stroke*,[28] which addresses the problem of heart disease and stroke in a clear and accessible format for a wide audience. This highly valuable reference material has been designed for use by policymakers, national and international organizations, health professionals, and the general public. This picturesque atlas is in six parts: CVD, risk factors, the burden, action, the future and the past, and world tables.[28]

In the West, major milestones in the management of angina pectoris and heart attack, including expensive or invasive interventions such as diagnostic coronary angiography, thrombolytic therapy, statins, IIb/IIIa platelet receptor blocker drugs, percutaneous transluminal coronary angioplasty, coronary artery stenting, coronary artery bypass grafting, and ventricular assist devices, have resulted in impressive declines in mortality from these conditions in the past 2 decades. The technologic future holds even more promise for CVD treatment. However, these diagnostic and therapeutic services are largely inaccessible to the majority of populations living in Asia, Africa, and Latin America. No matter what advances are made in high-technology medicine, major global reductions in death and disability from CVD will only come from preventive measures involving modification of risk factors—not from cure. The most cost-effective methods of reducing risk are population-wide interventions combining effective economic, educational, and broad health promotion policies and programs emphasizing reduction in the dietary intake of fats, cessation of smoking, and salt restriction.

HIV/AIDS

Much progress has been made since the early 1980s in improving our understanding of the etiology, epidemiology, natural history, and treatment of HIV/AIDS. Global efforts to combat the spread of AIDS have also become more organized and coordinated. In the last decade or so, more financial and pharmacologic resources have been made available to governmental and nongovernmental organizations internationally. For example, in 2004, only 700,000 people in low- and middle-income countries had access to antiretroviral treatment, but the number in 2011 had risen to 8 million (Figure 1-3). Since 2001, HIV incidence has fallen in 22 countries in sub-Saharan Africa and in 33 countries in the world. Also, the total number of AIDS-related deaths in the world fell from 2.2 million in 2005 to 1.8 million in 2010. In the developed world, the availability of antiretroviral treatment has led to a significant drop in morbidity, disability, and mortality resulting from AIDS. For example, the fixed-dose combination of two antiretroviral drugs, tenofovir and emtricitabine, is being used effectively to treat and prevent HIV infection. Combining the two agents

into one tablet reduces the pill burden and increases compliance with antiretroviral therapy.

In the early days of this pandemic, a patient could not expect to live more than 6 months after being diagnosed with AIDS. Now most patients who have access to adequate treatment can expect to live for many years if not a full lifespan. Aside from effectively managing and treating the disease, the real goal is the development and widespread availability of a vaccine. Limited prophylactic success has been achieved with the use of topical microbicides among women. However, their widespread use poses many practical and cultural challenges.[15-17]

According to UNAIDS data, at the end of 2010 an estimated 34 million people in the world were living with HIV, which represents a 17% increase from 2001. This increase is largely due to improved access for AIDS patients to antiretroviral therapy.[16,17] The UNAID 2011 World AIDS Day Report estimated that since 1997, 2.5 million deaths have been averted in low- and middle-income countries, and in 2010 alone, 700,000 AIDS-related deaths were averted. In 2010, there were 2.7 million new infections including 390,000 among children. The number of new infections was also down by 21% as compared with the peak in 1997. However, there were 7,000 new HIV infections every day in 2009 of which 97% were in low- and middle-income countries and 1,000 were in children under 15 years of age. Notably, between 2001 and 2010, AIDS-related deaths increased dramatically from 7,800 to 90,000 in Central Asia and Eastern Europe and from 24,000 to

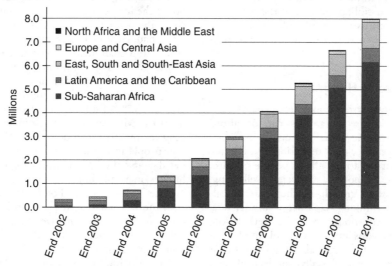

Figure 1-3. Number of people receiving antiretroviral therapy (ART) in low- and middle-income countries, by region, 2002–2011. World Health Organization. *http://www.who.int/hiv/topics/treatment/data/en/index1.html.* (*Reproduced with permission.*)

56,000 in East Asia. Also, the number of AIDS-related deaths in the Middle East increased 60% in the same period from 22,000 to 35,000.[7,15]

Since 2004, the U.S. Global AIDS initiative, also known as the President's Emergency Plan for AIDS Relief (PEPFAR), has made more than $30 billion available to combat the global HIV/AIDS epidemic. This program works in partnership with national governments and the private sector in more than 30 countries around the world, but primarily in Africa and the Caribbean. Despite many controversies about PEPFAR, by the end of 2008 the initiative is claimed to have supported, at least partly, antiretroviral treatment for more than 2 million people and averted 240,000 newborn infections and 1.1 million deaths worldwide.[29,30]

The HIV/AIDS epidemic has become a major obstacle in the fight against hunger and poverty in developing countries. Because most HIV-infected persons with AIDS are young adults who normally harvest crops, food production has dropped dramatically in countries with high HIV/AIDS prevalence rates. In half of the countries in sub-Saharan Africa, per capita economic growth is estimated to be falling by between 0.5% and 1.2% each year as a direct result of AIDS. Infected adults also leave behind children and elderly relatives who have little means to provide for themselves. In 2003, 12 million children were newly orphaned in sub-Saharan Africa, a number that rose to 14.8 million in 2010.[31] Since the epidemic began, 30 million people have died from AIDS, and more than 18 million children have lost at least one parent to the disease. The UNICEF term *child-headed households,* meaning minors orphaned by HIV/AIDS who are raising their siblings, illustrates the gravity of the situation.[31,32] Approximately 68% of the 34 million HIV-infected people in the world today live in sub-Saharan Africa.

Poverty and World Hunger

Hunger is the most extreme manifestation of poverty, where individuals or families cannot afford to meet their most basic need for food. It manifests itself in many ways other than starvation and famine. Undernourishment negatively affects people's health, productivity, sense of hope, and overall well-being. Lack of food can stunt growth, heighten susceptibility to illness, slow thinking, sap energy, hinder fetal development, and contribute to mental retardation. Economically, the constant securing of food consumes valuable time and energy, allowing less time for work and earning income. Socially, the lack of food erodes relationships and causes shame so that those most in need of support are often least able or willing to seek it.[33] It is estimated that every day more than 16,000 children die from hunger-related causes (one child every 5 seconds).

Poor nutrition and caloric deficiencies cause nearly one in three people to die prematurely or have disabilities, according to the WHO.[34] Pregnant women, nursing mothers, and children are among the groups most at risk for undernourishment. Every year, nearly 11 million children die before they reach their 5th birthday. Almost all of these deaths occur in developing countries, three fourths of them in sub-Saharan Africa and South Asia, the two regions that also suffer from the highest rates of hunger and malnutrition. Most of these deaths are attributed not to outright starvation but to diseases that opportunistically afflict vulnerable children with host defenses weakened by hunger. Each year, more than 20 million low-birthweight infants are born in developing countries. These infants are at a high risk of dying in infancy, and those who survive often suffer lifelong physical and cognitive disabilities.

The four most common childhood illnesses are diarrhea, acute respiratory illness, malaria, and measles. Each of these illnesses is both preventable and treatable. Yet poverty interferes with people's access to immunizations and medicines. Chronic undernourishment superimposed on inadequate treatment greatly increases a child's risk of death. In the developing world, 27% of children younger than 5 years are moderately to severely underweight, 10% are severely underweight, 10% are moderately to severely wasted or seriously below weight-for-height, and an overwhelming 31% are moderately to severely stunted or seriously below normal height-for-age.[35]

Proclaiming that freedom from hunger and malnutrition is the inalienable right of every man, woman, and child, the delegates at the World Food Conference in 1974 had set a goal to eradicate hunger, food insecurity, and malnutrition within a decade. In 1996, at the World Food Summit in Rome, a target was set to reduce the number of undernourished people in the world from 800 million to 400 million by the year 2015.[36,37] Endorsed by 189 countries in 2000, WHO's Millennium Development Goals to be achieved by 2015 include reducing by half the 1.2 billion people in the world who live on less than US$1 per day and the 852 million people who suffer from hunger on a daily basis.

The International Food Policy and Research Institute has noted that the world faces a new food economy that likely involves both higher and more volatile food prices. After the food price crisis of 2007–2008, food prices started rising again in June 2010, with international prices of maize and wheat roughly doubling by May 2011. The peak came in February 2011, in a spike that was even more pronounced than that of 2008, according to the food

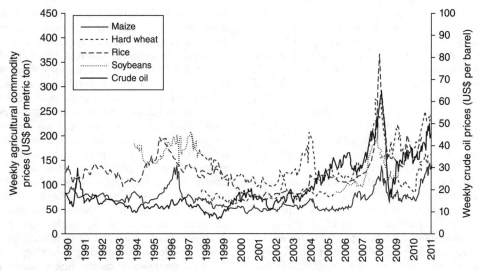

Figure 1-4. Major exporters' shares of global maize, wheat, and rice exports, 2008. *http://www.ifpri.org/node/8436.* (*Reproduced, with permission, from Torero M. "Food Prices: Riding the Rollercoaster." In 2011 Global Food Policy Report, Figure 1. Washington, DC: International Food Policy Research Institute, 2011.*)

price index of the Food and Agriculture Organization of the United Nations. When prices of specific commodities are adjusted for inflation, though, the 2011 price spike did not reach the levels of 2008 (Figure 1-4). As food prices have risen, the world hunger situation has become worse as witnessed by the famine in the horn of Africa in 2011–2012 resulting from a prolonged drought.

In 2005, the number of people in developing regions living on less than $1.25 per day was 1.4 billion, and it is expected that in 2015, 920 million people globally will be living below the International Poverty Line of $1 per day. More than half (51%) of the population in sub-Saharan Africa and 39% of those in Southern Asia in 2005 were living on less than $1.25 per day. The global financial crisis that began in 2008 in North America and Europe has also seriously affected the developing countries due to a decline in exports, trade, and investment and has pushed into extreme poverty an additional 64 million people worldwide. In 2005, 1.5 billion people in the world worked on their own or as unpaid family workers. In the period 2005–2007, 16% of the world population (830 million people), and 26% of the population in sub-Saharan Africa were undernourished; one of four children in developing countries was underweight. Children in rural areas are twice as likely to be undernourished as those in urban areas. However, there is a glimmer of hope resulting from improvements noticed in some of the developing countries. For example, the MDG Report 2010 noted that poverty in China will fall to only 5% of the population in 2015 and in India from

51% in 1990 to 24% in 2015. Also, it is projected that globally by the year 2015, the number of people in extreme poverty will decrease by 188 million.[38]

Maternal and Child Mortality

A hundred years ago, most obstetric deliveries and surgical interventions around the world were performed without appropriate sanitary and antiseptic measures. As a result, large numbers of maternal deaths were caused by sepsis following delivery or illegally induced abortion, with the remaining deaths primarily attributed to hemorrhage and toxemia. The complications of pregnancy and childbirth are still a leading cause of death and disability among women of reproductive age in the poorest regions of the world.[39,40] Severe bleeding, infections, unsafe abortions, and hypertensive disorders (preeclampsia and eclampsia) are responsible for 70% of global maternal deaths. Every year more than 136 million women worldwide—of which 16 million are girls between 15 and 19 years of age—give birth, and 20 million of them experience pregnancy and childbirth-related illnesses including infection, anemia, fistula, incontinence, and depression.

An estimated 287,000 women, nearly 800 every day, died worldwide in 2010 from maternal causes, and 99% of these deaths occurred in developing countries. The number of deaths in 2010 represents a 47% decline from an estimated 543,000 maternal deaths in 1990. Sub-Saharan Africa and South Asia accounted for 85% of maternal deaths in 2010 with India and Nigeria alone accounting for a third of all maternal deaths and

40 countries experiencing rates of 300 or more maternal deaths per 100,000 live births. In the same year, Chad and Somalia experienced extremely high rates of 1,000 or more maternal deaths per 100,000 live births. Currently, only 23 of 181 countries are on track to achieve the UN Millennium Development Goal of reducing global maternal mortality by 75% between 1990 and 2015. The most impressive gains have been in countries such as China where the maternal mortality rate dropped from 87 in 1990 to 40 in 2008, Vietnam where it dropped from 158 to 64, and Bolivia where it fell from 439 to 180 in the same period.

Like the rest of the world, maternal mortality declined dramatically in the United States in the last 100 years. However, the gains have not kept pace since 1990, and disparities between racial and socioeconomic groups have continued to persist in the 21st century. The maternal mortality rate in the United States reported for 1987 was 6.6 per 100,000 live births, whereas in 2007, the most recent year for which data are available from the CDC, the rate was reported as 12.7 deaths per 100,000 live births. Among non-Hispanic black women, the rate was 28.4, whereas it was 10.5 for non-Hispanic white women.

The foundations for maternal risk are often laid in girlhood. Women whose growth has been stunted by chronic malnutrition are vulnerable to obstructed labor. Anemia predisposes to hemorrhage and sepsis during delivery and has been implicated in at least 20% of postpartum maternal deaths in Africa and Asia. The risk of childbirth is even greater for women who have undergone female genital mutilation; an estimated 2 million girls are mutilated every year. Poor obstetric education and delivery practices are mainly responsible for the high numbers of maternal deaths, most of which are preventable. In many low-income countries, obstetric services are primarily provided by poorly trained or untrained medical practitioners. For example, in the Central African Republic only 44% of babies are delivered by skilled attendants. Most births occur at home with the assistance of midwives or traditional birth attendants. In much of the world, consistent access to antenatal and postnatal care, which benefits both mother and fetus, is inadequate or lacking.

Child mortality is closely linked to poverty and lack of education, and more than a third of under-5 deaths in the world are related to undernutrition.[41] It is important to emphasize that considerable progress has been made in reducing child mortality since 1990, with the number of under-5 deaths being reduced from nearly 12 million to 6.9 million in 2011, a drop of 41% (Figure 1-5). However, the

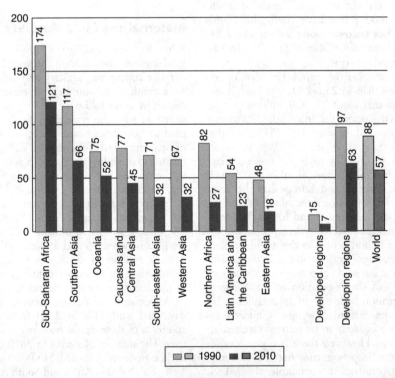

Figure 1-5. Under-5 mortality (deaths per 1,000 live births) declined in all regions between 1990 and 2010. *http://www.childinfo.org/files/Child_Mortality_Report_2011.pdf.* (*Reproduced with permission.*)

Table 1-4. Environmental and medical interventions contributing to the decline in infant mortality in the 20th century.

Improvements in standards of living
Reduction in vaccine-preventable diseases
Control of milkborne diseases
Improvements in nutrition
Declining fertility rates
Longer birth spacing
Advances in clinical medicine
Discovery of antibiotics and fluid and electrolyte therapies
Technologic advances in neonatal medicine
Improvements in access to health care
Increases in surveillance and monitoring of disease
Placing of infants on their back
Regionalization of perinatal services
Improvements in education levels

numbers for 2011 still indicate the largely avoidable deaths of 19,000 children in the world every day, or 51 deaths per 1,000 live births globally.[41] Similar to the trends in maternal mortality rate, much of the improvement in under-5 mortality has occurred in East Asia, North Africa, Latin America, and the Caribbean, with a reduction of more than 50% in under-5 mortality in these regions. In these regions, economic growth, better nutrition, and better access to health care have helped spur improvements in child survival (Table 1-4). However, in Sub-Saharan Africa 1 in 9 children and in South Asia 1 in 16 children dies before the age of 5 years. This is in stark contrast to developed countries where the rate is 1 death in 152 under-5 children. On the positive side, the rate of decline in under-5 mortality in sub-Saharan Africa has been much faster in the last 2 decades with the doubling of the rate between 1990 and 2000 and 2000 and 2011. One estimate has nearly half of all under-5 deaths in the world now occurring in only five countries: India, Nigeria, Democratic Republic of the Congo, Pakistan, and China. Most of these deaths are due to pneumonia (18%), preterm-birth complications (14%), diarrhea (11%), complications during births (9%), and malaria (7%). However, the rate of under-5 mortality per 1,000 live births, as estimated by the World Bank for 2011, was highest in Sierra Leone (185), Somalia (180), Mali (176), and Chad (169). In contrast, the number for under-5s in many of the developed countries such as Japan, Finland, Singapore, Germany, France, Denmark, and Belgium was only between 3 and 4 deaths per 1,000 live births.

The U.S. infant mortality rate declined more than 90% from 1915 through 1997 to 7.2 per 1,000 live births. The infant mortality rate in 2010 was 6.14 deaths per 1,000 live births, which represents a decrease of 3.9% from the rate of 6.39 in 2009. From 1958 to 2010, with the exception of 2002 and 2005, infant mortality rate in the United States has either declined or remained the same every successive year. Sadly, for black infants, the mortality rate in 2010 was 11.6 compared with the rate of 5.19 for white infants.

The achievement of the MDG4 entails reduction of under-5 mortality by two thirds between 1990 and 2015. However, almost 100 countries, including over 40 in sub-Saharan Africa, are not on track to reach this goal (Table 1-5). In fact, this MDG is lagging behind all other MDGs, particularly in Oceania, sub-Saharan Africa, and Central and Southern Asia. Improvements in public health services including safe drinking water, better sanitation, and education are critical to childhood survival throughout the world. (See Chapter 4 for more information on women and children.)

Obesity

In the last 3 decades, the rates of obesity, defined as a body mass index (BMI) of 30 kg/m^2 or more, in many developed countries have risen to the extent that obesity is fast becoming as serious a problem as undernourishment in most developing countries. Until 1980, less than 10% of the population in most developed nations was obese. Between 1980 and 2008, the global prevalence of obesity nearly doubled. Projections indicate that two of three persons in some of the Organization for Economic Cooperation and Development (OECD) countries will be obese or overweight by 2020. The OECD data for 2003 showed that 30.6% of the population in the United States and 24.2% in Mexico were obese. Additionally, women in all countries are more likely to be obese than men.

In 2008, more than 40 million preschool children and 1.4 billion adults worldwide were overweight (BMI 25 kg/m^2 or more), and more than 500 million (12% of the global population) were obese. Every year, 2.8 million people die as a direct result of being overweight or obese. Furthermore, 44% of cases of diabetes, 23% of ischemic heart disease, and 7% to 41% of some cancers are attributed to overweight or obesity. Globally, 1 in 6 adults is obese, 1 in 3 is hypertensive, and 1 in 10 is diabetic. On average, severely obese people are likely to die 8 to 10 years sooner than people of normal weight, and the risk of death increases by 30% with every 15 extra kilograms in body weight. In terms of societal costs, obesity is thought to be responsible for 1% to 3% of health care costs in most countries and 5% to 10% in the United States. Moreover, an obese person earns as much as 18% less in a given year than a person of

Table 1-5. Levels and trends in the under-5 mortality rate, by Millennium Development Goal region, 1990–2010 (deaths per 1,000 live births).

Region	1990	1995	2000	2005	2009	2010	MDG target 2015	Decline (percent) 1990–2010	Average annual rate of reduction (percent) 1990–2010	Progress towards Millennium Development Goal 4 target 2010
Developed regions	15	11	10	8	7	7	5	53	3.8	On track
Developing regions	97	90	80	71	64	63	32	35	2.2	Insufficient progress
Northern Africa	82	62	47	35	28	27	27	67	5.6	On track
Sub-Saharan Africa	174	168	154	138	124	121	58	30	1.8	Insufficient progress
Latin America and the Caribbean	54	44	35	27	22	23	18	57	4.3	On track
Caucasus and Central Asia	77	71	62	53	47	45	26	42	2.7	Insufficient progress
Eastern Asia	48	42	33	25	19	18	16	63	4.9	On track
Excluding China	28	36	30	19	18	17	9	39	2.5	On track
Southern Asia	117	102	87	75	67	66	39	44	2.9	Insufficient progress
Excluding India	123	107	91	80	73	72	41	41	2.7	Insufficient progress
South-eastern Asia	71	58	48	39	34	32	24	55	4.0	On track
Western Asia	67	57	45	38	33	32	22	52	3.7	On track
Oceania	75	68	63	57	53	52	25	31	1.8	Insufficient progress
World	88	82	73	65	58	57	29	35	2.2	Insufficient progress

Source: Reproduced, with permission, from http://www.childinfo.org/files/Child_Mortality_Report_2011.pdf. Copyright Childinfo, UNICEF.

14

normal weight but incurs 25% more in health expenditures.[42] Studies also show a link between childhood obesity, lower self-esteem, and lower academic performance.[43-45]

In some of the OECD countries, the obesity epidemic has either slowed or stabilized in the last 3 years.[42] These changes can be attributed to a number of factors including more aggressive public health measures and greater public awareness. One example of policy initiatives designed to achieve public health outcomes is a growing interest among developed countries in levying higher taxes on foods that are high in sugar and fat content.

To deal with this global tidal wave of obesity, comprehensive strategies involving communities and supportive environments are essential. Evidence shows that social and economic policies, both nationally and internationally, affect dietary habits and physical activity patterns. Therefore, population-based multisectoral public policy is critical for preventing and containing the obesity epidemic. In the United States, the "Let's Move" program led by First Lady Michelle Obama is beginning to have some impact. Close to 500 communities across the country have signed up for the "Let's Move Cities and Towns" initiative and made a commitment to bring about healthy changes in their communities. A number of organizations such as the American Academy of Pediatrics have lent their support to this program and are helping to spread the message and have pledged to have 100% of its doctors do BMI screenings during well-child visits. Other organizations including the National Football League, the National Hockey League, and major league baseball are supporting efforts to promote physical activity and active lifestyles.

Addiction

The online Merriam-Webster dictionary defines addiction as "*the compulsive need for and use of a habit-forming substance (as heroin, nicotine, or alcohol) characterized by tolerance and by well-defined physiological symptoms upon withdrawal*" or, more broadly, as "*the persistent compulsive use of a substance known by the user to be harmful.*" Often, the term is used in the limited context of physical dependence on a mood-altering substance such as cocaine, heroin, nicotine, or alcohol but, in fact, an individual can become physiologically, psychologically, behaviorally, or emotionally dependent on virtually anything; gambling is one such non-substance addiction.

To illustrate the magnitude of the problem of alcohol and illicit drug abuse in the world, it is estimated that about 2 billion people consume alcoholic beverages globally, and 76.3 million have a diagnosable alcohol abuse disorder. Every year, about 2.5 million people, including 320,000 young people between the ages of 15 and 29, die from alcohol abuse. In fact, alcohol abuse accounts for 9% of global deaths in the 15 to 29 age group, results in a loss of 58.3 million DALYs, and is causally related to more than 60 diseases and injuries including 20% to 30% of cases of esophageal cancer, liver cancer, liver cirrhosis, homicides, epileptic seizures, and motor vehicle accidents.[46] CDC data indicate that 1 in 13 pregnant women report consuming alcohol, and 0.2 to 1.5 cases of fetal alcohol syndrome are reported for every 1,000 live births.[47]

WHO also estimates that at least 15.3 million persons in the world have a drug abuse problem. The 2012 World Drug Report issued by the UN Office on Drugs and Crime (UNODC) indicates that in 2010 alone, 230 million people worldwide, or 1 in 20 adults, used an illicit drug at least once. The estimated number of individuals with a substance abuse problem is approximately 27 million, and about 200,000 people die each year as a result of illicit drug use.[48] Among injectable drug users, 20% are HIV infected, 47% have hepatitis C, and 15% have hepatitis B. UNODC reports that the most commonly used illicit drugs globally are cannabis and amphetamine-type stimulants excluding ecstasy. In 2010, the estimated global number of users of these substances was 119 to 224 million and 14 to 52 million, respectively. The production, distribution, and use of illicit drugs is closely associated with crime, prostitution, human trafficking, socioeconomic disruption, destruction of forests and agricultural land, strain on healthcare systems, and unraveling of family structures all over the world.

Research studies consistently demonstrate that the rates for alcoholism among first-degree relatives are significantly higher than among others in the population. One comparative study indicated that offspring of alcoholics are approximately three to five times more likely to develop alcoholism than offspring of nonalcoholics. An estimated 20% to 25% of sons of alcoholics and about 5% of daughters become alcoholics. Similarly, about 20% to 25% of male siblings of alcoholics and 5% of female siblings become alcoholics. These studies provide evidence that a family history of alcoholism represents the strongest known risk factor for the disease.[49]

Road Traffic Injuries and Deaths

Road traffic accidents are one of the leading causes of death and injury worldwide. Population growth, rapid urbanization, weak infrastructure, and increasing numbers of vehicles in low-and middle-income countries in particular has made road traffic accidents a pressing public health issue. Each year, road traffic accidents claim 1.3 million lives worldwide (more than

3,000 per day) and injure or disable as many as 50 million more.[50] Among persons 5 to 29 years of age, road traffic accidents are the second leading cause of death worldwide and 90% of road traffic deaths occur in low- and middle-income countries. The negative economic impact of automobile crashes is estimated to be in the range of 1% to 3% of the gross national product (GNP) of respective countries and globally reaching over $500 billion each year. Previous studies have shown that casualty and fatality rates in developing countries are much higher than in the West. Furthermore, in the Middle East gulf countries, injury and death rates are much higher than in developed countries with comparable vehicle ownership levels. For example, in the United Kingdom and United States in 2004, there were 0.72 and 1.51 road traffic fatalities per 100 million vehicle kilometers, respectively, whereas the United Arab Emirates recorded a disproportionate 3.33 deaths per 100 million kilometers.[51] In 2011, Oman experienced a total of 1,051 deaths in road traffic accidents, bringing the road traffic mortality rate to about 42 deaths per 100,000 population, far in excess of the global average of 19 per 100,000 persons. More than a third of those who died were younger than 25 years. The WHO 2009 Global Status Report estimated that in absolute numbers, India, with 105,725 fatalities, topped the list followed by China (96,611), the United States (42,642), and Russia (35,972). However, in terms of the rate of fatalities per 100,000 population, the top five countries were Eritrea (48.4), Cook Islands (45.0), Libya (34.7), South Africa (33.2), and Iran (32.2).

According to the WHO, with 29 deaths per 100,000 population, Saudi Arabia has one of the highest road accident mortality rates in the world.[52] Traffic injuries are now the principal cause of death for Saudi men between the ages of 16 and 36. Media reports have suggested that a third of all hospital beds in the country are occupied by victims of road accidents at an estimated annual cost of US $7 billion.[53] The Saudi General Directorate of Traffic reported in 2008–2009 that 17 people died in road accidents every day, with a total death toll of 6,485. Others have reported at the beginning of the last decade that 81% of deaths and 20% of bed occupancy in hospitals owned by the Saudi Ministry of Health were due to traffic accidents.[54]

Research over the last half century has provided a clear understanding of the circumstances surrounding motor vehicle injuries among children and factors that influence the likelihood that a child will be injured. Riding unrestrained is the single most important cause of death and injury among children involved in motor vehicle accidents. In the United States in 2010, there were 30,196 fatal crashes with 32,885 deaths. Of the 22,187 persons killed in passenger vehicles, 47.5% were not restrained, and of the 291 children younger than 5 years who were killed, 26.5% were not wearing restraining devices. In contrast, of the 35,149 survivors of fatal crashes of passenger vehicles, 74.4% were restrained, and among 1,469 children younger than 5 years who survived, 85.1% were restrained. In most developing countries the use of infant and child safety seats or booster seats is even lower.

During the past several decades, automobile design and use of safety features such as collision-absorbing materials, seat belts, rear-facing child seats, air bags, speed warning chimes and signals, rear-end cameras, and automatic braking systems have greatly reduced the risk of death and injury resulting from automobile crashes all over the world. Effective implementation of traffic rules including speed limits and better design of roads and highway systems have also contributed substantially in reducing the number of crashes per 100 million miles of driving. In the United States[55] in 2010, there were 1.09 fatalities per 100 million miles driven and 32,885 deaths compared with 1.46 fatalities per 100 million miles and 43,510 deaths in 2005, representing a 26% reduction in traffic deaths during the 5-year period.

Most of the positive change in fatality statistics in developed countries is attributed to safer automobiles and more frequent use of seat belts. It is believed that the number of fatalities would be even lower without distracted driving due to the use of cell phones and texting while driving. In the United States, the National Highway Traffic Safety Administration estimated that in 2010, 3,092 people (9.4% of all traffic fatalities) died due to crashes associated with distracted driving, and 12% (4,280 individuals) of traffic fatalities were among pedestrians. In response to the high numbers of injuries and fatalities attributed to pedestrian and driver behavior, a number of legislative and policing measures have been taken in various states. For example, 37 of the 50 U.S. states have banned texting on mobile phones or other electronic devices; 10 states have made illegal the use of handheld phones while driving (the use of phones while wearing headsets is exempt from this ruling). In comparison, road traffic fatalities have also steadily fallen in the last 10 years in the European Union (EU). For example, in the United Kingdom in 2010, only 1,905 people died in traffic fatalities compared with 3,598 deaths in 2001, an improvement of 43%.[56] (See Chapter 13 for more information on injuries.)

In 2010, the UN General Assembly proclaimed 2011–2020 to be the Decade of Action for road safety, and in 2011 the WHO, in partnership with the UN Road Safety Collaboration, produced a guiding document for member states to stabilize and reduce the number of road traffic fatalities worldwide.

Occupational Hazards and Workplace Safety

Workplace safety is a serious global concern because a formal workforce constitutes approximately 50% to 60% of a country's population. Workers in many occupations all over the world face many hazards. Consequently, specific laws, protocols, procedures, and safety measures in various countries are intended to minimize the level of risk to which workers are exposed. It is the responsibility of all stakeholders including workers, employers, regulators, and law enforcement agencies to fulfill their professional, ethical, and legal obligations to ensure the safety of all workers. In recognition of the importance of occupational health issues, in 1994, 31 WHO Collaborating Centers in Occupational Health in 27 countries adopted a proposal for a Global Strategy for "Occupational Health for All."[57] Likewise, on May 23, 2007, the 60th World Health Assembly of WHO endorsed a Global Plan of Action on Workers' Health 2008–2017 and requested the director general of WHO to promote the implementation of this plan of action at national and international levels. The assembly noted the existence of large gaps between and within countries with respect to the health status of workers and their exposure to occupational hazards.[58]

Work-related illnesses and injuries are often associated with equipment or environments that expose individuals to specific risks. Consequently, workers in some occupations are at a greater risk of disease and injury than others. The list of occupations at high risk for work-related diseases or injuries includes mining, construction, agriculture, fire fighting, commercial fishing, and transportation. In some countries an unsafe work environment and a lack of worker protection results in enormous amounts of unnecessary health burden, suffering, and economic loss. Globally, the cost of work-related injuries and deaths has been estimated to be in the range of 4% to 5% of GDP.[59] The WHO reports suggest that as many as 100 million workers are injured and 200,000 die each year due to work-related accidents and injuries. Occupational injuries and diseases are of much bigger concern in developing countries where 70% of all workers in the world live. Despite gross underreporting, the International Labor Organization estimates that every year 2.3 million individuals die as a result of work-related accidents and diseases around the world, and exposure to hazardous materials alone causes more than 650,000 deaths. Overall, approximately 340 million occupational accidents involving 160 million victims occur each year.[60]

In the United States, data from the National Safety Council from 1933 through 1997 indicate that deaths from unintentional work-related injuries declined 90%, from 37 per 100,000 workers to 4 per 100,000.[61,62] The corresponding annual number of deaths decreased from 14,500 to 5,100. During the same period, the workforce more than tripled, from 39 million to approximately 130 million. According to the U.S. Bureau of Labor Statistics, in 2010 there were 4,690 work-related fatalities, which were down from a high of 6,632 in 1994.[63] Of the deaths in 2010, 40% were related to transportation incidents, 16% involved contact with an object or equipment, 14% involved falls (38% of the falls were from ladders or roofs). Sadly, workplace assaults and violence accounted for 18% of the fatalities in 2010. Workplace fatal injuries in the private mining industry increased by 74% from 99 in 2009 to 172 in 2010 and from 12.4 per 100,000 full-time equivalent (FTE) of workers in 2009 to 19.9 per 100,000 FTES in 2010. Since 2007, fatal falls in the private construction industry in the United States have declined by 42%. However, fatal transportation-related incidents involving pedestrians have been on the rise. The data reported by the U.S. Bureau of Labor Statistics indicate that commercial fishing, with 116 and 129 deaths per 100,000 workers in 2010 and 2008, respectively, was the highest risk occupation.[63] Other high risk occupations are logging, aircraft pilots, farming, and mining. In the last 2 to 3 years there have been a number of widely reported mining-related incidents in the United States, Chile, China, South Africa, Australia, and the United Kingdom.

Displaced and Refugee Populations

Under the UN Convention on the Status of Refugees, a refugee is defined as a person who, "owing to a well-founded fear of being persecuted for reasons of race, religion, nationality, membership in a particular social group, or political opinion, is outside the country of his nationality, and is unable or, owing to such fear, is unwilling to avail himself of the protection of that country." Internally displaced persons (IDPs) are people who have similarly been forced from their homes but have not crossed an internationally recognized state border.

Due to unresolved conflicts and newly emerging crises in a number of countries, by the end of 2011 there were 42.5 million displaced people including 26.4 million IDPs and 15 million refugees.[64-66] In the same year, 22 countries admitted 79,800 individuals for resettlement. According to the Norwegian Refugee Council's Internal Displacement Monitoring Center, in 2011 there were 26.4 million IDPs in the world.[66] For example, in Iraq, more than a million people continue to be in a state of prolonged internal displacement. With 3.9 million IDPs in 2011 (nongovernmental sources place the number at 5.3 million), Colombia was the country with the most IDPs in the world. In Afghanistan, 60% of the millions of IDPs are children. The data reported by the UN High Commission for Refugees (UNHCR) indicate that at the beginning of 2011, there were 10.5 million refugees worldwide. Additionally, 4.8 million registered refugees continue to live in camps in the Middle East that were established in 1949 by the UN Relief and Works Agency for Palestine Refugees in the Near East to look after the displaced Palestinians.[65]

In addition to previously displaced individuals, conflicts in several African and Middle Eastern countries in 2011 including Libya, Syria, Sudan, and Mali caused the displacement of more than 4.3 million people of which almost a million fled to the neighboring countries. Although more than half of the refugees in the world are in Asia and 20% are in Africa, in 2011 Africa was still the region with the largest number of IDPs. The number of IDPs in sub-Saharan African alone was 9.7 million, an improvement on the number of 11.1 million IDPs in preceding years. Together, women and children make up approximately 80% of the refugee population.[67] The UNHCR reports that, on average, refugees will spend 17 years outside of their home country, and currently more than half of the world's refugees live in urban areas.

The internal conflict that started in early 2011 in Syria had, by the end of July 2012, resulted in the internal displacement of more than a million people and countless others who fled the country and sought refuge in Lebanon, Turkey, and Jordan. Previously displaced families and individuals from countries such as Iraq, Afghanistan, Colombia, and the Democratic Republic of Congo continue to live in temporary or semi permanent states of settlement in foreign lands including Iran, Jordan, Pakistan, and Kenya. Nearly all of the refugees originate from and more than 80% are hosted by developing countries. Rather than being camped in remote and rural border areas, more and more of the refugees and IDPs in recent years have lived in urban areas of the host or home countries and, in many instances, have been absorbed in the slums and shanty towns of big cities such as Kabul, Nairobi, Khartoum, and Bogota.

Refugees and IDPs face daunting economic, social, and health risks that accompany displacement (Table 1-6). Relief programs target the specific needs of women, children and adolescents, older refugees, and particular ethnic or social groups. Unaccompanied children and those with only one parent are at greatest risk because they lack the protection, physical care, and emotional support provided by the family.[68,69] Safety and well-being is especially difficult in the presence of armed elements among displaced or refugee populations. Furthermore, many IDPs and self-settled refugees are in countries where the government is either indifferent or actively hostile to their needs for assistance and protection. In at least 13 countries

Table 1-6. Factors that place refugees and internally displaced persons at risk for serious public health and humanitarian consequences.

Displacement and separation from families
Social instability
Increased mobility
Sexual and gender-based violence
Exploitation and abuse (including HIV/AIDS)
Poverty and food insecurity
Lack of access to health services, education, and basic assistance
Lack of linguistically and culturally appropriate health information
Forced labor or slavery
Forcible recruitment into armed groups
Trafficking
Abduction
Detention and denial of access to asylum or family-reunification procedures

in recent years, including Myanmar, Sudan, Uganda, and Zimbabwe, state forces or government-backed militia have attacked displaced and other civilian populations.

By putting strains on the local resources, IDPs and refugees pose many challenges for the host communities and countries but also for the national and international aid agencies. Now there is a growing recognition for the need to integrate IDPs and refugees into the existing health systems for their health care needs and to find new mechanisms for financing the health care of the IDPs and refugees including health insurance. An experimental model of health insurance for Afghan refugees was recently introduced in Iran with promising results in terms of close to 347,000 refugees, 40% of registered Afghan refugees in the country, being enrolled and given access to secondary and tertiary level health care.[64]

Population Growth

Human population increased in the 20th century at an unprecedented rate from 1.6 billion to 6.0 billion. In merely 13 years between 1999 and 2011, the world population grew from 6 to 7 billion; officially, we crossed the 7 billion mark on October 31, 2011. For the fourth time in the last 50 years, 1 billion more people were added to the world population in a span of 14 or fewer years. Growth projection by the United Nations indicates that at this rate, there will be 8 billion people on this planet by the year 2024 and more than 9 billion by the year 2042.[36] Because lack of education, poverty, and reliance on human labor as opposed to mechanized processes of production are closely linked with population growth; the developing countries of Africa and Asia have been the ones to experience the most rapid population growth. In contrast, because of smaller family size and aging populations, some of the most developed countries in Europe in recent years have actually experienced negative population growth.

In the coming years, continued population growth in developing countries will be accompanied by accelerated urbanization and international migration. These demographic shifts will put tremendous pressures on available resources and infrastructure. Unchecked human activity to exploit natural resources for human consumption is already exacting a heavy toll on the environment in terms of pollution, deforestation, and rapidly diminishing biodiversity. Given the rise in food and commodity prices and the challenges of economic productivity in the last 10 years, the prospects for the living standards of the poor and vulnerable masses in the developing world are more than worrisome.

Strong national and international measures to protect and conserve natural resources including water, land, forests, and environment will be necessary to avert the looming crises of worsening food shortages, hunger, and poverty. Population growth and evolving demographic characteristics will have profound implications for health care systems in the 21st century. In the ensuing decades, aging of the population in America, Japan, China, India, and elsewhere will have dramatic social, health, and economic ramifications. The ability of the world to feed itself will depend not only on food production but also on distribution of resources and patterns of human consumption.[11]

Environmental Pollution

Indoor Air Pollution

More than 3 billion people worldwide (42% of the total population, 21% of the urban population, and 76% of the rural population in 2007) continue to depend on solid fuels including coal and biomass fuels such as wood, dung, straw, and agricultural residues for their energy needs. Of the more than 3 billion people relying on solid fuels, 0.4 billion use coal and 2.7 billion use wood, animal dung, and crop waste.[70] Cooking and heating with solid fuels on open fires or traditional stoves result in high levels of indoor air pollution. In poorly ventilated housing units, indoor small particle levels can be 100 times greater than acceptable levels. Indoor solid-fuel smoke contains a range of health-damaging pollutants such as small particles, carbon monoxide, nitrous oxides, sulfur oxides (especially from coal), formaldehyde, and carcinogens (such as benzo[a]pyrene and benzene).

Close to 2 million premature deaths every year in the world are attributed to illnesses causally linked to indoor air pollution resulting from the use of solid fuels.[70]

The small particulate matter and other substances in the solid-fuel indoor smoke are known to affect the oxygen-carrying capacity of blood and cause inflammation of the airways and lungs. Emerging evidence suggests that indoor air pollution in developing countries may also increase the risk of other important child and adult health problems including asthma, otitis media and other acute upper respiratory infections, low birth weight and perinatal mortality, TB, nasopharyngeal and laryngeal cancer, cataracts (blindness), and CVD.

Further, open fires and poor quality stoves increase the risk of burns and injuries. WHO has reported that 50% of pneumonia deaths among children younger than 5 years of age are the direct result of inhaling particulate matter in the indoor air.[71] There is consistent evidence that exposure to indoor air pollution can lead to acute lower respiratory infections (ALRIs), particularly pneumonia, in children younger than 5 years. In fact, ALRIs are the single most important cause of death in children younger than 5 and account for at least 2 million deaths annually in this age group. Indoor air pollution resulting from coal burning is also linked to chronic obstructive pulmonary disease and lung cancer in adults. About 1.5% of lung cancers every year are attributed to carcinogenic substances in the smoke-laden indoor air.

According to the WHO, indoor air pollution is responsible for close to 2 million deaths, mostly of women and children, in developing countries, and is estimated to cause 3.1% of the overall burden of disease in developing countries and 2.7% globally (Figure 1-6).[70] In most societies, it is women who cook and spend time near the fire. In developing countries women are typically exposed to very high levels of indoor air pollution for 3 to 7 hours per day over many years. Young children are often carried on their mother's back during cooking. Consequently, many children from early infancy are also exposed to high levels of smoke in the indoor air. Clearly, some of the world's less developed regions rely heavily on solid fuel use at the household level, whereas other regions have made an almost complete transition to cleaner fuels, such as gas and electricity. For example, more than 75% of the population in India, China, and nearby countries and 50% to 75% of people in parts of South America and Africa continue to cook with solid fuels. These differences in household solid fuel use are correspondingly reflected in an unequal distribution of the burden of diseases related to indoor air pollution, with Africa, Southeast Asia, and the Western Pacific region shouldering the biggest death toll. More than half of the total DALYS

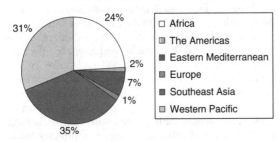

Deaths attributable to solid fuel use

24%
31%
2%
7%
1%
35%

- □ Africa
- ▨ The Americas
- ■ Eastern Mediterranean
- ▨ Europe
- ■ Southeast Asia
- □ Western Pacific

DALYs attributable to solid fuel use

26%
0%
2%
15%
3%
54%

- □ Africa
- ▨ The Americas
- ■ Eastern Mediterranean
- ▨ Europe
- ■ Southeast Asia
- □ Western Pacific

Figure 1-6. Deaths and disability-adjusted life years (DALYs) attributable to solid fuel use. From *http://www. who.int/mediacentre/factsheets/fs292/en/* (*Reproduced with permission.*)

lost due to exposure to indoor air pollution occurs in Africa, highlighting the urgent need to intervene. WHO has developed a comprehensive Program on Indoor Air Pollution to support developing countries. Many policymakers assert that addressing the indoor air pollution problem will help achieve MDGs related to child and maternal mortality (MDG 4 and 5), gender equality (MDG 3), and environmental sustainability (MDG 7).[70]

Water Pollution

In 2008, 78% of the rural population worldwide but only 48% of the rural population in the African Region had access to clean drinking water. Access to improved sanitation was even less with only 45% of the global rural population and 26% in the African Region having access to improved sanitation. In countries such as Ethiopia, the Democratic Republic of Congo, Angola, and Afghanistan, access to clean drinking water was only between 26% and 39%, and access to improved sanitation was between 8% and 30%.[72] According to some estimates, every day 2 million tons of human waste is disposed of into the world's watercourses, and in developing countries 70% of industrial wastes are also disposed of into watercourses. Altogether, every year 14 billion pounds

of waste including municipal waste, sludge, oil, and industrial waste is dumped into the world's oceans.[73,74]

A significant portion of the burden of water-related diseases (in particular, water-related vector-borne diseases) is attributable to the way in which water resources are developed and managed. Agriculture accounts for about 70% to 90% of freshwater use in the world, and about 7% to 8% of all energy produced in the world is used to lift, distribute, and treat ground water and wastewater.[75] In many parts of the world, the adverse health impacts of dam construction, irrigation development, and flood control include an increased incidence of malaria, Japanese encephalitis, schistosomiasis, lymphatic filariasis, and other diseases. Other health issues indirectly associated with water resource development include nutritional status, exposure to agricultural pesticides and their residues, and accidents/injuries.

Water-related infectious diseases are a major cause of morbidity and mortality worldwide. To address the global problem of waterborne diseases, the WHO's Water, Sanitation and Health Program focuses on the quality of drinking water, water resources, and wastewater management in various countries. Between 1972 and 1999, 35 new agents of disease were discovered, and many more have reemerged. Among these pathogens are several that may be transmitted through water. Newly recognized pathogens and new strains of established pathogens present additional challenges for both water management and public health sectors.

Climate Change and Natural Disasters

Despite the contentious debate and challenges by those not convinced by the evidence of global warming and its causes, cumulative data indicate that the surface of the earth has undergone unprecedented warming over the last century and more so in the last 2 decades. Every year since 1992 has been on the current list of the 20 warmest years on record. In the United States, a number of previous climatological records in terms of average temperature and number of consecutive days of triple-digit temperatures were broken in 2012 in a number of states. Moreover, numerous U.S. states have experienced widespread "exceptional" and/or "extreme" drought in the summer of 2012. In its 2001 report, the Intergovernmental Panel on Climate Change (IPCC) stated that "there is new and stronger evidence that most of the warming observed over the last 50 years is attributable to human activities"[76] and that global warming has altered natural patterns of climate.

Carbon dioxide from the burning of fossil fuels and clearing of land has been accumulating in the atmosphere, where it acts like a blanket keeping the earth warm and heating up the surface, oceans, and atmosphere (the greenhouse effect). Current levels of carbon dioxide are higher than at any time during the last 650,000 years. The world's oceans have absorbed about 20 times as much heat as the atmosphere over the past half century, leading to higher temperatures not only in surface waters but also in water 1,500 feet below the surface. Observed climatic, physical, and ecological changes include an increasing global average surface temperature of about 0.8°C (1.4°F) in the 20th century, a rise in global average sea level, an increase in ocean water temperatures, and increased rainfall and other precipitation levels in certain regions of the world.[77,78] Scientists predict that continued global warming on the order of 1.4°C to 5.8°C (2.5°F to 10.4°F) over the next 100 years (as projected in the IPCC's Third Assessment Report) is likely to result in the following:

- A rise in sea level between 3.5 and 34.6 inches (9 to 88 cm), leading to more coastal erosion, flooding during storms, and permanent inundation
- Severe stress on many forests, wetlands, alpine regions, and other natural ecosystems
- Greater threats to human health as mosquitoes and other disease-carrying insects and rodents spread diseases over larger geographic regions
- Disruption of agriculture in some parts of the world due to increased temperature, water stress, and sea-level rise in low-lying areas such as Bangladesh or the Mississippi River delta.

Natural disasters have been important sources of human morbidity and mortality throughout history in every region of the world. Floods, earthquakes, hurricanes, tornadoes, fires, and other disasters wreak havoc on global populations each year. The tsunami that struck 11 countries in South Asia in December 2004 resulted in devastation of staggering proportions: more than 150,000 people dead (especially in Indonesia and Sri Lanka), tens of thousands of people missing, thousands of miles of destroyed coastline, and loss of livelihood for millions of distraught survivors. Although this catastrophe was unusually vast, it was a classic natural disaster in several ways, uncomplicated by war or terrorism. The short-term public health needs of the surviving population were familiar (albeit massive): water, sanitation, food, shelter, and appropriate medical care administered to persons remaining in place and the thousands who were living in self-settled displaced communities.[79]

In addition to the immediate loss of life and property, in many natural disasters the number of casualties may increase by as much as twofold as a result of the spread of communicable diseases in the crowded communities that are often created in the aftermath. The public health model for natural disasters highlights a cycle of preparedness, mitigation, response, and recovery. Short-term interventions after large-scale natural disasters include supplying the recommended 20 liters of water per person per day and ensuring adequate, culturally appropriate sanitation facilities to prevent outbreaks of cholera, dysentery, and hepatitis A; targeted measles vaccination in unvaccinated populations, with vitamin A supplementation when indicated; control of vector-borne illnesses such as malaria and dengue through early treatment and mosquito-control measures; early diagnosis and treatment of acute respiratory and gastrointestinal infections, particularly among infants and young children; delivery of adequate amounts of culturally appropriate emergency food rations; counseling for survivors experiencing grief, loss, and guilt; and epidemic surveillance to detect the early appearance of communicable diseases. The longer-term recovery and rehabilitation needs in disaster-affected areas are less understood than the short-term needs but are typically strategic rather than logistic and involve a transition from emergency relief activities to sustainable reconstruction and development activities.

Landmines

In 2010, 79 countries or disputed territories in various regions of the world were affected by landmines, unexploded ordnance (UXO), or both. In the last decade, some of the most mine-contaminated countries have included Afghanistan, Angola, Bosnia and Herzegovina, Cambodia, Chechnya, Colombia, Iraq, Somalia, Sri Lanka, and Sudan.[80,81] However, data collection has been very inadequate or nonexistent in 64 of the 68 countries with recorded casualties.[82-84] Further, some of the affected countries such as Myanmar, India, and Pakistan choose to provide little public information about the extent of their problem.

Landmines indiscriminately kill or maim civilians, soldiers, peacekeepers, and aid workers alike. Over the past 5 or 6 decades, landmine deaths and injuries have totaled in the hundreds of thousands. According to the "Landmine Monitor 2011" report issued by the International Campaign to Ban Landmines (ICBL), a total of 4,191 casualties were reported in 2010 representing a 5% increase over the previous year's reported casualties of 4,010 but lower than the 5,502 casualties reported in 2008.[82] It has been estimated that 75% or more of the victims of landmines are civilians. In Cambodia, for example, over 45,000 landmine injuries were recorded between 1979 and 2005, and some 20,000 people were killed by landmines during the same period. More than 75% of the total casualties were civilians.

Antipersonnel landmines are still being produced and laid today and, together with mines from previous conflicts, claim victims each day in every corner of the globe. In 2010–2011, the "Landmine and Cluster Munition Monitor,"[82] an initiative of ICBL, identified Israel, Libya, and Myanmar as governments laying antipersonnel mines. Non-state armed groups in Afghanistan, Pakistan, Myanmar, and Colombia were also identified as users of antipersonnel landmines in the same period. Reports from the ongoing Syrian conflict in 2012 have indicated the use of landmines by both sides of the conflict. Twelve countries are identified in the "Landmine Monitor 2011" report as the current producers of antipersonnel mines: China, Cuba, India, Iran, Myanmar, North Korea, Pakistan, Russia, Singapore, South Korea, the United States, and Vietnam.

The precise number of still buried undetonated explosive devices is unknown. Approximately 200 square kilometers of mined areas were cleared by 45 different groups that destroyed more than 388,000 antipersonnel mines in 2010 alone. More than 80% of the cleared areas were in Afghanistan, Cambodia, Croatia, Iraq, and Sri Lanka. However, these achievements were partly, if not significantly, offset by continuing and emerging conflicts in various parts of the world. It is estimated that more than 160 million landmines are stored in stockpiles by various countries. In 1997, the International Committee of the Red Cross had estimated that while more than 100,000 mines were being removed each year, 2 million more were being planted every year, and an estimated 110 million active mines were scattered in more than 70 countries around the world. Although 160 countries have signed the 1997 Ottawa Ban Mine Treaty, 36 countries including China, Cuba, Egypt, India, Israel, Pakistan, the Russian Federation, Saudi Arabia, and the United States have not signed it.[81] It is estimated that it takes $3 to $30 to produce a landmine, but it can cost $300 to $1000 to remove one. In 1996, the UN secretary general had estimated that it would take about $50 billion to remove all existing mines; in the same year, total funding available for global demining operations was a meager $150 million. In 2010, ICBL reported that all donor and affected countries combined had provided about US$637 million in international and national support for demining operations. Given these statistics, it seems more than probable that antipersonnel mines and UXO will continue to be a global problem in the coming years and a mine-free world is still a long way off.

Biologic and Chemical Terrorism

Bioterrorism is the deliberate release of viruses, bacteria, or other biologic agents designed to cause large-scale illness or death in people, animals, or plants. Biologic agents can be spread through air, water, or food. Consequently, the protection of the food and water supply and distribution systems has been a source of concern for many countries. As demonstrated by the dissemination of anthrax spores via the U.S. postal service in 2001, even small-scale biologic or chemical attacks can cause tremendous socioeconomic disruption. Some potential bioterrorism agents such as smallpox virus and hemorrhagic fever viruses can be spread from person to person. Based on their transmissibility and the severity of health effects, these agents are classified into three categories (Table 1-7).[85] Category A agents are microorganisms or toxins that pose the greatest risk to public health and global security, whereas category C agents are those considered as emerging threats.

Category A agents (1) are easily transmitted from person to person, (2) result in high death rates and have the potential for major public health impact, (3) can cause public panic and social disruption, and (4) require special action for public health preparedness.

Category B agents (1) are moderately easy to spread, (2) result in moderate illness rates and low death rates, and (3) require specific enhancements of existing laboratory capacity and enhanced disease monitoring.

Category C agents (1) are easily available, (2) are easily produced and spread, and (3) have the potential for high morbidity and mortality rates and major public health impact.

Chemical terrorism refers to the intentional release of a hazardous chemical into the environment for the purpose of public harm. Types and categories of potential chemical warfare agents include biotoxins, blister agents/vesicants, blood agents, caustics (acids), choking/lung/pulmonary agents, incapacitating agents, long-acting anticoagulants, metallic poisons, nerve agents, organic solvents, toxic alcohols, and vomiting agents. Protection of the public from biologic and chemical terrorism involves well-orchestrated disaster preparedness including improved education, disease recognition, surveillance, and emergency notification by first responders, clinicians, laboratories, and public health workers.

In the last 12 years or so, there have been a number of incidents of terrorism including the September 11, 2001 attacks in the United States, the dissemination of lethal anthrax spores via mailed letters in the United States in 2001, the July 7, 2007 attack in the United Kingdom, and the November 26, 2008 attack in Mumbai, India. So far the number of incidents in which biologic or chemical agents were used by terrorists has been relatively few. One of the most notable cases was the use of the organophosphorus nerve gas sarin by the Aum Shinrikyo religious cult in Matsumoto, Japan in 1994 and again in 1995 in

Table 1-7. Microbial agents with bioterrorism potential.

Category A	Category B (cont.)
Bacillus anthracis (anthrax)	Bacteria
Clostridium botulinum (botulism)	Diarrheagenic *Escherichia coli*, pathogenic *Vibrio*
Yersinia pestis (plague)	spp., *Shigella* spp., *Salmonella* spp., *Listeria monocy-*
Variola major (smallpox) and other pox viruses	*togenes, Campylobacter jejuni, Yersinia enterocolitica*
Francisella tularensis (tularemia)	Viruses
Viral hemorrhagic fever viruses	Caliciviruses, hepatitis A virus
Arenaviruses	Protozoa
LCM, Junin, Machupo, Guanarito, and Lassa	*Cryptosporidium parvum, Cyclospora cayetanensis,*
fever viruses	*Giardia lamblia, Entamoeba histolytica, Toxoplasma*
Bunyaviruses	*gondii*, microsporidia
Hantaviruses	Viral encephalitis viruses
Rift Valley fever virus	West Nile, LaCrosse, California encephalitis,
Flaviviruses	Venezuelan equine encephalitis, Eastern equine
Dengue virus	encephalitis, Western equine encephalitis,
Filoviruses	Japanese B encephalitis, and Kyasanur forest viruses
Ebola virus	**Category C**
Marburg virus	Nipah virus and additional hantaviruses
Category B	Tickborne hemorrhagic fever viruses
Burkholderia pseudomallei (melioidosis)	Crimean-Congo hemorrhagic fever virus
Coxiella burnetii (Q fever)	Tickborne encephalitis viruses
Brucella species (brucellosis)	Yellow fever
Burkholderia mallei (glanders)	Multidrug-resistant *Mycobacterium tuberculosis*
Ricin toxin (of *Ricinus communis*)	Influenza
Epsilon toxin (of *Clostridium perfringens*)	Other rickettsiae
Staphylococcal enterotoxin B	Rabies virus
Rickettsia prowazekii (typhus fever)	Severe acute respiratory syndrome–associated
Food- and waterborne pathogens	coronavirus (SARS-CoV)

From National Institute of Allergy and Infectious Diseases (NIAID) Biodefense Research. NIAID category A, B, and C pathogens. http://www3.niaid.nih.gov/biodefense/bandc_priority.htm.

Tokyo. In the 1994 attack, 7 people were killed and more than 200 were injured, and in the 1995 attack on a subway train, 12 people died with hundreds more needing hospitalization.[86] In the past there have also been examples of deliberate contamination of food by non-state groups or individuals acting independently. For example, in 1984, members of a religious cult were responsible for contaminating salad bars in the United States that caused more than 750 cases of salmonella, and in 1996 a lab worker, acting alone, contaminated food with *Shigella dysenteriae* that resulted in 12 people getting sick.

The risk of smallpox as a biologic weapon for terrorism, although small, is a distinct possibility and an important reason for maintaining vaccine stocks and the virus itself in secure locations in the United States and Russia. After media reports suggesting that some governments such as North Korea, Russia, and Iraq had secretly kept smallpox virus in store, the U.S. government in June 2001 carried out a large-scale simulated smallpox attack exercise. This exercise

revealed that the country was quite ill prepared for such a threat. Since then, enhanced preparatory measures have been taken including the provision of hundreds of millions of additional doses of vaccine to the existing national stock. Since 2003, follow-up multi-country joint exercises have also been conducted to improve preparedness in the event of an attack.

STUDY QUESTIONS

1. Trace the rise and fall of the importance of infectious diseases to global health, and enumerate some of the new infectious threats in the world.

2. How have sanitation, environmental health, and attention to basic necessities such as food and water improved global health, and how are they threatened today?

3. Take one global health challenge from this chapter and expand on its causes, trends, and the corrective action(s) needed, taking into account limited resources in the developing world.

BOX 1-1. ZIMBABWE: A CASE STUDY OF AN HIV-RAVAGED COUNTRY

As is well known, public health results from the cumulative and interactive effects of scientific, social, cultural, economic, and political factors within a population. Because of its effect on the most economically and socially productive members of society, the ongoing HIV/AIDS pandemic has had an unprecedented impact on the fabric of individual nations and on the socioeconomic development of the planet as a whole. This case study of one country in sub-Saharan Africa, Zimbabwe, illustrates the interplay of a host of factors that can lead to a public health catastrophe.

With 14.3% of the adult population having HIV/AIDS, 1.2 million affected people, and 83,000 deaths in 2009, Zimbabwe ranks fifth in the world in HIV/AIDS prevalence and mortality statistics. In 2009, UNICEF reported that because of HIV/AIDS there were 1 million orphaned children in Zimbabwe. The overall HIV prevalence, which was as high as 34% in 2000, has declined in recent years. Yet close to 1,600 people die from AIDS each week, and AIDS-related illnesses account for about three fourths of hospital admissions. Approximately a third of all teachers and over half of Zimbabwe's soldiers were thought to be HIV seropositive.[87,88]

Zimbabwe (formerly Rhodesia) unilaterally declared its independence from Britain in 1965 and attained freedom and national statehood from the ruling white apartheid regime in 1980. Since then, the Zimbabwe African National Union-Patriotic Front has been in power under the presidency of Robert Mugabe. In 2009, Zimbabwe had a population of 12.52 million people with a median age of 19 years, 6% of the population above the age of 60, and 38% of the population living in urban areas. Total fertility rate per adult woman in 2009 was 3.4, and the adolescent fertility rate per 1,000 girls 15 to 19 years of age was 101. Currently, the average life expectancy of a Zimbabwean is only 52 years, about 9 years less than the historic high of 61 years in 1990. Also, the country has among the highest maternal deaths (730 deaths/1,000 live births) and infant mortality rate (51/1,000 live births) in the world.[7,87,88]

Since the 1990s, the decline of Zimbabwe's once flourishing economy has gravely affected a large segment of the population. The GDP per capita in 2009 was estimated to be $323, and in 2010 it was $500.[89] Approximately 56% of the population lives on less than US $1 a day, and 80% live on less than US $2 a day. In 2002, youth unemployment in the formal job sector among those 15 to 24 years of age was about 25%, but the overall unemployment rate including underemployment in 2009 was estimated to be as high as 95%. Approximately 68%

of the population in 2004 was below the poverty line. After a period of hyperinflation and a decade (1998–2008) of economic contraction, the economy now seems to be growing again with a real growth of 6% recorded in 2011. The change in monetary policy of 2009 that allowed currencies such as the South African rand and U.S. dollar to be used locally has helped curb further inflation and somewhat stabilized the economic situation. In fact, the Zimbabwean dollar effectively stopped circulating in early 2009.[87]

Before 2009, the GDP had drastically declined in the previous 10 years with annual inflation approaching a record 1000% in May 2006. Continued high inflation seriously hampered development, hitting the poor hardest. Agricultural production also plummeted in the last 10 years. For example, between 2000 and 2004, the national cattle herd shrank by 90%, and the production of flue-cured tobacco declined from 237 million kilograms to 70 million kilograms. The frequency of acute malnutrition declined in 2004, partly as a result of large-scale food aid, although the situation in some areas has continued to worsen. With a score of 0.376 on the Human Development Index, Zimbabwe currently ranks 173rd of 187 countries on the list and is below the regional index of 0.463 for sub-Saharan Africa.

Agriculture is the most important sector of the Zimbabwean economy but has been severely disrupted by the ill-advised land resettlement policies of President Mugabe. This has led to a collapse in investor confidence and the flight of capital. Lack of foreign exchange has led to critical shortages in fuel and other imported commodities including power. The cost of schooling has risen dramatically, posing serious challenges for low-income families. The decline in inward investment and development assistance is further compromising the prospects for economic recovery. Food shortages affect up to half the population of Zimbabwe. A national vulnerability assessment in November 2005 estimated that 2.8 million Zimbabweans would face food shortages in the "hungry season" (January through March) leading up to the next harvest. Following much better rains, the harvest in 2006 was expected to be better than that in 2005. Due to hyperinflation, even when food is available it is unaffordable to many. However, the impact of chronic illness, localized flooding, and the high price of seeds and fertilizer mean that many people require assistance later in the year.

The International Monetary Fund (IMF) suspended payments to Zimbabwe in 2000, following the government's decision to abandon IMF public

---

BOX 1-1. ZIMBABWE: A CASE STUDY OF AN HIV-RAVAGED COUNTRY (*Cont.*)

spending guidelines (including payments to war veterans, the cost of which amounted to 3% of GDP). The country went into arrears at the World Bank in 2000 and at the IMF the following year, effectively cutting off cooperation with either institution. The country is crippled by governmental corruption up to the presidential level. According to Transparency International's 2003 Corruption Perception Index, Zimbabwe ranked 106 of 133 on the global list of most corrupt nations.

Despite these obstacles, Zimbabwe is on track to achieve the MDG target on HIV and AIDS, namely, to "have halted by 2015, and begun to reverse, the spread of HIV/AIDS." Declining HIV prevalence

is likely to be a result of high mortality rates and changes in sexual behavior. Most of Zimbabwe's other MDGs are unlikely to be achieved by 2015 unless the political and social situation improves dramatically. Child and maternal mortality indicators show a steadily worsening situation, exacerbated by HIV/AIDS.[7]

Current foreign aid priorities include tackling HIV/AIDS (including increasing access to antiretroviral therapy), food insecurity (including increasing individuals' access to seeds and fertilizers, nutrition gardens, and safe water), and support for orphans and vulnerable children (including school feeding and home-based care programs).

REFERENCES

1. Beaglehole R, Bonita R. What is global health? *Global Health Action* 2010;3:5142. http://www.globalhealthaction.net/index.php/gha/article/view/5142.

2. Kickbush I. The need for a European strategy on global health. *Scandinavian J Public Health* 2006;34:561–565.

3. Macfarlane SB, Jacobs M, Kaaya EE. In the name of global health: trends in academic institutions. *J Public Health Policy* 2008;29:383–401.

4. Koplan JP, Bond TC, Merson MH, et al. Towards a common definition of global health. *Lancet* 2009;373(9679): 1993–1995.

5. Fried LP, Bentley ME, Buekens P, et al. Global health is public health. *Lancet* 2010;375:535–537.

6. Centers for Disease Control and Prevention. Ten great public health achievements—United States, 1900–1999. *MMWR* 1999;48:241–243.

7. World Health Organization. World Health Statistics, 2011. http://www.who.int/whosis/whostat/EN_WHS2011_Full.pdf.

8. Sachs J. Primary health care in low-income countries: building on recent achievements. *JAMA* 2012;307(19):2031–2032.

9. World Health Organization. The Global Burden of Disease: 2004 Update, 2008. http://www.who.int/healthinfo/global_burden_disease/GBD_report_2004update_full.pdf.

10. United Nations Department of Economic and Social Affairs. Changing Levels and Trends in Mortality: The Role of Patterns of Death by Cause, 2012. http://www.un.org/esa/population/publications/levelsandtrendsinmortality/Changing%20levels%20and%20trends%20in%20mortality.pdf.

11. Chen LC. World population and health. In: Institute of Medicine, ed. *2020 Vision: Health in the 21st Century.* New York: National Academies Press, 1996:16–23.

12. Hinman A. 1889 to 1989: a century of health and disease. *Public Health Rep* 1990;105:374–380.

13. Centers for Disease Control and Prevention. Achievements in public health, 1900–1999: control of infectious diseases. *MMWR* 1999;48:621–629.

14. United Nations Children's Fund/World Health Organization. Diarrhoea: why children are still dying and what can be done, 2009. http://whqlibdoc.who.int/publications/2009/9789241598415_eng.pdf.

15. World Health Organization. Global HIV/AIDS response: epidemic update and health sector progress towards Universal Access, 2011. http://www.who.int/hiv/pub/progress_report2011/en/index.

16. UNAIDS. UNAIDS Report on the Global AIDS Epidemic, 2010. http://www.unaids.org/documents/20101123_globalreport_em.pdf.

17. UNAIDS. World AIDS Day Report, 2011. http://www.unaids.org/en/media/unaids/contentassets/documents/unaidspublication/2011/JC2216_WorldAIDSday_report_2011_en.pdf.

18. World Health Organization. Influenza at the human-animal interface. Geneva: World Health Organization, 2012. http://www.who.int/influenza/human_animal_interface/en/.

19. National Center for Infectious Diseases. *Preventing Emerging Infectious Diseases: A Strategy for the 21st Century.* Atlanta: US Department of Health and Human Services, 1998. http://www.cdc.gov/mmwr/PDF/rr/rr4715.pdf.

20. Centers for Disease Control and Prevention. Achievements in public health, 1900–1999: impact of vaccines universally recommended for children—United States, 1990–1998. *MMWR* 1999;48:243–248. http://www.cdc.gov/mmwr/preview/mmwrhtml/00056803.htm.

21. Centers for Disease Control and Prevention. Recommended Immunizations for Babies, 2012. http://www.cdc.gov/vaccines/parents/rec-iz-babies.html.

22. World Health Organization. Global immunization vision and strategy: progress report and strategic direction for the decade of vaccines. Report by the secretariat, 2011. http://apps.who.int/gb/ebwha/pdf_files/WHA64/A64_14-en.pdf.

23. World Health Organization. Global immunization data, 2012. http://www.who.int/immunization_monitoring/Global_Immunization_Data.pdf.

24. World Health Organization. WHO immunization work: 2006–07 highlights. http://whqlibdoc.who.int/publications/2008/9789241596749_eng.pdf.

25. Mhatre SL, Schryer-Roy A. The fallacy of coverage: uncovering disparities to improve immunization rates through evidence. Results from the Canadian International Immunization initiative Phase 2 – Operational Research Grants. *BMC Int Health Human Rights* 2009;9(Suppl 1):S1. http://www.biomedcentral.com/1472–698X/9/S1/S1.

26. Duclos P, Okwo-Bele J, Gacis-Dobo M, et al. Global immunization: status, progress, challenges and future. *BMC Int Health Human Rights* 2009;9(Suppl):S2. http://www.biomedcentral.com/1472–698X/9/S1/S2.

27. Mackay J, Mensah GA. Global burden of coronary heart disease. In: WHO & CDC. *The Atlas of Heart Disease and Stroke.* Geneva: World Health Organization, 2004.http://www.who.int/entity/cardiovascular_diseases/en/cvd_atlas_13_coronaryHD.pdf.

28. World Health Organization. *The Atlas of Heart Disease and Stroke.* Geneva: World Health Organization, 2012.http://www.who.int/cardiovascular_diseases/resources/atlas/en/.

29. Bendavid E, Bhattacharya J. The president's emergency plan for AIDS Relief in Africa: an evaluation of outcomes. *Ann Intern Med* 2009;150(10):688–695. http://annals.org/article.aspx?volume=150&page=688.

30. United States President's Emergency Plan for Aids Relief. Celebrating Life: Fifth Annual Report to Congress, 2009. http://2006–2009.pepfar.gov/.

31. UNAIDS. UNAIDS report on the global AIDS epidemic, 2010 http://www.unaids.org/globalreport/global_report.htm.

32. World Health Organization. Central African Republic, 2004. http://www.who.int/disasters/repo/15100.pdf.

33. Food and Agriculture Organization of the United Nations. State of Food Insecurity in the World, 2005. ftp://ftp.fao.org/docrep/fao/008/a0200e/a0200e00.pdf.

34. United Nations Children's Fund. *State of the World's Children 2005: Childhood Under Threat.* New York: UNICEF, 2004. http://www.unicef.org/publications/files/SOWC_2005_(English).pdf.

35. United Nations Children's Fund. HIV/AIDS and children, 2003. http://www.unicef.org/aids/index_action.html.

36. World Population Institute. From 6 billion to 7 billion: how population growth is changing and challenging our world, 2011. http://www.populationinstitute.org/newsroom/news/view/45/.

37. Food and Agriculture Organization. World Food Summit 1996: Rome Declaration on World Food Security. http://www.fao.org/docrep/003/w3613e/w3613e00.htm.

38. United Nations Educational, Scientific and Cultural Organization: MDG Report, 2010. http://www.uis.unesco.org/Library/Documents/MDGR_2010_En.pdf.

39. WHO, UNICEF, UNFPA, and the World Bank. *Trends in Maternal Mortality 1990 to 2010.* Geneva: World Health Organization, 2012. http://www.unfpa.org/webdav/site/global/shared/documents/publications/2012/Trends_in_maternal_mortality_A4–1.pdf.

40. United National Population Fund. Maternal Mortality Estimates.2012. http://www.unfpa.org/public/home/mothers/MMEstimates2012.

41. United Nations Children's Fund. Levels and trends in child mortality, 2012.http://www.childinfo.org/files/Child_Mortality_Report_2011.pdf.

42. Organization for Economic Cooperation and Development. Obesity Update, 2012. http://www.oecd.org/health/healthpoliciesanddata/49716427.pdf.

43. Crosnoe R, Muller C. Body mass index, academic achievement, and school context: examining the educational experiences of adolescents at risk of obesity. *J Health Soc Behav* 2004;45(4):393–407.

44. Datar A, Sturm R. Childhood overweight and elementary school outcomes. *Int J Obes (Lond)* 2006;30:1449–1460.

45. Datar A, Sturm R, Magnabosco JL. Childhood overweight and academic performance: national study of kindergartners and first-graders. *Obes Res* 2004;12(1):58–68.

46. World Health Organization. Global Status Report on Alcohol, 2004. http://whqlibdoc.who.int/publications/2004/9241562722_(425KB).pdf.

47. Centers for Disease Control and Prevention. Fetal Alcohol Spectrum Disorders (FASDs), 2012. http://www.cdc.gov/ncbddd/fasd/index.html.

48. United Nations Office on Drugs and Crime. The World Drug Report, 2012. http://www.unodc.org/documents/data-and-analysis/WDR2012/WDR_2012_web_small.pdf.

49. National Institute on Alcohol Abuse and Alcoholism. Alcohol Alert, 1992. http://pubs.niaaa.nih.gov/publications/aa18.htm.

50. World Health Organization, Regional Office for the Eastern Mediterranean. *WHO Launches the World Report on Road Traffic Injury Prevention.* Geneva: WHOPress Release no. 10, July 12, 2005. http://www.searo.who.int/LinkFiles/whd04_Documents_summary_en_rev.pdf.

51. Bener A, Crundall D. Road traffic accidents in the United Arab Emirates compared to Western countries. *Adv Transport Studies* 2005; A6:5–12.

52. World Health Organization—Country Profiles, Saudi Arabia, 2010. http://www.who.int/violence_injury_prevention/road_safety_status/country_profiles/saudi_arabia.pdf.

53. Baxter E. Saudi hospitals struggling to cope with traffic victims, 2010. http://new.arabianbusiness.com/saudi-hospitals-struggling-cope-with-traffic-victims157591.html?tab = Article.

54. Ansari S, Akhdar F, Mandoorah M, Moutaery K. Causes and effects of road traffic accidents in Saudi Arabia. *Public Health* 2000; 114(1):37–39.

55. National Highway Traffic Safety Administration. *Traffic Safety Facts 2010 data.* Washington, DC: NHTSA, 2010. http://www-nrd.nhtsa.dot.gov/Pubs/811625.pdf.

56. European Commission. Road Fatalities in the EU since 2001. Directorate General for Mobility and Transportation, 2012. http://ec.europa.eu/transport/road_safety/specialist/statistics/index_en.htm.

57. World Health Organization. Declaration on Occupational Health for All, 1994. http://www.who.int/occupational_health/publications/declaration/en/index.html.

58. World Health Organization. Workers' Health: Global Plan of Action, 2007. http://www.who.int/occupational_health/WHO_health_assembly_en_web.pdf.

59. World Health Organization. Occupational Health, 2012. http://www.who.int/occupational_health/en/.

60. International Labor Organization. World Statistics: The Enormous Burden of Poor Working Conditions, 2011. http://www.ilo.org/public/english/region/eurpro/moscow/areas/safety/statistic.htm.

61. Centers for Disease Control and Prevention. Achievements in public health, 1900–1999: improvements in workplace safety—United States, 1900–1999. *MMWR* 1999;48: 461–469.

62. National Safety Council. *Accident Facts.* Itasca, IL: National Safety Council, 1998.

63. Bureau of Labor Statistics. National Census of Total Occupational Injuries in 2010 (Preliminary Results). U.S. Department of Labor, 2011. http://www.bls.gov/news.release/pdf/cfoi.pdf.

64. Guterres A, Spiegel P. The state of the world's refugees: adapting health responses to urban environments. *JAMA* 2012; 308(7):673–674.

65. United Nations High Commissioner for Refugees. *Global Trends 2011: A Year of Crises.* Geneva: UNHCR, 2011. http://www.unhcr.org/4fd6f87f9.html.

66. Internal Displacement Monitoring Centre. Global overview, 2011: People internally displaced by conflict and violence. http://www.internal-displacement.org/8025708F004CFA06/(httpPublications)/B7F783CA2B399F1EC12579E400579423?OpenDocument.

67. United Nations High Commissioner for Refugees. *UNHCR Global Appeal 2006.* Geneva: UNHCR, 2006. http://www.unhcr.org/4a0ad61f6.html.

68. Joint United Nations Programme on HIV/AIDS (UNAIDS) and the United Nations High Commissioner for Refugees. *Strategies to Support the HIV-Related Needs of Refugees and Host Populations.* Geneva: UNAIDS, 2005.

69. United Nations High Commissioner for Refugees. *Refugee Children.* Report of the Global Consultations on International Protection, 4th meeting. EC/GC/02/9, 25 April 2002, p.1.

70. World Health Organization. *Indoor Air Pollution and Health.* Geneva: WHO Media Center: FactSheet No. 292, 2011. http://www.who.int/mediacentre/factsheets/fs292/en/index.html.

71. World Health Organization. *Air Quality and Health.* Geneva: WHO Media Center: Fact Sheet 313, 2011. http://www.who.int/mediacentre/factsheets/fs313/en/.

72. World Health Organization. *Water Supply, Sanitation and Hygiene Development.* Geneva: WHO, 2012. http://www.who.int/water_sanitation_health/hygiene/en/.

73. World Health Organization. *Global Analysis and Assessment of Sanitation and Drinking Water.* Geneva: WHO, 2012. http://whqlibdoc.who.int/publications/2012/9789241503365_eng.pdf.

74. UN-Water. Statistics: Graphs and Maps. *Water Pollution, Environmental Degradation and Disasters.* New York: UN-Water, 2012. http://www.unwater.org/statistics_pollu.html.

75. United Nations Educational, Scientific and Cultural Organization. *Facts and Figures: Managing Water Under Uncertainty and Risk.* New York: UNESCO, 2012. http://unesdoc.unesco.org/images/0021/002154/215492e.pdf.

76. Intergovernmental Panel on Climate Change. *Climate Change 2001: IPCC Third Assessment Report.* New York: Cambridge University Press, 2002.

77. U.S. National Aeronautics and Space Administration Goddard Institute for Space Studies. *Global Temperature Trends: 2005 Summation.* New York: NASA GISS, 2006. http://data.giss.nasa.gov/gistemp/2005.

78. U.S. National Oceanic and Atmospheric Administration National Climate Data Center. *Climate of 2005: Annual Report.* Ashville: National Climate Data Center, 2005. http://www.ncdc.noaa.gov/oa/climate/research/2005/ann/global.html.

79. VanRooyen M, Leaning J. After the tsunami—facing the public health challenges. *N Engl J Med* 2005;352:435–438.

80. International Campaign to Ban Landmines. http://www.icbl.org/country.

81. International Campaign to Ban Landmines. *Landmine Monitor Report 2005: Toward a Mine-Free World.* Ottawa: Mines Action Canada, 2005. http://www.icbl.org/lm/2005/report.html.

82. International Campaign to Ban Landmines. *Global Landmine Overview 2010–2011.* Geneva:Landmine and Cluster Munition Monitor, International Campaign to Ban Landmines, 2011. http://www.the-monitor.org/index.php/publications/display?url=lm/2011/es/Major_Findings.html.

83. Canadian Red Cross. *The Landmine Epidemic.* Ottawa: Canadian Red Cross, 2008. http://www.redcross.ca/article.asp?id=1945&tid=006.

84. International Committee of the Red Cross. *Anti-personnel Landmines.* Geneva: International Committee of the Red Cross, 2010. http://www.icrc.org/eng/war-and-law/weapons/anti-personnel-landmines/.

85. National Institute of Allergy and Infectious Diseases (NIAID) Biodefense Research. *NIAID category A, B, and C pathogens.* Washington, DC: U.S. Department of HHS, NIH, 2003. http://www.niaid.nih.gov/topics/BiodefenseRelated/Biodefense/Documents/categorybandc.pdf.

86. World Health Organization. *Smallpox, Bioterrorism and the World Health Organization.* Geneva: WHO, 2006. http://www.who.int/global_health_histories/seminars/paper02.pdf.

87. United Nations Children's Fund. *Zimbabwe: Statistics.* New York: UNICEF, 2003. http://www.unicef.org/infobycountry/zimbabwe_statistics.html.

88. Central Intelligence Agency. *The World FactBook, Zimbabwe.* Washington, DC: CIA, 2012. https://www.cia.gov/library/publications/the-world-factbook/geos/zi.html.

89. United Nations. *World Statistics Pocketbook.* New York: The United Nations, 2010. http://unstats.un.org/unsd/pocketbook/PDF/Zimbabwe.pdf.

The Global Burden of Disease 2

Thuy D. Bui and William H. Markle

LEARNING OBJECTIVES

- *Recognize the rationale for summary measures of population health*
- *Understand the attributes of mortality, morbidity, and disability as they apply to burden of disease*
- *Describe various composite measures of burden of disease, their relative strengths and weaknesses, and how they are used in public health literature, World Health Organization reports, and the lay press*
- *Identify the changing global health risks and effective interventions to prevent disease and injury*
- *Understand how data on global health measures affect international development, policy change, and their limitations*
- *Apply the global burden of disease study to understanding poverty and global health inequalities*

RATIONALE FOR COMPOSITE INDICATORS

Measuring the impact of diseases on populations is a prerequisite for determining effective ways to reduce the burden of illness. Traditional methods of quantifying disease in populations, such as incidence, prevalence, mortality, birth rate, and infant mortality rate, do not capture nonfatal health outcomes. In the past 3 decades, significant international effort has been put into the development of composite indicators that

include both mortality and morbidity measures to make judgments about the health of populations and to identify which interventions would have the greatest effect.

The growth of aging populations and the increase of associated chronic diseases have provided an impetus to examine nonfatal health outcomes and the associated quality of life. Disability and suffering are difficult to quantify because they involve complex, subjective notions of pain, discomfort, and emotional distress that are interpreted within a social and cultural context. Prior work on health-related quality-of-life (HRQL) measures, measures of utility or preference-weighted measures, the 1980 International Classification of Impairment, Disability and Handicaps by the World Health Organization (WHO), and the later International Classification of Functioning, Disability and Health, a classification of health and health-related domains, laid the framework for the development of morbidity measures that would be incorporated into summary measures of population health.

The benefits of having a common currency to measure the magnitude of health problems include the following abilities:

- Comparing the health of populations
- Monitoring trends over time
- Conducting cost-effectiveness analyses
- Measuring the population-wide benefits of health interventions

Implicit in the applications of these measures is the ability to assess global health inequalities; to inform debates on priorities for health service delivery and for planning, research, and development in the health sector; and to improve public health curricula and training.[1]

Capturing timely accurate data is a particular concern, especially in resource-poor settings. Mortality information is probably the most widely available kind of health information, obtained through death certificates, vital registration, and verbal autopsy studies, but even this type of data is found to be incomplete and unreliable. An adult who presents with fever, diarrhea, and hypotension to a district hospital and dies before any definitive diagnostic testing may have died from malaria, dysentery, sepsis, and/or acquired immunodeficiency syndrome (AIDS). Data about morbidity presented in the literature are often based on self-perceived or observed assessments, household surveys, and interview information. As this chapter examines the methods used to assess the global burden of disease, keep in mind that all measures of population health involve choices and value judgments in both their construction and their application.[2]

HEALTH EXPECTANCIES AND HEALTH GAPS

The two types of composite measures are health expectancies and health gaps. Figure 2-1 illustrates a typical survivorship curve for a hypothetical population.[1] The area under the middle curve (black dashed line) is divided into two components: H, which represents health expectancy (time lived in full health), and D, which represents time lived at each age in some defined level of disability. Life expectancy at birth (the middle curve [black dashed line]) is simply H + D. The top curve (blue unbroken line) signifies an ideal goal of full health until death for the population. The area G between the middle curve (life expectancy) and the top curve is equivalent to premature mortality. A health gap is then area G and some

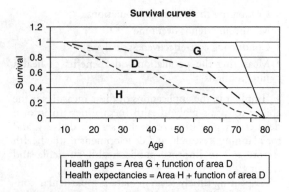

Survival curves

Figure 2-1. Health expectancy, health gap, and survivorship curves for a hypothetical population.
Source: Murray CJL, Salomon J, Mathers CD, Lopez AD, eds. *Summary Measures of Population Health.* Geneva: World Health Organization, 1999.

function of area D. How you define area D (disability weights) is a major issue wrestled with by the various composite measures. This chapter touches on quality-adjusted life year (QALY) and health-adjusted life expectancy (HALE) as examples of health expectancy measures and focuses on disability-adjusted life years (DALYs) as an example of a health gap measure.

Health Expectancies

Quality-Adjusted Life Year

QALY is a measure of health outcomes that incorporates both the quality and quantity of life lived into a single index number, originally developed over 30 years ago for cost-effectiveness analysis. The QALY calculation is derived from the change in utility value (individual preference for different nonfatal health outcomes) induced by the treatment multiplied by the duration of the treatment effect to provide the number of QALYs gained. A year of perfect health is considered equal to 1.0 QALY. The value of a year of ill health is discounted. For example, a year bedridden might have a value equal to 0.5 QALY. Extending someone's life for a year at one-half full health is equal to 0.5 QALY, which is also equal to extending two people's lives by a year at one-fourth full health! To permit aggregation of QALY changes, an improvement in health from 0.4 to 0.6 QALY is numerically equivalent to an improvement from 0.7 to 0.9. As another example, a woman who is healthy in her first 60 years of life with a HRQL valued at 0.95 experiences severe pneumonia with complications that decreases her HRQL to 0.7 until her death at age 62. Although she lives to age 62, she only attains 58 QALYs in her life path: $(0.95 \times 60) + (0.7 \times 2)$.

Traditional QALYs are built using HRQL weights that are *not* attached to any particular disease or condition but to individual health status. A number of approaches—standard gamble, time trade-off, or rating scales—have been used to generate quality-of-life valuations, also referred to as health utilities. The time trade-off method requires the respondents to value health states by making explicit what they would be willing to sacrifice in terms of time or risk of death to return to better or perfect health. The Health Utility Index, the EuroQoL EQ-5D, the WHO Quality of Life, and the SF-36 represent commonly used instruments for the measurement and valuation of HRQL, and they include key domains such as physical, psychological, and social role function, health perceptions, and symptoms (Table 2-1).

Finally, QALYs can then be incorporated with medical costs to arrive at a final common denominator of cost/QALY, or the cost-utility analysis. If, for example, a standard intervention allows a patient to live for 1 additional year than if no intervention had

Table 2-1. Key domains of utility measures.

HUI	SF-36	EuroQol EQ-5D	WHOQoL
Vision	Physical function (PF)	Mobility	Physical health
Hearing	Role—physical (RP)	Self-care	Psychological
Speech	Bodily pain (BP)	Usual activities	Level of independence
Ambulation	General health (GH)	Pain/discomfort	Social relations
Dexterity	Vitality (VT)	Anxiety/depression	Environment
Emotion	Social function (SF)		Spirituality/religion/ personal beliefs
Cognition	Role—emotional (RE)		
Pain	Mental health (MH)		

HUI, Health Utility Index; WHOQoL, World Health Organization Quality of Life project.

taken place, but only with a quality-of-life weight of 0.8, then the intervention confers $1 \times 0.8 = 0.8$ QALY to the patient. If a new intervention confers 2 extra years of life at a quality-of-life weight of 0.6, then it confers an additional $2 \times 0.6 = 1.2$ QALYs to the patient. The net benefit of the new over the standard intervention is therefore $1.2 - 0.8 = 0.4$ QALY. The difference in treatment costs ($10,000) is divided by the QALYs gained (0.4) to calculate the cost per QALY, or $25,000 per QALY.

Example: The Cost Effectiveness of Routine Voluntary Human Immunodeficiency Virus Screening in South Africa As of 2011, more than half of all South Africans living with human immunodeficiency virus (HIV) remained unaware of their infection and unable to access counseling and lifesaving care. Using a simulation model of HIV case detection and treatment, Walensky and colleagues examined three HIV screening scenarios in addition to current practice: one time, every 5 years, and annually.[3] They found a 16.9% HIV prevalence, a 1.3% annual incidence, a 49% test acceptance rate, HIV testing costs of $6.49/patient, and a 47% linkage-to-care rate (including two sequential antiretroviral therapy regimens) for identified cases. Annual routine HIV screening in South Africa increases the per person quality-adjusted life expectancy (LE) of an HIV-infected individual by 16.6 months, even when assuming highly constrained rates of acceptance and linkage to care. Annual screening is very cost effective ($1,720/QALY). This study has started to address the critical question of whether frequent HIV screening is clinically beneficial and economically viable for South Africa as researchers and policymakers tackle the bigger "HIV treatment as prevention" strategies globally.

Example: Cost Effectiveness of Treating Asymptomatic Hepatitis C US cohorts Using a Markov model, Salomon and colleagues estimated the incremental cost/QALY gained of $29,300 for men and $48,800 for women without fibrosis on biopsy using a combination therapy of interferon and ribavirin compared with no treatment in hepatitis C virus (HCV) infection.[4] The expected benefits of therapy are derived mostly from improvements in HRQL rather than from survival outcomes. Although considered reasonably cost effective, these results depend on assumptions about quality of life associated with mild HCV infection and treatment, and they vary widely among different patient subgroups. More information is needed on the quality weights associated with chronic liver disease and the decrements in quality of life associated with its treatment.

Healthy Life Expectancies

Healthy life expectancy (HLE) in combining the length and quality of life has become a standard summary measure of population health in many developed countries. Monitoring health expectancies allows countries to evaluate their population's health to see whether longer life is being spent in good health or ill health. Health expectancies can be created by adjusting LE for disability, specific disease, or for self-perceived health. Population health surveys assess self-perceived health or functional status. Levels of reported ill health are combined with mortality data to estimate the number of years of healthy life an individual will live. HLE, formerly known as disability-adjusted life expectancy, is also referred to as health adjusted life expectancy (HALE).

Various methods exist for calculating health expectancies. The Sullivan method is the only one for which data are widely available. It requires only a population life table that can be constructed for a population using the observed mortality rates at each age for a given time period, prevalence data for each type of disability at each age, and the weight assigned to each type of disability. Such prevalence rates can be obtained readily from cross-sectional health or disability surveys carried out for a population at a point in time. Levels of self-reported health vary systematically over time and social groups, making comparisons difficult. The Sullivan method, which uses observed prevalence estimates, is criticized for not producing a pure period indicator. The prevalence rates depend partly on earlier health conditions of each age cohort, and by not considering transition rates in and out of the health states, it is not capable of detecting rapid changes in population health.[5]

The International Network on Health Expectancies (Réseau Espérance de Vie en Santé [REVES]) has developed and promoted the concept and methods of health expectancies, which the European Union (EU) member states have adopted to monitor trends in health across the EU. The WHO uses data from the Global Burden of Disease (GBD) Study, the WHO Multi-Country Survey Study, and the World Health Survey to make independent estimates of severity-adjusted prevalence by age and sex for survey countries and life tables constructed with Sullivan's method to compute HALE for 193 countries. According to the WHO, in 2007 the range of healthy LE was more than twofold, ranging from 35 years in Sierra Leone to 76 years in Japan (Figure 2-2). Global HLE at birth was 58 years in 2002 and 59 in 2007.

The Global Burden of Disease Study 2010, published after most of this chapter was written, looked at

healthy life expectancy for 187 countries. It found that HALE had increased more slowly than LE over the past 20 years, with a 1 year increase in LE being associated with a 0.8 year increase in HALE. The global male HALE in 2010 was 58.3 years and the global female HALE was 61.8 years. Between 1990 and 2010, male HALE had increased by at least 5 years in 42 countries and female HALE had increased in 37 countries. However male HALE had decreased in 21 countries and female HALE had decreased in 11.[6]

It is difficult to relate health expectancies back to disease and risk factor causes because all disease and injury contribute to the risk of death or disability at each age, and the health expectancy is a weighted sum of these risks across all ages in a population life table. However, studies that involve decomposition of HLE into specific conditions, lifestyle, and health behaviors may lead to focused interventions to compress disability and/or reduce mortality with potentials for addressing health disparities across sociodemographic groups. In Europe, the United Kingdom, and Canada, HLE is playing an important role in a country's fiscal health planning, such as retirement/pension benefits and long-term care spending. In the United States, researchers and policymakers are starting to make the case for the adoption of HLE at the national, state, community, and health care system levels to guide health improvement efforts.[7]

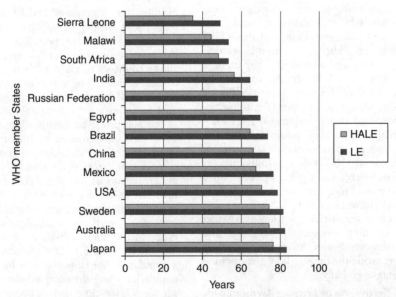

Figure 2-2. Healthy life expectancy at birth, 2007, for selected World Health Organization (WHO) member states. HALE, health-adjusted life expectancy; LE, life expectancy.
Source: World Health Statistics 2010, WHO.

Health Gaps

Potential Years of Life Lost

Potential years of life lost (PYLL) is a simple summary measure of premature mortality defined as the total number of years lost through the failure of individuals to live their expected number of years. The advantage of PYLL over crude mortality rates is that the crude mortality rate is weighted by the large number of deaths occurring in older people. PYLL allows decision makers and others to selectively evaluate leading causes of mortality in younger age groups. For example, if we define premature death as death before age 65, a person dying at age 52 from heart disease would represent 13 PYLL. The major limitation of the PYLL approach is that it does not count death at or above the potential (age 65 or 75 years) and hence cannot measure the benefits of health interventions in this age group. Moreover, morbidity and disability are not considered in this indicator. The US Centers for Disease Control and Prevention (CDC) has published statistics on years of potential life lost (YPLL, which is the same as PYLL) by race, sex, region/state, and by leading causes and risk factors (http://webappa.cdc.gov/sasweb/ncipc/ypll10.html).

Example: Global Burden of Injuries Attributable to Alcohol Consumption According to data on drinking indicators from the WHO's Comparative Risk Assessment Study, 851,900 deaths and 19,051,000 PYLL for people 15 years and older worldwide were due to injuries attributable to alcohol consumption in 2004.[8]

Example: According to the National Cancer Institute, on average, each person who died from cancer in 2007 lost an estimated 15.4 years of life. Cancer deaths were responsible for more than 8.6 million PYLL, which is more than heart disease and all other causes of death combined. Lung cancer accounted for nearly 2.4 million PYLL, the most by far for any cancer, partially because of the relatively low percentage of survival and the relatively early age of onset.[9]

Disability-Adjusted Life Years

The DALY metric was developed in the original GBD 1990 Study under the leadership of Murray and Lopez, the World Bank, WHO, and the Harvard School of Public Health to assess the burden of disease consistently across diseases, risk factors, and regions. Since 2000, the WHO has published regular GBD updates for 14 regions. The 2010 Global Burden of Diseases, Injuries, and Risk Factors Study, funded by the Bill and Melinda Gates Foundation and led by the Institute for Health Metrics and Evaluation, is the first major effort since the original GBD 1990 Study to carry out a complete systematic assessment of global data for 220 diseases and injuries and more than 60 risk factors for 21 regions of the world.

DALY belongs to the second group of composite indicators called health gaps and involves estimates of HRQL attached to specific diseases, rather than to health states (as in QALY). DALYs for a disease or health condition are calculated as the sum of the years of life lost (YLL) due to premature mortality for each disease and the years lost to disability (YLD) based on the *incidence* of cases of the health condition. DALY = YLL + YLD. YLL = N × L, where N is the number of deaths and L is standard LE at age of death in years. YLD = I × DW × L, where I is the number of incident cases, DW is disability weight, and L is the average duration of the case until remission or death in years. In the GBD Study 2010 YLDs are computed as the prevalence of different disease-sequelae and injury-sequelae multiplied by the DW for that sequela.

In the original study, severity scores for disability or disability preference weights for 22 sample diagnoses or indicator conditions were determined by an international panel of experts. An iterative "person trade-off" approach was used—participants chose whether it was more desirable to treat a given number of people with one condition than to treat a given number with another condition. They then created seven disability classes, and once preference scores for a set of index conditions were established, weights for hundreds of other conditions were mapped by extrapolation. Weights of 1 are equated with full disability or death, and 0 with no disability or full health on the DALY scale. These DWs are thought to be equal or universal across countries and cultures. With the Global Burden of Disease Study 2010[10], a reassessment of DWs was made with surveys in representative countries. 30,230 people participated in either household or web-based surveys. There was a high degree of consistency and the highest disability weights were given to schizophrenia and severe multiple sclerosis. The new weights were found in general to agree with the old weights, although in the mild range, many conditions were given lower rates than previously. See Table 2-2 for a comparison of sample sequelae and their DWs from the GBD 2004. An extensive list of disability weights for 220 unique health states can be found in the GBD Study 2010.[10]

The original DALY architects made two additional adjustments. The first of these is an age weighting that gives greater value to years lived in young adulthood and less to years lived at the beginning and end of life. The value of a healthy person's life peaks around age 25 by this calculation. The final adjustment to the DALY formula is to discount time in the future at a rate of 3%. The idea is that a future benefit is worth less than one you get now. A treatment that extends a person's lifespan from 65 to 75 is more cost effective

Table 2-2. Sample disability weights for diseases and conditions* (GBD 2004 update)

Sequela	Average disability weight	Range	Source
LBP, episode of limiting LBP	0.061		Netherlands study
AIDS cases on ART	0.167	0.165–0.469	GBD 2004
Glaucoma, low vision	0.170		GBD 2004
Unipolar depressive disorders, moderate depressive episode	0.350		Netherlands study
Ischemic heart disease, acute myocardial infarction	0.439	0.405–0.477	GBD 1990
COPD, severe symptomatic cases	0.530		Netherlands study
Cerebrovascular disease, first-ever stroke cases	0.920		GBD 1990

AIDS, acquired immunodeficiency syndrome; ART, antiretroviral therapy; COPD, chronic obstructive pulmonary disease; GBD, Global Burden of Disease; LBP, lower back pain.
From http://www.who.int/healthinfo/global_burden_disease/GBD2004_DisabilityWeights.pdf.

if provided to a 65-year-old than to a 50-year-old who sees no benefit for another 15 years.

Example: The National Burden of Road Traffic Injuries in Thailand Using road traffic injury (RTI) mortality estimates from verbal autopsy study, vital registration, and the proportion and severity of long-term disabilities from a Thai study, Ditsuwan and colleagues found the total loss of DALYs due to RTIs was 673,000 in 2004.[11] Mortality contributed 88% of this burden. The use of local data did lead to a significantly higher estimate of the burden of long-term disability due to RTIs (74,000 vs 43,000 DALYs) using standing GBD methods.

The GBD Study 2010[10] intended to address some of the criticisms of past burden of disease studies. Household surveys including face-to-face interviews in several countries and one made available on the Web allowed for a diverse set of cultural, demographic, and linguistic contexts. The surveys asked respondents to judge the relative severity of states of health in a series of paired comparisons and time trade-off questions, for example: "Imagine two people—the first person is completely blind, and the second person suffers from constant intense back pain. Who is healthier overall?" Answers are used to calculate a health state severity weight for each sequela. Comparisons could then be made between new and old DWs for around 120 sequelae common to the old and new GBD studies. The GBD Study 2010 identified 1160 sequelae of 291 diseases and injuries. For example, diabetic retinopathy is a sequela of diabetes mellitus. Researchers needed to establish a continuous ordinal scale between DW 0 (perfect health) and DW 1 (death) for each sequela.[12] The 2010 GBD team has benefited from new and improved methodologies since the last GBD Study including modeling missing data, DW estimation, cause of death attribution, and data collection techniques that provide better estimates

of mortality and the YLD globally. The base case for DALYs in this study has also been simplified to omit both discounting and age weighting. YLLs were calculated with reference to new reference–standard life expectancies at each age. For example, a death at 5 years counts as 81.4 YLLs and a death at 60 years counts as 27.8 YLLs.

Example: Global burden of human food-borne trematodiasis Through systematic review of literature, data on human prevalence, the morbidity and mortality of food-borne trematodiasis were extracted. Fürst, Keiser, and Utzinger developed simplified disease models and did meta-analyses on the proportions and odds ratios of specified sequelae and estimated that 56.2 million people were infected with food-borne trematodes in 2005; 7.9 million had severe sequelae and 7,158 died, mostly from cholangiocarcinoma and cerebral infection.[13] They estimate that the global burden of food-borne trematodiasis was 665,352 DALYs. This preliminary GBD Study 2010 was chosen to highlight the relevance of this group of neglected tropical diseases.

Table 2-3 offers a comparison of essential features of the various summary measures. DALYs are different from QALYs in their population perspective. From the work of the GBD Study, DALYs allow global comparisons of major diseases and risk factors. DALYs are additive in the sense that they can be additively decomposed with respect to causes and are a more sensitive measure of changes in burden. However, disability states in DALYs do not take account of comorbid conditions. There is no way to capture the burden of diabetes, hypertension, and coronary artery disease within the same individual. DALYs take 82.5 years for women and 80 years for men as their standard LE at birth, based on the average LE of Japanese people, who currently have the longest overall LE in the world. This will lead to

Table 2-3. Comparison of summary population health measures.

Features	QALYs	HALE	DALY
Origin and organizations	1976, Academia/research, North America and Europe	2000, REVES, EU, OECD, WHO	1993, WHO, World Bank
Type	Health expectancy	Health expectancy	Health gap
Health status instrument	Yes	Yes	No
Disability weights	Yes	Generic disability or handicap severity classes	Community and expert surveys; epidemiologic data
Disability measures	Yes	Self-report of disability	Derived for each health state linked to specific conditions
Estimating burden	No	Overall health status; hard to relate health expectancy back to disease and risk factors	Yes; more sensitive measure of changes in burden than gains in health expectancies through disease elimination
Level of use	Assess individual outcomes from interventions	Evaluate and compare national disease burdens	Compare disease burdens across populations
Causes additive	No	No	Yes
Prevalence vs incidence	Variable	Prevalent disability	Incidence based
Multicausality or comorbidities	Yes	Potential	No

Source: QALYs, quality-adjusted life years; HALE, health-adjusted life expectancy; DALYs, disability-adjusted life years; REVES, Réseau Espérance de Vie en Santé; EU, European Union; OECD, Organization for Economic Cooperation and Development; WHO, World Health Organization.

overestimation of YLL in high-mortality countries. Through these assumptions about social value of people at different ages and uniform LE in all different countries, Murray and Lopez tried to uphold a moral and political notion of equity and comparability for this population health measure.

The GBD Study 1990 presented estimates of mortality, YLL, and years lived with disability due to diseases and injuries for eight regions of the world. The GBD Study 2010 presented estimates in 21 distinct geographic regions. All diseases and health outcomes were categorized into the following three groups:

1. Communicable, maternal, perinatal, and nutritional
2. Noncommunicable
3. Accidents and injuries

Table 2-4a and 2-4b show that as you move from a low-, middle-, and then high-income country, group 1 causes of deaths and DALYs tend to decrease in importance, whereas group 2 causes tend to increase. However, group 2 causes are already of significant importance in most countries, and group 3 causes figure prominently in low- and middle-income countries. The importance of neuropsychiatric causes of DALYs is obvious. The use of age-standardized rates is necessary to compare rates of countries without being affected by the difference in age distributions from country to country.

GLOBAL HEALTH RISKS

Understanding risks to health is vital to preventing disease and injuries. The WHO's 2009 report *Global Health Risks* provides the latest estimates of the burden of disease and injury from exposure to risks, known as the "attributable" burden of disease and injury. The attributable burden is calculated by estimating the population attributable fraction (PAF), the proportional reduction in population disease or mortality that would occur if exposure to a risk factor was reduced to an alternative ideal exposure scenario. The number of deaths or DALYs attributed to a risk factor is quantified by applying the PAF to the total number of deaths or the total burden of disease. This report provides an update for the year 2004 of the comparative risk assessment (CRA) for 24 global risk factors. In the GBD Study to date, risk factor burden has been quantified according to counterfactual attribution as mentioned earlier; disease and injury burden has been reported according to the categorical

Table 2-4a. Deaths, death rates, and age-standardized death rates of 4 countries by groups 1, 2, and 3.

	Burkina Faso Low income			Egypt Lower middle income			Russian Federation Upper middle income			United States High income		
	Death	Death rate	Age std rate	Death	Death rate	Age std rate	Death	Death rate	Age std rate	Death	Death rate	Age std rate
All Causes	207.9	1364.9	1718.9	453.7	556.5	859.6	2083.7	1473.7	1027.0	2547.8	817.5	504.9
Group 1: Communicable, Maternal, and Perinatal	151.0	991.4	801.1	56.4	69.2	76.0	106.2	75.1	71.4	154.1	49.5	33.7
Infectious and parasitic	91.9	603.2	492.1	24.4	30.0	36.9	75.4	53.3	49.1	71.2	22.9	15.4
HIV/AIDS	8.2	53.7	72.7	0.4	0.5	0.6	45.0	31.8	30.0	11.6	3.7	3.4
Maternal	4.0	26.4	29.4	1.6	2.0	1.9	0.5	0.4	0.4	1.2	0.4	0.4
Perinatal	17.5	114.6	52.4	16.6	20.4	15.5	8.9	6.3	10.6	17.5	5.6	7.1
Nutritional deficiency	7.3	47.7	27.4	1.5	1.9	2.0	1.0	0.7	0.6	6.3	2.0	1.0
Group 2: Noncommunicable	43.2	283.9	810.1	371.1	455.2	749.3	1718.3	1215.3	796.8	2205.5	707.7	418.4
Malignant neoplasms	6.0	39.4	96.7	50.9	62.4	90.5	269.8	190.8	129.8	590.1	189.3	123.8
Diabetes	2.5	16.3	55.3	11.4	14.0	23.6	9.9	7.0	4.8	75.3	24.2	15.2
Neuropsychiatric	2.6	16.9	32.7	7.5	9.2	13.9	19.9	14.1	11.6	239.2	76.7	39.2
Cardiovascular	17.3	113.4	399.8	178.4	218.8	388.0	1264.5	894.3	568.4	872.4	279.9	155.7
Group 3: Injuries	13.7	89.6	107.7	26.2	32.1	34.3	259.2	183.3	158.8	188.1	60.4	52.8

Deaths in thousands; Death rate and age-standardized death rate is per 100,000 population. Data from WHO.

Table 2-4b. DALYs, DALY rates and age-standardized DALY rate of 4 countries by groups 1, 2 and 3.

	Burkina Faso Low income			Egypt Lower middle income			Russian Federation Upper middle income			United States High income		
	DALYs	DALY rate	Age standard rate	DALYs	DALY rate	Age standard rate	DALYs	DALY rate	Age standard rate	DALYs	DALY rate	Age standard rate
All causes	7,402	54,802	45,867	13,318	18,613	20,261	40,348	27,885	25,305	41,372	13,937	12,844
Group 1: Communicable, Maternal, and Perinatal	5,411	40,060	26,584	3,257	4,552	3,891	3,412	2,358	2,722	2,527	851	896
Infectious and parasitic	3,017	22,336	15,706	952	1,330	1,209	1,792	1,238	1,229	1,036	347	330
HIV/AIDS	254	1,881	2,456	11	15	16	533	368	378	368	124	121
Maternal	236	1,751	1,806	333	465	444	159	110	110	277	93	104
Perinatal	645	4,774	2,290	1,134	1,585	1,181	380	263	484	745	251	321
Nutritional deficiency	324	2,397	1,405	311	435	379	511	353	537	135	45	45
Group 2: Noncommunicable	1461	10,816	15,601	8,959	12,521	14,927	27,571	19,055	16,295	34,650	11,673	10,481
Malignant neoplasms	113	835	1,585	595	832	1,043	3,109	2,149	1,702	5,085	1,713	1,384
Diabetes	37	273	582	225	314	414	361	249	204	1,332	449	374
Neuropsychiatric	364	2,692	2,673	2,220	3,103	3,054	5,810	4,015	3,954	11,709	3,945	3,963
Cardiovascular	273	2,020	3,858	2,276	3,181	4,370	11,774	8,137	6,296	5,853	1,972	1,525
Group 3: Injuries	530	3,926	3,681	1,102	1,540	1,443	9,365	6,472	6,288	4,196	1,413	1,467

DALYs in the thousands, DALY rate and age-standardized rate per 100,000 population. Data from WHO.

attribution, primarily following the International Classification of Disease system.

A particular disease or injury is often caused by more than one risk factor. Similarly, most risk factors are associated with more than one disease, and targeting these factors can reduce multiple causes of disease. For example, the four noncommunicable diseases (NCDs) responsible for at least half of global deaths are cardiovascular diseases, diabetes, cancers, and chronic respiratory diseases. They share four underlying risk behaviors that could be targeted by public health interventions: tobacco use, physical inactivity, unhealthy diet, and the harmful use of alcohol that lead to raised blood pressure, overweight/obesity, elevated blood glucose, and raised cholesterol. Diabetes is an example of a disease whose total burden includes its directly attributable burden and its role as a risk factor for other diseases. Malaria, tuberculosis, hepatitis B and C, HIV, and sexually transmitted infections are also among a selected group of diseases subjected to counterfactual estimation and the CRA methods.[14]

Global health risks are in transition and driven by globalization, urbanization, longevity, declining fertility rates, climate change, and other social and lifestyle factors. Figure 2-3 shows the top leading global risks for mortality in the world including high blood pressure, tobacco use, physical inactivity, overweight, and obesity. The leading global risks for burden of disease (DALYs) in the world are underweight and unsafe

sex, followed by alcohol use and unsafe water, sanitation, and hygiene. Risks of chronic diseases cause the largest share of deaths and DALYs in high- and middle-income countries, although for middle-income countries risks such as unsafe sex and unsafe water and sanitation also cause a larger share of burden of disease, although not to the level noted for low-income countries (Figure 2-4a and 2-4b). In the GBD Study 2010, researchers made an estimate of cause-specific deaths and DALYs attributed to 67 risk factors and risk factor clusters in 21 regions. They estimated exposure distributions by systematically reviewing and synthesizing published and unpublished data. They found that in 2010, the three leading risk factors for disease burden were hypertension, tobacco smoking including secondhand smoke, and alcohol use. For comparison, in 1990 the leading risks were childhood underweight, household air pollution from solid fuels, and tobacco smoking.[15] Risks do vary substantially in different areas of the world but overall the contribution of risk factors to disease burden is shifting away from risks for communicable diseases in children and towards those for non-communicable diseases in adults.

Researchers and public health officials often study and address groups of diseases or conditions and their associated risk factors (cancers, cardiovascular diseases, childhood deaths) due to joint effects of those risk factors and potential synergistic prevention efforts. It is worth noting that the sum of the mortality or

Leading causes of attributable global mortality and burden of disease, 2004

	Attributable Mortality	%		Attributable DALYs	%
1.	High blood pressure	12.8	1.	Childhood underweight	5.9
2.	Tobacco use	8.7	2.	Unsafe sex	4.6
3.	High blood glucose	5.8	3.	Alcohol use	4.5
4.	Physical inactivity	5.5	4.	Unsafe water, sanitation, hygiene	4.2
5.	Overweight and obesity	4.8	5.	High blood pressure	3.7
6.	High cholesterol	4.5	6.	Tobacco use	3.7
7.	Unsafe sex	4.0	7.	Suboptimal breastfeeding	2.9
8.	Alcohol use	3.8	8.	High blood glucose	2.7
9.	Childhood underweight	3.8	9.	Indoor smoke from solid fuels	2.7
10.	Indoor smoke from solid fuels	3.3	10.	Overweight and obesity	2.3
	59 million total global deaths in 2004			1.5 billion total global DALYs in 2004	

Figure 2-3. Leading causes of attributable global mortality and burden of disease, 2004. DALY, disability-adjusted life years.

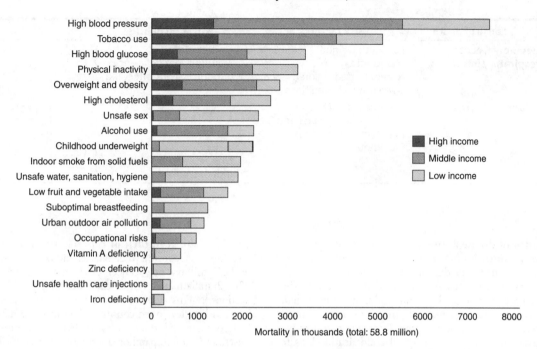

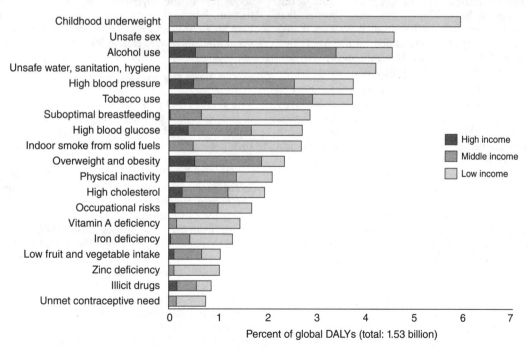

Figure 2-4. (a) Deaths attributed to 19 leading risk factors by country income level, 2004. (b) Percentage of disability-adjusted life-years (DALYs) attributed to 19 leading risk factors by country income level, 2004.

Table 2-5. Leading risk factors and causes of death in children: example of joint contribution of risk factors

Cause of death	Risk factors	% of child deaths		
Pneumonia, acute respiratory infections	Low birth weight Malnutrition Non-breastfed children Overcrowded conditions	Underweight Micronutrient deficiency Suboptimal breastfeeding	35%	
Childhood diarrhea	Non-breastfed children Unsafe drinking water and food Poor hygiene practices Malnutrition			39%
		Unsafe water & sanitation Indoor smoke	23%	

burden of disease attributable to each of the risk factors *separately* is often more than the combined mortality or burden of disease attributable to the groups of these risk factors. As illustrated in Table 2-5, the leading causes of death among children younger than 5 years are acute respiratory infections and diarrheal diseases. Malnutrition is the underlying contributing factor in over a third of all child deaths. Unsafe water, sanitation and hygiene, indoor smoke from solid fuels, together with the nutritional risks and suboptimal breastfeeding, caused 39% of child deaths worldwide in 2004. There is evidence, however, that the overall mortality rate for children younger than 5 years is declining according to new estimates for 2008 (8.795 million deaths from 10.6 million per year during 2000–2003 despite a population increase).

Example: Effect of physical inactivity on burden of disease and life expectancy Physical inactivity is known to increase the risk of heart disease, type 2 diabetes, and breast and colon cancers. Lee and colleagues calculated the PAFs associated with physical inactivity for each of the major NCDs by country to estimate how much disease could be averted if physical inactivity was eliminated.[16] They estimate that physical inactivity causes 6% of the burden of disease from coronary heart disease, 7% of type 2 diabetes, 10% of breast cancer, and 10% of colon cancer. Inactivity causes 9% of premature mortality, or more than 5.3 million of the 57 million deaths that occurred worldwide in 2008. Elimination of physical inactivity would increase the global LE by 0.68 years. The added years seem low, but they represent gains in the whole population including inactive and active people. *The gain for inactive people who become active would be greater.* These findings make inactivity similar to the established risk factors of smoking and obesity.

Example: Global burden of cancers attributable to infections According to de Martel and colleagues, of the 12.7 million new cancer cases that occurred in 2008, 2 million new cancer cases were attributable to infections.[17] This population attribution fraction was higher in less developed countries than in more developed countries. *Helicobacter pylori,* hepatitis B and C viruses, and human papilloma viruses were responsible for 1.9 million cases, mainly gastric, liver, and cervix uteri cancers. In women, cervix uteri cancer accounted for about half of the infection-related burden of cancer; in men, liver and gastric cancers accounted for more than 80%. Around 30% of infection-attributable cases occur in people younger than 50 years.

WHO PROJECTIONS FOR 2030

The WHO GBD project provides updated projections to the year 2030, and the global burden of disease per capita is projected to decrease. The decrease will be less than projected if favorable risk factor trends and economic growth are less than predicted in the model.

The five leading causes of death in 2030 are projected to be ischemic heart disease, stroke, chronic obstructive pulmonary disease (COPD), lower respiratory tract infections, and lung cancers (Table 2-6). Deaths from diarrheal diseases, HIV/AIDS, tuberculosis, maternal and perinatal conditions, and nutritional deficiencies are expected to decline. The impact of infectious diseases over the next 20 years will ultimately depend on control of microbial resistance, development of new antibiotics and vaccines, and national and global disease surveillance and response.

Table 2-7 shows the changes in the leading DALYs from 2004 to 2030. The leading causes of DALYs in 2030 are projected to be unipolar depressive disorder, ischemic heart disease, road traffic accidents,

Table 2-6. The top 10 causes of death worldwide, 2008 and 2030 projections.

Rank	Death or injury	% of deaths, 2008	Rank	Death or injury	% of deaths, 2030
1	Ischemic heart disease	12.8	1	Ischemic heart disease	14.1
2	Cerebrovascular disease	10.8	2	Cerebrovascular disease	12.1
3	Lower respiratory infections	6.1	3	COPD	8.6
4	COPD	5.8	4	Lower respiratory infections	4.2
5	Diarrheal diseases	4.3	5	Trachea, bronchus, lung cancers	3.4
6	HIV/AIDS	3.1	6	Diabetes mellitus	3.3
7	Trachea, bronchus, lung cancers	2.4	7	Road traffic accidents	3.2
8	Tuberculosis	2.4	8	Hypertensive heart disease	2.2
9	Diabetes mellitus	2.2	9	Stomach cancer	1.9
10	Road traffic accidents	2.1	10	HIV/AIDS	1.8

COPD, chronic obstructive pulmonary disease; HIV/AIDS, human immunodeficiency virus/acquired immunodeficiency syndrome. From World Health Organization The Global Burden of Disease: 2004 Update. Ranking of death causes for the 2030 projections are done by the authors and not the WHO.

cerebrovascular disorder, and COPD. Group 1 causes will represent only 20% of total DALYs lost in 2030; group 2 causes (noncommunicable diseases) will represent 66% of total DALYs lost in all income groups.[18] This is due in part to the demographic-epidemiologic transition and the convergence of morbidity and mortality patterns for low- to high-income countries. Ischemic heart disease was the leading cause of DALYs worldwide in 2010, followed by lower respiratory infections, stroke, diarrheal diseases and HIV/AIDS.[19] (Table 2-8)

The WHO and the Joint United Nations Programme on HIV/AIDS have down-adjusted AIDS mortality projections with increasing numbers of

Table 2-7. Leading causes of DALYs, 2004 and 2030.

2004 Disease or injury	As % of total DALYs	Rank	Rank	As % of total DALYs	2030 Disease or injury
Lower respiratory infections	6.2	1	1	6.2	Unipolar depressive disorders
Diarrheal diseases	4.8	2	2	5.5	Ischemic heart disease
Unipolar depressive disorders	4.3	3	3	4.9	Road traffic accidents
Ischemic heart disease	4.1	4	4	4.3	Cerebrovascular disease
HIV/AIDS	3.8	5	5	3.8	COPD
Cerebrovascular disease	3.1	6	6	3.2	Lower respiratory infections
Prematurity and low birth weight	2.9	7	7	2.9	Hearing loss, adult onset
Birth asphyxia and birth trauma	2.7	8	8	2.7	Refractive errors
Road traffic accidents	2.7	9	9	2.5	HIV/AIDS
Neonatal infections and other[a]	2.7	10	10	2.3	Diabetes mellitus
COPD	2.0	13	11	1.9	Neonatal infections and other[a]
Refractive errors	1.8	14	12	1.9	Prematurity and low birth weight
Hearing loss, adult onset	1.8	15	15	1.9	Birth asphyxia and birth trauma
Diabetes mellitus	1.3	19	18	1.6	Darrheal diseases

http://www.who.int/healthinfo/global_burden_disease/GBD_report_2004update_part4.pdf
[a]This category also includes other non-infectious causes arising in the perinatal period apart from prematurity, low birth weight, birth trauma and asphyxia. These non-infectious causes are responsible for about 20% of DALYs shown in this category.

Table 2-8. Global DALY rank with 95% uncertainty interval (UI) for the top 20 causes in 2010.

Disorder	Mean rank (95% UI)
1 Ischemic heart disease	1.0 (1 to 2)
2 Lower respiratory infections	2.0 (1 to 3)
3 Stroke	3.2 (2 to 5)
4 Diarrhea	4.9 (4 to 8)
5 HIV/AIDS	6.6 (4 to 9)
6 Low back pain	6.7 (3 to 11)
7 Malaria	6.7 (3 to 11)
8 Preterm birth complications	8.0 (5 to 11)
9 COPD	8.1 (5 to 11)
10 Road injury	8.4 (4 to 11)
11 Major depressive disorder	10.8 (7 to14)
12 Neonatal encephalopathy	13.3 (11 to 17)
13 Tuberculosis	13.4 (11 to 17)
14 Diabetes	14.2 (12 to 16)
15 Iron-deficiency anemia	15.2 (11 to 22)
16 Neonatal sepsis	15.9 (10 to 26)
17 Congenital anomalies	17.3 (14 to 21)
18 Self-harm	18.8 (15 to 26)
19 Falls	19.7 (16 to 25)
20 Protein-energy malnutrition	20.0 (16 to 26)

Data from Murray CJL, et al. Disability-adjusted life years (DALYs) for 291 diseases and injuries in 21 regions, 1990-2010: a systematic analysis for the Global Burden of Disease Study 2010. Lancet 2012; 380: 2197-2223.

people getting antiretroviral therapy and strengthening preventive measures. The latest WHO forecast expects AIDS deaths to decline to 1.2 million in 2030.[18] AIDS deaths were estimated to be 1.77 million in 2010 according to UNAIDS, 21% higher than the 1.47 million deaths estimated by the GBD Study 2010.[20] These projections are subject to change depending on available funding for universal access to treatment, new therapeutic options, and scaling up of programs such as treatment as prevention and preexposure prophylaxis. See Chapter 11 for more information on HIV/AIDS.

The WHO projected that tobacco use will cause 8.4 million deaths by 2020, 70% of which will occur in developing countries. The number of women who smoke (currently 9% of smokers) will continue to rise from 250 to 340 million by 2020.[21] According to another analysis, the worldwide tobacco mortality will increase to approximately 10 million per year, or 100 million per decade, around 2030.[22] Cardiovascular diseases, lung cancer, and COPD are the leading causes of death from smoking globally. Tobacco consumes a significant percentage of household expenditures, especially in low- and middle-income countries, diverting resources from education, food, and health care. Indeed, the link between tobacco and poverty is often ignored. Transnational tobacco companies are able to take advantage of trade liberalization and pursue massive marketing efforts in emerging market economies. More than ever, cost-effective tobacco control measures such as advertising control, price and tax increases, smoke-free area legislation, and other trade regulations as advocated by the WHO Framework Convention on Tobacco Control (http://www.who.int/fctc/en/) are absolutely critical to decrease tobacco consumption worldwide.

POVERTY AND THE GLOBAL BURDEN OF DISEASE

Public health officials have long recognized that human health is the foundation of economic growth and development. In the projections by the GBD Study, "diseases of poverty" such as malaria, tuberculosis, and AIDS will still affect low-income countries disproportionally more than affluent countries. This will perpetuate the never-ending cycle that starts with poor health status, underdevelopment of the workforce, and lack of economic growth and results in poverty and worsening of overall health status. Southeast Asia and Africa together bore 54% of the total global burden of disease in 2004, although they account for only about 40% of the world's population. Children bear more than half of the disease burden in low-income countries, and almost half of the disease burden in low- and middle-income countries is now from noncommunicable diseases.[18]

The eight Millennium Development Goals (MDGs) is a set of international development goals, agreed by 193 UN member states and several international organizations to tackle poverty, hunger, and disease by 2015. Four of the eight MDGs are particularly pertinent to the burden of disease and risk factors discussed in this chapter (http://www.un.org/millenniumgoals/).

MDG1: Eradicate extreme poverty and hunger includes clean drinking water and child malnutrition targets.

MDG4: Reduce child mortality. In 2004, among the 10.4 million deaths in children under 5 years worldwide, 4.7 million (45%) are in the African Region and 3.1 million (30%) are in the Southeast Asia Region. In other words, more than 7 of every 10 child deaths are in Africa and Southeast Asia, and of preventable causes such as diarrheal diseases, pneumonia, malaria, measles, and HIV/AIDS.

MDG5: Improve maternal health. Maternal mortality ratio in low-income country groups improved to 410/100,000 live births in 2010, slashed in half since 1990 but still 29 times the rate of high-income countries.

MDG6: Combat HIV/AIDS, malaria, and other diseases. There is need for more data on the burden of neglected and tropical diseases (NTDs), and the DALY has been criticized for underestimating DWs for chronic diseases such as the NTDs by not accounting for the importance of social, cultural, and environmental context of poverty in those health states.[23]

Collectively, the MDG-related causes of burden account for 29.8% of the total burden of disease in 2010. This reflects a decline by nearly 32.0% from 1990 and progress, although we are unlikely to achieve most of the targets by 2015.[19] According to analysis from the Center for Global Development, most of the world's poor (defined as living under US$1.25 per day) now live in middle-income countries (MICs). In fact, there are up to a billion poor people or a "new bottom billion" living not in the world's poorest countries but in MICs.[24] Most of the world's poor live in populous countries that have moved from low- to middle-income country status—China, Pakistan, India, Nigeria, and Indonesia. This has implications for international development policy by donors and public private partnerships such as the Global Fund and Global Alliance for Vaccine and Immunisation.

Researchers have long been interested in estimating the potential health benefits of eradicating poverty, with the belief that poverty is a major underlying determinant of health. In reality, the association of any specified socioeconomic factor with risk factors for disease or health is likely to be confounded by other variables such as education, age, and ethnicity, by contextual factors related to government and infrastructure development, and by time lags (i.e., the time it takes for income improvement to manifest as change in risk factor exposure).

Example: The Burden of Poverty To quantify the disease burden of socioeconomic position, Blakely, Hales, and Woodward used the "population-attributable risk" to estimate the impact of income poverty amelioration on child malnutrition as a health risk factor in Pakistan.[25] Based on the assumption that the relative risks of disease states are often comparable for different socioeconomic factors, they estimated that 60% of the population lives on US$1 to $2 per day. The counterfactual scenario requires that those people living on less than US$2 per day adopt the risk factor profile of those living on more than US$2 per day. The impact fractions or the population-attributable risk is then 50%. That is, 50% of childhood malnutrition is attributable to poverty by this calculation, reinforcing the importance of income poverty as a determinant of

risk factor prevalence (and as a proxy for health). The authors acknowledge that this may be an overestimate. Other studies suggest that both poverty eradication and public health programs targeted at poor communities are required to improve health and to reduce socioeconomic inequalities in health.

GLOBAL HEALTH DISPARITIES

The WHO is interested in measuring health inequalities separately from measuring the average levels of health as indications of a country's performance on health. The achievement of health equalities translates to equality of healthy lifespans and equality of health risks that involve unavoidable factors and individual choices. Health inequalities have typically been measured in a *bivariate* fashion, for example, different levels of health across income groups. Gakidou, Murray, and Frenk propose a framework to study health inequality as the distribution of health expectancy across individuals in the population.[26] These latter advocates of *univariate* health inequalities offer an overall picture of health inequality in the population in a way that is comparable across populations. A summary measure of health inequality has yet to be formalized at the time of this publication.

The burden of disease in the United States among racial or ethnic minorities disturbingly mirrors that in low-income countries and reflects global inequities in health. Compared with other high-income countries, its lack of universal health care coverage and resulting disparities in access to health care and preventive health services are well documented. The CDC's 2011 *Health Disparities and Inequalities* report outlines the persistent trends in health disparities by race and ethnicity, income and education, disability state, and other social characteristics.[27] In 2006, the US infant mortality rate was 6.68 infant deaths per 1,000 live births with the highest rate in non-Hispanic black women 2.4 times that of non-Hispanic white women. Black men and women also have higher death rates from coronary heart disease and strokes than men and women from other races. During the 9-year study period (1999–2007), homicide rates were consistently highest among young non-Hispanic black men. Similar disparities were found in obesity, asthma prevalence, HIV infection, diabetes, hypertension, hypertension control, cigarette smoking, adolescent pregnancy, binge drinking, environmental hazards, and social determinants of health.

The poorest and most vulnerable people in the world are still affected by infectious diseases that are largely treatable and preventable. Lower respiratory tract infections, tuberculosis, diarrheal diseases, HIV, neonatal infections, and malaria remain leading causes of death and burden of disease in low- and middle-income countries. At the same time, chronic diseases have become much more prominent due to social and economic development and the associated consumption of tobacco, alcohol, and high-sugar, high-fat foods. Such diseases further strain health care resources and infrastructure in these countries, which now have to deal with a double burden of disease. There is also evidence of a triple burden of disease that is referred to as communicable disease, noncommunicable disease, and sociobehavioral illness or the rising incidence of injuries particularly from road traffic accidents. Influenza-type pandemics have the potential to inflict catastrophic mortality and economic costs worldwide, especially in the poorest countries that have limited resources for surveillance coupled with poor health care infrastructure and health status.

We are at the critical junction in global health at which efforts to reform health systems and to control risk factors will require the commitment and coordination of policymakers, researchers, health ministries, the WHO, the World Bank, private donors, and nongovernmental organizations to improve the health of all citizens around the world. Summary measures of population health such as DALYs still need to prove their value in affecting health policy changes and resource allocation worldwide, especially in the poorest regions in the world. Such summary measures should also be sensitive to changes in the current health status and to changes in risk factors by particular interventions. Nevertheless, most experts believe in and advocate for better health data and disease surveillance as a first step to improving global health status and reducing health inequalities.

STUDY QUESTIONS

1. Try to obtain the latest mortality rates by age and sex of a low-income country. Could you decipher the data sources?

2. Examine the data in the World Health Statistics 2010. What is the LE at birth for a male in your country of interest in 2008? The HALE at birth in 2007? What is the average LE for the global population (both sexes)? How is LE calculated? It involves life tables and you can read more about it at http://www.who.int/en/

3. What information would you need to calculate the disease burden of HIV/AIDS for a specific country in a single year? Make up a hypothetical set of numbers for HIV/AIDS for an African country, and compute the burden as DALYs per 1,000 population per year. Dr. Neal Nathanson of the University of Pennsylvania has provided this

study question and a data set for HIV/AIDS for Botswana in year 2000. The data needed for this table are (1) the age distribution of the population for year 2000, (2) the age-specific incidence of HIV infections, (3) the LE after HIV infection and the weight for each year living with HIV/AIDS (arbitrary guesstimates), and (4) the LE for the healthy population (the average age of HIV infection is taken to be around 20 years of age, and a healthy LE of 65 years at age 20). The main guesstimate required is the conversion from age-specific prevalence of HIV infections to age-specific incidence of HIV infections because there were no direct measures of HIV incidence available in Botswana.

4. Scientists have tried to estimate the health impacts of climate change. What type of health outcomes or diseases would be associated with climate change? What knowledge gaps should be addressed to improve future assessments? (See http://www.who.int/globalchange/publications/climatechangechap7.pdf)

REFERENCES

1. Murray CJL, Salomon J, Mathers C. A critical examination of summary measures of population health. http://www.who.int/healthinfo/paper02.pdf.

2. Field MJ, Gold M; Institute of Medicine Committee on Summary Measures of Population Health. *Summarizing Population Health: Directions for the Development and Application of Population Metrics.* Washington, DC: National Academy Press,1998.

3. Walensky RP, Wood R, Fofana MO, et al. The clinical impact and cost-effectiveness of routine, voluntary HIV screening in South Africa. *J Acquir Immune Defic Syndr* 2011;56(1):26–35.

4. Salomon JA, Weinstein MC, Hammitt JK, Goldie SJ. Cost-effectiveness of treatment for chronic hepatitis C infection in an evolving patient population. *JAMA* 2003;290:228–237.

5. Jagger C, Reyes-Frausto S. Monitoring health by healthy active life expectancy—a user's guide. *Trent Public Health Observatory*, March 2003.

6. Salomon JA, Wang H, Freeman MK, et al. Healthy life expectancy for 187 countries, 1990-2010: a systematic analysis for the Global Burden of Disease Study 2010. *The Lancet* 2012;380(9859):2144-2162.

7. Stiefel MC, Perla RJ, Zell BL. A healthy bottom line: healthy life expectancy as an outcome measure for health improvement efforts. *Milbank Q* 2010;88(1):30–53.

8. Shield KD, Gmel G, Patra J, Rehm J. Global burden of injuries attributable to alcohol consumption in 2004. *Popul Health Metr* 2012;10:9.

9. National Cancer Institute. Cancer trends progress report—2011/2012 update. Person-years of life lost (through 2008). http://progressreport.cancer.gov/doc_detail.asp?pid=1&did=2007&chid=76&coid=730&mid=.

10. Salomon JA, Vos T, Hagan DR, et al. Common values in assessing health outcomes from disease and injury: disability weights measurement study for the Global Burden of Disease Study 2010. *The Lancet* 2012;380:2129-2143.

11. Ditsuwan V, Veerman LJ, Barendregt JJ, Bertram M, Vos T. The national burden of road traffic injuries in Thailand. *Popul Health Metr* 2011;9:2.

12. Institute of Health Metrics and Evaluation. GBG Study Operations Manual-Final Draft. 2009. Global Burden of Disease Study. http://www.globalburden.org/GBD_Study_Operations_Manual_Jan_20_2009.pdf.

13. Fürst T, Keiser J, Utzinger J. Global burden of human food-borne trematodiasis: a systematic review and meta-analysis. *Lancet Inf Dis* 2012;12:210–221.

14. World Health Organization. *Global Health Risks. Mortality and Burden of Disease Attributable to Selected Major Risks.* Geneva: World Health Organization, 2009.

15. Lim SS, Vos T, Flaxman AD, et al. A comparative risk assessment of burden of disease and injury attributable to 67 risk factors and risk factor clusters in 21 regions, 1990-2010: a systematic analysis for the Global Burden of Disease Study 2010. *The Lancet* 2012;380:2224-2260.

16. Lee IM, Shiroma EJ, Lobelo F, Puska P, Blair SN, Katzmarzyk PT. Effect of physical inactivity on major non-communicable disease worldwide: an analysis of burden of disease and life expectancy. *Lancet* 2012;380:219–229.

17. de Martel C, Ferlay J, Franceschi S, et al. Global burden of cancers attributable to infections in 2008: a review and synthetic analysis. *Lancet Oncol* 2012;13:607–615.

18. World Health Organization. *The Global Burden of Disease 2004 Update.* Geneva: World Health Organization, 2008.

19. Murray CJL, Vos T, Lozano R, et al. Disability-adjusted life years (DALYs) for 291 diseases and injuries in 21 regions, 1990-2010: a systematic analysis for the Global Burden of Disease Study 2010. *The Lancet* 2012;380:2197-2223.

20. Lozano R, Naghavi Mohsen, Foreman K, et al. Global and regional mortality from 235 causes of death for 20 age groups in 1990 and 2010: a systematic analysis for the Global Burden of Disease Study 2010. *Lancet* 2012;380:2095-2128.

21. World Health Organization. Trade, foreign policy, diplomacy and health. Tobacco. http://www.who.int/trade/glossary/story089/en/index.html.

22. Jha P. Avoidable global cancer deaths and total deaths from smoking. *Nat Rev Cancer* 2009;9:655–664.

23. King CH, Bertino AM. Asymmetries of poverty: why global burden of disease valuations underestimate the burden of neglected tropical diseases. *PLoS Negl Trop Dis* 2008:2(3):e209.

24. Glassman A, Duran D, Sumner A. Global health and the new bottom billion. Center for Global Development,October 2011. http://www.cgdev.org/files/1425581_file_Glassman_Duran_Sumner_MIC_global_health_FINAL.pdf.

25. Blakely T, Hales S, Woodward A. *Poverty: Assessing the Distribution of Health Risks by Socioeconomic Position at National and Local Levels.* Geneva: World Health Organization, 2004. http://www.who.int/quantifying_ehimpacts/publications/ebd10/en/index.html.

26. Gakidou EE, Murray CJ, Frenk J. Defining and measuring health inequality: an approach based on the distribution of health expectancy. *Bull World Health Organ* 2000;78(1):42–54.

27. Centers for Disease Control and Prevention MMWR supplement. Health disparities and inequalities reports—United States, 2011. Published January 14, 2011. http://www.cdc.gov/mmwr/pdf/other/su6001.pdf.

Epidemiology, Biostatistics, and Surveillance

3

Christopher Martin

LEARNING OBJECTIVES

- *Understand the important contributions of chance, bias, and confounding as potential sources of false epidemiologic associations and apply methods to control for these factors*
- *Describe commonly used measures of morbidity and mortality as they are used in the global setting*
- *Discuss the various types of epidemiologic study designs together with their relative strengths and weaknesses as well as the measures of association they provide*
- *Interpret test results within the context of screening and surveillance with attention to sensitivity, specificity, and predictive value*
- *Apply epidemiologic methods to the control of infectious disease*
- *Distinguish the two types of surveillance and describe the components of a useful surveillance program*

EPIDEMIOLOGY AND THE PUBLIC HEALTH APPROACH

Epidemiology is concerned with the identification, measurement, and analysis of factors that may be associated with differences in the health status of populations. The goal of such investigations is to modify these factors to improve the health status of individuals. *Classical epidemiology* is focused on populations, seeks to identify risk factors, and has been described as the "basic science" of public health. Therefore, some familiarity with epidemiologic methods is essential to the understanding of public and global health. The public health approach can be illustrated by the epidemiologic triad as applied to malaria (Figure 3-1).

According to this model, disease arises through interactions between a host, environment, and agent. In the case of many infectious diseases, a vector through which the agent is transmitted is also relevant. This model allows opportunities for the interruption of disease transmission to be clarified. For example, in the case of malaria, opportunities might include the use of insecticide-treated bednets for the host, reduced areas of standing water in the environment, destruction of the *Anopheles* mosquito vector through pesticides, and chemoprophylaxis targeted at the plasmodium.

Note that the public health model takes a very broad view of what constitutes a risk factor for disease. Whereas a traditional biomedical paradigm tends to focus on a small number of causes for a disease, such as a specific microorganism, public health considers more diverse social, economic, and environmental factors as playing a potentially causative role in disease development, each offering an opportunity for intervention.

Indeed, there are potentially an infinite number of causative factors, each acting at various points along a timeline as shown in Figure 3-2, which depicts two such factors for simplicity. For each factor, there is an *induction period* between when that factor acts and when the disease is initiated. After disease initiation, there follows a *latent period* corresponding to a preclinical phase before the disease is recognized. Preventive strategies can be placed into three groups based on this chronology. The preferred approach is always *primary prevention* because interventions are made prior to disease initiation, such as vaccination

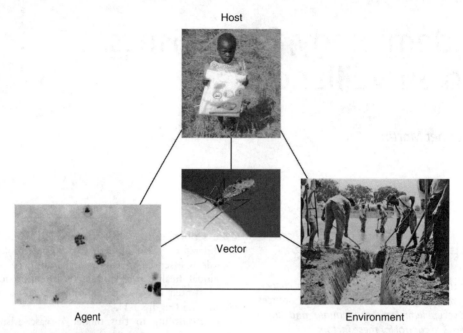

Figure 3-1. Epidemiologic triad for malaria.

to confer immunity to measles. Screening is by definition a form of *secondary prevention* as it attempts to identify asymptomatic individuals with disease with the intent of improving treatment outcomes through earlier intervention. Lastly, *tertiary prevention* does not alter the full manifestation of a disease but seeks to limit the long-term sequelae. Such measures might include physical and occupational therapy following a stroke resulting in hemiplegia.

Although the distinction between epidemiology and biostatistics is not always apparent, biostatistics has a relatively greater emphasis on data gathering and analysis. Accordingly, this field provides a variety of measures used to quantify both disease outcomes (morbidity) and

death (mortality). Further, biostatistics offers methods to examine the relationships between variables, especially whether such relationships could have arisen purely as a result of chance, a procedure known as *statistical inference*.

Chance, Bias, and Confounding

Before reviewing the methods of epidemiology and biostatistics, some understanding of the considerations in determining whether or not associations are valid and causal is needed. An *association* refers to a relationship in which a change in the frequency of one variable is associated with a change in the frequency

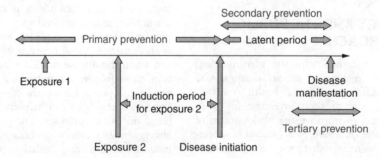

Figure 3-2. Disease timeline with levels of prevention.

of another. For example, x and y may be described as associated if an increase in x also results in an increase in y. *Causation* is a special type of association in which one condition precedes the other and must be present for the outcome to occur.

Although all causal relationships are forms of associations, the converse is not true; that is, there are many additional reasons that might account for any observed association. To illustrate the difference, epidemiologists classically refer to the example of storks and babies. It can be shown that for many parts of the world, birth rates are higher in those regions with higher populations of storks. However, although these two variables may be positively associated, this is clearly not a causal relationship. The distinction is important because statistics and epidemiology only provide insight into associations. Determining whether an association is causal depends on the application of nonepidemiologic principles. The most widely used are what have now come to be known as the Bradford Hill criteria.[1] The most important of these are listed in Table 3-1.

Other than causality, the three most important potential sources for a false association are chance, bias, and confounding. To critically interpret epidemiologic studies, it is essential to address the potential contribution of each of these three factors. If chance, bias, and confounding are not believed to account for an association, the findings are considered *valid*.

Chance refers to a fluke association. Whenever data are collected in an experiment, unusual results can be obtained in a random manner. For example, a coin may be flipped four times and yield heads on all occasions. Clearly, such unusual associations are more likely to occur when the sample size of an experiment is small. The role of chance is well handled by biostatistics, which provides information on the likelihood that any observed association could have arisen by chance through tests of statistical significance. Generally, a value of 0.05 (5%) is considered a key threshold in determining whether there is or is not an association.

Even when study results are reported as statistically significant, we must still determine whether the association is real. In some studies, a very large number of independent associations are explored. Often, these associations were not specified a priori as hypotheses under study. If 20 such comparisons were made, on average, one will appear to be statistically significant with the use of a 5% or 1-in-20 threshold for significance. Such findings are best described as *hypothesis generating* because they require further study in which the specific hypothesis is articulated before the data is collected to determine if the association is real.

However, a *negative study* refers to no association being observed in the study. Two potential

Table 3-1. Bradford Hill criteria.

Strength	Greater associations (large relative risks or odds ratios, generally above 1.5) are observed. In such instances, other influences, such as bias and confounding, are less likely to account for an association.
Consistency	The same association is observed repeatedly. Note that this criterion is only useful when different populations are studied using different experimental designs.
Specificity	One detailed association rather than claims of multiple outcomes for any one intervention. By this criterion, we often dismiss so-called cure-alls that are advocated for a plethora of ailments.
Temporality	The cause must precede the effect. This is the only mandatory criterion for causality.
Biological gradient	A dose-response relationship is observed in which the association becomes stronger with increases in the amount of the causal factor.
Plausibility	A mechanism can be advanced to explain the association.
Experimental evidence	Other types of investigations, such as animal studies, are supportive of the association.

From Bradford Hill A. *A Short Textbook of Medical Statistics*. 11th ed. 1977 London: Hodder and Stoughton. (Reproduced with permission.)

explanations must be considered in such a scenario. The first factor is insufficient sample size. A sample size justification should be included in any study that makes explicit the assumptions underlying the methods by which the number of participants was chosen. This sample size calculation depends on the magnitude of the effect under study (smaller effects require larger sample sizes) as well as information about the frequency of exposure and outcome in the study.

When a study is performed, investigators propose the so-called *null hypothesis*, denoted as H_0, which states there is no association between the risk factor and the outcome under study in the population from which the sample has been drawn. After the data are collected and analyzed, the null hypothesis will either be accepted (the findings are not statistically

Table 3-2. Types of error.

	H₀ is true	H₀ is false
Do not reject H₀ (not statistically significant)	Correct!	Type II error (beta)
Reject H₀ (statistically significant)	Type I error (alpha)	Correct! Statistical power

significant) or rejected (the findings are statistically significant). Therefore, four situations can arise, as depicted in Table 3-2. If the null hypothesis is accepted when it is true, a correct decision has been made. If the null hypothesis is accepted when in fact it is false, a type II error, denoted by beta, is committed. Beta is conventionally set at 20% in calculating an appropriate sample size.

Conversely, if one rejects the null hypothesis and concludes that there is a statistically significant relationship between two variables when in fact the null hypothesis is true, one commits a type I error, denoted by alpha. Alpha is set at 5%, again by convention, and corresponds to the threshold to which *p* values calculated from statistical tests of significance will be compared. If the calculated *p* value is less than alpha, the null hypothesis is rejected. Finally, if the null hypothesis is rejected when it is in fact false, a correct decision has been made.

Note that type I and type II errors are trade-offs because these are opposite actions. Therefore, a decrease in the likelihood of one increases the likelihood of the other. Because it is generally felt that errors involving incorrect rejection of the null hypothesis are worse, alpha is set at a lower level than that of beta. In planning a study, investigators want to be confident that they enroll a sufficient number of subjects so that if there truly is an association, it can be detected. As can be seen from Table 3-2, this refers to the statistical power of the study and is calculated as 1–beta.

What do these values of alpha and beta really mean? They provide distributions reflective of the values of statistical tests if there is no relationship between the two variables, that is, under the null hypothesis. The process of *statistical inference* involves the calculation of parameters such as z, t, or chi-square statistics, which all involve a difference between the observed results and those expected under the null hypothesis. As observed results become more extreme from those predicted under the null hypothesis, the likelihood of achieving statistical significance increases. Lower *p* values correspond to test statistics that fall near one end of this distribution and therefore to findings that are unlikely to have arisen by chance. It should always be borne in mind that the choice of a *p* value less than

0.05 as justification for statistical significance is both totally arbitrary and historic, with origins in publications dating back to the early 1900s.

Confounding occurs when there is a third variable that is independently linked to both the risk factor and the disease outcome under study. For example, epidemiologic studies published a number of years ago reported an association between consumption of coffee and the development of certain types of cancer. However, it was subsequently shown that the findings were confounded by failure to control for cigarette smoking. Those individuals who drink coffee are also more likely to smoke, and smoking is an independent risk factor for cancer. Although the investigators thought they were comparing groups who differed in the amount of coffee consumed, in reality, they were comparing groups with differing numbers of cigarettes consumed, and it was this latter risk factor that resulted in the observed difference in cancer between the groups.

Confounding can be handled using a variety of approaches, listed in Table 3-3. However, it is obvious that to control a confounder, one must be aware of it. The only method available to control for unknown confounders is *randomization* in a clinical trial. With appropriate randomization, groups will be the same with respect to every variable, including both known and unknown confounders, and differ only with respect to the intervention under study.

Finally, *bias* is a systematic error that affects one group preferentially in comparison with another. For example, *recall bias* refers to the observation that sick people tend to recall more of any exposures, even those that have nothing to do with disease. Many types of bias exist; some of the more common forms are listed in Table 3-4. Because bias is difficult to quantify or measure, it is not easily handled using statistical methods. Therefore, efforts are targeted at minimizing bias in study design through assessment tools that are objective and standardized. A clinical trial offers one of the most powerful methods to reduce bias through *blinding*. As the name suggests, with this technique a person (the study subject or investigator) is unaware of the intervention (if any) being allocated.

Table 3-3. Methods to control confounding.

Method	Example	Limitation
Matching	For each case with disease, a control is selected with the same level of confounder	Does not allow any measurement of the strength of the confounder
Stratification	Divide subjects into different levels of the confounder	Only practical for a small number of confounders
Randomization	Randomly allocate subjects to receive the intervention under study	Requires control of the intervention on the part of investigators
Multivariate analysis	Control influence of other variables using statistical software to isolate and examine the effect of one	Methods are complex
Restriction	A study of cardiovascular disease only enrolls men	Reduces the generalizability of the study findings

Table 3-4. Forms of bias.

Type of bias	Definition
Selection bias	Error in how subjects are enrolled in a study.
The healthy worker effect	Working populations appear to be healthier when compared with the general population due to out-migration of sick people from the workforce.
Volunteer bias	Subjects who agree to participate in a study differ from those who refuse, generally by being healthier.
Berkson's bias	Patients receiving medical treatment are different from those in the general population. For example, patients with comorbid conditions may be more likely to seek treatment than those with a single diagnosis, leading to false associations between the two diseases if only treated populations are studied.
Information or observer bias	Error in how data are gathered about exposure or disease.
Recall bias	Subjects who are sick recall more past exposures, independent of any causal role.
Interviewer bias	Investigators may preferentially elicit information about exposure or outcomes if aware of the subject's status in a study.
Systematic or differential misclassification	Errors in how exposure or outcome status is determined.
Loss to follow-up	Error introduced if loss to follow-up in a study is related to outcome under investigation.

If chance, bias, and confounding are not believed to account for an association, the findings are considered *valid*. However, many other factors must be considered before one can conclude that valid results are causal and relevant. These factors are discussed in the section on study design later in this chapter. Valid results may not apply to populations other than those included in the study. This consideration relates to the *generalizability* of the findings.

BASIC HEALTH INDICATORS

To study the causes of disease, it is necessary to begin by examining basic health indicators, which include measures of mortality and morbidity. In spite of the widespread use of such indicators, particularly to compare the health status of different countries, it is important to recognize that health involves much more than is reflected by such statistics. In 1948, the World Health Organization (WHO) defined health as "a state of complete physical, mental, and social well-being and not merely the absence of disease or infirmity." Although this definition has been criticized as utopian, it does highlight the concept that good health is a much more complex notion than simply not having a disease.

In a general sense, most of the measures of morbidity and mortality consist of a numerator such as the number of cases or deaths divided by a denominator representing the population at risk. To measure the size of the population, most countries perform a periodic census, usually every 10 years. Data on births and deaths are collected on a continuous basis and, together with marital status, are collectively referred to as *vital statistics*.

From a practical perspective, it is usually more difficult to obtain reliable data for the population at risk (denominator for the measures) relative to the number of cases or deaths (numerator). For example, according to the United Nations Statistics Division, the last census completed in the nation of Somalia was in 1987. This lack of information represents a major limitation in understanding the health status of such countries.

The WHO provides basic health indicators together with additional health statistics for all member states in the World Health Report, produced annually since 1995 and available in several languages online at http://www.who.int/whr/.

Measures of Morbidity

The two key measures of disease frequency are prevalence and incidence. Whereas *prevalence* refers to the number of existing cases at any one time, *incidence* is restricted to the number of new cases occurring over a defined period of time.

The two types of prevalence are point and period prevalence. The *point prevalence* is calculated as the number of existing cases divided by the population at risk at that same time. However, obtaining such instantaneous information is commonly quite difficult, especially for larger populations. In practice, it might require a prolonged period of time simply to assess the population for the number of cases. Suppose a survey was carried out in 2012 in a province of Indonesia to ascertain the number of cases of tuberculosis. The number of cases, divided usually by the mid-2012

population of the province, is a *period prevalence*. Note that for either type of prevalence, there are no units of time. Therefore, prevalence is not a rate.

The significant limitation in use of the prevalence with respect to understanding trends in disease is that it does not reflect differences in whether a case was recently diagnosed or diagnosed quite some time in the past. For this reason, it is usually preferable to examine the number of new cases by determining the incidence rather than the prevalence.

The denominator for incidence is usually expressed as *person-years*. This is a common metric that allows data from separate observations to be pooled when there is variable follow-up of each individual. For smaller populations, each subject may be considered separately rather than assuming that follow-up is uniform. In such situations, an *incidence density* is used when there is variable follow-up between subjects. Consider the example shown in Figure 3-3. Only subject A is followed for the entire duration of the study, contributing 8 person-years of disease-free time. However, each of the others can be added, for a total of 30 person-years. The incidence rate or incidence density is then calculated as 4 cases divided by 30 person-years, or 0.13 case per person-year.

There is a clear relationship between incidence and prevalence, namely, prevalence equals incidence times duration, $P = I \times D$. Therefore, factors that increase the duration of disease will increase the prevalence, independent of any change in incidence. The many

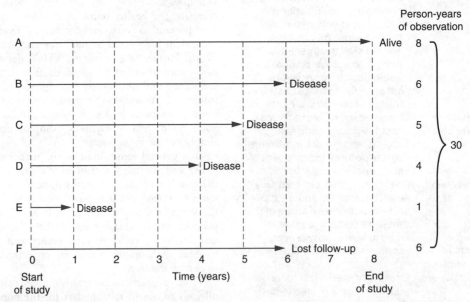

Figure 3-3. Calculation of incidence rate or density in an 8-year study of six persons (A through F).

Table 3-5. Factors that may increase incidence and prevalence independent of changes in the number of new cases.

Factors increasing both incidence and prevalence	Factors increasing prevalence only
Greater case ascertainment	Improved (noncurative) treatment
Enhanced diagnostic methods	Out-migration of healthy people from population.
More liberal criteria in disease definition (examples: AIDS; body mass index thresholds for obesity in the United States)	In-migration of people with disease into population

factors that can influence prevalence and incidence other than changes in the frequency of new cases are shown in Table 3-5.

Measures of Mortality

Measures of mortality offer the obvious practical advantage of being based on an objective, easily recognized outcome. Three generic measures—rates, ratios, and proportions—are generally used (Figure 3-4). However, incorrect usage of these terms (especially *rate*) is very common in the health literature.

The most simple death measure is what is usually referred to as the *crude death rate,* which, because it contains no unit of time, is not actually a rate. Because the calculated number is usually very small, the figure is conventionally expressed per 1,000 people. For example, the WHO reported that the crude death rate for Botswana was 12.6 deaths per 1,000 persons in 2010. In contrast, the corresponding figure for Brazil was reported to be 6.4 deaths per 1,000 persons.

Obviously, these figures cannot be directly compared because many other differences between these two countries may independently influence mortality. Perhaps most important, Brazil has an older population than Botswana, a confounder that precludes a meaningful direct comparison of rates. In other words, comparing crude death rates may actually *underestimate* the true difference in health status of these two populations. A variety of approaches can be used to address this limitation. One is to compare age-specific death rates (such as deaths in those 25 to 30 years of age) or cause-specific death rates (such as deaths from pneumonia).

Another method is *standardization,* which can be done either directly or indirectly. Both types involve the same calculation but are performed in different directions, as illustrated using hypothetical data in Table 3-6. Note that the crude death rate of town A is lower than that of town B. However, closer inspection of the rate within each age stratum shows that all are higher in town A than B. The explanation for this paradox lies in the differing age structure of the two towns: more people are in the older age groups

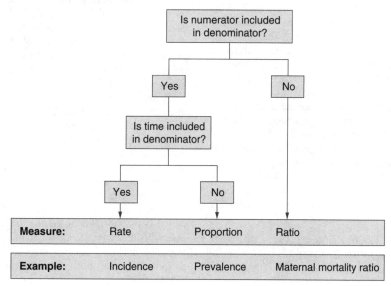

Figure 3-4. Distinguishing between rates, proportions, and ratios.

Table 3-6. Data for standardization example. (see text)

	Town A			Town B		
Age	Population	Deaths	Death rate per 1,000	Population	Deaths	Death rate per 1,000
0–14	500	2	4	400	1	2.5
15–29	2,000	8	4	300	1	3.3
30–44	2,000	12	6	1,000	5	5
45–59	1,000	10	10	2,000	18	9
60–74	500	20	40	2,000	70	35
75+	100	15	150	400	50	125
Total	6,100	67	11.0	6,100	145	23.8

From Bradford Hill A. *A Short Textbook of Medical Statistics.* 11th ed. London: Hodder and Stoughton. (Modified with permission.)

in town B. With direct standardization, the death rate from town A is multiplied by the number of people in that age stratum in town B. The number that arises is the number of deaths given town A's death rate for each age stratum but using town B's overall population structure. This is the directly standardized death rate for town A, using town B as a standard. This figure is calculated as follows:

$$(4/1,000) \times 400 = 1.6 \text{ deaths}$$
$$(4/1,000) \times 300 = 1.2 \text{ deaths}$$
$$(6/1,000) \times 1,000 = 6 \text{ deaths}$$
$$(10/1,000) \times 2,000 = 20 \text{ deaths}$$
$$(40/1,000) \times 2,000 = 80 \text{ deaths}$$
$$(150/1,000) \times 400 = 60 \text{ deaths}$$

Total of 168.8 deaths per 6,100 = 27.7 deaths per 1,000 persons

This figure is now higher than the rate of 23.8 in town B. The conclusion is that, when corrected for age, the mortality is higher in town A than B. This disappearance or reversal of an observed difference when data are stratified and standardized by different levels of a confounder illustrates a concept epidemiologists refer to as *Simpson's paradox.*

An alternative approach is to take the death rates of town B and apply them to the age structure of town A. The deaths for each stratum can then be added to yield the number of "expected" deaths if people in town A were dying at the same frequency as those in town B. The observed number of deaths divided by the expected number of deaths yields the *standardized mortality ratio* (SMR). In this case, the calculation is as follows:

$$(2.5/1,000) \times 500 = 1.25$$
$$(3.3/1,000) \times 2000 = 6.6$$
$$(5/1,000) \times 2000 = 10$$
$$(9/1,000) \times 1000 = 9$$
$$(35/1,000) \times 500 = 17.5$$

$$(125/1,000) \times 100 = 12.5$$
$$\text{Total} = 56.9$$
$$\text{SMR} = 67/56.9 = 1.18$$

The SMR of 1.18 (sometimes multiplied by 100 and expressed as 118) is an indirectly standardized ratio for town A using town B as a standard. Because this figure is greater than 1 (or 100), it provides the same result as the directly standardized rates: the mortality appears to be greater in town A than B when corrected for the different age structures. In general, indirect standardization is used when study populations are smaller. Moreover, the SMR provides an intuitive comparison within one figure, rather than two contrasting rates.

As noted earlier, because it is difficult to obtain denominator data, the *proportional mortality ratio* (PMR) is frequently used because it only requires more readily available death data. The PMR is calculated as the number of deaths from a specific cause divided by the total number of deaths in the same population. If there are 4,000 total deaths in a population and 200 of these are as the result of injury, the PMR is 0.05, or 5%. The obvious disadvantage of this measurement is that a decline in one significant cause of death must elevate the PMR of another, which can lead to misleading impressions. For example, a successful campaign to reduce injury rates might increase the PMR for cancer only because many individuals who previously might have died at a young age from injuries might now be living long enough to develop an alternative cause of death.

It is also useful to know the *case-fatality rate,* which is the number of people diagnosed with a disease who die from it. Lastly, a number of reproductive and perinatal fatality rates are commonly used in global health, both because these indicators are quite sensitive to significant disruptions affecting the health status of populations and because deaths in the

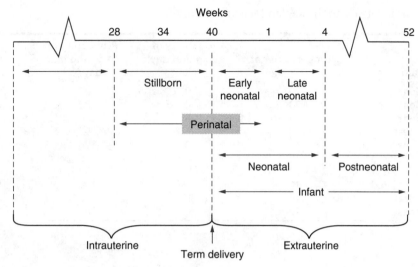

Figure 3-5. Overlapping time periods for fetal and infant deaths.

very young have an enormous public health impact. Figure 3-5 illustrates the eight overlapping fetal and infant periods used to calculate these death rates. Note that for practical reasons, the denominator used is the total number of live births, not the number of pregnancies. Therefore, a woman who dies during the delivery of live-born twins would constitute a maternal mortality ratio of 50%.

Survival Analysis

The concept of case-fatality rate is really only meaningful for shorter periods of observation, that is, for acute diseases. In other situations, it is important to have a more refined measurement that factors in how long each person lived prior to dying. The technique used is referred to as *survival analysis,* which involves following a group of individuals over a period of time to determine the mortality experience.

In the largest sense, this can be done from birth to death. However, such data would be very difficult to obtain because of the length and effort of follow-up required. As a surrogate, populations at any one time are divided into smaller age groups to create a *life table.* The WHO provides life tables for all member countries at http://www.who.int/countries/. In this type of survival analysis, the population is divided into the smaller interval of the first year of life because of increased mortality in this group and subsequently is divided into 5-year intervals.

Column e_x is the life expectancy at a specified age and the most frequently cited number from a life table. This is clearly a hypothetical number because it is drawn from a cross-section of people all born at different times and assumes that conditions affecting mortality will be stable during a person's entire lifetime. If e_x is taken from the first row of a life table, it represents the overall life expectancy for someone born in that year. If e_x is taken from the lower rows of a life table, the number must be added to the age group for that row to calculate the overall life expectancy. For example, the additional life expectancy of a 50-year-old (e_{50}) might be listed as 30.3 years, meaning that the overall life expectancy is 80.3 years (50 + 30.3 years). Note that within each age stratum, there is always an additional period of life expectancy, even in the row for those over 100 years of age. The overall life expectancy is therefore always increasing for each successive age category and is greater than that at birth because those causes of death that might affect younger populations, such as perinatal causes, no longer apply to older populations.

Rather than dividing a large population into arbitrary time intervals and examining how many survived to the beginning of each interval, one can examine a smaller population and determine the exact duration of survival for each member of the group. The procedure is much the same as that used to calculate an incidence density, shown earlier. Instead of birth as used in a life table, the starting point can be the time at diagnosis of a disease or the time when a treatment was administered. Outcomes other than death can also be considered, in which case the term *time to event analysis* is used. For example, following treatment of breast cancer with mastectomy, time to event analysis may be used with an endpoint of tumor recurrence.

Whenever a group is followed in survival analysis, there will always be those who are lost to follow-up,

Table 3-7. Survival data using the Kaplan-Meier method.

Day	Outcomes	Number at risk at start of day	Probability of dying that day (%)	Probability of surviving that day (%)	Cumulative probability of survival (%)
1	None	20	0	100	100
2	None	20	0	100	100
3	None	20	0	100	100
4	1 death	20	5	95	95
5	None	19	0	100	95
6	1 censored	19	0	100	95
7	2 deaths	18	11	89	85
8	1 censored	16	0	100	85
9	3 deaths	15	20	80	68
10	4 deaths	12	33	67	46

which might occur either if a subject is lost prior to the end of the study or for those subjects who are still alive at the conclusion of the study. In either instance, we do not know the status of such individuals when they are no longer under observation. In survival analysis, such individuals are referred to as being *censored*. However, the refinement of survival analysis is that the contribution of survival time prior to censoring is preserved for each subject.

In the example in Table 3-7, 20 subjects are followed for 10 days. On day 4, one subject dies, on day 6 one subject is lost to follow-up, on day 7 there are two more deaths, on day 8 another is lost to follow-up, on day 9 there are three deaths, and on day 10 four more deaths occur. We can generate a Kaplan-Meier curve (Figure 3-6) showing the successive probability of survival for each of these time spans. According to

this analysis, an individual's cumulative probability of survival for this period is 46%. Multiple survival curves can be compared to allow a visual inspection of the different survival experiences.

STUDY DESIGN

Recognition of study design is an important precondition for critical interpretation of any study's findings. Although the randomized double-blind clinical trial is clearly the most superior, application of this study design may be constrained by practical limitations or ethical concerns. Perhaps more so than other fields, global health uses a wide variety of additional epidemiologic study designs to provide essential and valuable information.

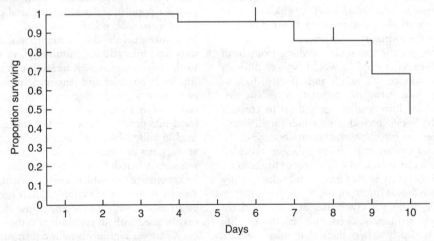

Figure 3-6. Kaplan-Meier curve using data from Table 3-7.

For example, different countries show marked variation in the prevalence of disease. One of the greatest differences has been observed for cancer of the esophagus, which has a much higher prevalence in Iran than in other parts of the world.[2] These types of studies are referred to as *descriptive studies* because they are simply initial attempts to describe the general characteristics of disease. They do not involve an explicit hypothesis because the investigators do not test specifically why one country might have more disease than another.

The findings from descriptive studies usually need to be investigated further using more rigorous *analytical study* designs that articulate and explore a specific relationship between disease and exposure. In the previous example, suppose there was a suspicion that consumption of very hot tea was a potential reason for the high prevalence of esophageal cancer in Iran. A variety of different analytical study designs could be applied that involve comparing differences in cancer of the esophagus among individuals with different levels of consumption of hot tea.

Descriptive Epidemiologic Studies

Case Reports and Case Series

A *case report* is a description of one case of the disease, whereas a *case series* consists of more than one case of the same disease. This type of study is simply a careful description of the disease and the circumstances in which it occurred. Case reports or case series can be drawn from clinical experience or from routine surveillance.

It is worth remembering that some of the first evidence of the human immunodeficiency virus pandemic arose from a case series reported by a clinician and through surveillance data.[3] Therefore, although definitive conclusions can seldom be drawn by this type of study design, it may be the first indication of a new disease. Frequently, when control groups for comparison are logistically difficult, such as for surgical interventions, the only available studies may be case series.

Correlational Studies

Correlational studies compare disease frequency with respect to another demographic factor, such as place or time. The example provided earlier of a study noting a much higher prevalence of cancer of the esophagus in northern Iran is an example of a correlational or ecological study.

These studies are inexpensive and can be performed rapidly, without the need to examine or follow individuals. Correlational studies have provided the first evidence of important new disease risk factors. However, the results must be interpreted with caution. Because the data are aggregate and at a population level, we do not know what is occurring at the level of individuals within the study population. The reason northern Iranians seem to experience more esophageal cancer may be as a result of genetic or environmental factors, or both. Moreover, these findings do not preclude the possibility that there may be smaller subpopulations in northern Iran who have a much lower risk of esophageal cancer. The essential point is that associations observed for populations do not necessarily hold true for individuals. When such incorrect inferences are made, one is said to commit the *ecological fallacy*.

Cross-Sectional Studies

In a *cross-sectional study* design, the cross-section is through time, with exposure and disease status (prevalence) in a population ascertained simultaneously. Frequently, this is accomplished through surveys of large numbers of individuals.

Cross-sectional studies are the most important type of study design for understanding the current magnitude of a public health problem and for planning interventions. One of the most well-known cross-sectional studies is the National Health and Nutritional Examination Survey (NHANES) in the United States. NHANES provides current statistical data on "the amount, distribution and effects of illness and disability in the United States" through a sample of 5,000 people taken over 12 months.[4] The sample includes a home interview and a health examination, with investigations and examination by a physician.

Successive cross-sectional studies performed at intervals on the same population may demonstrate what is known in epidemiology as a *cohort* or *generation effect* (not to be confused with cohort studies, discussed later). Consider the data shown in Figure 3-7 for mortality from gastric ulcer, duodenal ulcer, and ulcerative colitis in the United Kingdom, which show that mortality for gastric ulcer peaked for those born around 1880.[5] Some shared environmental exposure at birth was predictive of death many years later. This finding was observed in the 1960s, long before any knowledge of the important contribution of *Helicobacter pylori*. Although the explanation for these observations remains incompletely understood, these studies were the first to draw attention to environmental risk factors for these diseases.

The obvious limitation of cross-sectional studies is a chicken or egg dilemma. Because exposure and disease are studied at the same time, it is not necessarily clear which came first. Additionally, because of the large number of individuals included, cross-sectional studies may become expensive and are inefficient because they are usually performed without regard for

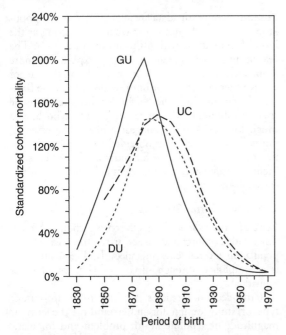

Figure 3-7. Birth cohort effects for gastric ulcer (GU), ulcerative colitis (UC), and duodenal ulcer (DU). From Sonnenberg A, Cucino C, Bauerfeind P. Commentary: the unresolved mystery of birth-cohort phenomena in gastroenterology. *Int J Epidemiol* 2002;31(1):23–26. (*Reproduced with permission.*)

disease or exposure status. For this reason, the assessment methods are often limited to simple, inexpensive measurement tools such as questionnaires.

Analytical Epidemiology

Analytical studies are often needed to test hypotheses definitively that may have been generated by earlier descriptive approaches. In *observational analytical studies,* the investigator has no control over which group in the study population received the exposure under study. In contrast, *interventional analytical studies* (clinical trials) involve the deliberate administration of an exposure to study subjects. The two types of observational analytical studies are the case-control study and cohort study.

Case-Control Studies

In case-control studies, as the name suggests, subjects are selected on the basis of having the disease under study (cases) or not having the disease under study (controls). The investigators then look back in time to determine whether there are any differences in previous exposures between the two groups.

Table 3-8. Results of a study investigating disease and exposure.

	Disease present	Disease absent
Exposure present	a	b
Exposure absent	c	d

It is important that a clear definition of a case be provided and consistently applied. Inclusion criteria must be described in detail and should generally be very strict to avoid misclassifications of controls as cases. Exclusion criteria may also be needed; these should also be explicit and applied both in the selection of cases and controls. Cases can be derived from disease registries, clinic or hospital populations, or from the general population. Selection of controls is an important consideration to reduce bias and confounding. The general rule is that controls should resemble cases in every way other than having the disease under study.

If the disease under study is rare, more controls than cases may be enrolled as a way to increase the statistical power of the study. The greatest gain occurs at a ratio of four controls per case; beyond this, the additional costs usually do not justify the modest gain in statistical power.

The results of a study investigating an exposure and a particular disease are depicted in Table 3-8. If this is a case-control study, it is meaningless to calculate a prevalence from this data. The apparent prevalence is artificial because it depends entirely on the ratio of cases to controls selected by the investigators. Instead, the measure of association used in case-control studies is the *odds ratio* (OR). Most people have some familiarity with odds from gambling, although the concept is used in a slightly different way in epidemiology. If the odds for a horse are given as 4-1, this means that if you wagered $1 on the horse and it won the race, you would receive $4. Note that, as stated, this was because the horse was believed to be four times more likely not to win the race than to win it. Therefore, the odds in gambling represent the likelihood of an event not happening to the likelihood that it will happen. In terms of probability (p), this type of odds can be expressed as $(1 - p):p$. Thus the horse has a 20% probability of winning the race because 80%:20% = 4:1.

In a case-control study, instead of connecting a horse to winning, investigators use the OR to connect disease to exposure. Second, instead of the odds expressing the likelihood of the event not happening to the likelihood of it happening, the ratio is calculated the other way around: epidemiologists calculate the odds that an individual will have exposure relative to not having exposure. This is done separately for cases and controls, and the results are compared as a ratio.

Using Table 3-8, the odds of exposure for cases are simply a/c and the odds of exposure for controls, b/d. The ratio is therefore

$$\frac{a/c}{b/d} = \frac{ad}{bc}$$

An OR greater than 1 means the disease is associated with more exposure, a value equal to 1 means there is no association, and a value less than 1 indicates the disease is associated with less exposure. The calculation of a measure of association such as an OR should not be confused with the concept of statistical inference or significance, discussed later. Even if one observes a greatly elevated OR, it does not necessarily mean that the findings are considered statistically significant.

Case-control studies are chosen for diseases that have lengthy induction periods between a causative exposure and the onset of disease, such as cancer or cardiovascular disease. Because investigators enroll people who currently have the disease, they do not need to wait until disease develops, and future follow-up is not required. By similar reasoning, this type of study design is most suitable for rare diseases. Multiple different exposures can be studied for any one disease. Case-control studies are also less expensive than other analytical studies.

The major disadvantage of a case-control study is the potential for bias, both on the part of participants and investigators, because disease status is known prior to the determination of exposure status.

Cohort Studies

In cohort studies, individuals are selected who are free of the disease under study at the time that observation begins. Their exposure status is then established, and they are followed forward in time to determine their subsequent disease status. Cohort studies can either be prospective or retrospective.

In a prospective cohort study, subjects are currently free of the disease under study and are followed into the future to determine who later develops disease. A well-known prospective cohort study is the Framingham Heart Study, which was initiated in 1948 with the enrollment of 5,209 adult residents of Framingham, Massachusetts. To be eligible to participate, these individuals had to have been free of cardiovascular disease in 1948. Ever since, each of them has undergone a standardized biannual cardiovascular examination. Daily surveillance of hospital admissions, deaths, and information from other health care providers is performed

to determine disease status. A wealth of important information, including much of our current insight about standard coronary heart disease risk factors, arose from this study. The very obvious practical limitation of this study is that years, or in most instances decades, elapsed before sufficient numbers of subjects developed cardiovascular disease to provide a large enough sample size for statistical analysis. One solution to this problem is to apply a retrospective cohort study design. In this case, some of the study subjects have developed disease at the present time. However, the investigators perform the steps in the same order by taking advantage of historical information to avoid the need for future follow-up. A cohort of disease-free individuals is identified from past records and subsequently followed forward in time for a defined period to determine who later developed disease. However, all of these events have occurred in the past relative to the time of the study.

For example, investigators in China were interested in learning whether the use of chimneys to provide ventilation of coal stoves would reduce the incidence of chronic obstructive pulmonary disease. They examined historical data on individuals from 1976 until 1992 who had switched from an unvented to a vented stove and identified a reduction in the incidence of chronic obstructive pulmonary disease. Because the development of disease occurred prior to the onset of the study, this cohort study is retrospective.[6]

Returning to Table 3-8, if these results are from a cohort study, the incidence can be directly calculated because all individuals are disease free at enrollment. The measure of association from a cohort study, known as the *relative risk* (RR), is simply the incidence of disease in those exposed divided by the incidence of disease in those who are unexposed:

$$\frac{a/(a+b)}{c/(c+d)}$$

In many ways, cohort studies represent a mirror image of case-control studies. The unexposed and exposed people should resemble each other in every way other than having the exposure under study. Cohort studies are good for rare exposures, and many diseases can be studied for any one exposure. Because exposure status is determined prior to disease status, bias is less of a concern than in a case-control study.

However, cohort studies are obviously not suitable for rare disease outcomes. Prospective studies are more expensive and prolonged because future follow-up is required. For retrospective cohort studies, data quality when the cohort is assembled from historical sources may be a concern. Finally, subjects may always be lost to follow-up, which may influence the findings.

Clinical Trials

An intervention study or clinical trial is the gold standard study design in epidemiology. Because the investigators determine who receives the exposure under study, there is a greater degree of experimental control than in any other epidemiologic study.

Broadly speaking, the two goals of any clinical trial are to determine the efficacy and the safety of the intervention under study. As with a cohort study, a homogeneous group without the outcome under study is first assembled. If the clinical trial involves a pharmaceutical agent, the studies occur in four phases (Table 3-9). Although the distinction between phases is not always clear, there is a relatively greater emphasis on efficacy and less on safety in progressing from phase 1 to 4. Regulatory approval of a pharmaceutical for clinical use usually occurs following satisfactory phase 3 study outcomes.

Before subjects receive the intervention, several considerations are important. Because subjects will receive a deliberately applied intervention, there are significant ethical issues involved in a clinical trial; appropriate oversight must be in place, and informed written consent must be obtained from all participants. It is essential that a clinical trial include a sample size justification to ensure it is of appropriate statistical power. This justification should be explicit about the assumptions made in choosing a particular number of participants. Finally, because the investigators can determine who receives the exposure of interest, it allows them to apply two very powerful tools: randomization and blinding.

The importance of *blinding* was first appreciated by Benjamin Franklin in 1784. He recognized that if individuals had an expectation of improvement, beneficial effects could falsely be ascribed to ineffective interventions, a phenomenon now referred to as the *placebo effect*. Accordingly, an essential feature of any clinical trial is an appropriate control group for comparison. The control group may receive standard therapy when it would be unethical for any participant to remain untreated during the study. If the control group receives an inactive intervention, this is referred to as a *placebo* for a pharmaceutical agent or a *sham* treatment for a procedural intervention. To maximize the effect of blinding, an *active placebo* may be chosen that has similar side effects to the drug under study.

In single blinding, study subjects are not aware of whether they are being allocated treatment or placebo/sham intervention. If the investigators are similarly unaware, the study is described as double blind. Triple blinding includes those individuals performing analysis of data. Clearly, blinding is the ultimate method to deal with bias in study design.

Randomization in clinical trials offers the great benefit that study subjects differ only with respect to receiving the intervention under study. Therefore, randomization is the most desirable method to deal with the problem of confounders because all such variables will equal out between groups of sufficient size with appropriate randomization.

Three general designs are used in an intervention study: simple or parallel (Figure 3-8a), crossover (Figure 3-8b) or factorial (Figure 3-8c). In a *crossover study*, each subject serves as his or her own control, and the variation between those in the intervention and control arms is eliminated. Accordingly, this design is the most efficient and requires the smallest sample size. Similarly, it is also the most robust design because the results are affected to a lesser extent when subjects are lost to follow-up. Obviously, the main disadvantage of a crossover design is a *carry-over effect* in which a residual influence may persist after subjects have crossed over. Such an effect can obscure the

Table 3-9. Phases of a clinical trial of a pharmaceutical agent.

Phase	Number of subjects	Type of subjects	Goals
I	<100	Healthy volunteers or end stage disease patients in inpatient setting	Determine safety, investigate pharmacokinetics, determine appropriate dosage
II	Hundreds	Healthy volunteers; patients with less severe disease	Further investigate safety, begin to determine preliminary efficacy
III	Hundreds to thousands	Patients	Compare new pharmaceutical with existing therapy
IV	Hundreds to tens of thousands	Patients in long-term studies	Investigate other indications for treatment, explore longer-term and rarer adverse effects

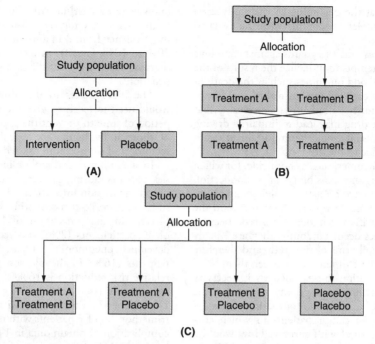

Figure 3-8. Three general designs of intervention studies. (a) Simple or parallel intervention study. (b) Crossover intervention study. (c) Factorial intervention study of two treatments.

differences between the two treatments studied in a crossover study.

Further reflection will indicate that a carry-over effect may also occur in simple or parallel studies because clinical trials are frequently performed on individuals receiving some sort of treatment prior to enrollment in the study. One method to deal with this problem is to include a *washout period* before or in between study treatments, during which subjects receive placebo only.

The *factorial design* allows interactions between two treatments to be studied, which may be either synergistic or antagonistic. In either instance, this is important additional information. A well-known example of a factorial study design is the Physicians' Health Study. The first Physicians' Health Study, which ended in 1995, examined the use of aspirin and beta-carotene to prevent cardiovascular disease and cancer. The Physicians' Health Study II, completed in December 2007, was a clinical trial of vitamins C and E, beta-carotene, and multivitamin supplementation in a factorial design with 16 different study groups.[7]

Noncompliance and Dropouts Once a study group of appropriate size is assembled and randomized, and blinding is applied to participants and investigators, the only remaining threats to validity are noncompliance and dropouts.

A variety of methods are available to deal with noncompliance. A run-in period may be included prior to randomization during which all participants receive a placebo. Only those subjects who comply with instructions are randomized and included in the study. Obviously, such an approach cannot be used for treatments that must be given acutely. Furthermore, this method will influence the generalizability of the findings because a selected group showing greater compliance than the general population has been enrolled in the study. Where possible, compliance can be monitored using pill counts or direct measurement of the pharmaceutical agent in subjects. High-risk subjects, who will presumably be more motivated to comply with the study protocol, can be selected for enrollment. Financial incentives and regular contact with the participants can also be used to maintain compliance throughout the study.

Subjects who are lost to follow-up while the study is under way represent another dilemma. Suppose, for example, that a woman enrolled in the drug arm of a study comparing this drug with a placebo is killed in a car collision while the study is under way. Although it may seem intuitive to exclude her death from the study, according to a widely used approach known as *intention-to-treat analysis,* her death is attributed to the drug. This approach requires all subjects in each group to be followed up and analyzed according to their assignment at the beginning of the study even if they do not complete or comply with the assigned therapy.

Intention-to-treat analysis guards against conscious or unconscious attempts to influence the results of the study by excluding odd outcomes such as the death of the woman in the car collision. In reality, we do not know the reason for her death. It is conceivable that a side effect of the drug may lead to impaired driving ability, in which case it would be important to retain her death as one due to the drug.

What about outcomes, such as homicide, for which there is absolutely no possibility of a connection with the study protocol? Again, applying intention-to-treat analysis, those deaths are counted toward the arm of the study in which they occurred. Because such odd outcomes occur randomly, they are equally likely to occur in all arms of the study and therefore should not create false differences between them.

Ultimately, intention-to-treat analysis is necessary to preserve the baseline homogeneity achieved at the outset of the study through randomization. Consider a study of advanced cancer patients in which chemotherapy is compared with surgery. How would a death that occurred prior to the patient reaching the operating room be handled for a patient randomized to receive surgery? Intention-to-treat analysis tells us that this death would be ascribed to the surgery. If all patients who died prior to reaching the operating room were excluded, the benefit of randomization would be lost. Rather than comparing two groups that differ only in the treatment received, we would be comparing a group of those with less aggressive disease in the surgical arm because these individuals had to have survived long enough to reach the operating room.

Intention-to-treat analysis also provides a greater reflection of how a treatment will perform in the general population by ignoring adherence when the data are analyzed. This relates to a distinction made by epidemiologists between effectiveness and efficacy. *Efficacy* refers to a treatment working under the idealized conditions of the randomized clinical trial. The ability of a treatment to work in the real world is referred to as *effectiveness*. Intention-to-treat analysis therefore provides a closer approximation of effectiveness.

Number Needed to Treat   To complete what has been termed "the three E's" of an intervention, one needs to consider the *efficiency*, or the cost versus benefit, of a particular treatment. One way to measure efficiency is the *number needed to treat* (NNT), a very useful concept in global health given scarce resources. To understand the NNT, it is essential to appreciate the distinction between absolute and relative risk (see the example given later). A very dramatic relative risk reduction cannot be interpreted without some

knowledge of baseline risk. For example, a twofold relative risk reduction is consistent both with a change in prevalence from 2 in a million to 1 in a million, or 20% to 10%. Clearly, in terms of the efficiency of a therapy, there is a great difference between these two situations.

The NNT refers to the number of people who would need to receive a given treatment for a defined period of time to prevent the specific outcome in one of those individuals. The calculation is simply the reciprocal of the absolute risk reduction.

In a randomized double-blind study of 84 measles patients during an epidemic in Guinea-Bissau, prophylactic administration of a 7-day course of sulfamethoxazole-trimethoprim was compared with placebo in the prevention of complications.[8] One of 46 participants (2%) who received the antibiotic developed pneumonia, compared with 6 of 38 participants (16%) in the placebo group. Whereas the relative risk reduction is 16%/2%, or 8, the absolute reduction in risk is 16% − 2% = 14%. The NNT is 1/0.14, or 7. Prophylaxis with sulfamethoxazole-trimethoprim of 7 patients with measles will prevent a complication of pneumonia in 1 of them. Table 3-10 lists the NNTs for a variety of interventions used in different countries.

Finally, criteria need to be considered for stopping a clinical trial. Because blinding is frequently involved, an independent data monitoring group is needed to continuously follow the results while the study is under way. Termination prior to the end of the study may be required if there has been a clear demonstration of benefit or an unacceptably high level of adverse effects.

Because of the great advantages offered by randomization and blinding, there are no inherent disadvantages to a clinical trial with respect to epidemiology. Rather, the use of this design is limited by practical constraints or ethical concerns. For example, in the study of a surgical treatment, it may not be possible to blind the control subjects appropriately. Blinding these subjects might mean subjecting them to invasive procedures that, even though they are sham therapies, may nevertheless be painful or otherwise risky.

Systematic Reviews and Meta-Analysis

Summaries of the best available evidence concerning a therapy are termed *systematic reviews*. All such reviews include a statement of the question to be addressed as well as an explicit and transparent description of how the evidence was selected and evaluated. Systematic reviews may be either qualitative or quantitative, the latter method being a meta-analysis. *Meta-analysis* an approach in which many smaller studies are pooled together and handled statistically as if all the subjects were in one larger study. The steps include identification

Table 3-10. Number needed to treat (NNT) for a variety of interventions.

Intervention	Number needed to treat	Reference
Biweekly phone calls to promote adherence with asthma therapy in Brazil	4.5	Chatkin JM, Blanco DC, Scaglia N, Wagner MB, Fritscher CC. Impact of a low-cost and simple intervention in enhancing treatment adherence in a Brazilian asthma sample. *J Asthma* 2006;43(4):263–266.
Lifestyle modification to prevent type 2 diabetes among those with impaired glucose tolerance in India	6.4	Ramachandran A, Snehalatha C, Mary S, et al. The Indian Diabetes Prevention Programme shows that lifestyle modification and metformin prevent type 2 diabetes in Asian Indian subjects with impaired glucose tolerance (IDPP-1). *Diabetologia* 2006;49(2):289–297.
Prophylactic sulfamethoxazole-trimethoprim in measles patients to prevent pneumonia in Guinea-Bissau	7	Garly ML, Bale C, Martins CL, et al. Prophylactic antibiotics to prevent pneumonia and other complications after measles: community based randomised double blind placebo controlled trial in Guinea-Bissau. *BMJ* 2006;333 (7581):1245.
Telephone counseling of parents who smoke and have children younger than 5 years in Hong Kong	13	Abdullah AS, Mak YW, Loke AY, Lam TH. Smoking cessation intervention in parents of young children: a randomised controlled trial. *Addiction* 2005;100(11):1731–1740.
Sulfamethoxazole-trimethoprim to prevent tuberculosis in HIV-positive adults in South Africa	24	Grimwade K, Sturm AW, Nunn AJ, et al. Effectiveness of cotrimoxazole prophylaxis on mortality in adults with tuberculosis in rural South Africa. *AIDS* 2005;19(2):163–168.

of studies, a critique of the quality of each study, and the performance of summary statistical analysis on the aggregate data.

The search strategy used should be explicit. In addition to electronic databases such as Medline, it may also be important to search so-called *fugitive literature* such as dissertations, unpublished manuscripts, or abstract presentations. Therefore, a meta-analysis may also include expert consultations, hand searches, and articles identified through reference lists.

However, published studies may provide a distorted view of the true measure of an association. This effect arises because published articles are more likely to contain positive rather than negative findings, a phenomenon known as *publication bias*.

To determine if publication bias is present in a meta-analysis, it is useful to examine a *funnel plot*. In the absence of publication bias, a funnel plot should have a pyramid-type distribution. Smaller studies have more variable results; as the sample size of the study increases, the estimate of effect should narrow down closer to the true value. However, with publication bias, there may be asymmetry to the pyramid, with an absence of smaller negative studies. In Figure 3-9a, the results of published studies are shown with the ○ symbol. Note that as the sample size of each study

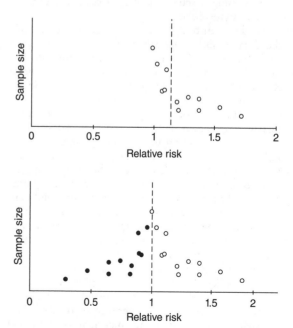

Figure 3-9. Funnel plots. (a) Publication bias with falsely elevated relative risk. (b) Graphically corrected plot with hypothetical small studies inserted.

Table 3-11. Criteria for the evaluation of a meta-analysis.

Study design: clinical trials generally preferred
Year of publication
Language
Sample size
Adequacy of follow-up
Similarity of exposure or treatment
Similarity of outcome measures
Completeness of data
Multiple publication bias: the results of one study may be published in more than one paper

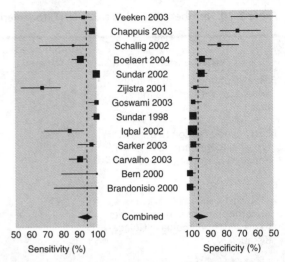

Figure 3-10. Ladder plot showing the results of a meta-analysis. From Chappuis F, Rijal S, Soto A, Menten J, Boelaert M. A meta-analysis of the diagnostic performance of the direct agglutination test and rK39 dipstick for visceral leishmaniasis. *BMJ* 2006;333(7571):723. (*Reproduced with permission.*)

increases, the results move closer to a relative risk of 1, suggestive of no difference. However, the plot suggests there are many small studies showing a reduction in relative risk that were not published. To correct for this observation, a number of such hypothetical studies have been added and denoted with the • symbol, simply as a mirror image of the smaller positive studies in Figure 3-9b. Failure to correct for publication bias can lead to misleading results if the meta-analysis relies solely on the results of published studies. In this example, publication bias would have resulted in the false conclusion of an elevated relative risk.

Each of the studies must be evaluated both for quality as well as suitability for inclusion in the meta-analysis using a standardized approach. Table 3-11 provides some of the criteria.

Finally, statistical analysis must be performed on the data to summarize the results. There are three components to this analysis. The first is the calculation of a summary measure of effect, which may be a RR, an OR, or some change in an important widely used parameter, such as blood pressure. The results of a meta-analysis on two tests used for visceral leishmaniasis are shown in Figure 3-10 as a ladder plot. Sensitivity is shown on the left and specificity on the right. These two concepts are discussed in a later section. For each individual study, the sample size is reflected in the size of the box used to denote the point estimate. The 95% confidence interval is the solid line extending out horizontally. Note that as the sample size of the study increases, the 95% confidence interval becomes narrower. The summary measure of effect is shown at the bottom as a diamond.

Second, statistical tests, known as *tests of homogeneity*, are applied to determine if the individual studies are similar enough to be pooled together. Finally, a *sensitivity analysis* should be performed to determine to what extent alterations in important assumptions influence the final results. The results of a meta-analysis are more likely to be valid if similar findings are found, even when assumptions are modified.

EPIDEMIOLOGY OF INFECTIOUS DISEASE

Infectious disease is of particular importance in global health, and it is therefore appropriate to discuss specifically how epidemiologic methods can be applied for investigation and control. Although many of the same epidemiologic principles already discussed apply, there are some additional and unique considerations because of the involvement of an infectious agent. Several definitions are provided in Table 3-12.

Reservoirs

Infectious agents may be present in *reservoirs*, which represent environments where the microorganism can survive and replicate on a long-term if not indefinite basis. The reservoir may be an inanimate object (soil, water, or contaminated food), animals, or humans. As will be seen, whether or not an infectious agent can persist in a reservoir has enormous implications for control measures.

From the reservoir, the infectious agent can be transmitted to host. For any given infectious agent, both the number of reservoirs and the routes of transmission are limited because the microbe has evolved to replicate and be transmitted under highly specific conditions. Nevertheless, because of rapid reproduction, the ability of these microorganisms to undergo

Table 3-12. Definitions used in infectious disease epidemiology.

> *Infection:* Presence of a microbe in a host to the bene-fit of the microbe, with some detectable response on the part of the host either clinically or serologically.
>
> *Colonization:* Presence of microbe in a host without a response by the host. Example: GI flora.
>
> *Latent infection:* Persistence of a microbe in the host with the possibility of clinical disease in the future *without* shedding of the microbe in the interval. Example: shingles from *Varicella zoster*.
>
> *Inapparent infection:* Persistence of a microbe in a host without clinical disease with shedding of the microbe. Example: typhoid fever carrier.
>
> *Infectivity:* The ability of the microbe to cause infec-tion in those exposed. Calculated as the number of people with infection (clinically or serologically) divided by the number exposed.
>
> *Pathogenicity:* The ability of the microbe to cause clinically apparent disease, generally used without regard for the severity of that disease. Calculated as the number of cases with clinical signs and symp-toms divided by the number of those infected.
>
> *Virulence:* The degree of severity of disease in diag-nosed cases of an infectious disease. Calculated as the number of fatalities divided by the number of diagnosed cases.
>
> *Epidemic:* A sudden increase in the frequency of infec-tion in a particular population or region.
>
> *Pandemic:* An epidemic that affects populations in large regions—continents or the entire globe.
>
> *Endemic:* An infection that occurs at a stable, elevated rate in a particular population or region.

alterations in genetic material to allow adaptation to new hosts and new modes of transmission is well recognized.

Methods of Transmission

A foodborne infection, such as salmonella, results from ingestion of the microorganism and subsequent estab-lishment of the microbe in the host. In such cases, ill-ness occurs beginning approximately 24 hours after ingestion of the contaminated food and is accompanied by constitutional signs and symptoms such as fever. Conversely, other microorganisms, such as staphylo-cocci, produce a toxin while growing on food products causing a more rapid illness (after about 6 hours) with-out constitutional symptoms. Strictly speaking, this is not an infection but rather what is commonly called food poisoning.

Infections may be spread by respiratory tract secre-tions containing the microorganism, which becomes

airborne as a result of sneezing, coughing, or even talking. With evaporation of water, small respirable residual particles, known as *droplet nuclei*, may be formed, which can remain suspended in air for many hours. Droplet nuclei spread some diseases such as tuberculosis over great distances from the source.

A *zoonosis* is an infection normally present in other vertebrate animals that can, under some circum-stances, spread and cause disease in humans. Because the infectious agent has evolved to infect, replicate, and spread in a nonhuman host, transmission to humans generally requires extensive exposure, person-to-person spread is rare, and disease in otherwise healthy humans is usually mild.

A *nosocomial infection* is one acquired in a hospital. Because this term is too narrow, the preferred termi-nology is now *healthcare–associated infection*. In such cases, clinical disease usually may occur more fre-quently or with greater severity in immune compro-mised hosts, and pathogens may be resistant to one or more antimicrobial therapies.

Infectious Disease Control

There are different time courses with respect to the ability of a host to spread an infectious disease (infec-tiousness) and the associated clinical course for the same infectious disease as depicted in Figure 3-11. The time between infection and the development of symptomatic disease is referred to as the *incuba-tion period,* whereas the time between infection and the ability of a host to spread the infectious agent to others is defined as the *latent period.* Note that the infectious period precedes the symptomatic period.

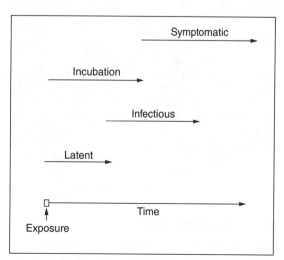

Figure 3-11. Timeline for an infectious disease.

Therefore, efforts to control the spread of an infectious disease based on the prompt identification of clinically affected individuals are usually unsuccessful because such individuals have already had the opportunity to spread disease prior to developing symptoms.

Basic Reproductive Number

The basic reproductive number (R_0) is an essential calculation for understanding how infectious diseases spread through a population and serves as an important metric by which to assess the effectiveness of control strategies. R_0 is the average number of persons in a totally susceptible population infected by one case during that case's entire infectious period. R_0 is influenced by the number of contacts that an infectious person has per unit of time, the probability of transmission with each contact, and the duration of infectiousness in units of time.

For example, R_0 during one point of a measles outbreak may have a value of 8, meaning that one person with measles introduced into a nonimmune population will produce eight new *secondary infections* of measles before that individual recovers or dies. Subsequent infections (known as waves or generations) are not included in the calculation of R_0. Instead, reproductive numbers are formulated for each subsequent wave and denoted as R_1, R_2, R_3, and so on.

Note that R_0 is a highly dynamic number; it will change over time and with changes in circumstances. An R_0 of 1 represents a critical threshold and target for control measures. If R_0 can be kept below 1, the spread of infection is being reduced and the outbreak will eventually end.

One of the principal determinants of R_0 is the pool of susceptible hosts. Typically, as an infectious disease spreads, the number of susceptible hosts declines, either from death or the development of immunity until R_0 falls below 1 and the epidemic dies out. When R_0 is high, epidemics will have explosive increases but, for the same reason, deplete the reservoir of susceptible individuals just as rapidly and have proportionately precipitous declines. Conversely, when R_0 is low, outbreaks are more prolonged.

Referring back to Figure 3-4, it is clear that R_0 is not a rate (even though it is frequently called the basic reproductive rate) because the measure does not contains units of time. Therefore, although R_0 tells us about trends in the spread of an infection, it provides no information on the duration or time course of an outbreak.

Epidemic Investigation

The first step in any investigation of an infectious disease outbreak is to define a case. In this context, a case definition is an operational one, suitable for rapid use in field conditions. Two approaches may then be taken. The first is based on seeking a common exposure variable in an outbreak. In such instances, the difference in attack rates is calculated between those who were and those who were not exposed. This method is commonly used in the investigation of foodborne illness to determine what specific food is the source of illness.

If it is not clear how the disease is spreading, it may be useful to generate an epidemic curve by plotting the number of cases on the *y*-axis against time on the *x*-axis to guide preventive efforts. Several different types of epidemic curves are recognized. The first is a *point source outbreak* (Figure 3-12a), which typically occurs when there is one common source of infection without person-to-person transmission. In a *propagated epidemic* (Figure 3-12b), person-to-person transmission occurs, with successive peaks in the number of cases observed. The time between these peaks corresponds roughly to the mean incubation period for the infectious agent. Finally, *continuous,* also referred to as *intermittent* or *common epidemic,* curves (Figure 3-12c) consist of a relatively stable number of elevated cases over time. By definition, this corresponds to the typical pattern seen for an endemic. Epidemic curves are not mutually exclusive. For example, an infection may start as a point source outbreak and then become propagated with subsequent transmission between hosts.

Herd Immunity

R_0 provides useful insight into how to control an infectious disease. It is not necessary to completely halt transmission of the agent (reduce R_0 to zero), merely to maintain an R_0 level less than 1 for a sufficient period of time to halt the spread of the agent.

To appreciate the role of control measures, it is important to understand the significance of *herd immunity* (Figure 3-13). In the population to the left, a person with infection is introduced into a population with a low level of immunity. So long as each infected person has a reasonably high likelihood of coming into contact with a susceptible host, the disease can spread. Conversely, in the population to the right, because of a sufficiently high prevalence of immunity, the probability of contact with a susceptible person is so low that the disease cannot propagate. Many susceptible individuals in this population are protected from infection by the preponderance of immune members.

Herd immunity tells us that an entire population can be protected from an infectious disease if a sufficiently high number of members of that population have immunity. It is therefore not necessary to vaccinate 100% of a population, but rather a sufficiently high number to achieve herd immunity.

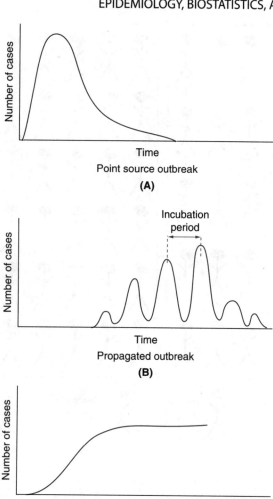

Figure 3-12. Types of epidemic curves. (a) Point source epidemic curve. (b) Propagated epidemic curve. (c) Continuous epidemic curve.

Ring treatment is a method of infection control based on herd immunity. Using this approach, when a case is identified, aggressive efforts are made to immunize all those individuals who may come into contact with the case. In effect, a ring of immunity is created to prevent the infection from spreading to susceptible individuals. Ring treatment was successfully used in the final stages of the smallpox eradication effort.

Control Measures

Two basic strategies are targeted to the host to control an infectious disease. The first is *quarantine*, which refers to the restriction of the activities of healthy people on the basis of exposure. In addition, quarantine frequently includes measures for the early detection of infection, such as periodic measurements of temperature. Quarantine can follow a spectrum from *absolute quarantine* with complete restriction of activities to a *modified quarantine*, which might involve confining individuals to their homes. The latter approach was used by public health authorities in Toronto during the severe acute respiratory syndrome outbreak, which involved a modified quarantine with over 15,000 people confined to their homes.

In contrast, *isolation* refers to the restriction of activities of an individual on the basis of having infection for the duration of the infectious period.

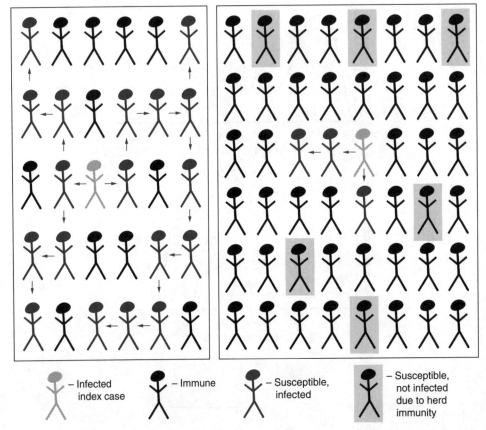

Figure 3-13. Herd immunity.

Isolation may be complete or specific to the mode of transmission of the infectious agent (respiratory isolation, enteric precautions, etc.).

Disease Eradication

Eradication means a permanent reduction to zero incidence for a disease. Because treatment and preventive measures will never be needed in the future, eradication is of tremendous long-term benefit relative to cost. It is intuitive that the only diseases that can be eradicated are those due to an infectious cause. Other types of diseases, such as silicosis, can be reduced to the lowest feasible levels, a status the WHO refers to as *elimination*.

Disease eradication efforts involve nonsustainable campaigns, with enormous amounts of resources dedicated for a defined period of time in the hope of permanent control. Two infectious diseases have been declared eradicated to date, smallpox in 1980 and rinderpest, a viral infection of cattle, in 2011.

A variety of considerations must be taken into account in selecting an infectious disease for eradication:

- The disease should be easily recognizable on the basis of signs and symptoms.
- A control intervention conferring long-term protection and suitable for widespread application in the field must be available.
- All populations experiencing or at risk for the infectious disease must be accessible.
- There must be no nonhuman reservoir for the disease.

The WHO is currently attempting to eradicate polio and has successfully done so in Europe, the Americas, and the western Pacific. Most cases are currently reported in Nigeria, periodically spilling over to neighboring countries. Local transmission also persists in Afghanistan and Pakistan.

The only other disease currently targeted by the World Health Assembly for eradication is dracunculiasis, or guinea-worm disease, with efforts centered around the use of filters and a larvicide for drinking water. In this case, almost all locally transmitted disease is in South Sudan. Steady progress has been made in recent years, and, if current trends continue, this disease is likely to be the second human pathogen to be declared eradicated.

EPIDEMIOLOGY OF TESTS

Correct interpretation of any medical test requires an understanding of both the properties of the test and the setting in which the test is applied.

Test Properties

The *accuracy* of a test is defined as how close the measured value is to the true value of the parameter under measurement. *Reliability* or *reproducibility* refers to consistency in test results when repeated measurements are made on the same sample. *Validity* refers to the extent to which a test really measures what it purports to measure. For example, it is possible to measure a variety of metals in hair. However, because it is difficult to wash off metals that may be sources of external contamination, this is generally not considered a valid measure of human exposure.

In evaluating a test, it is important to consider how it compares with a given gold standard. The gold standard represents the closest one can come to the truth for a particular test. The reason the gold standard cannot be used relates to practical limitations. For example, the gold standard test to diagnose dementia of the Alzheimer type is to obtain brain tissue for neuropathologic examination. Clearly, such an approach cannot be used routinely. Therefore, one might compare the results of a noninvasive battery of neuropsychological tests to the gold standard obtained postmortem. Results are usually dichotomized as either positive (abnormal) or negative (normal), generating the contingency or 2×2 table depicted in Table 3-13. Those individuals in cell a are true positives; in cell b, false positives; in cell c, false negatives; and in cell d, true negatives. Four essential calculations can then be obtained: sensitivity, specificity, positive predictive value, and negative predictive value.

Sensitivity is calculated as $a/(a+c)$ and refers to the ability of the test to correctly identify those with disease. *Specificity* is calculated as $d/(b+d)$ and refers to the ability to correctly rule out disease or to identify those who are healthy. Although it is obvious that both properties should be maximized in a test, an increase in one means a decrease in the other and vice versa.

Consider the extreme example of a new test used to diagnose death. Because the developers did not want to ever miss a case of death, the sensitivity was maximized to 100% by having the test always indicate that a person was dead. Examination of the table indicates that because the test is always positive, the value of cell c is zero, and the sensitivity $(a/[a+c])$ becomes a/a, or 100%. The test will never fail in identifying a dead person. However, the value of cell d is also zero, so the specificity is 0%, meaning that the test will never be able to correctly identify a living person.

Sensitivity and specificity are fixed properties of the test and do not change when the same test is applied in different settings. Suppose the test just discussed was used in a typical outpatient clinic and then brought to a morgue. In either location, the test always indicates that a person is dead and therefore will never fail in correctly identifying death, yet will always mistakenly classify live people as dead (100% sensitivity, 0% specificity, respectively). However, although the test always provides wrong answers in the clinic, it is always correct in the morgue, even though the test itself has not changed.

The change in the performance of the test is a result of the prevalence or *pretest likelihood* of the outcome in the population being tested. In this case, when the prevalence increases from 0% to 100%, the test went from generating only false-positive results in the office to generating only true-positive results. This property of the test is known as the *positive predictive value* and is calculated as $a/(a+b)$. It measures the proportion of positive test results that are correct.

As the example shows, the positive predictive value will increase as the prevalence of disease in the population tested increases, a phenomenon of enormous clinical significance. Tests must be carefully selected to be used on individuals for whom a clinical assessment identifies a sufficiently high likelihood of disease such that positive test results are more likely to be true rather than false positives.

The *negative predictive value* is calculated as $d/(c+d)$ and measures the proportion of negative test results that are correct. As the prevalence of disease increases, the negative predictive value declines. The prevalence or pretest likelihood of disease is $a+c/(a+b+c+d)$. Finally, the accuracy of the test is calculated as $a+d/(a+b+c+d)$.

Table 3-13. Contingency table.

	Gold standard positive	Gold standard negative
Test positive	a	b
Test negative	c	d

Applications of Tests

A medical test can be performed in three different contexts: diagnosis, screening, and surveillance. In this section, only screening and surveillance are considered.

Screening

The object of any screening test is to identify disease at an earlier point in time than when signs and symptoms develop. Returning to Figure 3-2, by advancing forward knowledge of disease status, screening tests shorten the latent period. The amount of time by which knowledge of disease status is advanced is known as the *lead time*. In other words, the lead time is the difference between the period of time when disease is detected on clinical grounds and when the disease is detected through a positive screening test result. Individuals identified by a screening test usually undergo additional tests to either confirm that they have the disease or identify false-positive test results (Figure 3-14). Therefore, screening tests should have high sensitivity, even at the expense of specificity. In clinical practice, many of the diseases we screen for are rare, meaning that the pretest likelihood of disease is low. Consequently, most positive screening tests are found to be false positive results upon additional investigation.

A variety of practical considerations are important before screening tests are applied. These include the following:

- High sensitivity
- Low cost
- Acceptability
- Suitable for outpatient or community application

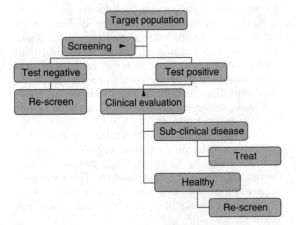

Figure 3-14. Application of a screening test.

- Screened disease has significant adverse impact
- Early identification leads to improved outcomes in screened individuals or prevents further spread of disease to others
- Sufficient resources are available to provide appropriate follow-up for those testing positive

In terms of validity, the two types of bias specific to screening tests are lead time bias and length bias. These are both sources of error that may result in screened populations falsely appearing to have improved survival when compared with unscreened populations.

By definition, for any individual who screens positively, we will have knowledge of his or her disease status earlier than an unscreened individual. Part of this time is simply the lead time. Therefore, a demonstration that a screened population survives for a longer period of time than an unscreened population *from the time of diagnosis* does not mean that the screening was necessarily useful when the starting point for the screened population is the positive screening test and, for the unscreened population, the development of symptoms. Such comparisons must show that the increased survival is beyond that which arises solely because of the lead time.

Length bias arises because not all cases of the same disease follow the same natural history; some are more aggressive and some milder. Because the time between development of symptoms and death may vary between diseases, so too the preclinical phase can vary proportionately. Because the preclinical phase represents the window of opportunity for an individual to screen positive on a test, it follows that those individuals screening positive are more likely to have milder courses of disease. The most extreme form of length bias is overdiagnosis. This identifies individuals who would have never known they had the disease if not for screening positively on a test.

Surveillance

Surveillance involves performing tests on populations to identify outbreaks of disease. Therefore, while screening targets individuals, surveillance targets populations. The aim of surveillance is the prompt identification of shared exposures to prevent additional cases of disease. Ultimately, surveillance is a form of primary prevention; the goal is to prevent new cases of disease.

There are four essential components to any surveillance program:

1. Case reporting
2. Data analysis
3. Communication of results
4. Application of findings

Case Reporting *Passive surveillance* systems rely on the reporting of cases by health care providers. Most jurisdictions have specified lists of conditions that must be reported to public health authorities. These lists are mostly, but not exclusively, infectious diseases. Other potentially reportable conditions include diseases resulting from overexposure to toxic substances, such as lead poisoning, or certain types of cancer. Although reporting of these conditions is required by law and failure to comply is punishable by fines, compliance is generally very poor.

Active surveillance seeks to improve ascertainment through supplemental measures to prompt case reporting. Public health authorities may contact health care providers to encourage reporting, or large-scale surveys may be undertaken. Although case ascertainment is superior using active surveillance, such programs are more time consuming and costly.

Data Analysis Data must be continuously compiled and analyzed by a central agency to ensure that important trends are promptly recognized. For infectious diseases, this is an essential precondition for effective containment measures. In some cases, such as Ebola virus, even a single case is noteworthy. However, in the case of diseases such as influenza that occur at a regular background rate, the key determination is whether the number of cases is greater than expected, a parameter known as the *epidemic threshold*.

Communication of Results The results of the analysis of surveillance data must be both rapidly and widely disseminated to all who need to know. Therefore, a properly functioning surveillance system involves a bidirectional flow of information: case reporting to a central public health agency and reporting of results from the agency back to health care providers and others. In the United States, an important vehicle for communicating the results of surveillance is the *Morbidity and Mortality Weekly Report* from the Centers for Disease Control and Prevention, which is circulated both electronically and in hardcopy formats.

In a global context, surveillance systems should also be designed for stability because they may be most needed during times of substantial disruptions in society and infrastructure. Flexibility is another important consideration and can be illustrated by the concept of *syndromic surveillance*, an approach that has been applied in response to bioterrorism concerns. Rather than reporting specific diseases, each of which may be extremely rare, systems to report shared symptoms are implemented.

Application of Findings Surveillance systems have a variety of uses including the following[9]:

- Triggering rapid interventions as appropriate
- Measuring the burden of disease
- Guiding control measures
- Evaluating health-related policy
- Prioritizing resource allocation
- Characterizing the natural history of disease
- Initiating further research

SUMMARY

Epidemiology is often described as the basic science of public health, and some familiarity with this field is essential to the understanding of causes of disease in global health and to guide preventive strategies. Biostatistics provides important measures of morbidity and mortality that serve as indicators of the overall health status of populations and countries. However, a variety of different techniques are needed, such as stratification and survival analysis, to provide greater insight when comparisons are made.

Several study designs are available, each with advantages, disadvantages, and practical limitations. When a disease association is reported by a study, it is important to first address the roles of chance, bias, and confounding as potential explanations. If these three factors are not felt to account for the association, in whole or in part, the association is considered valid. Additional criteria are applied to determine if the association is causal.

Epidemiology has important applications in the management of infectious disease and the early detection of disease through screening and surveillance. Because primary prevention of disease is always preferred, epidemiology and biostatistics provide very powerful tools in global health.

STUDY QUESTIONS

1. A disease has an annual incidence rate of 50 cases per year, mortality of 10 cases per year, and prevalence of 200 cases (all per 1 million people). What is the average duration of the disease?

2. You are working in a hospital in Africa that admits approximately 50 patients a day. There is a concern that deaths from malaria have risen sharply in the past year, and you are asked to analyze data to explore this suspicion. You are told that fairly good-quality mortality data have been kept for several years that include age and gender of the decedent. However, morbidity data are extremely limited. Moreover, a census has not been carried out in the country in over 25 years. Under these circumstances, what measure of mortality for malaria would you recommend be calculated? What is the limitation of this measure?

3. The minister of health of a Central American country is concerned that a great many citizens have a poor diet and is wondering about spending additional funds in next year's budget on a community-based dietary education effort that has been shown to be very successful in other parts of Central America. He is well aware of the known adverse health effects of a poor diet but really wants to know how much money will be needed. What is the best choice of study design you could recommend to assist the minister in such circumstances?

4. A medical student unfamiliar with epidemiology proposes to do a case-control study involving in-person interviews with chemotherapy patients (cases) and patients with nonmalignant chronic disease (controls). You point out that some of the signs of chemotherapy, such as hair loss, are very obvious. Thus determining exposure status in this way may introduce what threat to the validity of the findings?

5. A study is performed examining the relationship between vitamin A consumption and measles. A total of 140 children are enrolled at birth, and the mothers are interviewed. Based on this interview, each child's diet is categorized as either vitamin A adequate or vitamin A deficient. The children are then followed until age 5, and the number of cases of measles is recorded. What is the risk of measles as a result of a vitamin A–deficient diet?

	Measles	No Measles
Vitamin A–deficient diet	20	20
Vitamin A–appropriate diet	40	60

6. Three hours following a picnic, 30 of 100 people develop vomiting and diarrhea without fever. All food is immediately disposed. What type of epidemic curve would be seen for this outbreak?

7. Investigators are studying the use of a new rapid field test to identify patients with cysticercosis.

The accompanying table summarizes the results of initial research involving 200 subjects.

	Cysticercosis present	Cysticercosis absent	Total
Test result positive	60	40	100
Test result negative	20	80	100
Total	80	120	200

What is the sensitivity of this test for cysticercosis?

REFERENCES

1. Bradford Hill A. *A Short Textbook of Medical Statistics*. 11th ed. London: Hodder and Stoughton, 1977.

2. Kmet J, Mahboubi E. Esophageal cancer in the Caspian littoral of Iran: initial studies. *Science* 1972;175(4024):846–853.

3. Centers for Disease Control and Prevention. *Pneumocystis* pneumonia—Los Angeles. *MMWR* 1981;30(21):1–3.

4. Centers for Disease Control and Prevention, National Center for Health Statistics. *National Health and Nutrition Examination Survey Data*. Hyattsville, MD: U.S. Department of Health and Human Services, Centers for Disease Control and Prevention, 2012. http://www.cdc.gov/nchs/about/major/nhanes/DataAccomp.htm.

5. Sonnenberg A, Cucino C, Bauerfeind P. Commentary: the unresolved mystery of birth-cohort phenomena in gastroenterology. *Int J Epidemiol* 2002;31(1):23–26.

6. Chapman RS, Hex, Blair AE, Lan Q. Improvement in household stoves and risk of chronic obstructive pulmonary disease in Xuanwei, China: retrospective cohort study. *BMJ* 2005;331(7524):1050.

7. Christen WG, Gaziano JM, Hennekens CH. Design of Physicians' Health Study II—a randomized trial of beta-carotene, vitamins E and C, and multivitamins, in prevention of cancer, cardiovascular disease, and eye disease, and review of results of completed trials [abstract]. *Ann Epidemiol* 2000;10(2):125–134.

8. Garly ML, Bale C, Martins CL, et al. Prophylactic antibiotics to prevent pneumonia and other complications after measles: community based randomized double blind placebo controlled trial in Guinea-Bissau. *BMJ* 2006;333(7581):1245.

9. Centers for Disease Control and Prevention. Updated guidelines for evaluating surveillance systems. *MMWR* 2001;50(RR13): 1–35.

The Health of Women/Mothers and Children

4

Judy Lewis, Monika Doshi, Deyanira Gonzalez de Leon, and Amany Refaat

LEARNING OBJECTIVES

- *Understand the basic terms and definitions of indicators*
- *Understand the main causes of mortality and morbidity through the lifecycle of women and children*
- *Describe the social, economic, and cultural context of maternal and child health*
- *Distinguish maternal health issues and interventions from other women's health issues and describe the relationships between them*
- *Identify low-cost, effective community-based approaches to interventions*

INTRODUCTION

Global Context

Maternal and child health (MCH) refers to the health status and health services provided to women and children. The traditional focus of the disciplines of MCH has been on women in their roles as mothers (childbearing and child rearing) and on children (primarily the healthy survival of infants and young children). MCH indicators are often used to measure the social, economic, and educational status of women as well as community-level access to primary care. MCH was the mainstay of international health and development programs until human immunodeficiency virus/ acquired immunodeficiency syndrome (HIV/AIDS) became an epidemic in many parts of the world.

Remarkable achievements have been made in reducing child and maternal mortality and morbidity. However, of the eight Millennium Development Goals (MDGs), the only three that will not be achieved by 2015 are those related to MCH: MDGs 3, promote gender equality and empower women; 4, reduce child mortality; and 5, improve maternal health.[1]

There continues to be a large disparity in MCH indicators between high- and low-income countries. The highest levels of mother and child health can be found in European and higher income countries in Asia. These are also countries that provide high-quality and accessible health and social services. Infant mortality rates (IMR) of less than 4/1,000 are found in Singapore, Iceland, Japan, Sweden, Finland, and Norway, and maternal mortality rates (MMRs) less than 5/100,000 can be found in Estonia, Greece, Singapore, Italy, Austria, and Sweden. Although there has been great improvement in MCH indicators in low income countries in the last 10 years, the rates remain much higher. In 2000, 18 countries had MMRs higher than 1,000/100,000, but there were only 2 in 2010. These were 1,100/100,000 in Chad and 1,000/100,000 in Somalia. Sierra Leone, which had the highest rate in 2000 (2000/100,000), was reduced to 890 by 2010. There were eight other countries with very high MMRs (above 600)—all in sub-Saharan Africa (Sierra Leone, Central African Republic Burundi, Guinea-Bissau, Liberia, the Sudan, Cameroon, and Nigeria).[2,3] Most of the countries with the highest mortality rates are also those experiencing war and conflict. Almost all (99%) of maternal deaths occur in low-income countries. The regions with the highest maternal deaths are Africa and the poorer parts of Asia (Table 4-1).[2] Two countries, India and Nigeria, account for a third of global maternal deaths.[2] Infant mortality disparities show the same trend, although not to the same extreme level. The highest infant mortality rates (IMRs) are found in the same countries with high maternal mortality, with the highest reported in 2011 in Sierra Leone at 119/1,000—which was a significant

Table 4-1. Comparison of 1990 and 2010 maternal mortality ratio and number of maternal deaths by UN MDG region.

Region	1990[a]		2010[a]		% change in MMR between 1990 and 2010[a]	Average annual % change in MMR between 1990 and 2010[a]
	MMR	Maternal deaths	MMR	Maternal deaths		
World	400	543,000	210	287,000	−47	−3.1
Developed regions	26	4,000	16	2,200	−39	−2.5
Developing regions	440	539,000	240	284,000	−47	−3.1
Northern Africa	230	8,500	78	2,800	−66	−5.3
Sub-Saharan Africa	850	192,000	500	162,000	−41	−2.6
Eastern Asia	120	30,000	37	6,400	−69	−5.7
Eastern Asia excluding China	53	610	45	400	−15	−0.8
Southern Asia	590	233,000	220	83,000	−64	−4.9
Southern Asia excluding India	590	70,000	240	28,000	−59	−4.4
Southeast Asia	410	50,000	150	17,000	−63	−4.9
Western Asia	170	7,000	71	3,500	−57	−4.2
Caucasus and Central Asia	71	1,400	46	740	−35	−2.1
Latin America and the Caribbean	140	16,000	80	8,800	−41	−2.6
Latin America	130	14,000	72	7,400	−43	−2.8
Caribbean	280	2,300	190	1,400	−30	−1.8
Oceania	320	620	200	510	−38	−2.4

MDG, Millennium Development Goal; MMR, maternal mortality rate. Source WHO [2].
[a]MMR estimates have been rounded according to the following scheme: less than100, no rounding; 100 to 999, rounded to the nearest 10; and more than1,000, rounded to the nearest 100. The numbers of maternal deaths have been rounded as follows: less than 1,000, rounded to the nearest 10; 1,000 to 9,999, rounded to the nearest 100; and more than 10,000, rounded to the nearest 1,000. Negative values for % changes indicate a decreasing MMR from 1990 to 2010; positive values indicate an increasing MMR. Percentages have been calculated using unrounded estimates.

reduction from 2003 when the IMR was 166. Four countries (Sierra Leone, Somalia, Democratic Republic of Congo, Central African Republic) had IMRs higher than 100/1,000, compared with 24 in 2003. Twenty-one countries had rates higher than 70/1,000.[4,5]

The means to improve MCH outcomes have been well demonstrated in high-income countries. It is not just a matter of technology; the health of mothers and children is inexorably linked to women's status and education, and the general socioeconomic well-being of communities. This chapter explores some of the reasons for the disparities that exist between developed and developing regions, and it examines some of the emerging women's health issues. It provides an emphasis on interventions that have made a difference.

A BASIC PRIMER OF MATERNAL AND CHILD HEALTH INDICATORS AND TERMS

Prior to an exploration of the issues, it is important to have a basic understanding of some of the terms and indicators used in maternal and child health.

- **Maternal mortality rate:** The number of maternal deaths per 100,000 births. The formal definition of maternal mortality is death while pregnant or within 42 days of the termination of pregnancy, regardless of the duration or site of the pregnancy. Death may be from any cause related to or aggravated by the pregnancy or its management, but not from accidental or incidental causes.
- **Infant mortality rate:** The number of infant deaths per 1,000 births. This is defined as a death of a child from birth up to 1 year of age.
- **Perinatal mortality rate (PNMR):** The number of perinatal deaths per 1,000 births. Perinatal deaths are defined as occurring during late pregnancy (at 22 completed weeks of gestation and over), during childbirth, and for up to 7 completed days of life.
- **Neonatal mortality rate (NMR):** The number of deaths during the first month of life per 1,000 births.
- **Postneonatal mortality rate (PNNMR):** The number of postnatal deaths (1 month through 12 months) per 1,000 births.
- **Child mortality rate (CMR):** The number of deaths among children younger than 5 years per 1,000 births.

This is also referenced as the under-5 mortality rate (U5MR).

- **Preterm birth:** Birth at gestational age of less than 37 weeks.
- **Low birth weight (LBW):** Less than 2,500 grams, as defined by the World Health Organization (WHO); may be due to preterm delivery or smallness for gestational age (intrauterine growth retardation), or to a combination of both.
- **Very low birth weight (VLBW):** Less than 1,500 grams; these infants are too small and physiologically undeveloped to survive in most developing countries.
- **Total fertility rate (TFR):** The number of children that would be born to each woman if she was to live to the end of her childbearing years and bear children at each age at the same rate as the existing age-specific fertility rate. TFR is used to estimate population growth rates.
- **Contraceptive prevalence rate (CPR):** The percentage of married women of reproductive age (15 to 49) who are using or whose partners are using contraception.
- **Traditional birth attendant (TBA):** A person who assists the mother during childbirth and delivery. This person, who may be male or female, depending on the country and culture, is usually trained through apprenticeship. A *trained TBA* refers to a TBA who has had some formal training in hygienic delivery, often through the provision of WHO birthing kits.
- **Skilled birth attendance:** Delivery by a nurse, nurse midwife, or doctor who is licensed to practice and has undergone specific training.

A warning about mortality and morbidity data: Measurement issues are often a problem; many countries' vital statistics are not reliable or consistently collected. In these situations, there are two approaches to estimating mortality: very large sample sizes and interviews to determine maternal or child deaths; and methods that use smaller sample sizes, such as the Sisterhood Method that was developed in the 1980s for MMR estimation. The Sisterhood Method inquires about deaths of sisters in pregnancy, childbirth, and postpartum and has been used in many parts of the world to provide data.[6] If mortality data are difficult to determine, obviously morbidity data are even less reliable.

HISTORICAL PERSPECTIVE

MCH has always been used as an indicator of the overall health of a society. MCH really began to improve around the beginning of the 20th century in developed countries when general public health improvements reduced the spread of infectious diseases and economic development increased access to food and better housing. This overview focuses on the period after World War II when global efforts were initiated after the founding of the United Nations (UN).

Prior to World War II, the health care systems of developed and developing countries were more or less similar. A gradual increase in the standard of living among developed countries led to the betterment of health services, including those that revolved around MCH. After World War II, the health care systems of many developing countries emphasized tertiary care, modeled after the systems that existed in industrialized nations. This resulted in increasing medical specialization and a hierarchy in health care systems in which most of the resources went to tertiary care and technology. The major emphasis for international development agencies during this time was on the eradication of specific diseases such as smallpox, TB, and malaria. Although there were some successes with this approach, it did not do much to improve health care access at the community level, and MCH health indicators did not greatly improve. Furthermore, the overall disease burden of the poor was not being addressed. The limitations of vertical disease programs were eventually recognized. In 1978, the Declaration of Alma-Ata established the importance of a holistic approach to health (complete physical, mental, and social well-being) and identified the role of economic and social development, and individual and government responsibility. Primary health care was proposed as the means to reach the goal of Health for All by 2000.[7] Unfortunately, this laudable goal was not accomplished, but the striving continues.

Many global initiatives have focused on MCH issues: White Ribbon Alliance, Saving Newborn Lives, Family Care International, The Partnership for Maternal, Newborn and Child Health, Women Deliver, The Global Campaign for the Health Millennium Development Goals, and Saving Newborn Lives, to mention just a few. This also includes maternal, newborn, and child health streams within larger initiatives such as the Global Fund to Fight AIDS, Tuberculosis and Malaria.

EARLY AGE AT MARRIAGE

A woman's age at first marriage is an important indicator of her social, educational, and economic status and has significant implications for her reproductive health, specifically with respect to childbearing. Pregnancy and childbirth closely follow the start of marriage. In many developing countries, between 50% and 75% of all births to married women occur less than 2 years after women enter their first union.[8] Early marriage, therefore, coincides with childbearing at a young age. Early pregnancy creates a number of health risks for a young woman and her infant, if she carries the pregnancy to term. Moreover, for women who marry young, motherhood limits opportunities for education, employment, and personal growth. Early age at first marriage is often associated with a higher probability of divorce and separation. With the dissolution of marriage, women face economic and social challenges because they either assume full responsibility for dependent family members or are expelled from the family of origin as well as their family of marriage, leaving them without support.

Prevalence of Early Marriage

Although the situation varies greatly by country and region, marriage during the teenage years is common in developing countries with 20% to 50% of women marrying or entering a union by age 18, and 40% to 70% doing so by age 20.[8] Singh and colleagues have done extensive work on early marriage and provide the data for the information in the rest of this paragraph. Women are most likely to marry at a young age in sub-Saharan Africa where 60% to 92% of all women ages 20 to 24 had entered their first union by age 20. A high prevalence of early marriage was also found in a few countries in other regions. In Bangladesh, Guatemala, India, and Yemen, 60% to 82% of all women 20 to 24 had married by age 20. Compared with sub-Saharan Africa, marriage during teenage years is less common in Latin America, Asia, North Africa, and the Middle East. About 20% to 33% of 20- to 24-year-olds in those regions had entered their first marriage by age 18, and 33% to 50% had married by age 20. Even in France and the United States, 11% of all 20- to 24-year-olds were married or cohabiting by age 18, and 32% of these by age 20. The only exception to such high rates of marriage during adolescence can be found in Japan, where only 2% of 20- to 24-year-olds had married by age 20.[8]

Determinants of Early Marriage

The data clearly indicates that there are variations in the timing of marriage within and between regions. There are three factors, however, that are thought to be closely correlated and relevant to a woman's age at first marriage: women's acquisition of formal education, their participation in the labor force, and urbanization. Exposure to formal schooling helps shape values and ideas, often resulting in the adoption of Western values and behavior. Additionally, exposure to and attainment of education often leads to better jobs and higher wages, which, in turn, increases economic stability and reduces motivation for early marriage. With access to higher education and with knowledge in areas such as reproduction, women often have an increased ability to regulate their own fertility.

Another key variable relevant to a woman's age at first marriage is her participation in the formal work sector. A woman's participation in the formal work sector often exposes her to new ideas and norms that discourage early marriage. Economic stability and/or independence as a result of participation in the labor force may enhance a woman's ability to postpone marriage. There is an economic incentive for parents to encourage their daughters to remain single and continue work. Therefore, the family pressure to get married often subsides or disappears.

Urbanization is the third factor that influences a woman's age at first marriage. Research shows that there are significant differences in the age at marriage between women who live in urban settings compared with those who live in rural settings. Women living in urban areas marry at a later age. Possible explanations for this include a sense of independence gained from greater access to the labor force, increased accessibility to higher education, distance from community- and kinship-based social control, and exposure to modern values and beliefs.

Child Marriage

Child marriage is used to describe a legal or customary union between two people, of whom one or both of the spouses are under the age of 18.[9] Child marriage curtails educational opportunities and impacts the social development of young girls. Because it affects girls in greater numbers and with graver consequences compared with boys, child marriage brings additional dimensions that further exacerbate the health status of women. In addition to the lack of access to information regarding basic reproductive health issues, the social isolation, limited social support, and powerlessness pose greater reproductive health risks. Lack of autonomy in movement and decision making among young wives can aggravate the risks of maternal mortality and morbidity for pregnant adolescents who already face high-risk pregnancies. There is a strong correlation between the age of the mother and maternal mortality and morbidity. Girls ages 10 to 14 are five times more likely to die in pregnancy or childbirth than women ages 20 to 24.[10] Girls ages 15 to 19 are twice as likely to die (Figure 4-1).[10] In addition, girls who have children before their bodies are fully developed are at greater risk for obstetric fistula, a debilitating medical condition often caused by prolonged or obstructed labor. The ability to negotiate sexual relations, contraception, and childbearing, as well as other aspects of domestic life, diminishes as the age of first marriage decreases. Vulnerability to HIV and other sexually transmitted infections also

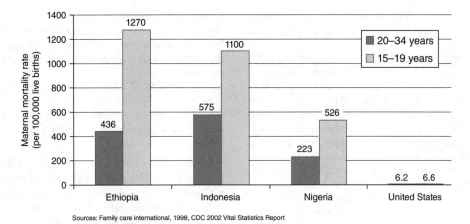

Sources: Family care international, 1998, CDC 2002 Vital Statistics Report

Figure 4-1. Child marriage and maternal mortality: maternal mortality by age.[10]

increases with the lack of ability to negotiate condom use with an older, sexually experienced partner. Women who marry at a younger age are more likely to be victims of domestic violence, and more likely to believe that the violence is justified.[10]

Although most countries have declared 18 as the minimum legal age of marriage, in a few developing countries, marriage before age 18 remains common. Child marriages remain common in rural areas and among groups with the least economic resources. For the years 2000 to 2011, just over a third of women ages 20 to 24 years in developing regions were married or in union before their 18th birthday, equivalent to approximately 67 million women in 2010. About 12% of them were married or in union before age 15. The prevalence of child marriage varies substantially among countries, ranging from only 2% in Algeria to 75% in Niger. In 41 countries, 30% or more of women ages 20 to 24 were married or in union when they were still children.[9] Child marriage is most common in South Asia and in West and Central Africa, where two of five girls marry or enter into union before age 18 (46% and 41%, respectively). Over the last 10 years, child marriage at the global level has remained relatively constant (about 50% in rural areas and 23% in urban areas).[9] If current trends continue, by 2030 the number of child brides marrying each year will have grown 14% since 2010, from 14.2 to 15.1 million.[9]

A number of factors perpetuate the practice of child marriage. Risk factors such as poverty and low levels of education are directly correlated with higher rates of child marriage. In parts of Africa and Asia, marriage of children is valued as a means of consolidating powerful relations between families, for sealing deals over land or other property, or even for settling disputes or feuds between families or clans.[11]

Child marriage may also be valued as an economic coping strategy to reduce the costs of raising daughters. The economic benefits of bride price (money, livestock, or property given to the bride's family by the groom's family) may act as further motivation for child marriage in regions of sub-Saharan Africa. In many regions around the world, child marriage is traditionally recognized as necessary for controlling girls' sexuality and reproduction. Social, traditional, and cultural norms around child marriages often lead to pressure on families to conform. Lastly, the desire to secure the future of a girl child in situations of insecurity and acute poverty, particularly during disasters such as war and famine, contribute further to the practice of child marriage.[11]

Approaches to address and eventually eliminate child marriages include increasing education and income, creating safe spaces, and reducing isolation of girls/women. Using social media and behavior change techniques to empower girls by helping them understand their rights, providing access to family planning and reproductive health knowledge and services, and working within communities to change attitudes and behaviors are also promising approaches.

WOMEN'S EMPOWERMENT AND EDUCATION

Empowerment

The UN has identified five components of women's empowerment: (1) the sense of self-worth; (2) the right to have and to determine choices; (3) the right to have access to opportunities and resources; (4) the right to have the power to control their own lives, both within and outside the home; and (5) the ability to influence the direction of social change to create a more just social and economic order, nationally and internationally.[12]

The United Nations Development Program (UNDP) focuses on gender equality and women's empowerment not only as human rights, but also because they are a pathway to achieving the MDGs and sustainable development.[13] The nature of empowerment renders it difficult to define. It is often referred to as a goal for development programs/projects, but it is also an individual development process that contributes to the attainment of rights identified by the UN. Empowerment is a complex issue with varying interpretations in different societal, national, and cultural contexts. Indicators have been developed for societal, community, family and individual levels. Indicators for family and individual levels include participation in crucial decision-making processes; women's control of their reproductive functions and decisions on family size; women's control of expenditures of their own incomes; a sense of pride and value in their work; building self-confidence and self-esteem; the ability to prevent violence; and men's participation in domestic work.

Empowering Women through Education

"Education is one of the most important means of empowering women with the knowledge, skills and self-confidence necessary to participate fully in the development process."[14] Education is important for everyone, but especially for girls and women. As discussed earlier, education and early marriage are closely related. But there are many health and economic factors that are influenced by women's education.

Women's education has been associated with better health outcomes for mothers and children, delayed age at marriage, and increased family income. In terms of women's health, increasing levels of women's education has been related to reductions in maternal mortality. Women ages 25 to 44 in sub-Saharan Africa showed an increase in education from 1.5 years in 1980 to 4.4 in 2008 and concomitant declines in MMR.[15] Other studies have shown the relationship between lower levels of maternal education and higher maternal mortality exists even among women who are able to access facilities providing intrapartum care. In a 2004-2005 study of 287,000 women giving birth in facilities in 24 countries in Africa, Asia, and Latin America, the risk of maternal mortality was greatest for women with no education (2.7 times higher). Those with between 1 and 6 years of education had twice the risk of maternal mortality compared with women with more than 12 years of education.[16,17] Gender inequality also contributes to a woman's risk of acquiring HIV. Nearly half of those living with the

virus worldwide are women, and women's subordination to men not only increases their risk of infection but also limits access to treatment.[18] In many parts of the world a woman's greatest risk for HIV is being married.

The UNESCO 2011 Report, "Education Counts: Towards the Millennium Development Goals,"[19] clearly documents the many benefits of girls' and women's education. Higher levels of women's education have been associated with:

- Lower fertility rates, increased facility deliveries, better birth spacing, and higher levels of prenatal care.
- Greater knowledge about HIV and higher utilization of retrovirals when HIV positive.
- Lower IMRs and CMRs, higher rates of vaccination, and less stunting from malnutrition.
- Reduced poverty; each additional year of schooling can increase income by 10%.

Education and empowerment are strongly linked to women's and children's health, and they are mutually reinforcing. Children of mothers with higher education are more likely to complete school. Educated mothers are more likely to be aware of the benefits of schooling and to contribute to the costs of schooling through their participation in the labor force.[20]

Improving women's education, workforce participation, and social and political opportunities are crucial to strengthening their health.[21] It is generally believed that women's lack of decision-making power may restrict their use of modern contraceptives. In a study using Demographic Health Survey (DHS) data from Namibia, Zambia, Ghana, and Uganda, positive associations were found between the overall empowerment score and contraception use.[22]

Although some studies have shown that domestic violence against women is negatively associated with the educational level, this is not universally true. Educational discrepancies between spouses may also play a role. In a recent study in India and Bangladesh, wives with higher education than their husbands were less likely to experience violence compared with when both spouses had lower education. Equally high-educated couples revealed the lowest likelihood of experiencing violence.[23] Another study in Egypt found that higher levels of education had a 28-fold positive effect in improving women's lives and empowerment. Uneducated women were five times more likely to be exposed to violence. Uneducated husbands were four times more likely to hurt their wives.[24] An older study in Finland suggested that life expectancy as well as disability-free life expectancy showed a direct relationship with level of education: the higher the level of education, the higher the life expectancy and disability-free life expectancy.[25]

OVERVIEW OF MAJOR WOMEN'S AND CHILDREN'S HEALTH ISSUES

This section addresses the major problems in women's and children's health. It presents information about epidemiology, causation, health care delivery, and basic treatment and interventions. These topics are organized around a life cycle approach that begins with family planning and ends with old age. The major issues that affect both maternal and child health are anemia, pregnancy, childbirth, and perinatal, infant, child, and adolescent health.

Access to Family Planning

Reproductive choice is a basic human right. The aim of family planning programs is to enable individuals to decide freely and responsibly the number and spacing of their children, to have the information and means to do so, to make informed choices, and to choose from a full range of safe and effective methods of contraception.[26] However, access to relevant information and high-quality services is limited in many regions of the world. Most family planning programs have been targeted at women; therefore, this section concentrates on them.

During the 1994 International Conference on Population and Development, 180 nations adopted a program of action that included, among its major goals, improving reproductive health and making family planning services universally available.[26]

Women between the ages of 15 and 49 years are considered to be women of reproductive age (WRA), and this group is the population base used to estimate need and utilization of family planning. In 2012, there were an estimated 1.5 billion WRA. Of these, 645 million were using modern contraceptive methods. This represents a 42% increase from 2008. However, the unmet need increased in most of Africa, Latin America, and the Caribbean. There are 220 million women, mostly in developing countries and the former Soviet republics, who are not using contraception in spite of an expressed desire to space or limit the numbers of their births.[27] These women are considered to have an "unmet need for family planning."

Before examining the global estimates as well as the impact of unmet need on MCH, it is important to understand how the unmet need for family planning is estimated. It has conventionally been estimated from representative population-based surveys of currently married women as the sum of currently pregnant women who report that their pregnancy was unintended (those who wish to limit their births) and the number of currently nonpregnant women who are not using contraception and would not like to have any more children or none in the next 2 years (those who wish to space their births).[28] This method to estimate unmet need has been criticized because it is thought to underestimate the actual numbers. Furthermore, it excludes both currently married women who are not pregnant and who are using ineffective or unsatisfactory methods of contraception and sexually active women who are not currently married and who do not wish to become pregnant, at least in the next 2 years.

The debate about expanding the definition of unmet need continues. Ross and Winfrey used an expanded definition to offer an updated estimate of unmet need in the developing world and the former Soviet republics.[29] Under their definition, the group includes all fecund women, married or living in union, who are not using any method of contraception and who either do not want to have any more children or who want to postpone their next birth for at least 2 more years. The group also includes all pregnant married women and women who have recently given birth and are still amenorrheic. They are included if their pregnancies or births were unwanted or mistimed because they were not using contraception. This approach may still underestimate the number of women with unmet need because the group does not include users of traditional methods who may have an unmet need for modern methods. Their inclusion would result in considerably larger estimates, especially in regions where the use of traditional methods is popular.

Table 4-2 shows the number and percentage of women with an unmet need for contraception in various regions and the changes between 2008 and 2012.[27] The number of women in the reproductive-age group varies by region, with 63% of the total for the developing world in Asia, which contains 140 million WRA with unmet need. It is important to keep in mind that Asia contains several countries with very large populations (India, Indonesia, Pakistan, and Bangladesh). Sub-Saharan Africa contains 53 million WRA with unmet need (26% of the total). Latin America contributes 23 million WRA with unmet need (10%), nearly half of whom live in Mexico and Brazil. The 69 poorest countries in the world have 162 million women with unmet need (73% of the total), which suggests that unmet need will continue to have a major impact on population growth in those countries.

Regional variations in the prevalence among women who wish to space or limit births are evident. Ross and Winfrey found that in sub-Saharan Africa, 65% of unmet need is for spacing, in contrast to Latin America, where it is only 42%. In other regions, such as Asia, spacing and limiting needs are nearly equal. Unmarried women add to unmet need, accounting for 7% of the developing world total.[29]

Table 4-2. Number of women with unmet need for modern methods and proportion with unmet need by region for the 69 lowest-income countries, 2008 and 2012.

Region and subregion	Women ages 15 to 49 with unmet need for modern methods, millions			% of women ages 15 to 49 in need of contraception who have unmet need for modern methods		
	2008	2012	Annual % change	2008	2012	Annual % change
Developing world	226	222	−0.5	27	26	−1.5
Africa	55	58	1.6	54	53	−0.5
Sub-Saharan Africa*	50	53	1.6	62	60	−0.9
Eastern Africa	19	20	0.4	63	54	−3.5
Middle Africa	10	10	1.3	82	81	−0.1
Southern Africa	2	2	−6.2	25	17	−8.1
Western Africa	18	19	2.6	74	74	0.0
Northern Africa	6	8	5.8	25	32	7.8
Asia	147	140	−1.1	23	21	−1.9
Eastern Asia	24	16	−7.8	8	6	−7.7
Central Asia	3	2	−3.1	30	28	−1.4
South Asia	79	83	1.1	34	34	−0.4
Southeast Asia	25	25	−0.6	33	28	−4.2
Western Asia	15	14	−2.8	54	50	−1.8
Oceania	<1	1	2.1	39	49	6.8
Latin America	24	23	−1.4	25	22	−2.8
Caribbean	2	2	−2.4	31	30	−0.8
Central America	5	5	1.3	23	23	0.0
South America	17	16	−2.0	25	21	−3.8
69 poorest countries	153	162	1.5	40	39	−0.6

*Sub-Saharan Africa includes Sudan and South Sudan, both of which are in the Northern Africa region.
Source: Singh S and Darroch JE[27]. Adding it Up: Costs and Benefits of Contraceptive Services - Estimates for 2012. New York: Guttmacher Institute and United Nations Population Fund (UNFPA), 2012, Table 2.

The proportion of unmarried women who are sexually active varies by region, ranging from 4% in Asia to 16% in sub-Saharan Africa. These differences in demand affect the kinds of contraceptive supplies needed as well as budgetary allocations.

A number of proven benefits are associated with family planning including maternal health, child survival, gender equality, and HIV prevention. Additionally, family planning can improve family well-being, raise female economic productivity, and lower fertility, thereby reducing poverty and promoting economic growth.[26] Despite these outcomes, the unmet need for family planning still persists. The causes for this include lack of accessible services; shortages of equipment, commodities, and personnel; lack of method choices appropriate to the situation of the woman and her family; lack of knowledge about the safety, effectiveness, and availability of choices; lack of community or spousal support (social opposition); misinformation and rumors; health concerns about possible side effects; and financial constraints.[26,30]

A number of social, cultural, and gender-related obstacles can prevent a woman from realizing her childbearing preferences. At the policy level, for example, decision makers may not place high priority on funding contraceptive services because they view them as "women's programs." Laws may require the woman to seek her husband's approval to use some methods. At the health facilities level, service providers' bias may limit options for contraception. At the community level, contraceptives may be considered as contributing to female promiscuity. Furthermore, men often have a greater decision-making power to determine family size. Social norms regarding fertility and virility, and the overall low status of women, keep many women and men from seeking family planning.[31]

Over the years, the WHO and the U.S. Agency for International Development (USAID) have made varying recommendations on birth spacing. These recommendations, which have traditionally been based on pregnancy outcomes, have caused confusion due to the differences in the time interval recommended between births by each agency. A 2006 WHO report, supported by USAID, recommends an interval of at least 24 months following a live birth to the next pregnancy to reduce the risk of adverse maternal, perinatal, and infant outcomes. An interval of at least 6 months to the next pregnancy is recommended following a miscarriage or induced abortion.[32]

The unmet need for spacing has multiple consequences on MCH. First, maternal depletion, defined as a broad pattern of maternal malnutrition resulting from the combined effects of dietary inadequacy, heavy workloads, and energy costs of repeated pregnancy, can result in increased maternal morbidity and mortality. There is, however, limited empirical evidence to support the theory of maternal depletion. The consequences for infants born after a short birth interval can include poor intrauterine growth and an increased risk of preterm birth.[33] Second, close birth spacing may further burden already limited family resources. Third, a child born after a short birth interval can also suffer from nutritional deficits as the mother interrupts breastfeeding to focus on the newborn. Fourth, the likelihood of transmission of infectious diseases is increased as a result of overcrowding and the presence of children of similar ages.

As with the unmet need for spacing, a number of consequences are associated with the unmet need to limit births. The WHO estimates that approximately 38% of all pregnancies occurring around the world every year are unintended. In 2012, an estimated 80 million unintended pregnancies occurred in the developing world due to contraceptive failure and nonuse among women with unmet need. About 6 of 10 such unplanned pregnancies result in induced abortion. Unintended pregnancies increase the lifetime risk of maternal mortality. They can also lead to unsafe abortion, poor infant health, and lower investment in the child. The prevention benefits of contraception are well documented. In 2012, modern contraception prevented 218 million unintended pregnancies, 55 million unplanned births, 138 million induced abortions (40 million of which were unsafe), 25 million miscarriages, 118 million maternal deaths, 1.1 million neonatal deaths, and 700,000 neonatal deaths.[27]

Anemia

Anemia is a global public health problem. It is the decreased ability of red blood cells to provide adequate oxygen to body tissues and is characterized by a hemoglobin (Hb) concentration below the established cut-off levels (Table 4-3). Hb is the oxygen-carrying molecule of red blood cells. Anemia affects both developing and developed countries with the greatest burden felt in resource-poor areas where significant proportions of young children and women of childbearing age are assumed to be anemic. In 2002, iron deficiency anemia (IDA) was considered to be among the most important contributing factors to global burden of disease.[34]

It is important to differentiate between anemia, iron deficiency, and iron deficiency anemia (Box 4-1).[35] Dietary iron deficiency is the most common cause of anemia; however, it is not the sole contributor. Factors that lower blood Hb concentrations, such as heavy blood loss due to menstruation or parasitic infections, are among other causes of anemia. Acute or chronic infections, such as malaria, cancer, TB, and HIV, can also lower blood Hb concentrations. In fact, anemia is recognized as an independent risk factor for early death among HIV/AIDS-infected individuals.[36] Micronutrient deficiencies, other than iron, including vitamins A, B_{12}, folate, riboflavin, and copper, can increase the risk of anemia. Within some populations, the impact of hemoglobinopathies on anemia also needs to be considered.

Measuring Hb concentration is the most reliable, easy, and inexpensive way to assess anemia. Estimates of prevalence rates of IDA often use rates of anemia as a proxy because Hb concentration is relatively easy to determine. However, because anemia can be caused by factors other than iron deficiency, the etiology of anemia should be interpreted with caution if the only indicator used is Hb concentration.

Prevalence

The WHO estimates that anemia affects 1.6 billion people globally, almost one-fourth of the world's

Table 4-3. Cut-offs for WHO definition of anemia.

Age or gender group	Hemoglobin below,g/dl	Hematocrit below,%
Children, 0.50–4.99 years	11.0	33
Children, 5–11.99 years	11.5	34
Children,12–14.99 years	12.0	36
Nonpregnant women, ≥15.00 years	12.0	36
Pregnant women	11.0	33
Men, ≥15.00 years	13.0	39

From United Nations Children's Fund. Prevention and control of iron deficiency anaemia in women and children. Geneva: Report of the UNICEF/WHO regional consultation, 1999.

BOX 4-1. DEFINITIONS AND DISTINCTIONS: ANEMIA, IRON DEFICIENCY, AND IRON DEFICIENCY ANEMIA

Anemia: Abnormally low hemoglobin level due to pathologic condition(s). Iron deficiency is one of the most common, but not the only cause of anemia. Other causes of anemia include chronic infections, particularly malaria, hereditary hemoglobinopathies, and other micronutrient deficiencies, particularly folic acid deficiency. It is worth noting that multiple causes of anemia can coexist in an individual or in a population and contribute to the severity of the anemia.

Iron deficiency: Functional tissue iron deficiency and the absence of iron stores with or without anemia. Iron deficiency is defined by abnormal iron biochemistry with or without the presence of anemia. Iron deficiency is usually the result of inadequate bioavailable dietary iron, increased iron requirement during a period of rapid growth (pregnancy

and infancy), and/or increased blood loss such as gastrointestinal bleeding due to hookworm or urinary blood loss due to schistosomiasis.

Iron Deficiency Anemia: Iron deficiency, when sufficiently severe, causes anemia. Although some functional consequences may be observed in individuals who have iron deficiency without anemia, cognitive impairment, decreased physical capacity, and reduced immunity are commonly associated with iron deficiency anemia. In severe iron deficiency anemia, capacity to maintain body temperature may also be reduced. Severe anemia is also life threatening.

Source: Yip R, Lynch S. *Iron Deficiency Anemia Technical Consultation.* New York: UNICEF, October 1998.

---

population, and that approximately 50% of all cases can be attributed to iron deficiency.[37] Globally, the highest prevalence of anemia is found among preschool-age children (47.4%) and the lowest prevalence among men (12.7%); global prevalence among men is based on regression-based estimates because limited data are available for this population group (Table 4-4). Nonpregnant women represent the population group with the greatest number of individuals affected, although the prevalence rate is lower among this group compared with pregnant women.[37] Regional estimates for preschool-age children and pregnant and nonpregnant women by the WHO, based on a systematic review of all data collected and published between 1993 and 2005, indicate that

the highest proportion of individuals affected are in Africa (44% to 64%) (Table 4-5). The greatest number affected are in Asia where 520 million individuals in these three population groups are affected:[37] 60% of all anemic preschool-age children and pregnant women, and 70% of all anemic nonpregnant women.

The main cause of anemia in developed countries is iron deficiency. However, in developing countries, factors such as malaria and parasitic infections often play a role. Anemia rates are further impacted, especially in developing countries, by consequences of low socioeconomic status such as lack of food security, inadequate or lack of access to health care, and poor environmental sanitation and personal hygiene.

Table 4-4. Prevalence of anemia by population group.

Population group	Prevalence of anemia		Population affected	
	%	95% CI	Number, millions	95% CI
Preschool-age children	47.4	45.7–49.1	293	283–303
School-age children*	25.4	19.9–30.9	305	238–371
Pregnant women	41.8	39.9–43.8	56	54–59
Nonpregnant women	30.2	28.7–31.6	468	446–491
Men*	12.7	8.6–16.9	260	175–345
Elderly*	23.9	18.3–29.4	164	126–202
Total population	**24.8**	**22.9–26.7**	**1620**	**1500–1740**

CI, confidence interval.
Source: World Health Organization[37]
*Prevalence for these populations is based on regression-based estimates.

Table 4-5. Prevalence of anemia by region.

UN region[a]	Preschool-age children[b]		Pregnant women[b]		Nonpregnant women[b]	
	Prevalence, %	No. affected, millions	Prevalence, %	No. affected, millions	Prevalence, %	No. affected, millions
Africa	64.6	93.2	55.8	19.3	44.4	82.9
Asia	47.7	170.0	41.6	31.7	33.0	318.3
Europe	16.7	6.1	18.7	1.4	15.2	26.6
LAC	39.5	22.3	31.1	3.6	23.5	33.0
NA	3.4	0.8	6.1	0.3	7.6	6.0
Oceania	28.0	0.7	30.4	0.2	20.2	1.5
Global	**47.4**	**293.1**	**41.8**	**56.4**	**30.2**	**468.4**

Source: World health Organization.[37]
[a]UN regions: Africa, Asia, Europe, Latin America, and the Caribbean (LAC), Northern America (NA), and Oceania.
[b]Population subgroups: Preschool-age children (0.00 to 4.99 years); Pregnant women (no age range defined); non-pregnant women (15.00 to 49.99 years).

Health Consequences

The consequences of IDA in the general population include increased morbidity from infectious diseases because anemia adversely affects the immune system. It also reduces the body's ability to monitor and regulate body temperature when exposed to cold. Additionally, cognitive performance is impaired at all stages of life, and physical work capacity is significantly reduced as a result of iron deficiency.

Women, in particular, are at risk of anemia due to periodic menstrual blood loss and an increased need for iron during pregnancy.[38-40] Anemia affects approximately 42% (over 56 million) of the pregnant women in the world.[41] IDA during pregnancy has serious clinical consequences. It is associated with multiple adverse outcomes for both mother and infant, including intrauterine growth retardation, an increased risk of hemorrhage, sepsis, maternal, infant, and perinatal mortality, increased stillbirths, low birth weight, and prematurity. Forty percent of all maternal perinatal deaths are linked to anemia.[42] Favorable pregnancy outcomes occur 30% to 45% less often in anemic mothers, and their infants have less than half of normal iron reserves.[42] Pregnant women who are severely anemic are less able to withstand blood loss and may require transfusions. The availability and safety of blood poses a dilemma in poorer countries, which usually have a higher prevalence and a more complex etiology of anemia.

Long-term health consequences, such as the development of chronic noncommunicable diseases in adulthood (e.g., cardiovascular diseases, diabetes mellitus, hypertension, and cancer), have been linked to early nutritional deficiencies and intrauterine growth retardation among infants born to mothers with anemia.[43] Furthermore, infants who become anemic may experience permanent impairment of cognitive development. Lower cognitive test scores have been observed in young children with anemia. These outcomes do not improve when anemia is corrected or as development continues.

Prevention and Control

A range of strategies are used to control and prevent anemia. Increasing awareness and knowledge among health care providers and the general public concerning the health risks associated with anemia is a key strategy. Additional strategies include food-based approaches, food fortification, and iron supplementation. These strategies may not be feasible or sustainable, especially in low-resource settings, where challenges such as food security and low social status of women are still problems.

Pregnancy and Childbirth

Pregnancy and childbirth are a natural part of the human life cycle. However, pregnancy and delivery can be very dangerous for women who have complications and do not have access to emergency care. Delivery and the immediate newborn period is a similarly dangerous time for infants. Two factors that play major roles in both maternal and neonatal birth outcomes are where and by whom a woman is delivered. Whereas hospital deliveries with a doctor in attendance is the norm for high-income countries, most women, especially in the lowest income countries, deliver at home with assistance from unskilled caregivers. Meeting MDG 5 requires improving many indicators, as shown in Figure 4-2.

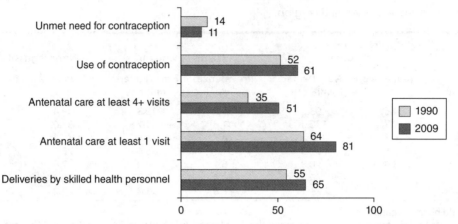

Figure 4-2. Reproductive health indicators in developing regions, 1990 and 2009 (percentage). (*Reproduced from WHO, UNICEF, UNFPA, World Bank.* Trends in Maternal Mortality, 1990–2010. *Geneva: World Health Organization, 2012: 28.*)

Prenatal Care

The relationship between early and frequent provision of prenatal care and better MCH outcomes has been documented but is subject to ongoing review regarding the number and content of visits.[44]

The WHO recommends a minimum of four antenatal visits with skilled health professionals (nurses, nurse midwives, or doctors) and that the basic minimum services should include measurement of blood pressure, blood tests for syphilis and anemia, and urine testing for bacteriuria and proteinuria.[45] The purpose of these visits is to provide early access to health care with immunization, maternal monitoring, screening, treatment, and referral. Early and more frequent contact with health care provides the opportunity to increase health knowledge and improve health behaviors, as well as access to the following services:

- Maternal monitoring, including nutrition and weight, and the identification and treatment of other problems such as anemia and hypertension. In some programs prenatal care includes food supplements.
- Screening and treatment for sexually transmitted infections (STIs) and HIV, and giving HIV-positive pregnant women antiretroviral treatment to prevent mother-to-child transmission.
- Treatment of malaria, TB, and other diseases that may cause problems for a pregnant woman and her fetus.

Prenatal care can identify women at high risk based on their obstetric history, complications, and general health status. It is important to note that approximately 40% of all pregnant women experience some type of complication, and 15% have a serious problem requiring immediate obstetric attention.[46] In most cases the risks cannot be adequately predicted, which requires that all women receive skilled care to prevent maternal and neonatal deaths. In 2010, only 55% of women in developing regions had the recommended four prenatal visits.[1]

The Role of Traditional Birth Attendants

Traditional birth attendants (TBAs) are usually apprenticed with an experienced TBA to learn the skills of delivering babies. In some countries, training in more sanitary delivery techniques, such as the use of new razors, and in the recognition of danger signs and when to refer, has been provided to TBAs, who are then called trained TBAs. The WHO has provided home delivery kits (soap, new razors, gauze, and other materials) to many programs that work with TBAs. These kits can also be assembled locally. TBAs provide accessible community-based care that incorporates local beliefs and traditions. Many women prefer to deliver at home with their family, where they can follow traditional practices regarding care of the mother and baby and the disposition of the placenta.

TBAs typically do not provide prenatal care, although this has been incorporated in TBA training so that they can identify women at risk. However, there has been considerable controversy about the role of TBAs and whether it is possible to improve maternal and prenatal outcomes during home deliveries by TBAs.[47–49] A major issue is that even trained TBAs observing best practices are unable to refer and transport mothers and babies to higher-level care when emergencies occur.[50]

As a result, the WHO recommends that women be delivered by skilled health personnel (an accredited health professional, nurse midwife, doctor, or nurse who has been educated and trained to manage normal pregnancies and deliveries and to refer complications). These goals were incorporated in the MDGs, which set the objective of 80% of all births assisted by skilled attendants by 2005; however, this goal has not been reached, nor is it likely that the goal of 95% will be reached by 2015 (see Figure 4-3).[1]

Currently, 65% of women in developing countries deliver with skilled attendance, but this does not reflect the situation in countries such as Haiti or regions such as sub-Saharan Africa, where 80% to 90% of deliveries occur at home with TBAs. The MDGs also set the goal of reducing maternal mortality by 75% between 1990 and 2015. Although maternal mortality was reduced by 47%, as of 2010 the MMR

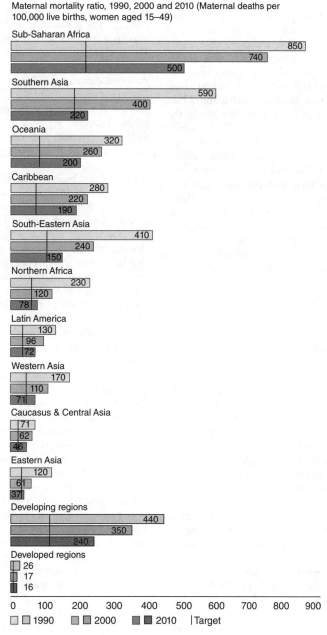

Maternal mortality ratio, 1990, 2000 and 2010 (Maternal deaths per 100,000 live births, women aged 15–49)

Figure 4-3. Maternal mortality ratio, 1990, 2000, and 2010 (women ages 15–49).[1]

for developing regions was 240/100,000 and seems unlikely to reach the target by 2015.[1]

Limited Access to Primary Care and Hospital Services   Related to the issue of home delivery by TBAs is access to primary care and hospital services. Prenatal care, especially tetanus immunization and iron supplementation, has been demonstrated to improve pregnancy outcomes, but it requires that women have access to basic primary care services. As noted earlier, the recommendation is that women have a minimum of four prenatal visits. At least 27% of women in developing countries receive no antenatal care during pregnancy, and 35% give birth without a skilled attendant.[1] Less information is available about postpartum care, which is important for mothers and newborns. It has been estimated that 42% of maternal deaths, 32% of stillbirths, and 23% of neonatal deaths occur in the period between birth and the period immediately following birth. Most women and babies do not receive postpartum care, and this is especially true of those without skilled attendance at delivery.[51] This lack of care is most life threatening during childbirth and the days immediately after delivery because these are the times when sudden life-threatening complications are most likely to arise. WHO recommendations call for mothers and infants to be seen within 72 hours of delivery, but recent data from the 47 countries of sub-Saharan Africa shows that only 51% of them track postnatal care for nonfacility deliveries. None of these had rates of coverage higher than 32%, and most were below 15%.[52]

Delivery Care

As mentioned previously, most maternal complications occur within 24 hours of delivery, requiring access to immediate care. Although the percentage of births with skilled attendance has increased in all regions of the world, there is still a large gap between high-income and low-income countries (Figure 4-4).[1]

It is important that delivery sites have the appropriate medications and technology, and well-trained staff. These sites should be affordable and accessible, and emergency transport should be provided for women who do not live near the facilities. One approach has been the development of maternal waiting homes, where women who are having problems during pregnancy, and those who are very young or very old, can stay near a hospital, receiving treatment and good nutrition.

An intermediate intervention when skilled attendance at a hospital or clinic is not possible has been to train TBAs to provide better services during delivery and to recognize complications and refer. This has been the subject of considerable controversy because some research found no difference between trained

and untrained TBAs.[47–49] Even skilled attendance is not necessarily enough to make a difference and is contingent on other systemic factors.[53]

Where skilled delivery is available in sterile clinic sites, midwives and nurses as well as doctors are able to provide more appropriate interventions, such as active management of the third stage of labor. This includes both physiologic and drug management to limit labor time and reduce maternal and infant complications such as postpartum hemorrhage and infant death. This can be done with relatively inexpensive medications (oxytocics) and simple physical maneuvers in a hospital setting and does not require extensive equipment or training.

Financial resources are not the only answer to reducing maternal mortality. Sri Lanka and Malaysia are examples of early interventions in the 1950s when they were both low-income countries with low MMRs.[54] Other, more recent, examples are Bolivia, China, Egypt, Honduras, Indonesia, Jamaica, and Zimbabwe.[55] These examples suggest that there are many ways to improve maternal mortality in resource-poor settings. Another factor that must be considered is the inequality between income groups in accessing and receiving services.[56]

Almost 6 million women developed serious complications from pregnancy and childbirth in 2012, and 287,000 died.[57] Hemorrhage and hypertensive disorders are the most common contributors to maternal deaths in the developing world.[58] The most common causes of maternal morbidity and mortality were hemorrhage (24%), infections (15%), unsafe abortions (13%), hypertensive disorders (12%), obstructed labor (8%). These five conditions account for over 70% of the MMR. Inadequate health care, poor health status, and inadequate nutrition are the major underlying causes.[2]

With limited resources and deficient health care systems, many preventable emergencies occur because of lack of treatment or a delay in care.[59] The "three delays model" was developed by Thaddeus and Maine to describe the complex issues preventing pregnant women from receiving adequate care.[60] Phase 1 involves delay in the decision to seek care (unawareness of complications, acceptance of maternal death, and sociocultural factors such as beliefs, practices, and women's decision-making ability), phase 2 involves delay in reaching care (due to poor roads, geographic barriers, and poor service organization), and phase 3 involves delay in receiving adequate care (because of health care system problems including lack of facilities and personnel and lack of a family's ability to pay for services). These complex delays led to the causes of maternal death listed previously, resulting in 287,000 maternal deaths in 2012.[2] Figure 4-5 illustrates the proportion of deaths attributable to these causes and interventions that have been developed to prevent or treat them.

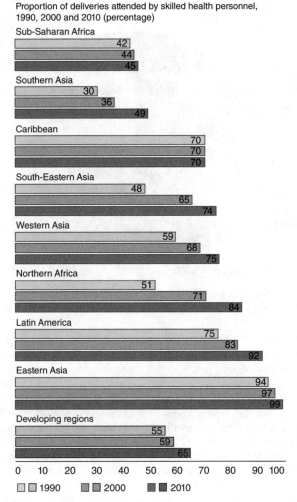

Proportion of deliveries attended by skilled health personnel, 1990, 2000 and 2010 (percentage)

Figure 4-4. Deliveries attended by skilled health personnel.[1]

- **Hemorrhage:** Severe bleeding/postpartum hemorrhage (PPH) has been identified as the most important cause of maternal death. Most (60%) of maternal deaths occur during childbirth, and half of these are within 24 hours of delivery,[61] with most of these deaths due to hemorrhage. Anemia is a major contributor to maternal deaths from hemorrhage. Because the risk for hemorrhage cannot be predicted with high accuracy, skilled attendance and access to hospital services are recommended for all women. Women should be monitored for complications of hemorrhage during the immediate postpartum period. If severe bleeding occurs, women should be stabilized and referred to the next level of care.[31] Uterotonics and Active Management of the Third Stage of Labor (AMTSL) provide effective interventions to prevent PPH. Uterotonics include oxytocin that is used at the facility level and misoprostol, which has been shown to be effective for home deliveries. A recent survey of 37 countries found that use of uterotonics and AMTSL had increased. Oxytocin was available in 87% of the countries and AMTSL was part of the national service guidelines for 99% of the countries (although only 48% met all the requirements). Misoprostol was less commonly accepted with only 57% of countries having it on the essential medicines list, and only a few countries actively promoting its use.[62]

- **Infection:** Postpartum endometritis, puerperal sepsis, and urinary tract infection are the most common infections following childbirth. These infections can be prevented by good prenatal, delivery, and postpartum care, especially by maintaining sterile delivery techniques. Infections must be treated immediately

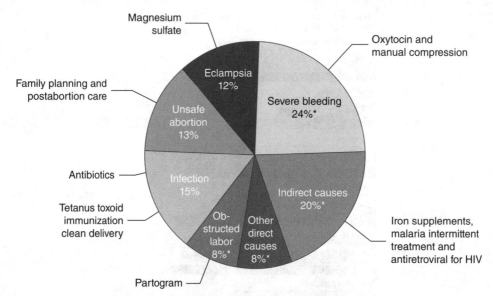

Figure 4-5. Causes of maternal mortality and effective interventions. (*Reproduced from Maternal and Child Health. USAID. http://transition.usaid.gov/our_work/global_health/mch/mh/techareas/maternal_mortality.html.*)

after occurrence to prevent chronic problems including infertility and death from generalized sepsis.[63]

- **Unsafe abortion:** In 2008, there were 43.8 million abortions, of which 49% were unsafe, resulting in 47,000 maternal deaths in developing countries.[64,65] Unsafe abortion is a procedure for terminating an unwanted pregnancy by persons lacking the necessary skills or in an environment lacking the minimal medical standards, or both.[64] The risks are determined by the health of the woman, the method used, and the hygiene of the instruments and the setting. Severe complications such as infection, hemorrhage, perforated uterus, and poisoning due to ingestion of harmful substances may result in death or permanent disability.[66]

- **Obstetric fistula:** *Fistula* refers to any abnormal connection between two bodily organs. The two types of obstetric fistula are vesicovaginal and rectovaginal. A vesicovaginal fistula is a hole between the wall of the vagina and the bladder, resulting in urinary incontinence. A rectovaginal fistula is a hole between the wall of the vagina and the rectum, resulting in fecal incontinence. Both types of obstetric fistula are caused by abnormal pressure of the fetal head during obstructed labor, which interrupts the flow of blood to nearby tissues in the mother's pelvis. Early childhood marriage is the most common cause of obstructed labor resulting in fistula.[67] Very young women are not physically developed enough to allow the easy passage of a baby. The result is that the child dies in childbirth

and the mother suffers a lifetime of ostracism and neglect due to chronic infections, poor hygiene, and social stigma. Another contributing factor is female genital cutting or mutilation when the cutting of the vaginal wall goes too deep.[68]

- **Eclampsia:** Eclampsia and preeclampsia are hypertensive disorders of pregnancy. Eclampsia is a seizure or coma in a pregnant woman with preeclampsia. Preeclampsia is characterized by high blood pressure and proteinuria. Preeclampsia occurs in 5% to 8% of pregnancies; symptoms include swelling, sudden weight gain, headaches, and changes in vision, although some women may be asymptomatic. The specific cause of these conditions is not well understood.[69] Two major collaborative research projects in the past 12 years examined the effectiveness of treatment. The first project, the Collaborative Eclampsia Trial, found that magnesium sulfate was the most effective treatment for controlling eclamptic convulsions.[70–72] More recently, the Magpie Trial conducted a randomized controlled trial of magnesium sulfate versus a placebo in 33 countries and found a 50% reduction in eclampsia in response to magnesium sulfate.[73] A commentary in the same issue of *Lancet* made a call for global implementation of magnesium sulfate treatment for women with preeclampsia, stating that it is safe, effective, and relatively inexpensive, costing no more than US$5 per patient.[74] Magnesium sulfate was part of the regimen of all 37 countries surveyed in a recent study, although it was not routinely available in facilities for over 50% of countries responding.[62]

In addition to the loss of women's lives, maternal deaths directly affect children's health and well-being. According to a 2004 WHO report, an estimated 1 million children die as a result of their mother's death every year. Large numbers of orphans become the responsibility of extended families and communities, which often lack resources to provide proper care.[67]

On the continuum of maternity care, antenatal and perinatal care often take precedence over postpartum/postnatal care. However, 77% of maternal deaths and 40% of neonatal deaths occur in the 48 hours after labor and birth; therefore, care of the mother and child should not stop after delivery.[75] Postpartum/postnatal care and follow-up are essential for the health of the mother and her child. There must be collaboration between parents, families, caregivers (trained or traditional), health professionals, health planners, health care administrators, and other related sectors such as community groups, policymakers, and politicians.[75] Basic postpartum/postnatal care includes the warmth and cleanliness of the newborn, treatment for complications such as birth asphyxia, hygienic cord care, and infections. Also important are immunizations, exclusive breastfeeding, proper maternal nutrition (including micronutrient supplementation), counseling, and other family planning services such as birth spacing and interventions for the prevention of mother-to-child transmission of infections.[76]

Perinatal and Neonatal Mortality

Perinatal deaths occur during childbirth and the first week of life; *neonatal mortality* occurs during the first 28 days of life and includes perinatal mortality. These periods are also referred to as early and late neonatal mortality. The causes of death in the first week and the first month are similar, although the role of infectious diseases increases with age in the first month.

Perinatal Deaths

There were 6.7 million perinatal deaths in 2004. This was almost evenly divided between stillbirths (3 million) and neonatal (3.7 million), and 75% of the neonatal deaths were in the first week of life.[77] Almost 98% of deaths occurred in developing countries, with 30% of these in the least developed countries. Africa had the highest regional perinatal death rate (56/1,000), followed by Asia (47/1,000), Oceania (42/1,000), the Caribbean (29/1,000), and Latin America (19/1,000).[77,78] In reality, the situation is even worse. In developing countries, many infants who die in the womb or soon after birth are not reported. Only a third of the world's countries have reliable vital registration, and stillbirths and early neonatal deaths are least likely to be reported.[79]

The most common causes of perinatal mortality are unexplained intrauterine death in pregnancy, intrauterine death due to maternal complications, intrapartum death due to obstetric complications, inadequate management of birth, birth asphyxia, preterm birth, sepsis, congenital anomalies, and low birth weight. Deaths in the early neonatal period (during the first week of life) are largely the result of inadequate or inappropriate care during pregnancy, childbirth, or the first critical hours after birth.[75]

Perinatal mortality is generally high in most developing countries because of low socioeconomic conditions and the lack of emergency obstetric and neonatal services.[44] The PNMR is used as an indicator of the quality of antenatal and perinatal care and of the general health status of pregnant women, new mothers, and newborns.[80] This indicator is a major marker of maternal care, maternal health, and nutrition; it is also affected by the availability and quality of in-hospital care for neonates.

Perinatal mortality varies by country and region. Some developing countries have reduced the PNMR by regular mortality review and auditing of delivery and postpartum practices. Effective technical and community interventions are important to reduce the incidence and severity of major complications associated with pregnancy and childbirth including perinatal mortality.[2] Other serious newborn morbidity results from neonatal tetanus, disturbance in thermoregulation, jaundice, ophthalmia neonatorum, neonatal herpes infection, hepatitis B, and HIV; the last two result from vertical transmission. Figure 4-6 illustrates the relative proportion of neonatal deaths by cause.[80]

Maternal health factors that play a role in neonatal deaths include access to family planning and prenatal care (syphilis screening, folate and nutrition supplementation, vaccination against tetanus, malaria treatment, and promotion of exclusive breastfeeding). Access to health interventions such as safe delivery practices, eye care, kangaroo care (discussed later in this chapter), and treatment of infections is also critical for the newborn. Some of the most important recent developments in MCH address these issues in a comprehensive way.

Postneonatal and Infant Mortality

Postneonatal mortality refers to infant deaths during the period of 1 to 12 months. Deaths in this age group are primarily due to infection, malnutrition, and dehydration. These conditions are similar to those of early childhood and are addressed in the following section. It is important to note that in the first year of life the severity of these conditions is often greater and more likely to result in death. Nutrition is critical during the first year of life, both in terms of the promotion of exclusive breastfeeding in the first

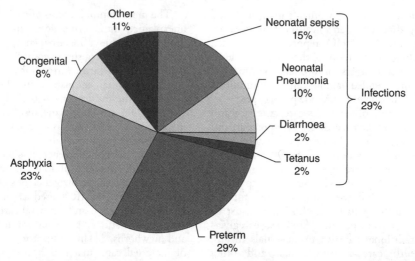

Figure 4-6. Main causes of neonatal deaths.[80]

6 months of life and the transition to other foods, which is often a time of decreasing growth for infants due to the poor quality of weaning foods. These issues are addressed more fully in Chapter 7. *Infant mortality* refers to all deaths of children younger than 1 year of age and thus is the sum of neonatal and postneonatal mortality.

Early Childhood

Early childhood is defined as the period from birth to 8 years old, although most statistics focus on children under 5 because this is the period when most vaccinations and other interventions take place. During this time, children undergo rapid growth, and this is the most intensive period of brain development; therefore, adequate stimulation and nutrition are essential. However, every year more than 200 million children under 5 years old fail to reach their full cognitive and social potential.[81] Most of these children live in South Asia and sub-Saharan Africa. Poor development during these crucial years has far-reaching negative outcomes in adult society. Mental health problems, obesity/stunting, heart disease, criminality, and competency in literacy and numeracy have all have been linked to early childhood development.[82] Many factors can disrupt early child development; however, 20% to 25% of infants and young children in developing countries are affected by the following four:

- Malnutrition that is chronic and severe enough to cause growth stunting
- Inadequate stimulation or learning opportunities
- Iodine deficiency
- Iron Deficiency Anemia

Other risk factors are malaria, intrauterine growth restriction, maternal depression, exposure to violence, and heavy metals.[81,83]

In 2011, 6.9 million children under the age of 5 died, and more than half of these deaths were due to conditions that could be prevented or treated with access to simple, affordable interventions.[84] The risk of death during the neonatal period is the greatest, with 43% of child deaths under the age of 5 taking place during this period.[84] Geographic disparities in early child deaths are apparent because children in sub-Saharan Africa are 16.5 times more likely to die before the age of 5 years than children in developed regions.[84] With the highest levels of under-5 mortality, one in eight children in sub-Saharan Africa die before the age of 5 (129 deaths per 1,000 live births) and one in 14 children die in South Asia, which has the second highest rate (69 deaths per 1,000 live births). In these countries child mortality is higher in rural areas and among the poorer and less educated families.[85] In 2000, world leaders committed to reducing the under-5 mortality rate by two thirds between 1990 and 2015 through MDG 4. Substantial progress has been made as the under-5 mortality rate has been reduced to 41%, from 87 deaths per 1,000 live births in 1990 to 51 in 2011; however, the rate of reduction is still insufficient to reach the MDG target for 2015.[86] Success in impacting child survival will require further action to address the leading causes of death.

Major Causes of Mortality and Morbidity

Preterm birth, intrapartum-related complications (birth asphyxia or lack of breathing at birth), and infections cause most neonatal deaths. Pneumonia, diarrhea,

Table 4-6. Leading causes of death in children under 5 years in the world, 2011.

	Death of children under 5 years
Pneumonia	18
Preterm birth complications	14
Diarrhea	11
Birth asphyxia	9
Malaria	7
Other causes	41

Source: World Health Organization.[84]

and malaria are the main causes of death from the end of the neonatal period and through the first 5 years of life (Table 4-6). Malnutrition is the underlying contributing factor in over a third of all child deaths, making children more vulnerable to severe diseases.

Malnutrition (undernutrition), the underlying cause of over a third of deaths among children under 5 years of age, results in 2.6 million child deaths every year.[87] The nutritional status of a woman during adolescence, pregnancy, and lactation has a direct impact on child health, as well as her own. In many developing countries, the nutritional status of large segments of the population, especially women, is inadequate. Undernutrition of women can be attributed to discrimination in terms of food allocation, to the heavy burden of physical labor, and to reproduction.[75] Nutritional indicators such as low birth weight, wasting, stunting, and underweight are discussed in Chapter 7. Micronutrient malnutrition also has public health significance. Micronutrient deficiencies account for a third of all malnutrition-related child deaths and 10% of all children's deaths. Nearly all deaths linked to micronutrient deficiency are due to a lack of vitamin A, zinc, or iron.[87] Ensuring proper nutrition for both mother and child is essential. With respect to infant feeding practice, the WHO and UNICEF recommend exclusive breastfeeding for the first 6 months. Thereafter, infants should receive complementary foods with continued breastfeeding up to 2 years of age or beyond or 12 months for mothers known to be HIV-infected in regions where mothers receive antiretrovirals (ARVs) and national authorities promote breastfeeding.[88,89] Breastfeeding promotes sensory and cognitive development. Furthermore, infants who are exclusively breastfed are likely to experience only a quarter as many episodes of diarrhea and respiratory infection as those who are not breastfed.[88] Breastfeeding also contributes to the health and well-being of mothers. It helps to space children and reduces the risk of ovarian and breast cancer.

Acute respiratory infections (ARIs) are the most important cause of infant and young child mortality, accounting for about 2 million deaths each year.[90] Although upper respiratory infections (URIs) occur more frequently, lower respiratory infections (LRIs) are responsible for more severe illnesses such as influenza, pneumonia, TB, and bronchiolitis. Pneumonia is responsible for about 18% of all deaths in children under 5 years of age, with an estimated 1.4 million children dying every year.[91] The risk of getting pneumonia increases if the child is low birth weight, malnourished, or has not been breastfed. The risk is also increased among children living in overcrowded conditions. Children and families worldwide are affected by pneumonia, but it is most prevalent in South Asia and sub-Saharan Africa. Treatment is possible with antibiotics. However, accessibility and affordability of health care is an issue in many developing countries.

Diarrheal disease is the second leading cause of child deaths, killing 1.5 million children every year, more than AIDS, malaria, and measles *combined*.[92,93] As with ARI, the greatest burden of diarrheal diseases is in the developing world; Africa and South Asia account for over half the cases of childhood diarrhea and more than 80% of child deaths due to diarrhea.[93] Diarrhea, defined as the passage of three or more loose or liquid stools per day (or more frequent passage than is normal for the individual), is both preventable and treatable. The causes of diarrhea include bacterial, viral and parasitic infections, contaminated water and food, and malnutrition (malnourished children are more likely to fall ill from diarrhea). Diarrhea can last for several days, depleting the body of essential salts and water. Most diarrhea-related deaths result from severe dehydration and fluid loss. Dehydration from diarrhea can be prevented by giving extra fluids at home.[94] With the exception of severe cases, diarrhea can be treated with oral administration of an adequate glucose-electrolyte solution. Oral rehydration therapy (ORT), giving fluids to prevent or treat dehydration, combined with guidance on appropriate feeding practices, is the main strategy recommended by the WHO to achieve a reduction in diarrhea-related mortality and malnutrition in children. ORT can be delivered by village health workers and practiced in the home by mothers with some guidance. In 2006, the WHO and UNICEF announced a new formula for oral rehydration salts (ORS), which better combats acute diarrheal diseases and advances the MDG of reducing child mortality by two thirds before 2015. In addition, zinc supplements reduce the duration and severity of diarrheal episodes as well as reducing stool volume and the need for advanced medical care.[94]

Malaria, caused by parasites transmitted to people through the bites of infected mosquitoes, is another leading cause of mortality among children under

5 years of age. Ninety percent of the over 1 million deaths due to malaria each year occur in sub-Saharan Africa, mostly among young children.[95] Pregnant women and their unborn children are also particularly vulnerable to malaria, which is a major cause of perinatal mortality, low birth weight, and maternal anemia. The tragedy is that if people can reach care, this is a preventable, treatable, and controllable disease through effective low-cost strategies. Vector control (e.g., insecticide-treated mosquito nets, indoor spraying with residual insecticides) is the main way to reduce malaria transmission at the community level. For individuals, personal protection against mosquito bites represents the first line of defense. Antimalarial medicines can also be used. The WHO recommends intermittent preventive treatment for pregnant women who live in high transmission areas. For infants who live in these areas, the WHO also recommends intermittent preventive treatment alongside routine vaccinations. The best available treatment is artemisinin-based combination therapy. However, the rapid spread of resistance to antimalarial drugs, especially to the previous generations of medicines, coupled with widespread poverty and a weak health infrastructure, means that mortality from malaria continues to rise in developing countries. See Chapter 9 for more information on this subject.

Measles, caused by a highly contagious virus, remains a leading cause of death among children under 5 years of age in developing countries despite the availability of a safe and effective vaccine. In 2010, an estimated 139,300 people died from measles, most of them children under the age of 5.[96] More than 95% of measles deaths occur in low-income countries that have a weak health infrastructure. Poorly nourished young children, especially those who are vitamin A deficient or whose immune systems have been weakened by HIV/AIDS or other diseases, are more vulnerable to experiencing severe measles. Suffering, complications, and death caused by measles can be easily prevented through immunization, which is important in reducing child mortality and morbidity. Measles vaccination resulted in a 74% drop in measles deaths between 2000 and 2010 worldwide.[96] Beside measles, immunizations against TB, diphtheria, tetanus, pertussis, poliomyelitis, and hepatitis B are also recommended. There are internationally accepted immunization schedules that should be followed during the prenatal and postnatal period. However, in the developing world, there are many obstacles in realizing these schedules.

Middle Years and Adolescence

The uses and meanings of the terms *young people, youth, teenager,* and *adolescence* vary according to region and depend on the political, economic, and sociocultural context. The following definitions are most commonly accepted[97]:

- Adolescence: Period between ages 10 and 19 years
- Youth: People aged between 15 and 24 years
- Teenager: People aged between 13 and 19 years
- Young people: People aged between 10 and 24 years
- 10 to 14 years (early adolescence)
- 15 to 19 years (late adolescence)
- 20 to 24 years (young adulthood)

According to the WHO, young people (10 to 24 years old) comprise more than a quarter of the world's population,[97] making this cohort larger than ever before. Of the 1.8 billion young people worldwide, 86% live in low-income and middle-income countries.[98] Adolescents (10 to 19 years old) make up 18% of the world's population. Of the 1.2 billion adolescents, more than half live in Asia (Figure 4-7); around 243 million live in India, 201 million live in China, and 90 million in other countries in South Asia.[99]

The greatest proportion of adolescents, 23% of the region's population, is found in sub-Saharan Africa. The two countries with the highest proportion of adolescents in the world (26%) are Swaziland and Zimbabwe. Adolescents comprise 23% of the population in least developed countries, 19% in developing countries, and 12% in industrialized countries. The differences among regions are explained by the demographic transition that occurs when a decline in mortality rate is later followed by a decline in fertility rate; the interim period of lower mortality rates and still-high fertility rates results in a large proportion of youth in a population, sometimes termed a *youth bulge*.[99]

Generally speaking, adolescents are thought to be healthy because they have survived the diseases of early childhood and have many years before the onset of health problems associated with aging. Yet, more than 2.6 million young people ages 10 to 24 die each year.[100] Even a greater number experience illnesses that impact their ability to grow and develop. Many young people engage in behaviors (e.g., tobacco, alcohol and drug use, physical inactivity, unprotected sex) that jeopardize their current and future health; nearly two thirds of premature deaths and one third of the total disease burden in adults are associated with conditions or behaviors that began in their youth.[99] Trends in adolescent morbidity and mortality have shifted from predominantly infectious to social etiologies.[101]

Trends and Challenges

A global increase in child survival has led to a growth in the youth population. The distribution of youth has begun to drift toward developing countries with

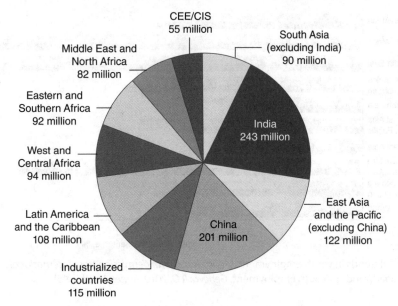

Figure 4-7. Population of adolescents by region, 2010.[99] CEE/CIS, Central Eastern Europe/Commonwealth of Independent States.

the greatest concentration in sub-Saharan Africa and Asia. A demographic shift, resulting from both rural-to-urban and cross-national migration, has also been evident over the last 25 years. Youth migration is a major cause of the rural-to-urban migration and predisposes youth to significant behavioral health risks that stem from unemployment and poverty, such as violence, prostitution, STIs/HIV, and substance abuse.[101] (See Chapter 5 for more information.)

Other trends that have a major impact on the health of adolescents include marriage, education, and globalization. The prevalence and consequences of early marriage and education have already been addressed. The cultural aspects of globalization have a large influence on adolescents' values and lifestyles. As a result of rapid globalization over the last decade or so, new patterns of disease have emerged in the world. For example, tobacco-related morbidities have risen owing largely to multinational cigarette companies targeting adolescents in developing countries, where fewer restrictions are placed on marketing and distribution.[101] The increasing prevalence of obesity worldwide, partially stemming from the greater availability of cheap vegetable oils and fat, is another impact of globalization on adolescent health.[101] One of the most detrimental effects of globalization has been the AIDS epidemic that has spread to every part of the world through travel and migration.

With massive advances in information and communication technology (e.g., mobile phones, the Internet, social networking sites) and its related access, young people in low-, middle- and high-income regions have ways to actively engage with one another through means that are less traditional and/or less controlled.[97] Health risks for young people, as a result of intense engagement with media, include decreased physical activity, sleep disturbance, cyber-bullying, pornography, and sexting (the act of sending sexually explicit messages or photographs by mobile phone).[97]

A major challenge faced by many young people is finding adequate employment. In 2009, 81 million youth worldwide were unemployed, and in 2010, young people ages 15 to 24 formed around a quarter of the world's working poor (Figure 4-8). In addition, many adolescents are leaving school with skills that do not match the needs of the global economy. More than 20% of the international companies operating in developing countries that have been recently surveyed cited the inadequate education of workers to be a significant obstacle to higher levels of corporate investment and faster economic growth.[102] Furthermore, the recent global economic crisis has exacerbated prospects of finding employment for everyone, but especially for adolescents.

Causes of Mortality

In comparison with younger children, the health of adolescents has improved to a lesser extent in the past 50 years.[97] Each year, 1.4 million deaths occur among 10- to 19-year-olds.[103] Risks to adolescent health stem from several causes including accidents, AIDS, early

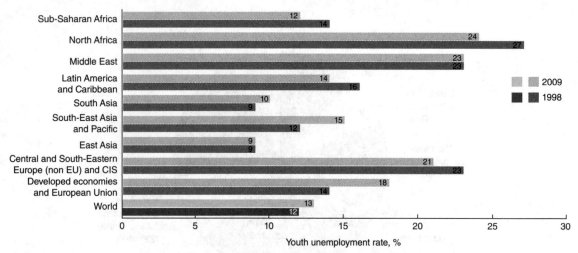

Figure 4-8. Global trends in youth employment. (*Reproduced with permission from International Labour Organization. Global Trends in Youth Employment. Geneva: ILO, 2010. Annex 1, Table A5*).

pregnancy, unsafe abortions, risky behaviors such as tobacco consumption and drug use, mental health issues, and violence. Injuries are the leading causes of death among 10- to 19-year-olds, accounting for almost 400,000 deaths per year.[102] These include road traffic injuries, injuries from recreational and sports accidents, falls, burns, poisoning and drowning, and injuries from violence including armed violence.[99,101] The poor in low- and middle-income countries experience the greatest burden of fatalities related to injuries. Boys are more prone than girls to injury and death from accidents and violence.[102] An estimated 430 young people ages 10 to 24 die every day through interpersonal violence. For every death, an estimated 20 to 40 youth require hospital treatment for a violence-related injury.[100]

About 16 million girls ages 15 to 19 give birth every year, roughly 11% of all births worldwide.[4] Complications related to pregnancy and childbirth account for the deaths of approximately 50,000 adolescent girls each year. In Africa, childbirth is the leading killer of adolescent girls, with maternal causes accounting for the largest proportion of deaths among women in all age groups. In contrast, in middle- and high-income countries, cars are the biggest killers, with road traffic injuries a leading cause of death among adolescent girls.[99]

Suicide is a major cause of death among adolescents worldwide. Globally, an estimated 71,000 adolescents commit suicide annually; up to 40 times as many make suicide attempts.[102]

One of the most important challenges for adolescent survival and health is preventing the transmission of HIV. AIDS is estimated to be the eighth leading cause of death among adolescents ages 15 to 19, and the sixth leading cause among 10- to 14-year-olds; however, it takes a disproportionately high toll in high-prevalence countries.[102] In 2009, young people (15- to 24-years-old) accounted for 40% of all new HIV infections among adults. Globally, about 2.2 million (2.0 to 2.5 million) adolescents were living with HIV in 2010.[99] Due to the sheer scale of the epidemic in East and South Africa, AIDS is the prominent cause of death for women ages 15 to 29 worldwide, as well as one of the leading causes of death for men in this age group.[102] Adolescent girls and young women are more at risk for contracting HIV than boys and young men. This is a result of their greater physiologic susceptibility and also because they may have older sexual partners, who may be exposed to the virus. They also face a high risk of sexual violence and rape and are not able to negotiate condom use. Currently, only 36% of young men and 24% of young women have the comprehensive and correct knowledge they need to protect themselves from acquiring the virus.[100]

The risk of death increases as adolescents grow older. In 2004, for example, the mortality rate for adolescents ages 10 to 14 was 95 deaths per 100,000 persons, among 15- to 19-year-olds, it was 139, and among 20- to 24-year-olds, 224.[99]

Causes of Morbidity

For adolescents, causes of morbidity center on reproductive health issues (pregnancy and early childbearing, abortion, STIs, and various traditional reproductive practices). Other causes include violence (sexual coercion and abuse), mental health, and tobacco/substance abuse. Pregnancy and early childbirth were addressed earlier in this chapter, as was abortion. According to WHO estimates, 1 in 20 adolescents worldwide acquires a STI each year. However, in the wake of the HIV and AIDS epidemic, very little attention has been focused on other STIs, even though they can lead to serious reproductive morbidity and mortality. Because STIs frequently go undetected and untreated, they are considerably underreported. The actual prevalence among adolescents worldwide is not known. Other reproductive health issues that specifically affect adolescents are traditional reproductive practices, such as female genital mutilation (FGM). FGM is examined in detail later in this chapter.

Sexual coercion and abuse has not been well studied due to the sensitive nature of the topic. Although girls are more likely to be victims of sexual abuse or coercion, several studies show that large numbers of boys also experience it. Sexual abuse and coercion can lead to a wide variety of negative health consequences including behavioral and psychological problems, sexual dysfunction, low self-esteem, relationship problems, thoughts of suicide, alcohol and substance abuse, and sexual risk taking. In addition, sexual violence has been linked to many serious physical health problems, such as injuries, chronic pain syndromes, and gastrointestinal disorders.[101]

Every year, an estimated 20% of adolescents experience a mental health problem.[100] According to WHO estimates, by the year 2020 adolescent psychiatric disorders will increase more than 50% worldwide to become one of the five leading causes of disability among adolescents.[101] Depression and anxiety are the most common mental disorders affecting adolescents and young people worldwide. The primary concern with depression among adolescents is that it is often combined with substance abuse, which puts adolescents at even greater risk for suicide.[101]

Tobacco and substance abuse (alcohol and drug abuse) is quite prevalent among adolescents, particularly among young men. Recent trends show an even earlier age of initiation and rising smoking prevalence rates among children and adolescents.[101] Worldwide, 150 million young people use tobacco. This number is increasing, particularly among young women. Based on the data available, alcohol use is also initiated at a young age; 14% of adolescent girls and 18% of boys ages 13 to 15 years in low- and middle-income countries are reported to have used alcohol.[100] It is the primary cause of injuries, violence, and premature deaths.[100] Marijuana appears to be the most widely used illicit substance worldwide. Similar to tobacco and alcohol use, studies have also shown that more boys than girls engage in illicit drug use.[101]

Domestic Violence/Intimate Partner Violence

The UN defines violence against women as "any act of gender-based violence that results in, or is likely to result in, physical, sexual or mental harm or suffering to women, including threats of such acts, coercion or arbitrary deprivation of liberty, whether occurring in public or in private life." The UN reported that violence against women remains widespread around the world, exacerbated by traditions and customary practices that determine the way women are treated in families, places of work, and communities.[104]

Until recently, most governments and policymakers viewed violence against women as a relatively minor social problem, particularly "domestic" violence by a husband or other intimate partner. Since the 1990s, however, the efforts of women's organizations, experts, and committed governments have resulted in a profound transformation in public awareness about this problem. Such violence is now widely recognized as a serious human rights and public health problem that concerns all sectors of society.[105] The term *domestic violence* is now being replaced by *intimate partner violence* (IPV), which refers to behavior in an intimate relationship that causes physical, sexual, or psychological harm including physical and verbal aggression and sexual coercion. A WHO multi-country study found that between 15% and 71% of women ages 15 to 49 years reported physical and/or sexual violence by an intimate partner at some point in their lives.[106,107]

Types

IPV includes different types of physical, emotional/psychological, and sexual forms. Physical abuse, which is the most observed type, occurs when the husband/partner is slapping, hitting, pushing, kicking, beating, biting, or throwing things at the woman. It can reach severe levels such as burning, choking, or using a weapon. Emotional/psychological abuse includes belittling, insulting, or threatening to cause serious problems for the woman or those she cares about such as her children. Sexual violence includes forced sexual acts or behaviors.

Risk Factors for the Experience of Domestic Violence

Violence is a forced control of one person by another. Therefore, it is always directed toward the weaker or more fragile person. Poorer, uneducated, and less empowered women are more likely to be victims of IPV. Women who married at a young age and those who have many children are also more likely to report having experienced violence. A nine-country (Cambodia, Colombia, Dominican Republic, Haiti,

Egypt, India, Nicaragua, Peru, and Zambia) study used DHS data for 164,295 women to examine prevalence and risk factors for domestic violence.[108] Women who have ever experienced violence from their husbands ranged from 17.5% in Cambodia to 48.4% in Zambia. Women who experienced violence in the past 12 months ranged from 10.6% in India to 26.5% in Zambia. Most women did not seek help for the abuse (77.5% in Cambodia; 40.5% in Nicaragua). The primary reason was "there is no use," followed by embarrassment and not knowing where to go. In all countries, women who had been married more than once or who were divorced or separated reported higher rates of violence than women who were currently married and had married only once.[108] This is not surprising because domestic violence can be an important reason for marriage dissolution. The wealth of a household has an inconsistent and often nonlinear relationship with the experience of violence. The perpetrators are more likely to be men who are less educated, unemployed, or under the influence of alcohol and other intoxicating substances.[109–114]

Health Consequences of IPV

The role of IPV in women's injury and ill health has become a major concern in public health.[115] Substantial literature provides an overview of the different health consequences for women exposed to IPV. These include increased physical health problems (e.g., injury, chronic pain, gastrointestinal, and gynecologic problems including sexually transmitted diseases) and psychological health problems (e.g., depression, posttraumatic stress disorder, and suicide attempts).[116–118] There is no standard way of classifying the severity of injuries. Studies using the DHS use one approach and other types of research use others. Injuries range from bruises, abrasions, cuts, punctures, and bites to broken bones, injuries to ears, eyes, or internal organs. Pregnancy increases the risk of IPV and results in adverse pregnancy outcomes including low birth weight and maternal and infant mortality.[119, 120]

Cycle of Violence

Research has demonstrated that children who grow up in an abusive family are more likely to use violence as a solution for disputes or conflicts. Children who experience abuse and neglect are more likely to abuse their own children when they become parents. Women exposed to IPV are more likely to abuse their children. In many countries, women are exposed to violence not only from their husbands but also from their in-laws and even their own families. Having a family history of domestic violence significantly increases the likelihood of experiencing violence oneself.[121–123]

Screening and Management of IPV

Women who have been abused usually seek care for other complaints when they go to emergency departments or clinics. They are ashamed or frightened to admit that their injuries were a result of IPV. Routine screening for IPV is endorsed by numerous health professional organizations. Screening rates in health care settings, however, remain low. Barriers to IPV screening, as perceived by health care providers, include lack of provider education regarding IPV, no time, lack of effective interventions and patient-related factors such as unwillingness to disclose and fear of offending the patient.[124–127]

Most research on screening and referral has been conducted in developed countries, but a few studies have examined provider training in IPV, screening, and referral in developing countries. These studies have demonstrated the importance of training, of understanding women's perspectives, and the availability of resources for intervention and support. A recent pilot intervention in an outpatient clinic in Tanzania found that IPV screening was feasible and that health care workers viewed it as useful, some saying that "just asking feels good."[128] Another study at Kenyatta National Hospital in Kenya had similar results in terms of feasibility and acceptability of screening. This research found that patients and families defined IPV more broadly than health care providers. This broader definition will be incorporated in future training. Kenyatta Hospital has one of several one-stop Gender-Based Violence Recovery Centres (GBVRC) in Kenya. GBVRCs provide medical, social, legal, and other support for women who have experienced IPV.[129]

Sex Selection

Another form of gender-based violence is sex selection before birth. Over 180 countries are signatories to the 1994 Programme of Action of the International Conference on Population and Development that includes agreement to *"eliminate all forms of discrimination against the girl child and the root causes of son preference, which result in harmful and unethical practices regarding female infanticide and prenatal sex selection.* (United Nations (1994); paragraph 4.16).[130]

Even though sex determination for the purpose of sex selection is illegal in the two countries where it is most common (India and China), sex determination and abortion continue creating a major disparity in sex ratios. The number of male babies born per 100 female babies is called the sex ratio at birth. Normally this is a ratio of 102 to 106 males per 100 females.[130] In affected countries this ratio is 110 to 120, and because of ethnic and cultural variation reaches 130 in some regions (Table 4-7). It has been estimated

Table 4-7. Most recent estimates of sex ratio at birth in various countries, 2007–2011.

Country/Regions	SRB	Period	Data source
East and Southeast Asia			
China	117.8	2011	Annual estimate
Anhui Province	128.7	2010	2010 census
Fujian Province	125.6	2010	2010 census
Hainan Province	125.5	2010	2010 census
Hong Kong	116.2	2011	Birth registration*
Taiwan	108.4	2009	Birth registration
Singapore	107.5	2009	Birth registration
South Korea	106.7	2010	Birth registration
Vietnam	111.2	2010	Annual demographic survey
Red River Delta Region	116.2	2010	Annual demographic survey
South Asia			
India	110.5	2008–10	Sample registration
Punjab State	120.3	2008–10	Sample registration
Haryana State	117.9	2008–10	Sample registration
Uttar Pradesh State	114.9	2007	Population and demographic survey
Pakistan	109.9	2007	Population and demographic survey
West Asia			
Azerbaijan	116.5	2011	Birth registration
Armenia	114.9	2010	Birth registration
Georgia	113.6	2009–11	Birth registration*
Southeast Europe			
Albania	111.7	2008–10	Birth registration*
Montenegro	109.8	2009–11	Birth registration

Source: National Statistical Offices, Eurostat. Sex Imbalances at Birth: Current Trends, consequences and policy implications. UNFPA Asia and the Pacific Regional Office. 2012. http://www.unfpa.org/public/home/publications/pid/12405
*Provisional data.

that 1.5 million girls are missing at birth every year. A shortage of girls does not lead to an increase in their status as individuals even if it does increase their value as a commodity. Rather, girl shortage often contributes to greater family control and more restrictions on girls' movement and behavior, as well as increases in female trafficking and early and forced marriages.[131]

Three factors influence sex selection before birth: son preference, sex selection technology, and low fertility levels. Son preference is the key determinant because many countries have low fertility and access to sex selection technology but do not experience these extreme sex imbalances.[132] Son preference is so strongly rooted in some cultures that it is not influenced by increased income, education, or urbanization. This suggests that regulating access to ultrasound and other sex determination technology will not decrease sex selection and may adversely affect access to important medical interventions during pregnancy. It has been suggested that addressing sex selection requires the same approach used for FGM—involving a broad range of actors in a concerted effort working at many levels of action.[130] This approach should also address the factors that lead to further loss of girls after birth including infanticide and neglect.

Female Genital Mutilation

FGM, as defined by the WHO, "comprises all procedures involving partial or total removal of the external female genitalia or other injury to the female genital organs for non-medical reasons. It is mostly performed on girls less than 15 years, but this varies from one community to another. It has no health benefits and harms girls and women in many ways. It involves removing and damaging healthy and normal female genital tissue, and hence interferes with the natural function of girls' and women's bodies."[133] Amnesty International backed by the UN defined FGM as a human rights violation.[134] On December 20, 2012, the UN General Assembly unanimously passed a resolution banning the practice of FGM. This was widely hailed as a first step toward the cultural and attitudinal changes required to eliminate this practice.[135] FGM affects 100 to 140 million women and girls, and every year 3 million more girls are at risk.

FGM is sometimes referred to as female circumcision (FC). The term FC was widely used for many years to describe the practice; however, it has been largely abandoned because it implies equivalence with male circumcision. In contrast to male circumcision, which is seen as affirming manhood according to many religious and health regulations, FC is often used to limit premarital sexual activities. In the mid-1990s, many local practicing communities and activists decided to shift to the use of the more neutral term, female genital cutting (FGC), because they considered FGM to be judgmental, pejorative, and not conducive to discussion or collaboration on abandonment of the practice.[136] FGM is the term most commonly used by women's rights and health advocates who wish to emphasize the damage caused by the procedure.

FGM is not based on a requirement of religious observance, although parents usually seek it for their daughters in good faith. It is directed to the social control of women's sexuality or with the preservation of virginity, as a kind of "rite of passage." The procedure reduces the sexual desire of a female, thereby helping maintain a girl's virginity prior to marriage and her fidelity subsequently. The main motivations seem to be in controlling women's sexual urges and the belief that it makes a woman more feminine.[137,138] The practice predates the founding of both Christianity and Islam. Although confined mainly to Muslims, it is also practiced by some Christian communities in Africa and among Ethiopian Jews (Falashas). The practice seems to be rooted in both African tradition and Islamic beliefs, although many Islamic countries do not practice female circumcision.[139]

In most of the countries where FGM is practiced, it is performed by traditional circumcisers, TBAs, and sometimes health care personnel. Evidence has shown that a trend of medicalization of the practice, whereby it is performed by trained health care professionals, is increasing in a number of countries such as Egypt, Kenya, and Guinea. In Egypt, for example, 77.4% of all FGMs were performed by trained health care professionals in 2008 compared with 17% in 1996, according to data from the Egypt Demographic and Health Survey.[140,141] It is likely that several factors are influencing the medicalization of the practice including cultural influence and pressure from the community, as well as physicians' desire to reduce negative health consequences from the procedure and benefit financially.[142]

Classification

In 2008, WHO/UNICEF/UNFPA reiterated the four types of female genital mutilation in their Joint Statement first developed in1997.[143]

- Type I: Clitoridectomy: partial or total removal of the clitoris and, in very rare cases, only the prepuce.
- Type II: Excision: partial or total removal of the clitoris and the labia minora, with or without excision of the labia majora.

- Type III: Infibulations: narrowing of the vaginal opening through the creation of a covering seal. The seal is formed by cutting and repositioning the inner, or outer, labia, with or without removal of the clitoris.
- Other: All other harmful procedures to the female genitalia for nonmedical purposes (e.g., pricking, piercing, incising, scraping, and cauterizing the genital area).

Prevalence and Trends

The 100 to 140 million women who have been subjected to FGM are in 27 countries in Africa as well as immigrants in Europe, Australia, Canada, New Zealand, and the United States. FGM is also practiced in some countries in Asia, especially among certain populations in India, Indonesia, and Malaysia.[144] The practice has also been reported in Western Asia, particularly in Iraq, southern Jordan, northern Saudi Arabia, and Yemen. According to UNICEF,[145] approximately 3 million girls are at risk of being mutilated/cut each year. Prevalence of FGM/C among women ages 15 to 49 varies widely (Figure 4-9), from 98% in Somalia to 1% in Uganda, and Cameroon.[146]

UNICEF reported that the prevalence of FGM in general has declined, with variations among countries.[147] Younger generations are less likely to have undergone any form of FGM than women in the older age groups, and fewer daughters are circumcised compared with mothers (Figure 4-10). In some countries, low support for FGM by mothers is correlated with higher prevalence among daughters. This is probably due to decision making about FGM being controlled by older generations, mothers-in-law, and grandmothers. Mothers may truly oppose FGM, but they might not be able to prevent it by themselves due to the complex set of beliefs and social constraints that surround the practice.

Health Consequences

There is a substantial amount of literature covering the different physical and psychosexual health complications of this harmful practice:

- Physical complications: Immediate complications can include severe pain, shock, hemorrhage, tetanus or sepsis, urine retention, open sores in the genital region, and injury to nearby genital tissue. Long-term consequences can include recurrent bladder and urinary tract infections; cysts; infertility; an increased risk of childbirth complications and newborn deaths; and, the need for later surgeries. For example, the FGM procedure that seals or narrows a vaginal opening (type III) needs to be cut open later to allow for sexual intercourse and childbirth. Sometimes it is stitched again several times, including after childbirth; hence the woman goes through repeated

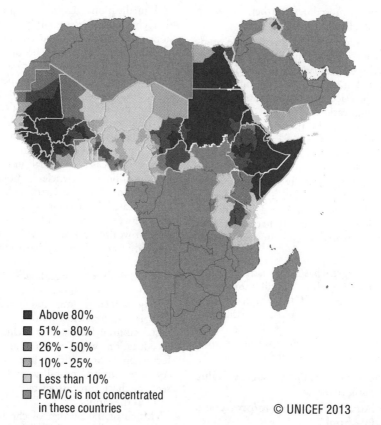

© UNICEF 2013

Figure 4-9. Percentage of girls and women aged 15-49 years who have undergone FGM/C, by regions within countries. Map not to scale. Source: United Nations Children's Fund (UNICEF). Female Genital Mutilation/Cutting: A statistical overview and exploration of the dynamics of change. UNICEF. New York, NY: 2013. (Reproduced with permission.)

Legend:
- Above 80%
- 51% - 80%
- 26% - 50%
- 10% - 25%
- Less than 10%
- FGM/C is not concentrated in these countries

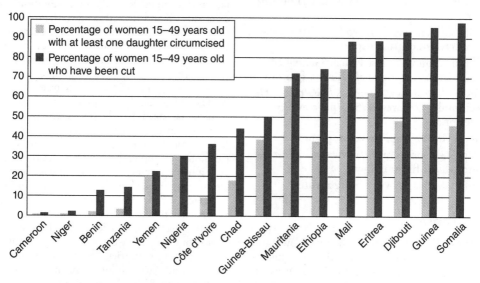

Figure 4-10. Percentage of women 15 to 49 years old who have been cut and the percentage of women 15 to 49 years old with at least one daughter circumcised, in selected countries with available data.[147]

opening and closing procedures, further increasing both immediate and long-term risks.[148–154]

- Psychosocial and sexual consequences: Some studies have shown an increased likelihood of fear of sexual intercourse, posttraumatic stress disorder, anxiety, depression, and memory loss. The cultural significance of the practice might not protect against psychological complications. The pain, shock, and the use of physical force by those performing the procedure are mentioned as reasons why many women describe female genital mutilation as a traumatic event. Removal of, or damage to highly sensitive genital tissue, especially the clitoris, may affect sexual sensitivity and lead to sexual problems, such as decreased sexual pleasure and pain during sex. Scar formation, pain, and traumatic memories associated with the procedure can also lead to such problems.[155–159]

Although much progress has been made in reducing this harmful practice, there is still more to be done to completely eliminate FGM. The recent UN Resolution to ban the practice may lend further support to advocacy and policy initiatives.

Suggested sites of advocacy groups and international nongovernmental organizations:

1. WHO: **http://www.who.int/reproductivehealth/publications/fgm/en/**
2. UNICEF: **http://www.unicef.org/protection/57929_58002.html**
3. UNDP: **http://www.undp.org/content/undp/en/home/ourwork/womenempowerment/overview.html**
4. Equality Now: **http://www.equalitynow.org/fgm**
5. FGM Education and Networking: **http://www.fgmnetwork.org/index.php**
6. Global Alliance Against Female Genital Mutilation: **http://www.global-alliance-fgm.org/**
7. Tostan: **http://www.tostan.org/web/page/586/sectionid/547/parentid/585/pagelevel/3/interior.asp**
8. Stop FGM/C: **http://www.stopfgmc.org/**
9. Stop FGM now: **http://www.stop-fgm-now.com/who-is-fighting-fgm**
10. End FGM: **http://www.endfgm.eu/en/**

Chronic Diseases

The burden of chronic diseases is rapidly growing in most low- and middle-income countries. The underlying causes are high levels of poverty, social exclusion, adverse living conditions, increased exposure to health risks, and limited access to quality health care and medications. Despite common misconceptions that chronic diseases mainly affect old people, millions of young adults and children of both sexes are vulnerable to developing chronic diseases early in life. These result in long-term preventable complications and early death compared with people in high-income countries. About 25% of global deaths from chronic diseases occur before the age of 60. Of the estimated 57 million deaths in 2008, almost two thirds—36 million—were attributed to chronic diseases.[160] This figure is double the number of deaths due to infectious diseases, maternal and perinatal conditions, and nutritional deficiencies combined. Currently, 80% of the mortality associated with chronic diseases is concentrated in developing countries. The relationship between poverty and chronic diseases is also evident in wealthy countries, where social inequalities in morbidity and mortality have increased over the last decades.[161]

Chronic diseases, including obesity, currently account for an excessive burden of morbidity and mortality among women in low- and middle-income countries. This is due to socioeconomic disparities and gender-based cultural factors that include inequitable access to education, work, income, and health care. Other factors are poor nutrition, low control over household resources, limited mobility, and delayed decisions to seek medical care associated with their care giving roles in the family.[160,161]

Much of the burden of chronic diseases faced by women could be prevented by addressing six critical risk factors: high blood pressure, high blood glucose, physical inactivity, tobacco use, overweight and obesity, and high blood cholesterol. In 2004, these six risk factors accounted for 63% of deaths from cardiovascular disease and diabetes, more than 75% of deaths from ischemic heart disease, and a substantial number of deaths from several types of cancer and chronic respiratory diseases (see Table 4-8). Most deaths attributed to chronic diseases occur at older ages, but most of the exposure to risk factors begins earlier in life.[162]

The high burden of chronic diseases affecting women has been largely neglected, despite the fact that women are exposed to more of the risk factors for chronic diseases than men.[163] Cardiovascular diseases, for example, have been traditionally considered a male problem, and women have been excluded from most clinical trials to develop new treatment approaches. However, coronary heart disease (CHD) is currently the leading cause of death among women in most wealthy countries and is becoming a major health problem for women in an increasing number of developing countries.[164] Global estimates indicate that around 3.6 million women died from CHD in 2005, and 80% of these deaths were in low- and middle-income countries.[165]

Table 4-8. Deaths in women ages 20 years and older attributable to six leading risk factors for chronic diseases, 2004.

Risk	World	Low-income countries	Middle-income countries	High-income countries
% of Deaths				
High blood pressure	18	13	22	19
High blood glucose	8	8	8	7
Physical inactivity	8	6	8	8
Tobacco use	7	2	8	14
Overweight and obesity	7	4	9	9
High cholesterol	6	5	6	6

Source: World Health Organization. *Women and Health: Today's Evidence Tomorrow's Agenda.* Geneva: WHO, 2009. http://www.who.int/gender/documents/9789241563857/en/index.html

It is clear that chronic diseases and their effects on women should receive more attention. An analysis of data from nine countries—Argentina, Chile, Colombia, Ecuador, Mexico, Peru, South Africa, China, and India—found that, except for India and South Africa, three chronic diseases (cardiovascular disease, cancer, and diabetes) accounted for more than 20% of overall deaths for women age 15 to 34 years; maternal causes and HIV/AIDS accounted for around 10%. Among older women, ages 35 to 44 years in all countries but India, chronic diseases accounted for over four times the deaths caused by reproductive conditions and HIV/AIDS. In light of these results and other relevant evidence on the increasing rates of chronic diseases among women, the authors of this study called for expanding the concept of women's health beyond the traditional focus on reproductive health.[163]

Reproductive Cancers

Breast Cancer

Breast cancer is the most common cancer in women worldwide. Despite misconceptions that breast cancer is mostly a problem of industrialized countries, currently it accounts for an increasing proportion of cancer-related morbidity and mortality in all developing regions. According to the most recent global estimates[166]:

- More than 1 million new cases occur each year worldwide; 1.38 million new cases were diagnosed in 2008, representing 23% of all cancers.
- The incidence is almost equal in both developed and developing regions—with around 690,000 new cases for each—but rates vary from 19.3 per 100,000 women in East Africa to 89.7 per 100,000 women in Western Europe.
- Breast cancer accounted for 458,000 deaths in 2008; of these deaths, 269,000—more than 50%—occurred in low- and middle-income countries.

- Breast cancer survival is directly related to country income levels, with estimated 80% survival in high-income countries, 60% in middle-income, and 40% in low-income countries.[167]

The causes for an increase in the global incidence of breast cancer are unknown, although many cases are associated with genetic factors and individual susceptibility.[168] Evidence has shown that the risks for developing breast cancer include long menstrual history, with early menarche and late menopause; never having children, or having one's first child after age 30; being overweight or obese; use of postmenopausal hormone therapy, in particular combined estrogen and progestin therapy; low physical activity; and alcohol consumption. Among these factors, those related to reproduction have been primarily associated with the higher rates of postmenopausal breast cancer among women in developed regions.[169] Recent global estimates show that a large proportion of cases in low- and middle-income countries are in premenopausal women. One example is Latin America and the Caribbean, where half of all new cases and 40% of deaths occur among women younger than 54 years.[168] In addition, overweight and obesity, along with reproductive factors, have also been suggested as relevant risk factors for breast cancer among postmenopausal women in some developing countries such as Brazil[170] and Mexico.[171]

Breast cancer has not been recognized as a priority of health policies in low- and middle-income countries, and most women are diagnosed when the disease is advanced. Early detection includes breast self-examination, clinical breast examination, and screening mammography. Breast self-examination has not been proven effective in reducing mortality rates, and both clinical breast examination and screening mammography require well-trained personnel and expensive technology that puts them out of reach for most women in developing countries. Treatment for breast cancer is always expensive, especially when the disease is detected at advanced stages. Breast cancer rates have continued to increase all over the world, but survival rates have also increased in places where women have access to mammography and early quality treatment.[167,168,172,173]

Cervical Cancer

Cervical cancer is the third most common cancer in women worldwide—after lung and breast cancer—and the first or second most common cancer among women in developing countries. Cervical cancer is associated with poverty and lack of access to quality reproductive health services. Disparities in the burden of cervical cancer persist in some developed countries where women of the lower income groups are disproportionately affected.[174] The last estimates from the International Agency for Research on Cancer (2008) show the following:[166]

- More than half a million new cases occur each year, 530,232 in 2008. More than 85% of cervical cancer is in developing countries, where it accounts for 13% of all female cancers.
- Cervical cancer accounted for 275,000 deaths in 2008.
- Each year more than 88% of the total deaths occur in developing countries; by 2030, this proportion will reach 98%.
- The regions with the highest rates of deaths from cervical cancer are eastern, western, middle, and southern Africa, south central Asia, Latin America, and the Caribbean.

Human papillomavirus (HPV), a widely disseminated sexually transmitted virus, is the underlying cause of cervical cancer. The 13 most common oncogenic types of HPV account for 98% of all new cases of cervical cancers worldwide, of which types 16 and 18 are the most prevalent. Most HPV infections are short term and resolve spontaneously, but chronic infection may lead to precancerous lesions. The slow progress from infection to invasive cancer—10 to 20 years—allows for the detection of cervical cancer at early stages, and survival rates are high in places where women have access to screening and prompt quality treatment.[174–176] HPV infection seems necessary for cervical cancer to develop, but additional factors are also associated with progression of precancerous lesions to invasive cancer. These include early start of sexual activity, older age, long-term use of oral contraceptives, high parity, tobacco smoking, multiple sexual partners, and HIV infection. Other factors that may increase the risk for cervical cancer are previous infections with *Chlamydia trachomatis* and herpesvirus type 2.[175]

Cervical cancer is one of the most preventable and treatable cancers, but it has not been a priority for public health policies. The chance for a woman to survive depends greatly on the stage at which her diagnosis occurs. Treatment is usually quick and effective at the earliest stages of the disease, but in more advanced stages it is always expensive and mostly unobtainable for women in developing countries. Therefore, early diagnosis and treatment are crucial to give women greater chances for recovery and survival.[173,174,177]

Cytology-based screening programs using the Papanicolaou test—the Pap smear—have been highly effective in industrialized countries, but in most developing countries these programs have been ineffective due to the high costs associated with providing wide coverage and the technologies needed to assure quality screening standards.[174,176–178]

Extensive evidence suggests that the morbidity and mortality from cervical cancer could be substantially reduced in low-resource settings by using simpler and cost-effective options for early screening and treatment. Options for screening include visual inspection with acetic acid or Lugol (known as VIA or VILI) followed immediately by cryotherapy for treating precancerous lesions. Early treatment with cryotherapy has been proven to be safe and effective, resulting in success rates of at least 85%. A great advantage of these options is that screening and treatment can be performed in a single visit at primary-level clinics by both skilled physicians and midlevel providers including nurses and midwives. The *single-visit approach* is especially appropriate for low-resource settings because women often face difficulties getting to clinics and to additional visits.[176,177,179]

Many studies have concluded that HPV DNA testing alone will eventually become the best option for screening women over age 30 for cervical cancer. An effective, portable, and low-cost technology for screening HPV DNA, the *care*HPV, has been tested for its use in low-resource settings and will become available in the coming years. In the meantime, visual inspection, especially VIA, can be used as a highly effective method to reduce the incidence of cervical cancer until low-cost HPV DNA testing becomes affordable.[176,177]

Recently introduced HPV vaccines are a safe and effective means of preventing cervical cancer when given to girls age 9 to 13 before they initiate sexual activity. Available vaccines have proven highly effective in preventing infection from HPV types 16 and 18 that account for more than 70% of all cervical cancers.[175,180,181] HPV vaccines, however, have been a matter of intense debate. Implementation of these vaccines for vulnerable populations in developing countries faces multiple barriers such as high cost, poor delivery infrastructure, and limited and inequitable coverage and access. Public information about these vaccines is focused on girls and cervical cancer, suggesting that HPV infection is only a women's issue and ignores the fact that these vaccines can also be useful to prevent other cancers. In fact, HPV infections affect heterosexual women and men as well as lesbian, gay, bisexual, and transgender people and may cause other types of cancers including in the vulva, throat, anus, and penis. Additionally, HPV types 6 and 11 cause genital warts that are nonlethal but painful and difficult to treat. One of the available vaccines is effective against these viruses.[182],* Recent recommendations from the Centers for Disease Control and Prevention include vaccination for boys for their own protection as well as for their future sexual partners.[183]

It must be remembered that HPV vaccines cannot replace screening. The WHO and other global agencies recommend that countries improve the quality and coverage of the screening programs for women older than 30 years, the most vulnerable to develop cervical cancer, even when a vaccination program is in place. Finally, available vaccines only protect against HPV types 16 and 18, so early screening for cervical cancer caused by other oncogenic types of HPV must continue.[175]

Aging Women

The WHO has stated that between 2000 and 2050, the proportion of the world's population over 60 years will double from about 11% to 22%, with the absolute number increasing from 605 million to 2 billion. On average, women live 6 to 8 years longer than men.[184] As they age, women and men share basic needs and concerns related to the enjoyment of human rights: shelter, food, access to health services, dignity, independence, and freedom from abuse. The evidence shows, however, that when judged in terms of the likelihood of being poor, vulnerable, and lacking in access to affordable health care, older women merit special attention. Approximately 80% of chronic disease deaths occur in middle- and low-income countries, where most of the world's aging women live. Although women do not experience more mental illness than men, they are more prone to certain types of disorders including depression and anxiety. The onset of depression in the later years of

life may be related to psychosocial factors (such as socioeconomic status) and stressful life events (such as bereavement and caring for chronically ill family members and friends).

Like aging men, women can remain sexually active until the end of life, but they may have fewer opportunities because most outlive their partners. Many STIs are physically transmitted more efficiently at all ages from males to females than from females to males. The HIV/AIDS epidemic has had devastating economic, social, health, and psychological impacts on older women especially in sub-Saharan Africa. Older women who care for those who are ill with HIV/AIDS and then for their orphaned children are themselves at risk of infection. Studies show that older caregivers are under severe financial, physical, and emotional stress arising from financial hardships leading to an inability to pay for food, clothing, essential drugs, and basic health care. They lack information about self-protection while providing care to their infected children and grandchildren.[185]

The health of women residing in developing countries is not limited to reproductive health conditions or infectious diseases. These illnesses remain serious threats to a healthy life, but as the population ages, chronic conditions are of increasing importance. Health-related quality of life among older women living in developing countries was found to be less than men, especially in terms of physical limitations for those living in rural areas.[186–190]

Frailty in many physiologic systems is prevalent in older ages, and it is characterized by increased vulnerability to disability and mortality.[191] Deficits in anabolic hormones are theorized to contribute to aging and frailty among women.[192]

Menopause

Menopause is a normal change in a woman's life when her menstrual period stops. A woman has reached menopause when she has not had a period for at least 12 continuous months. During menopause a woman's body slowly makes less of the hormones estrogen and progesterone. This often happens between the ages of 45 and 55 years.[193] There is great variation in the experience of menopause and postmenopausal symptoms in women around the world. The variation in women's experiences of menopause indicates that different cultural groups of women have different understandings and needs during the menopausal transition.[194–200] Management plans also differ around the world. Hormone replacement therapy (HRT), also called menopausal hormone therapy, is often used to relieve these symptoms. HRT is considered an effective treatment option for menopause-related symptoms and prevention of osteoporosis in many developed countries. But HRT also has risks for increasing breast cancer and

*The two available vaccines for the primary prevention of HPV oncogenic types 16 and 18 are Gardasil or Silgard, produced by Merck and distributed since 2006, and Cervarix, produced by GlaxoSmithKline and distributed since 2007. Gardasil also protects against HPV nononcogenic types 6 and 11, which cause genital warts. In 2006, the U.S. Food and Drug Administration licensed the use of Gardasil for males ages 9 to 26.[182]

cardiovascular disease, stroke, thromboembolic disorders, gallbladder disease, and urinary incontinence.[201]

Women in developing countries are less likely to use any medications for postmenopausal symptoms; one example is Egypt where fewer than 2% of women reported medication use.[202] As concern about the risk of HRT has increased, women and their physicians in developed countries prefer to use alternative approaches such as phytoestrogens and dietary interventions to alleviate postmenopausal symptoms. These treatments avoid the risks of HRT and are low cost. Support groups have also been effective.[203–205]

Elder Maltreatment

Elder maltreatment is a single or repeated act, or lack of appropriate action, occurring within any relationship where there is an expectation of trust that causes harm or distress to an older person. This type of abuse is a violation of human rights and includes physical, sexual, psychological, and emotional violence; financial and material abuse; abandonment; neglect; and serious loss of dignity and respect. Although there is little information regarding the extent of maltreatment in elderly populations, especially in developing countries, it is estimated that 4% to 6% of elderly people in high-income countries have experienced some form of maltreatment at home. Older people are often afraid to report cases of maltreatment to family, friends, or to the authorities. Risks at the individual level include dementia and disability in the victim, a shared living situation, and caretaker mental disorders, plus alcohol and substance abuse. Older men are also at risk of abuse, but in cultures where women have inferior social status, widowed elderly women are at high risk of neglect through abandonment and property seizure. Women may also be at higher risk of more persistent and severe forms of abuse and injury.[206]

INNOVATIVE COMMUNITY-BASED APPROACHES TO MCH

Although many facility-based interventions contribute to improved women's health and MCH outcomes, this section focuses on community-based approaches with the understanding that they need to be closely linked to high-quality facility-based care. These approaches have the potential for the greatest impact on a population basis. Improved technology, supplies, proper equipment, and staff training are required for clinic- and hospital-based facilities to reduce mortality and morbidity for women and children.

Community Case Management

Community Case Management (CCM) is a major new initiative for reaching children in communities within 24 hours of the onset of illness. It focuses on the three major causes of mortality and morbidity in young children: diarrheal diseases, pneumonia, and malaria. CCM is based on the community/family level of the Integrated Management of Childhood Illnesses (IMCI) strategy, which is the foundation of most child health policy and national programs in developing countries; it has been adopted by more than 100 countries.[207] IMCI was developed by the WHO, UNICEF, and other partners in the mid-1990s to reduce under-5 mortality. It was a response to vertical disease-specific programs that separately addressed the major causes of child death. The basic principle of IMCI is to assess all of a child's health and development needs whenever they come to a first-level health facility, rather than only treating the presenting symptoms. A series of algorithms was developed to help frontline health workers follow the guidelines.[208] IMCI has three main components:

- Health system support for child health (including essential drugs and vaccines, supervision, and health information systems)
- Improving the performance of first-level facility health workers through training
- Strengthening family practices to prevent disease, ensure early treatment, and improve home care[207]

Community level IMCI (C-IMCI) evolved from this facility-based integrated approach to reducing child mortality. C-IMCI utilizes community health workers to reach larger numbers of children and newborns, especially where clinics are hard to reach. CCM treatments include antibiotics for dysentery, ORS and zinc for diarrhea, antibiotics for pneumonia, and antimalarials for malaria. Assessment and treatment protocols are based on scientific evidence.[209] CCM is provided by a broad range of frontline community health workers (CHWs) from paid full-time workers to part-time volunteers. CHWs also represent a range of requirements and skills. In some countries they must be literate (which often means they are male). The quality and extent of supervision of CHWs, linkages to health facilities, and availability of medications are critical to the success of CCM. See Box 4-2 for examples of types of CHWs in different countries.

There have many examples of programs implementing CCM, which have resulted in data about CHW retention of knowledge after training and the adequacy of treatment for malaria, pneumonia, diarrhea, and neonatal infections.[209] The significance of CCM in treating the children most in need has been acknowledged in several recent reports and studies. Several international meetings have been devoted to this approach, and the global CCM Operations Research Group (ccm.org) was formed to develop evidence. In June 2012, WHO and UNICEF issued a joint statement advocating for Integrated Community Case Management as an equity-focused strategy to improve access to essential treatment for children.[210] In November 2012, the *American Journal of Tropical Medicine and Hygiene* published a special supplement, *Evidence for the Implementation, Effects, and Impact of the Integrated Community Case Management Strategy to Treat Childhood Infection.*[211] The research presented in this supplement documented a reduction in mortality[212], the use of rapid diagnostic tests to prevent overtreatment of fever,[213] a lower cost of pneumonia treatment,[214] and a quality of treatment equivalent to health facilities[215] with a higher uptake of services.[215, 216]

The research also raised questions about the overuse of antibiotics for fever,[213] problems with medication stock outs,[217] CHW motivation and retention,[218] and limitations on what CHWs can do in terms of assessment and treatment.[219] CCM will remain a major strategy for reducing child mortality in countries with the highest rates and greatest need.

Enhancing the Role of Men in Maternal and Child Health

MCH services have traditionally focused on women and children to the exclusion of men as partners and fathers. This focus occurred because maternity care during pregnancy appropriately focuses on the health and risks of the woman, and because women are the primary caregivers for infants and children. Another reason, especially in reproductive health services, was to provide women a degree of self-determination in male-dominant societies. Although it was important to establish the importance of women's roles in their own health and that of their children, this approach ignored the role of men in families and the fact that they are often the decision makers about when, where, and what health services the family members access. These facts were recognized at the 1994 International Conference on Population and Development in Cairo in the Program of Action, and at the 1995 Conference on Women in Beijing, resulting in action plans that had sections on male responsibilities in reproductive health, parenthood, and maternal and child care. However, it took another decade for the UN secretary general to issue a report on *The Role of Men and Boys in Achieving Gender Equity.*[220] This was followed by a major WHO review of the evidence for engaging men and boys in gender-based equity for health in 2007.[221] USAID and several other partners have begun using the terminology *constructive men's engagement*, with a special focus on reproductive health.[222] Another recent report reviewed the evidence for the involvement of men and grandmothers, and found that for many MCH behaviors, grandmothers played a critical role and fathers a more distant supportive one. Awareness and incorporation of culture and family structure are critical for successful programs.[223]

In 2009, the Rio Declaration was endorsed by over 500 participants at a Global Symposium on Engaging Men and Boys. It set a broad and comprehensive advocacy agenda for reducing gender inequality.[224]

BOX 4-2. WHO ARE THE CCM WORKERS?

Strategies to deliver lifesaving interventions to poor children require local adaptation. Thus community-based providers—the CCM workers—have varying characteristics and many different titles. Many are volunteers; others receive salaries or some other form of financial compensation. Examples of CHWs who provide CCM include:

- *Agents de santé communitaire* (volunteer community health agents) in Rwanda and Senegal
- *Brigadistas* (volunteer MOH health promoters) in Nicaragua
- Female community health volunteers in Nepal
- Lady Health Workers, salaried employees of MOH in Pakistan
- Traditional healers (bonesetters, circumcisers, herbalists) in semi-pastoralist Ethiopia

- Accredited Drug Dispensing Outlet dispensers in Tanzania
- Village drug-kit managers in Mali

Usually, but not always, CCM workers are literate. Increasingly they are the lowest level of paid health worker in the national health system, such as the Health Surveillance Assistants of Malawi and the Health Extension Workers of Ethiopia.

Source: Connell RW. The Role of Men and Boys in Achieving Gender Equity. Brasilia, Brazil: United Nations, 2003.

MenEngage is one of the many organizations working to improve the health of women, children, and men through full participation of women and men. Others include MenEngage Alliance, Men as Partners, and Sonke Gender Justice Network. GBC Health is a global business alliance that has advocated working to improve family health by reaching men through the workplace.[225]

Although research on programs involving men in MCH continues to evolve, there is evidence of effectiveness in several countries. The Men in Maternity study was conducted in India and South Africa to examine the effectiveness of involving the male partners of women in their care during the antenatal and postpartum periods. These two sites offered different challenges in male participation. In India, women's husbands (and their husbands' mothers) were the key decision makers determining their access to health services. In the South African communities, women were unlikely to be married or have live-in partners, and men often had several female partners. Women were more likely to access health care independently, with little involvement by their partners. Both programs focused on involving the men in prenatal care, delivery, postnatal care, and family planning. Different levels of success were achieved, due in part to the local culture of male roles and also to the type of service integration. Both interventions provided valuable insights into incorporating men in maternity care and family planning. In Delhi, India, the clinic sites were linked to men's places of work, and men frequently accompanied their wives to initial prenatal visits; therefore, it was easier to recruit them. In KwaZulu, South Africa, there was little precedence for men's involvement in their partner's care, and their employers were not committed to the program. In India, the results showed that couples in the program group were more likely to communicate about family planning, engage in joint decision making, and continue use of family planning 6 months postpartum. This program is expanding to 34 clinics and 5 hospitals in Delhi. In KwaZulu, men have traditionally not played any role in prenatal care and delivery because of the cultural view that this activity makes them weak. Initially, involving men was also strongly opposed by health providers. In spite of these barriers, about a third of the male partners in the intervention group participated in the counseling sessions. Men felt that they learned something useful from the counseling, and women felt that the main benefit was that their partner became more helpful and supportive. Communication about STIs, sexual relations, immunization, and breastfeeding increased.[226,227] A recent study in Malawi found that involving couples in maternal health care worked better with urban and better educated families, whereas peer outreach and community mobilization was more effective in rural areas. Facility-based factors included scheduled appointments so that men did not have to devote a whole day to a maternal health visit.[228]

Other examples of involving men in MCH are the formation of Fathers' Clubs (to parallel Mothers' Clubs) at the Haitian Health Foundation in Jeremie, Haiti,[229] a study of gender and family dynamics in El Alto, Bolivia,[230] and a major National Institutes of Health study of men's sexual health in relation to women's health in Mumbai, India.[231] A review of 58 studies of men's involvement in programs focused on sexual and reproductive health, fatherhood, gender-based violence, and maternal, newborn, and child health found that the most effective programs were those that were "gender transformative"—those that address the root causes of MCH problems regardless of the topic focus. These were integrated approaches that work to transform gender roles and promote gender-equitable relationships between men and women.[221]

Home Based Life Saving Skills

Home Based Life Saving Skills (HBLSS) is a training and intervention program developed by the American College of Nurse-Midwives (ACNM) to address the needs of mothers and newborns in situations where skilled attendance at birth is not immediately available. Although the standard for maternal delivery is skilled attendance for all deliveries, the reality for much of the developing world is that women deliver at home by themselves, or with family members and TBAs. Although the goal is to improve the quality of referral facilities and upgrade the training in emergency obstetric care (EMOC) as well as to increase access to hospital and clinic delivery by skilled health professionals, this will take years to achieve in many countries. HBLSS is a community-based approach to complement EMOC, also called essential lifesaving skills (LSS) at the facility level. It was designed to provide education, motivation, and mobilization of pregnant women, families, and communities. It is a community- and competency-based program focused on reducing maternal and newborn mortality by increasing access to basic lifesaving skills in the home and community and to decrease delays in reaching facility-based care in an emergency.

The concept for this program emerged in the mid-1990s and was developed by ACNM staff and consultants with extensive field experience in developing countries. They worked for several years to create the materials and conduct baseline studies. The materials were pretested in India and Ethiopia in 2001 and are currently in use in many high-mortality countries, including Afghanistan, Haiti, Liberia, Guatemala, Pakistan, Bangladesh, Kenya, and Zambia. A second edition of HBLSS was published in 2010. The revised edition modules can be downloaded from http://www.midwife.org/Home-Based-Life-Saving-Skills-HBLSS.

HBLSS consists of 12 topic modules organized into three domains: core topics (introduction, mother and baby problems, preventing problems and referral), maternal problems (too much bleeding, birth delay, sickness and pain with fever, pregnancy swelling and fits, too many children), and newborn problems (trouble breathing at birth, born too small, baby is sick). The program is based on a Training of Trainers model, with selection of TBAs and other health providers who work through all the modules with ACNM-certified trainers and then practice by teaching the modules to others in the community with ACNM supervision. The initial emphasis of training was on the birth team at the home level: mother, family members, and TBA. The continued expansion of HBLSS implementation has resulted in some other models, such as community-level training of the population through mothers' groups and other representative groups, as well as community health workers and TBAs. Each module uses a stepwise process of problem identification, problem solving, negotiation, and practice and incorporates a respectful discussion of existing community practices and how to apply new strategies. The modules are accompanied by pictorial "Take Action" cards for the steps appropriate to each problem. The materials are well suited to communities with low literacy and include a pregnancy and birth tracking system that can be completed by TBAs or other community residents.

Preliminary research in Ethiopia demonstrated improved management of postpartum hemorrhage but less impact on the management of newborn infections. This approach is being implemented in several countries, and further research will enhance understanding of the program operation and outcomes in other field sites.[232,233] Community health worker knowledge retention of HBLSS was demonstrated in an evaluation in Bangladesh, where there was actually an increase in knowledge a year after training (from 77.8% to 97.7%).[234] A USAID Child Survival project at the Haitian Health Foundation found that HBLSS was a highly effective community mobilization method, raising awareness of danger signs, supporting village-level emergency evacuation committees, and supervision of TBA deliveries by community members to ensure the safety of mothers and newborns.[235] Data from a cluster-randomized controlled trial at seven sites in six countries (Argentina, Guatemala, India, Kenya, Pakistan, Zambia) through the Global Network for Women's and Children's Health is being analyzed and will provide outcome measures for three interventions: community mobilization, home-based lifesaving skills for communities and birth attendants, and facility-based provider training.[236]

Helping Babies Breathe and Kangaroo Mother Care

Birth asphyxia is a major cause of newborn death. Helping Babies Breathe (HBB) was designed to address this problem in low-resource settings. It is an initiative of the American Academy of Pediatrics (AAP) in collaboration with the WHO, USAID, Saving Newborn Lives, the National Institute of Child Health and Development, and other global health organizations. HBB is an evidence-based curriculum that is being used at hospitals, clinics, and with home-based birth attendants.[237]

Much like HBLSS, the goal is to have all women deliver with skilled birth attendants but addresses the reality that this is not always possible. It utilizes pictorial educational materials and has easily adaptable messages. The key messages are that all newborns need to be kept clean and warm, mothers should be encouraged to breastfeed, and that an infant who does not breathe within the first minute after delivery needs extra help. The extra help comes by clearing the airway and using bag-mask ventilation to stimulate breathing. The HBB curriculum is hands on, utilizing a special manikin and the actual suction device. The decision-making chart is also a key element (Figure 4-11) for training and implementation. It focuses on the "golden minute" within which interventions should begin.

Kangaroo mother care (KMC) is care of preterm infants carried skin to skin with the mother to prevent hypothermia (low body temperature and poor temperature regulation), promote breastfeeding, mother-infant bonding, and infant health.[238] Preterm and LBW infants are at a greater risk for hypothermia, malnutrition, and infection. Health consequences of hypothermia include hypoxia, cardiorespiratory complications, and acidosis. These can progress to neurologic complications, hyperbilirubinemia, clotting disorders, and death.[239]

In developed countries, the infant is placed in an incubator in the hospital nursery, and, although this approach is effective, it has been criticized for disrupting mother-infant attachment. The kangaroo care method was first developed in a hospital in Bogota, Colombia, in 1979, primarily because the hospital had limited resources and a high mortality rate for premature infants. This approach demonstrated reduced mortality and morbidity.[240] Since the early 1980s, research and implementation of this approach has demonstrated its effectiveness in thermal control, breastfeeding, and bonding for all newborns.[241] Two recent meta-analyses have demonstrated lower mortality for KMC in hospital settings after LBW infants have been stabilized. Lawn et al found a 51% reduction in mortality and a significant reduction

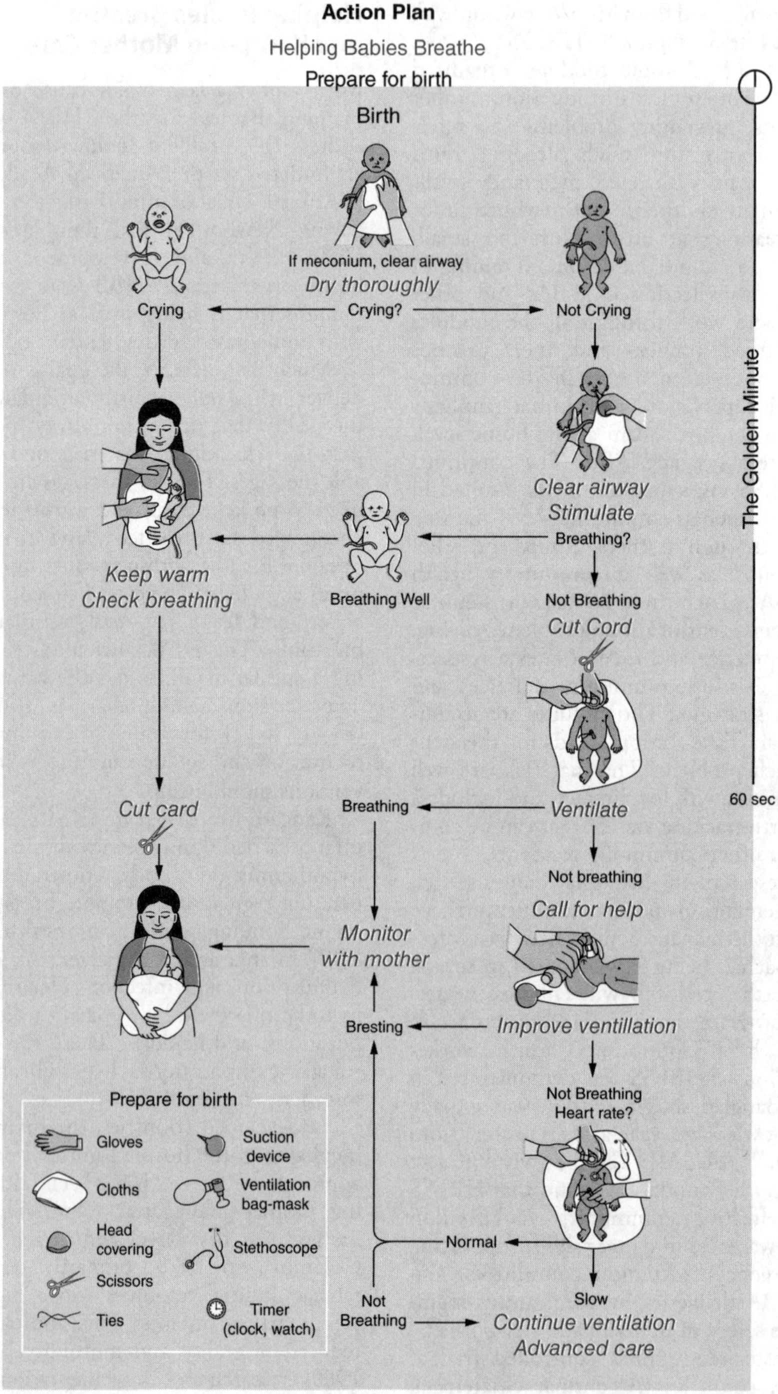

Action Plan

Helping Babies Breathe

Prepare for birth

Figure 4-11. Helping Babies Breathe Action Plan. (*Reproduced with permission from Little GA, Keenan WJ, Niermeyer S, Singhal N, Lawn JE. Neonatal nursing and helping babies breathe: an effective intervention to decrease global neonatal mortality. Newborn Infant Nurs Rev 2011;11(2):82–87.*)

in serious morbidity for infants born less than 2000 grams.[242] A 2011 revision of a 2003 Cochrane Review that found no evidence of KMC's reduction in mortality did find a significant reduction in both mortality and morbidity as well as an increase in some indicators of infant growth, breastfeeding, and mother-infant attachment.[243]

In developing countries, KMC has been implemented by trained community health workers in home settings. For some infants this provides adequate treatment; for those at higher risk, it can be used to stabilize them until they can be transferred to a hospital. Kangaroo mother care has also been expanded from "mother care" to include fathers and grandmothers. Unfortunately there have been few randomized controlled studies of KMC initiation in community settings. One trial in Bangladesh did demonstrate a substantial reduction in mortality for LBW infants.[244] Further study of community KMC is required as it continues to be used in many countries.

CONCLUSION

The health outcomes for mothers and children continue to be poor in many parts of the world. The interconnectedness of MCH with women's roles, education, and poverty makes single-focus disease or health promotion initiatives of limited value. The inclusion of maternal and child mortality as the focus of two MDGs, as well as the integration of MCH into the goals of reducing poverty, increasing access to primary education, and improving nutrition is a first step. The MDGs provide evidence that a holistic approach to MCH is critical for global health and development.

Maternal mortality and morbidity and maternal health services pertain to all aspects of women's health related to her role as a mother including pregnancy and after delivery, breastfeeding, and child care. Child health services have primarily focused on infants and children younger than 5, although there is increasing awareness of the health needs of neonates, older children, and adolescents. The emphasis on women as mothers is a strength because it helps to focus primary health care services on improving the quality of life of the next generation as well as saving the lives of women in their reproductive roles. However, it can be criticized for neglecting the health of women in roles other than that of a mother. The emphasis on women as baby carriers and baby/child caregivers results in a lack of attention to other important health issues of women including preconceptual health, infectious diseases other than STIs or those that might have an effect on the child, violence against women, and health of women past the age of childbearing. Because many of the determinants of a pregnant woman's health begin well before childbearing, attention to the nutrition, education, development, and treatment of illnesses of girls must become a priority for MCH in addition to the traditional services.

The health and well-being of women and children also depends on the involvement of families and communities. The inclusion of men in MCH is often neglected; however, their role as decision makers often supersedes that of women. The challenge is how to involve men in MCH without undermining the goal of gender equity. Community-based interventions provide the opportunity for a gender-inclusive participatory approach.

STUDY QUESTIONS

1. Why is it difficult to reduce maternal mortality in low-income countries?

2. How do maternal factors influence child health?

3. What are the determinants of marriage at an early age? What are the consequences?

4. How can men be more effectively engaged in MCH?

5. Describe and discuss several low-cost interventions that reduce maternal and child mortality. Focus on sustainability as well as impact.

REFERENCES

1. United Nations. *The Millennium Development Goals Report 2012.* New York: The United Nations, 2012.

2. World Health Organization. *Trends in Maternal Mortality: 1990 to 2010.* Geneva: WHO, 2012.

3. World Health Organization. *Maternal Mortality in 2000: Estimates Developed by WHO, UNICEF, UNFPA.* Geneva: WHO, 2004

4. The World Bank. *Level & Trends in Child Mortality.* Report 2011.http://data.worldbank.org/indicator/SP.DYN.IMRT.IN

5. United Nations Statistics Division. *Infant Mortality Rate per 1000 Live Births.* (UN Pop. Div. quinquennial estimates and projections) [code 13620].http://unstats.un.org/unsd/demographic/sconcerns/mortality/mort2.htm

6. World Health Organization. *The Sisterhood Method for Estimating Maternal Mortality: Guidance Notes for Potential Users.* Geneva: WHO, 1997. WHO/RHT/97.28.

7. International Conference on Primary Health Care. Declaration of Alma-Ata. Paper presented at: International Conference on Primary Health Care; September 6–12, 1978; Alma-Ata, USSR. http://www.who.int/publications/almaata_declaration_en.pdf.

8. Singh S, Samara R.Early marriage among women in developing countries. *Int Fam Plann Perspect* 1996;22:148–157,175.

9. United Nations Population Fund. *Marrying too Young: End Child Marriage.*New York: UNFPA, 2012.

10. Child Marriage Fact Sheet. http://www.unfpa.org/swp/2005/presskit/factsheets/facts_child_marriage.htm;http://www.unfpa.org/public/site/global/search-results?q=child%20marriage.

11. IPPF and the Forum on the Marriage and the Rights of Women and Girls. *Ending Child Marriage: A Guide for Policy Action*. London: IPPF, 2006.

12. Guidelines on Women's Empowerment. http://www.un.org/popin/unfpa/taskforce/guide/iatfwemp.gdl.html.

13. http://www.undp.org/content/undp/en/home/ourwork/womenempowerment/overview.html.

14. International Conference on Population and Development (1994) Program of Action, paragraph 4.2. http://www.unfpa.org/public/icpd/.

15. Hogan MC, Foreman KJ, Naghavi M, et al. Maternal mortality for 181 countries, 1980–2008: a systematic analysis of progress towards Millennium Development Goal 5. *Lancet* 2010;375(9726):1609–1623.

16. Karlsen S, Say L, Souza JP, et al. The relationship between maternal education and mortality among women giving birth in health care institutions: analysis of the cross sectional WHO global survey on maternal and perinatal health. *BMC Public Health* 2011;11(1):606.

17. Ehrhardt AA, Sawires S, McGovern T, Peacock D, Weston, M. Gender, empowerment, and health: what is it? How does it work? *J Acquir Immune Defic Syndr* 2009;51(Suppl 3): S96–S105.

18. World Health Organization. *Global HIV/AIDS Response: Epidemic Update and Health Sector Progress toward Universal Access*. Geneva: WHO, 2011.

19. Education Counts: Towards the Millennium Development Goals. Paris: UNESCO, 2010. http://unesdoc.unesco.org/images/0019/001902/190214e.pdf.

20. Promoting Gender Equality. Empowering Women through Education. UNFPA. http://www.unfpa.org/gender/empowerment2.htm.

21. Dalal K, Shabnam J, Andrews-Chavez J, Mårtensson LB, Timpka T. Economic empowerment of women and utilization of maternal delivery care in Bangladesh. *IntJ Prevent Med* 2012;3(9):628–636.

22. Do M, Kurimoto N. Women's empowerment and choice of contraceptive methods in selected African countries. *Int Perspect Sex Reprod Health* 2012;38(1):23–33.

23. Rapp D, Zoch B, Khan MMH, Pollmann T, Krämer A. Association between gap in spousal education and domestic violence in India and Bangladesh. *BMC Public Health* 2012; 12:467.

24. Refaat A, Simister J. Effects of Education on Gender-Based Violence in Egypt. Presented at APHA 137 Annual Meeting & Exposition; November 2009; Philadelphia, PA.

25. Valkonen T, Sihvonen AP, Lahelma E. Health expectancy by level of education in Finland. *Soc Sci Med* 1997;44(6):801–808.

26. United Nations Population Fund. Summary of the ICPD programme of action. March 1995. http://www.unfpa.org/public/home/publications/pid/1973.

27. Singh S, Darroch JE. *Adding It Up: Costs and Benefits of Contraceptive Services. Estimates for 2012*. New York: Guttmacher Institute/United Nations Population Fund, 2012.

28. World Health Organization. *Measuring Access to Reproductive Health Services: Report of WHO/UNFPA Technical Consultation 2–3 December 2003*. Geneva: WHO, 2005. WHO/RHR/04.11.

29. Ross JA, Winfrey W. Unmet need for contraception in the developing world and former Soviet Union: an updated estimate. *Int Fam Plann Perspect* 2002;28(3):138–143.

30. Casterline JB, Sinding SW. Unmet need for family planning in developing countries and implications for population policy. *Popul Develop Rev* 2000;26(4):691–723.

31. United Nations Population Fund. *Reproductive health: a measure of equity. In: United Nations Population Fund. State of World Population 2005. The Promise of Equality: Gender Equity, Reproductive Health, and the Millennium Development Goals*. New York: UNFPA, 2005.

32. World Health Organization. *Report of a WHO technical consultation on birth spacing*. Geneva: WHO, 2006.

33. Rawlings JS, Rawlings VB, Read JA. Prevalence of low birth weight and preterm delivery in relation to the interval between pregnancies among white and black women. *N Engl J Med* 1995;332(2):69–74.

34. World Health Organization. *The World Health Report 2002: Reducing risks, promoting healthy life*. Geneva: WHO, 2002.

35. Yip R, Lynch S. *Iron Deficiency Anemia Technical Consultation*. New York: UNICEF, October 1998.

36. International Nutritional Anemia Consultative Group (INACG). *Integrating programs to move iron deficiency and anemia control forward. Report of the 2003 International Nutritional Anemia Consultative Group Symposium, 6 February 2003, Marrakech, Morocco*. Washington, DC: ILSI Press, 2003. http://www.ilsi.org/researchfoundation/publications/inacgfinal.pdf.

37. De Benoist B, McLean E, Egli I, Cogswell M. *Worldwide Prevalence of Anaemia 1993–2005. Who Global Database on Anaemia*. Geneva: WHO, 2008.

38. Scholl TO, Hediger ML. Anemia and iron-deficiency anemia: compilation of data on pregnancy outcome. *Am J Clin Nutr* 1994;59 (Suppl): 492s–501s.

39. Tolentino K, Friedman JF. An update on anemia in less developed countries. *Am J Trop Med Hyg* 2007;77(1):44–51.

40. Black RE, Allen LH, Bhutta ZA, et al. Maternal and child undernutrition: global and regional exposures and health consequences. *Lancet* 2008;371:243–260.

41. World Health Organization. *World Health Report*. Geneva: WHO, 2005. http://www.who.int/whr/2005/en/index.html.

42. World Health Organization, UNICEF and UNU. *Iron Deficiency Anaemia: Assessment, Prevention and Control. A Guide for Programme Managers*. Geneva: WHO, 2001.

43. World Health Organization. *Nutrition for Health and Development: A Global Agenda for Combating Malnutrition*. Geneva: WHO, 2000.

44. Dowswell T. Carroli G, Duley L, et al. Alternative versus standard packages of antenatal care for low-risk pregnancy. *Cochrane Database Syst Rev* 2010:CD000934.

45. Antenatal care. ChildInfo, UNICEF, 2012. http://www.childinfo.org/antenatal_care.html.

46. Maternal Health. Women Deliver. http://www.womendeliver.org/knowledge-center/facts-figures/maternal-health/.

47. Bergström S, Goodburn E. The role of traditional birth attendants in the reduction of maternal mortality. In: De Brouwere V, Van Lerberghe W, eds. *Safe Motherhood Strategies: A Review of the Evidence*. Antwerp: ITG Press, 2001.

48. Ray AM, Salihu HM. The impact of maternal mortality interventions using traditional birth attendants and village midwives. *J Obstet Gynaecol* 2004;24(1):5–11.

49. Garces A, McClure EM, Chomba E, et al. Home birth attendants in low income countries: who are they and what do they do? *BMC Pregnancy Childbirth* 2012(12);34.

50. Graham W, Bell JS, Bullough CHW, et al. Can skilled attendance at delivery reduce maternal mortality in developing countries? In: De Brouwere V, Van Lerberghe W, eds. *Safe Motherhood Strategies: A Review of the Evidence.* Antwerp: ITG Press, 2001.

51. Lawn JE, Kinney M, Lee AC, et al. Reducing intrapartum-related deaths and disability: can the health system deliver? *Int J Gynaecol Obstet* 2009;107(Suppl 1): S123–S140, S140–S142.

52. World Health Organization. *The Partnership for Maternal, Newborn and Child Health, Opportunities for Africa's Newborns.* Geneva: WHO, 2006.

53. World Health Organization. *Technical Consultation on "Guidelines for Monitoring the Availability and Use of Obstetric Services."* Geneva: WHO/UNFPA/UNICEF/AMDD, 2006.

54. Liljestrand J, Martins JM, Rajapaksa LC, et al. *Investing in Maternal Health: Learning from Malaysia and Sri Lanka.* Washington, DC: The World Bank, 2003.

55. Koblinski M, ed. *Reducing Maternal Mortality: Learning from Bolivia, China, Egypt, Honduras, Indonesia, Jamaica, and Zimbabwe (Health, Nutrition, and Population Series).* Washington, DC: The World Bank, 2003.

56. Victora GVC, Aluisio JDB, Axelson H, et al. How changes in coverage affect equity in maternal and child health interventions in 35 countdown to 2015 countries: an analysis of national surveys. *Lancet* 2012;380:1149–1156.

57. UNFPA Safe Motherhood Fact Sheet 2012. http://www.unfpa.org/public/mothers.

58. Khan KS, Wojdyla D, Say L, Gülmezoglu AM,Van Look PFA. WHO analysis of causes of maternal death: a systematic review. *Lancet* 2006;367:1066–1074.

59. Barnes-Josiah D, Myntti C, Augustin A. The three delays as a framework for examining maternal mortality in Haiti. *Soc Sci Med* 1998;46(8):981–993.

60. Thaddeus S, Maine D. Too far to walk: maternal mortality in context. *Soc Sci Med* 1996;38:1091–1110.

61. Rogo KO, Oucho J, Mwalali. Chapter 16. In: Jamison DT, Feachem RG, Makgoba MW, et al., eds. *Maternal Mortality in Disease and Mortality in Sub-Saharan Africa.* 2nd ed. Washington, DC: World Bank, 2006.

62. Smith J, Currie S, Perri J, Bluestone J, Cannon T. *National Programs for the Prevention and Management of Postpartum Hemorrhage and Pre-Eclampsia/Eclampsia: A Global Survey, 2012.* Washington, DC: USAID and MCHIP, 2012.

63. World Health Organization. Management of STIs/RTIs. 2005. http://www.who.int/reproductive-health/publications/rtis_gep/infection_childbirth.htm.

64. World Health Organization. *Unsafe Abortion: Global and Regional Estimates of the Incidence of Unsafe Abortion and Associated Mortality in 2008.* 6th ed. Geneva: WHO, 2011.

65. Sedgh G, Singh S, Shah IH, Åhman E, Henshaw SK, Bankole A. Induced abortion: incidence and trends worldwide from 1995 to 2008. *Lancet* 2012;379:625–632.

66. Singh S. Hospital admissions resulting from unsafe abortion: estimates from 13 developing countries. *Lancet* 2006;368(9550): 1887–1892.

67. World Health Organization. *Maternal Mortality in 2000: Estimates Developed by WHO, UNICEF, UNFPA.* Geneva: WHO, 2004.

68. United National Population Fundand Engender Health. *Fistula Needs Assessment Report: Findings from Nine African Countries.* New York: UNFPA, 2003

69. Castro LC. Hypertensive disorders of pregnancy. In: Hacker N, Moore JG, eds. *Essentials of Obstetrics and Gynecology.* 3rd ed. Philadelphia: WB Saunders, 1998: 196–207.

70. The Eclampsia Trial Collaborative Group. Which anticonvulsant for women with eclampsia? Evidence from the collaborative eclampsia trial. *Lancet* 1995;345(8963): 1455–1463.

71. Reproductive Health Supplies Coalition. Product Brief: Magnesium Sulfate. Updated January 2012. http://www.path.org/publications/files/RHSC_ms_br.pdf.

72. The Magpie Trial Collaborative Group. Do women with pre-eclampsia, and their babies, benefit from magnesium sulphate? The Magpie Trial: a randomised placebo-controlled trial. *Lancet* 2002;359(9321):1877–1890.

73. Sheth SS, Chalmers I. Magnesium for preventing and treating eclampsia: time for international action. *Lancet* 2002; 359(9321): 1872–1873.

74. The Eclampsia Trial Collaborative Group. Which anticonvulsant for women with eclampsia? Evidence from the collaborative eclampsia trial. *Lancet* 1995;345(8963):1455–1463.

75. World Health Organization. *Department of Making Pregnancy Safer. WHO Technical Consultation on Postpartum and Postnatal Care.* Geneva: WHO, 2010.

76. USAID. Maternal and child health: technical areas. Postpartum and newborn care. 2005. http://www.usaid.gov/our_work/global_health/mch/mh/techareas/post.html.

77. Åhman E, Zupan, J. *Neonatal and perinatal mortality: country, regional and global estimates 2004.* Geneva: WHO, 2007.

78. Lawn J, Shibuya K, Stein C, Åhman E, Zupan J. *Neonatal and perinatal mortality: country, regional and global estimates 2004.* Geneva: WHO, 2007: Global estimates of intrapartum stillbirths and intrapartum-related neonatal deaths. *Bull World Health Organ* [online] 2005;83(6): 409–417. ISSN 0042-9686.

79. World Health Organization. *Neonatal and Perinatal Mortality: Country, Regional and Global Estimates.* Geneva: WHO, 2006.

80. Lawn JE, Kerber K, Enwernu-Laryea C, Cousens S. 3.6 million neonatal deaths—what is progressing and what is not? *Semin Perinatol* 2010;34(6): 371–386. http://dx.doi.org/10.1053/j.semperi.2010.09.011.

81. World Health Organization. *Early Child Development.* Geneva: WHO, 2009. http://www.who.int/mediacentre/factsheets/fs332/en/index.html.

82. Early Child Development Knowledge Network. *Early child development: a powerful equalizer.* Tech. Rep., The Early Child Development Knowledge Network of the Commission on Social Determinants of Health. Geneva: World Health Organization, 2007. http://www.who.int/social_determinants/publications/earlychilddevelopment/en/index.html

83. Walker S, Wachs T, Meeks Gardner J, et al. Child development: risk factors for adverse outcomes in developing countries. *Lancet* 2007;369:145–157.

84. World Health Organization. *Children: Reducing Mortality.* Geneva: WHO, 2012. http://www.who.int/mediacentre/factsheets/fs178/en/index.html.

85. United Nations. Millennium Development Goals Report 2011, June 2011, ISBN 978-92-1-101244-6. http://www.unhcr.org/refworld/docid/4e42118b2.html.

86. UNICEF, WHO, The World Bank, UN DESA/Population Division. *Levels and Trends in Child Mortality—Report 2012.* Geneva: UNICEF, 2012.

87. Save the Children. *A Life Free from Hunger: Tackling Child Malnutrition*. London: Save the Children, 2012.

88. World Health Organization. *Essential Antenatal, Perinatal and Postpartum Care*. Training modules. EUR/03/5035043. Geneva: WHO, 2003.

89. WHO, UNICEF, UNFPA, UNAIDS.Guidelines on HIV and Infant Feeding 2010: Principles and recommendations for infant feeding in the context of HIV and a summary of evidence. 2010. http://www.who.int/maternal_child_adolescent/documents/9789241599535/en/.

90. World Health Organization. *Initiatives for Vaccine Research. Acute Respiratory Infections*. Geneva: WHO, 2012. http://www.who.int/vaccine_research/diseases/ari/en/.

91. World Health Organization. *Pneumonia*. Geneva: WHO, 2012 http://www.who.int/mediacentre/factsheets/fs331/en/index.html.

92. World Health Organization. *Diarrheal Disease*. Geneva: WHO, 2009. http://www.who.int/mediacentre/factsheets/fs330/en/index.html.

93. UNICEF/World Health Organization. *Diarrhoea: Why Children Are Still Dying and What Can Be Done*. Geneva: UNICEF, 2009.

94. World Health Organization. *Oral Rehydration Salts: Production of the New ORS*. Geneva: WHO, 2006.

95. UNICEF. *Malaria*. Geneva: UNICEF, 2012. http://www.unicef.org/health/index_malaria.html.

96. World Health Organization. *Measles*. Geneva: WHO, 2013. http://www.who.int/mediacentre/factsheets/fs286/en/.

97. Sawyer SM, Afifi RA, Bearinger LH, et al. Adolescence: a foundation for future health. *Lancet* 2012;379:1630–1640.

98. United National Population Fund. *The state of the world population 2011*. New York: UNFPA, 2011.

99. United National Children's Fund. *Progress for children: a report card on adolescents*. New York: UNICEF, 2012.

100. World Health Organization. *Young People: Health Risks and Solutions*. Geneva: WHO, 2011. http://www.who.int/mediacentre/factsheets/fs345/en/index.html.

101. Blum RW, Nelson-Mmari K. The health of young people in a global context. *J Adolesc Health* 2004;35:402–418.

102. United Nations Children's Fund. *State of the world's children 2011: Adolescence—an age of opportunity*. New York: UNICEF, 2011.

103. World Health Organization, *Child and Adolescent Health and Development Progress Report 2009*. Geneva: WHO, 2009: Highlights, p. 16.

104. United Nations. *Violence Against Women: A Global Phenomenon*. New York: UN report, 2010. http://www.un.org/apps/news/story.asp?NewsID=36513&Cr=gender+equality&Cr1#.UNXatWdmWBo.

105. World Health Organization. *Violence Against Women: WHO Consultation*. Geneva: WHO, 1996.

106. World Health Organization. *Multi-Country Study on Women's Health and Domestic Violence Against Women: Summary Report of Initial Results on Prevalence, Health Outcomes and Women's Responses*. Geneva: WHO, 2005.

107. Garcia-Moreno C, Jansen HAFM, Ellsberg M, Heise L, Watts CH. Prevalence of intimate partner violence: findings from the WHO multi-country study on women's health and domestic violence. *Lancet* 2006; 368(9543):1260–1269.

108. Kishor S, Johnson K. *Profiling Domestic Violence—A Multi-Country Study*. Calverton, MD: ORC Macro, 2004.

109. Abramsky T, Watts CH, Garcia-Moreno C, et al. What factors are associated with recent intimate partner violence? Findings from the WHO multi-country study on women's health and domestic violence. *BMC Public Health* 2011; 11:109.

110. Centers for Disease Control and Prevention. *Understanding Intimate Partner Violence*. Atlanta: CDC, 2012. http://www.cdc.gov/ViolencePrevention/pdf/IPV_Factsheet2012-a.pdf.

111. Domestic Violence Statistics. http://domesticviolencestatistics.org/domestic-violence-statistics/.

112. Stöckl H, Heise L, Watts C. Factors associated with violence by a current partner in a nationally representative sample of German women. *Sociol Health Illness* 2011;33(5):694–709.

113. Murphy CM, Ting L. The effects of treatment for substance use problems on intimate partner violence: a review of empirical data. *Aggression Violent Behav* 2010;15(5):325–333.

114. Seifert D, Lambe A, Anders S, Pueschel K, Heinemann A. Quantitative analysis of victim demographics and injury characteristics at a metropolitan Medico-Legal Center. *Forensic Sci Int* 2009;188(1–3):46–51.

115. Chrisler JC, Ferguson S. Violence against women as a public health issue. *Ann NY Acad Sci* 2006;1087:235–249.

116. Dutton, MA, Kaltman S, Goodman LA, Weinfurt K, Vankos N. Patterns of intimate partner violence: correlates and outcomes. *Violence Victims* 2005;20(5):483–497.

117. Narula A, Agarwal G, McCarthy L. Intimate partner violence: patients' experiences and perceptions in family practice. *Family Pract* 2012;29(5):593–600.

118. Devries K, Watts C, Yoshihama M, et al. Violence against women is strongly associated with suicide attempts: evidence from the WHO multi-country study on women's health and domestic violence against women. *Soc Sci Med* 2011;73(1):79–86.

119. Makayoto LA, Omolo J, Kamweya AM, Harder VS, Mutai J. Prevalence and associated factors of intimate partner violence among pregnant women attending Kisumu District Hospital, Kenya. *Matern Child Health J* 2013;17(3):441–447.

120. Osinde MO, Kaye DK, Kakaire O. Intimate partner violence among women with HIV infection in rural Uganda: critical implications for policy and practice. *BMC Women Health* 2011;11:50.

121. Rodriguez CM, Tucker MC. Behind the cycle of violence, beyond abuse history: a brief report on the association of parental attachment to physical child abuse potential. *Violence Vict* 2011;26(2):246–256.

122. Schluter PJ, Tautolo ES, Paterson J. Experience of physical abuse in childhood and perpetration of physical punishment and violence in adulthood amongst fathers: findings from the Pacific Islands Families Study. *Pac Health Dialog* 2011;17(2):148–162.

123. Thornberry TP, Knight KE, Lovegrove PJ. Does maltreatment beget maltreatment? A systematic review of the intergenerational literature. *Trauma Violence Abuse* 2012;13(3):135–152.

124. Nelson HD, Bougatsos C, Blazina I. Screening women for intimate partner violence: a systematic review to update the U.S. Preventive Services Task Force recommendation. *Ann Intern Med* 2012;156(11):796–808.

125. Krasnoff M, Moscati R. Domestic violence screening and referral can be effective. *Ann Emerg Med* 2012;40(5):485–492.

126. Chapin JR, Coleman G, Varner E. Yes we can! Improving medical screening for intimate partner violence through self-efficacy. *J Inj Violence Res* 2011;3(1):19–23.

127. Umhau JC, Trandem K, Shah M, George DT. The physician's unique role in preventing violence: a neglected opportunity? *BMC Med* 2012;10(1):146.

128. Laisser RM, Nyström L, Lindmark G, Lugina HI, Emmelin M. Screening of women for intimate partner violence: a pilot intervention at an outpatient department in Tanzania. *Global Health Action* 2011;4:7228.

129. Undie C, Maternowska MC, Mak'anyengo M, Birungi H, Keesbury J, Askew I. *Routine Screening for Intimate Partner Violence in Public Health Care Settings in Kenya: An Assessment of Acceptability*. New York: Population Council, 2012.

130. World Health Organization. *Preventing Gender-biased Sex Selection: An Interagency Statement*. Geneva: WHO, 2011.

131. Giles K, Feldman-Jacobs C. *When Technology and Tradition Collide: From Gender Bias to Sex Selection*. Washington, DC: Population Reference Bureau, Policy Brief, September 2012.

132. Guilmoto C. *Sex Imbalances at Birth: Trends, Consequences, and Policy Implications*. Bangkok: UNFPA, 2012.

133. World Health Organization.*Female genital mutilation*. Geneva, WHO, 2013. http://www.who.int/mediacentre/factsheets/fs241/en/.

134. Amnesty International. *Fight against female genital mutilation wins UN backing*. New York: Amnesty International, 2012. http://www.amnestyusa.org/news/news-item/fight-against-female-genital-mutilation-wins-un-backing.

135. United Nations Women. *UN bans female genital mutilation*. New York: UN, 2012. http://www.unwomen.org/2012/12/united-nations-bans-female-genital-mutilation/;http://www.un.org/News/Press/docs/2012/sgsm14742.doc.htm.

136. Population Reference Bureau. Abandoning female genital cutting: prevalence, attitudes, and efforts to end the practice. http://www.prb.org/pdf/AbandoningFGC_Eng.pdf.

137. Mackie G. Female genital cutting: a harmless practice? *Med Anthropol Q* 2003;17(2):135–158.

138. El-Gibaly O, Ibrahim B, Mensch BS, Clark WH. The decline of female circumcision in Egypt: evidence and interpretation. *Soc Sci Med* 2002;54(2):205–220.

139. Wiens J. Female circumcision is curbed in Egypt. *BMJ* 1996;313(7052): 249.

140. EI-Zanaty, Way A. *Egypt Demographic and Health Survey 1995*. Calverton, MD: National Population Council [Egypt] and Macro International Inc., 1996.

141. El-Zanaty F, Way A. *Egypt Demographic and Health Survey 2008*. Cairo, Egypt: Ministry of Health, El-Zanaty and Associates, and Macro International, 2009.

142. Refaat A. Medicalization of female genital cutting in Egypt. *East Mediterr Health J* 2009;15(6):1379–1388.

143. World Health Organization. *Eliminating Female Genital Mutilation: An Interagency Statement*. Geneva: WHO, 2008. http://www.un.org/womenwatch/daw/csw/csw52/statements_missions/Interagency_Statement_on_Eliminating_FGM.pdf.

144. World Health Organization. *Female Genital Mutilation and Other Harmful Practices: Prevalence of FGM*. Geneva: WHO. http://www.who.int/reproductivehealth/topics/fgm/prevalence/en/index.html.

145. United Nations Children's Fund. *Female Genital Cutting: A Statistical Exploration*. Geneva: UNICEF, 2005. http://www.unicef.org/publications/files/FGM-C_final_10_October.pdf.

146. United Nations Children's Fund, Female Genital Mutilation/Cutting: A statistical overview and exploration of the dynamics of change, UNICEF, New York, 2013.

147. United Nations Children's Fund. *Child Info Progress*. Geneva: UNICEF, 2013. http://www.childinfo.org/fgmc_progress.html.

148. Ekenze SO, EzegwuiHU, AdiriCO. Genital lesions complicating female genital cutting in infancy: a hospital-based study in south-east Nigeria. *Ann Trop Paediatr* 2007;27(4):285–290.

149. Bjälkander O, Bangura L, Leigh B, Berggren V, Bergström S, Almroth L. Health complications of female genital mutilation in Sierra Leone. *Int J Womens Health* 2012;4:321–331.

150. Kaplan A, Hechavarría S, Martín M, Bonhoure I. Health consequences of female genital mutilation/cutting in the Gambia, evidence into action. *Reprod Health* 2011;8:26.

151. Merritt DF. Genital trauma in pre-pubertal girls and adolescents. *Curr Opin Obstet Gynecol* 2011;23(5):307–314.

152. Raouf SA, Ball T, Hughes A, Holder R, Papaioannou S. Obstetric and neonatal outcomes for women with reversed and non-reversed type III female genital mutilation. *Int J Gynaecol Obstet* 2011;113(2):141–143.

153. Hamoudi A, Shier M. Late complications of childhood female genital mutilation. *J Obstet Gynaecol Can* 2010;32(6):587–589.

154. Bishai D, Bonnenfant YT, Darwish M, et al; FGM Cost Study Group of World Health Organization. Estimating the obstetric costs of female genital mutilation in six African countries. *Bull World Health Organ* 2010;88(4):281–288.

155. El-Defrawi, Lotfy G, Dandash KF, Refaat AH, Eyada M. Female genital mutilation and its psychosexual impact *J Sex Marital Ther* 2001;27(5):465–473.

156. Shah G, Susan L, Furcroy J. Female circumcision: history, medical and psychological complications, and initiatives to eradicate this practice. *Can J Urol* 2009;16(2):4576–4579.

157. Utz-Billing I, Kentenich H. Female genital mutilation: an injury, physical and mental harm. *J Psychosom Obstet Gynaecol* 2008;29(4):225–229.

158. Alsibiani SA, Rouzi AA. Sexual function in women with female genital mutilation. *Fertil Steril* 2010;93(3):722–724.

159. Catania L, et al. Pleasure and orgasm in women with female genital mutilation/cutting (FGM/C). *J Sex Med* 2007;4(6):1666–1678.

160. World Health Organization. *Global Status Report on Noncommunicable Diseases 2010: Description of the Global Burden of NCDs, Their Risk Factors and Determinants*. Geneva: WHO, 2011.

161. World Health Organization. *Obesity and overweight*. Fact sheet N°311. Geneva: WHO, May 2012.

162. World Health Organization. *Women and Health. Today's Evidence Tomorrow's Agenda*. Geneva: WHO, 2009.

163. Raymond SU, Greenberg HM, Leeder SR. Beyond reproduction: women's health in today's developing world. *Int J Epidemiol* 2005;34:1144–1148.

164. Wenger N. You've come a long way, baby. Cardiovascular health and disease in women. Problems and prospects. *Circulation* 2004;109:558–560.

165. World Health Organization. *Preventing chronic diseases. A vital investment*. Geneva: WHO, 2005.

166. International Agency for Research on Cancer. *Breast cancer incidence, mortality and prevalence worldwide in 2008*. Lyon, France: GLOBOCAN Fast Stats, 2008. IARC/WHO. http://globocan.iarc.fr/factsheets/cancers/breast.asp.

167. Coleman MP, et al. CONCORD Working Group. Cancer survival in five continents: a worldwide population-based study (CONCORD). *Lancet Oncol* 2008;9:730–756.

168. Knaul F, Bustreo F, Ha E, Langer A. Breast cancer: why link early detection to reproductive health interventions in developing countries? *Salud Publica Mex* 2009;51(S2):S220–S227.

169. Porter PL. Global trends in breast cancer incidence and mortality. *Salud Publica Mex* 2009;51(S2):S141–S146.

170. De Vasconcelos AB, Azevedo e Silva Mendonça G, Sichieri R. Height, weight change and risk for breast cancer in Rio de Janeiro, Brazil. *Sao Paulo Med J* 2001;119(2):62–66.

171. Romieu I, Lajous M. The role of obesity, physical activity and dietary factors on the risk of breast cancer: the Mexican experience. *Salud Publica Mex* 2009;51(S2):172–180.

172. Anderson BO, Yip C, Smith RA, et al. Guideline implementation for breast healthcare in low- and middle-income countries. Overview of the Breast Health Global Initiative Global Summit 2007. *Cancer* 2008;113(S8):S2215–S2371.

173. Berer M. Reproductive cancers: high burden of disease, low level of priority. *Reprod Health Matters* 2008;16(32):4–8.

174. World Health Organization. *Comprehensive Cervical Cancer Control. A Guide to Essential Practice.* Geneva: WHO, 2006.

175. Murray M. Progress in preventing cervical cancer: updated evidence on vaccination and screening. *Outlook* 2010;27(2).

176. Alliance for Cervical Cancer Prevention. *Recent Evidence on Cervical Cancer Screening in Low-Resource Settings.* Seattle: ACCP, 2011.

177. Sherris J, Wittet S, Kleine A, et al. Evidence-based, alternative cancer screening approaches in low-resource settings. *Int Perspect Sex and Reprod Health* 2009;35(3):147–154.

178. Gakidou E, Nordhagen S, Obermeyer Z. Coverage of cervical cancer screening in 57 countries: low average levels and large inequalities. *PLoS Med* 2008;5(6):863–868.

179. Blumenthal PD, Lauterbach M, Sellors JW, Sankaranarayanan R. Training for cervical cancer prevention programs in low-resource settings: focus on visual inspection with acetic acid and cryotherapy. *Int J Gynecol Obstet* 2005;89:S30–S37.

180. Cohen S. A long and winding road: getting the HPV vaccine to women in the developing world. *Guttmacher Policy Rev* 2007;10(3):15–19.

181. World Health Organization. *Strengthening Cervical Cancer Prevention and Control.* Report of the GAVI-UNFPA-WHO meeting. Geneva: WHO, 2010.

182. Graham JE, Mishra A. Global challenges of implementing human papillomavirus vaccines. *Int J Equity Health* 2011; 10:27.

183. Centers for Disease Control. Recommendations on the use of quadrivalent human papillomavirus vaccine in males—Advisory Committee on Immunization Practices (ACIP). *MMWR Morb Mortal Wkly Rep* 2011;60(50):1705–1708.

184. World Health Organization. *Aging and Life Course. Interesting Facts About Aging.* Geneva: WHO, 2012. http://www.who.int/ageing/about/facts/en/index.html.

185. World Health Organization. *Women Aging and Health: A Framework for Action, Focus on Gender.* Geneva: WHO, 2007. http://www.who.int/ageing/publications/Women-ageing-health-lowres.pdf.

186. Duda RB, Anarfi JK, Adanu RM, Seffah J, Darko R, Hill AG. The health of the "older women" in Accra, Ghana: results of the Women's Health Study of Accra. *J Cross Cult Gerontol* 2011;26(3):299–314.

187. Aghamolaei T, Tavafian SS, Zare S. Health related quality of life in elderly people living in Bandar Abbas, Iran: a population-based study. *Acta Med Iran* 2010;48(3):185–191.

188. Gómez F, Curcio CL, Duque G. Health care for older persons in Colombia: a country profile. *J Am Geriatr Soc* 2009;57(9):1692–1696.

189. Tabloski PA. Global aging: implications for women and women's health. *J Obstet Gynecol Neonatal Nurs* 2004;33(5): 627–638.

190. Mwanyangala MA, Mayombana C, Urassa H, Charles J, Mahutanga C, Abdullah S, Nathan R. Health status and quality of life among older adults in rural Tanzania. *Global Health Action* 2010;3.

191. Szanton SL, Allen JK, Seplaki CL, Bandeen-Roche K, Fried LP. Allostatic load and frailty in the women's health and aging studies. *Biol Res Nurs* 2009;10(3):248–256.

192. Cappola AR, Xue QL, Fried LP. Multiple hormonal deficiencies in anabolic hormones are found in frail older women: the women's health and aging studies. *J Gerontol Ser A: Biol Sci Med Sci* 2009;64A(2):243–248.

193. Centers for Disease Control and Prevention. *Menopause: Women's Reproductive Health.* Atlanta: CDC, 2012. http://www.cdc.gov/reproductivehealth/WomensRH/Menopause.htm.

194. Jones EK, Jurgenson JR, Katzenellenbogen JM, Thompson SC. Menopause and the influence of culture: another gap for Indigenous Australian women? *BMC Women's Health* 2012;12(1):43.

195. Hunter MS, Gupta P, Chedraui P, et al. The International Menopause Study of Climate, Altitude, Temperature (IMS-CAT) and vasomotor symptoms. *Climacteric* 2012; September 4.

196. Aggarwal N, et al. Prevalence and related risk factors of osteoporosis in peri- and postmenopausal Indian women. *J Midlife Health* 2011;2(2):81–85.

197. Sweed HS, Elawam AD, Nabeel AM, Mortagy K. Post menopausal symptoms among Egyptian geripausal women. *East Mediterr Health J* 2012;18(3):213–220.

198. Avis, et al. Longitudinal changes in sexual functioning as women transition through menopause: results from the Study of Women's Health Across the Nation. *Menopause* 2009;16(3):442–452.

199. Ayatollahi SMT, Ghaem H, Ayatollahi SAR. Sociodemographic factors and age at natural menopause in Shiraz, Islamic Republic of Iran. *East Mediterr Health J* 2005;11(1/2):2005.

200. Loutfy I, Abdel Aziz F, Dabbous NI, Hassan MH. Women's perception and experience of menopause: a community-based study in Alexandria, Egypt. *East Mediterr Health J* 2006;12(Suppl 2): S93–S106.

201. Nelson HD, Walker M, Zakher B, Mitchell J. Menopausal hormone therapy for the primary prevention of chronic conditions: a systematic review to update the U.S. Preventive Services Task Force Recommendations. *Ann Intern Med* 2012;157:104–113.

202. Dandash, K, Abd El AllH, Refaat A. *Final Report of Women's Health Problems in Egypt Focusing on Cancer Cervix.* Cairo: National Population Council, Egypt, 2005. http://www.popcouncil.org/countries/egypt.asp.

203. Meherishi S, Khandelwal S, Swarankar ML, Kaur P. Attitudes and practices of gynecologists in Jaipur toward management of menopause. *J Midlife Health* 2010;1(2):74–78.

204. Saleh F, Afnan F, Ara F, Yasmin S, Nahar K, Khatun F, Ali L. Phytoestrogen intake and cardiovascular risk markers in Bangladeshi postmenopausal women. *Mymensingh Med J* 2011;20(2):219–225.

205. Yazdkhasti M, et al. The effect of support group method on quality of life in post-menopausal women. *Iran J Public Health* 2012;41(11):78–84.

206. World Health Organization. *Elder Maltreatment.* Geneva: WHO, 2011. http://www.who.int/mediacentre/factsheets/fs357/en/index.html.

207. Bryce J, Victora CG, Habicht JP, Black RE, Scherpbier RW. Programmatic pathways to child survival: results of a multi-country evaluation of integrated management of childhood illness. *Health Policy Plan* 2005;20(Suppl):5s–17s.

208. World Health Organization. *IMCI: Model Chapter for Textbooks.* Geneva: WHO, 2001. WHO/FCH/CAH/00.40.

209. CORE Group, Save the Children, BASICS, MCHIP. *Community Case Management Essentials: Treating Common Childhood Illnesses in the Community. A Guide for Program Managers.* Washington, DC: CORE Group, 2010.

210. WHO/UNICEF. *Integrated Community Case Management.* New York: United Nations Children's Fund, 2012.

211. Marsh DR, Hamer DH, Pagnoni F, Peterson S. Evidence for the implementation, effects, and impact of the integrated community case management strategy to treat childhood infection. *Am J Trop Med Hyg* 2012;87 (5 Suppl):2–5.

212. Chinbuah MA, Kager PA, Abbey M, et al. Impact of community management of fever (using antimalarials with or without antibiotics) on childhood mortality: a cluster-randomized controlled trial in Ghana. *Am J Trop Med Hyg* 2012;87(5 Suppl):11–20.

213. Mukanga D, Tiono AB, Anyorigiya T, et al. Integrated community case management of fever in children under five using rapid diagnostic tests and respiratory rate counting: a multi-country cluster randomized trial. *Am J Trop Med Hyg* 2012;87(5 Suppl):21–29.

214. Sadruddin S, Shehzad S, Bari A, et al. Household costs for treatment of severe pneumonia in Pakistan. *Am J Trop Med Hyg* 2012;87(5 Suppl):137–143.

215. Nsona H, Mtimuni A, Daelmans B, et al. Scaling up integrated community case management of childhood illness: update from Malawi. *Am J Trop Med Hyg* 2012;87(5 Suppl):54–60.

216. Guenther T, Sadruddin S, Chimuna T, et al. Beyond distance: an approach to measure effective access to case management for sick children in Africa. *Am J Trop Med Hyg* 2012;87 (5 Suppl):77–84.

217. Chandani Y, Noel M, Pomeroy A, Andersson S, Pahl MK, Williams T. Factors affecting availability of essential medicines among community health workers in Ethiopia, Malawi and Rwanda: solving the last mile puzzle. *Am J Trop Med Hyg* 2012;87(5 Suppl):120–126.

218. Strachan DL, Kallander K, ten Asbroek AHA, et al. Interventions to improve motivation and retention of community health workers delivering integrated community case management (iCCM): stakeholder perceptions and priorities. *Am J Trop Med Hyg* 2012;87(5 Suppl):111–119.

219. George A, Young M, Nefdt R, et al. Community health workers providing government community case management for child survival in sub-Saharan Africa: who are they and what are they expected to do? *Am J Trop Med Hyg* 2012;87(5 Suppl):85–91.

220. Connell RW. *The Role of Men and Boys in Achieving Gender Equity.* Brasilia, Brazil: UN, 2003. E/CN, 6/2004/9. http://www.un.org/womenwatch/daw/egm/men-boys2003/Connell-bp.pdf.

221. World Health Organization. *Engaging Men and Boys in Changing Gender-Based Inequity in Health: Evidence from Programme Interventions.* Geneva: WHO, 2007.

222. Population Reference Bureau. *Engaging Men for Gender Equality and Improved Reproductive Health.* Washington, DC: PRB, 2009.

223. IYCN. USAID. *The Roles and Influence of Grandmothers and Men Evidence Supporting a Family-Focused Approach to Optimal Infant and Young Child Nutrition.* Washington, DC: PATH, 2011.

224. Engaging men and boys in achieving gender equality. Rio de Janeiro, Brazil: 2009. http://www.menengage.org/images/files/declaracao-rio-ingles-para.pdf.

225. GBCHealth. *Engaging Men for Family Health: Why it Matters.* Issue Brief. December 2011. www.gbchealth.org.

226. Population Council. Mixed success involving men in maternal care worldwide. *Pop Briefs* 2005;11(1).

227. Mullick S, Kunene B, Wanjiru M. Involving men in maternity care: health service delivery issues. *Agenda: Special Focus Gender, Culture Rights* 2005;(special issue):124–134. http://www.popcouncil.org/pdfs/frontiers/journals/Agenda_Mullick05.pdf.

228. Kululanga LI, Sundby J, Malata A, Chirwa E. Striving to promote male involvement in maternal health care in rural and urban settings in Malawi—a qualitative study. *Reprod Health* 2011;8:36. http://www.reproductive-health-journal.com/content/8/1/36.

229. Gebrian B, Tobing S, Lowney M, Anderson F, Bourdeau R. Madonna Project. Innovations in maternal-newborn and child health. Unpublished manuscript, 2002.

230. Population Council/Bolivia. The involvement of men in perinatal health in El Alto. 2006. http://www.popcouncil.org/countries/bolivia.asp.

231. Schensul SL, Sharma S, Maitra S, Pinto N. Gender concepts, marital relationships and sexual risk behavior in Mumbai, India. September 2003. http://www.igwg.org/pdf/AgendaGlobalConference.pdf.

232. Sibley L, Buffington S, Haileyesus D. The American College of Nurse-Midwives' home-based lifesaving skills program: a review of the Ethiopia field test. *J Midwifery Womens Health* 2004;49(4):320–328.

233. Sibley L, Buffington S, Beck D, Armbruster D. Home based life saving skills: promoting safe motherhood through innovative community-based interventions. *J Midwifery Womens Health* 2001;46(4):258–266.

234. Dynes M, Rahman A, Beck D, Moran A. Home-based life saving skills in Matlab, Bangladesh: a process evaluation of a community-based maternal child health programme. *Midwifery* 2011;27(1):15–22.

235. Rosales A. HHF/KOMBIT PROJECT Innovations in Maternal-Newborn and Child Health Award No. GHS-A-00-04-00020-00 OCTOBER 1, 2004–SEPTEMBER 30, 2009, Final Evaluation Report.

236. Pasha O, Goldenberg RL, McClure EM, et al. Communities, birth attendants and health facilities: a continuum of emergency maternal and newborn care (the global network's EMONC trial). *BMC Pregnancy Childbirth* 2010;10:82. http://www.biomedcentral.com/1471-2393/10/82.

237. American Academy of Pediatrics. Helping Babies Breathe. Elk Grove, IL: AAP, 2012. http://www.helpingbabiesbreathe.org/about.html.

238. World Health Organization. *Kangaroo Mother Care: A Practical Guide.* Geneva: WHO, 2003.

239. Hackman PS. Recognizing and understanding the cold stressed term infant. *Neonatal Netw* 2001;20(8):35–41.

240. Bosque EM, Affonso DD, Wahlberg V. Physiologic measures of kangaroo versus incubator care in a tertiary-level nursery. *J Obstet Gynecol Neonatal Nurs* 1995;24(3):219–226.

241. World Health Organization. *Thermal Control of the Newborn: A Practical Guide.* Geneva: WHO, 1993. WHO/FHE/MSM/93.2.

242. Lawn JE, Mwansa-Kambafwile J, Horta BL, Barros FC, Cousens S. 'Kangaroo mother care' to prevent neonatal deaths due to preterm birth complications. *Int J Epidemiol* 2010;39.

243. Conde-Agudelo A, Belizan JM, Diaz-Rossello J. Kangaroo mother care to reduce morbidity and mortality in low birthweight infants. *Cochrane Database Syst Rev* 2010: CD002771.

244. Sloan NL, Ahmed S, Choudhury N, Chowdhury M, Rob U, Winikoff B. Community-based kangaroo mother care to prevent neonatal and infant mortality: a randomized, controlled cluster trial. *Pediatrics* 2008;121(5):e1047–e1059.

Human Trafficking

Clydette Powell

LEARNING OBJECTIVES

- *Describe the global burden, causes, forms, and impact of human trafficking*
- *Identity the health implications (public and individual) of human trafficking*
- *Describe the interventions used to combat human trafficking, and give examples of public health prevention approaches*
- *Identify some key initiatives and partners in anti-human trafficking*
- *Describe the role of demand reduction in combating human trafficking*

CASE EXAMPLES[1]

Case 1: Bopah: Cambodia

Bopah lived in a rural village and married at age 17. Her husband took her to a hotel in another village in Cambodia and left her. Bopah discovered the hotel was a brothel and tried to escape, but she was forcibly detained and told she must pay off her price. Bopah's "debt" increased due to charges for her food, clothing, and other necessities. Bopah could not leave. Several years later, ravaged by disease, she was thrown out on the street.

Case 2: Alin: Romania to Italy

Alin is a 14-year-old boy from Romania who is sexually exploited by his father and sold to foreign tourists who frequent a section of Milan known for child prostitution. Alin's father receives 40 euros each time his son is picked up. He uses the money for food and cigarettes. Under the Trafficking Victim's Protection Act of 2000 and international covenants,

child prostitution is, by definition, a form of human trafficking.

Case 3: Boy sewing sari

Young men sew beads and sequins in intricate patterns onto saris and shawls at a "zari" workshop in Mumbai, India (Figure 5-1). The boys who arrive by train from impoverished villages across India often work from 6 in the morning until 2 in the morning the next day. Some sleep on the floor of the workshop. If they make the smallest mistake, they might be beaten. All say they work to send money back to their families, but some employers are known to withhold their meager pay.

Case 4: Street child with flowers

Street kids, runaways, or children living in poverty can fall under the control of traffickers who force them into begging rings (Figure 5-2). Children are sometimes intentionally disfigured to attract more money from passersby. Victims of organized begging rings are often beaten or injured if they do not bring in enough money. They are also vulnerable to sexual abuse.

Case 5: American teen[2]

Debbie was a 15-year-old when she was abducted from her suburban Phoenix, Arizona, home. Shortly thereafter, she was threatened, raped, and crammed into a small dog crate. Her captors forced her to work as a prostitute. Finally local police followed up a tip and found Debbie, shaking, locked in a drawer under a bed.

INTRODUCTION

Every year as many as 27 million men, women, and children around the world, including the United States, may be subject to force, fraud, or coercion for

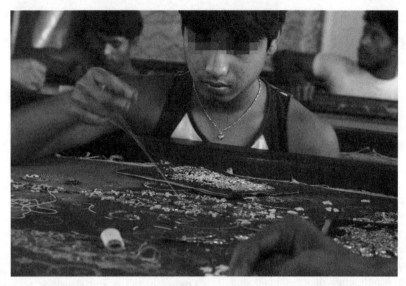

Figure 5-1. Young men sew beads and sequins in intricate patterns onto saris and shawls at a "zari" workshop in Mumbai, India. (*Courtesy of Kay Chernush for the U.S. State Department. http://www.gtipphotos.state.gov.*)

the purposes of sexual exploitation or forced labor.[3] A modern-day form of slavery, human trafficking is sometimes referred to as an epidemic that is "hidden in plain sight." The International Labor Organization (ILO) conservatively estimates that some 21 million persons are labor trafficked around the world.[4] Trafficking victims are of all ages, races, nationalities, socioeconomic status, sexual orientation, and educational levels. Their perpetrators come from the same categories. No group is exempt from the risk of being trafficked or the choice of being a trafficker.

Human slavery has a long history around the world. Written accounts of labor trafficking date back to thousands of years before Christ when a young man named

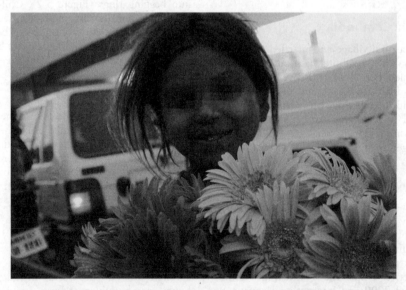

Figure 5-2. Street kids, runaways, or children living in poverty can fall under the control of traffickers who force them into begging rings. (*Courtesy of Kay Chernush for the U.S. State Department. http://www.gtipphotos.state.gov.*)

Joseph was sold by his brothers to travelers en route to Egypt and then resold by those buyers to other traders for slave labor. Over the centuries, warring tribes captured people and sold them to others; slave traders in the 1700s and 1800s plied the waters between Europe, Africa, and the Caribbean; the history of the United States is marred with tragic years of slavery; and today traffickers still troll inner cities, impoverished areas, and highways, looking for someone to entrap and then sell. Indeed, the for-profit sale of a person as a commodity is not limited to time, geography, ethnicity, economic status, or gender.

BOX 5-1

Those who traffic in persons are not limited to men. Women can be traffickers and perpetrators, too.

Over the decades, various countries, parliaments, legislative bodies, as well as individuals in the public eye and those working quietly and covertly, have sought to rid their world of this injustice. Nevertheless, the reality of the 21st century is that slavery in the form of human trafficking still exists. It would seem inconceivable that people today would still enslave others or be subject to exploitation by others for profit. Yet unscrupulous employers, pimps, and other opportunists recruit, control, transport, hold hostage, and torture other human beings against their will. Their victims have been made vulnerable by poverty, civil conflict and war, unemployment, corruption, discrimination, gender inequities, or just the hope for a better future. Deception, force, or coercion change their dreams and another's false promises to harsh realities from which physical, emotional, and psychological escape is very difficult.

In some countries, the pressures for economic survival or the need to break out of poverty can be the risk factor for being trafficked. People may be approached by a relative, neighbor, or business person proposing that they or a family member, often a child, could benefit from an educational opportunity, vocational training, or employment—for example, on a cocoa plantation, on a fishing boat, in the entertainment world, hospitality business, or textile industry. The recruiter pays the family for that person and then arranges for transport to a larger place, the capital city, or even another country. Once there, the trafficked person may be initially placed in a hotel or restaurant setting but transitioned out to a brothel or forced to labor in a garment or carpet factory or as a camel jockey. The buyer of the trafficked person may just be an intermediary, reselling the victim, or may be the end beneficiary of the sex or labor services. Wages earned are retained by the employer or trafficker for payment of expenses in transit, such as transport, visas, and lodging, and then for recurring costs (e.g., shelter, food, clothing) from which the trafficked person can rarely recover, thereby indenturing him or her indefinitely.

It is a common misperception that to be trafficked, a person must cross borders. Trafficking can be a very local phenomenon. Children can be trafficked for agricultural or fishing labor within the environs of their home village. Teen runaways can be deceived by a neighborhood boyfriend, then forced to have sex with his friends, who pay her boyfriend for the opportunity to rape; they can abuse her in the house next door. Roving armies and guerrilla bands can forcibly conscript children living in the path of civil conflict and war-torn areas to be cooks, soldiers, sex slaves, or murderers.

Why would people buy and sell each other? Unlike drugs and arms, people are commodities that can be used over and over again, without final transfer to the buyer. Human trafficking is very profitable. It is estimated to be the third most profitable "business" after trafficking in drugs and arms. The ILO estimates that transnational criminal networks and local gangs take as much as US$32 billion in profits from labor and sex trafficking enterprises. Hidden from authorities, these profits are not taxed or regulated. Like drugs, arms, and any other commodity, there is a so-called shelf life. Humans who have been trafficked repeatedly can reach their expiration date through homicide or suicide, a disabling injury or illness, or by virtue of having reached an age where their usefulness is exhausted. For example, their fingers are no longer able to weave carpets, their body weight is too much for a camel jockey, their sexual organs diseased or damaged from many customers, or their backs broken by heavy loads or occupational hazards. They have been called "disposable people."[5] The trafficker goes back to his market for a new supply, and the cycle starts over again.

DEFINITIONS OF TERMS

Although the term *trafficking* might suggest transportation, trafficked persons can be born into a state of servitude, placed in an exploitative situation, or have consented initially to a job, only to find that they are forced to work without wages, rights, or decent working conditions. In 2000, the UN Protocol to Prevent, Suppress, and Punish Trafficking in Persons, especially Women and Children (the Palermo Protocol) and the U.S. government's Trafficking Victims Protection Act

(TVPA) of 2001 describe this compelled service as "force, fraud, or coercion." The TVPA defines "severe forms of trafficking in persons" as:

1. Sex trafficking in which a commercial sex act is induced by force, fraud, or coercion, or in which the person induced to perform such an act has not attained 18 years of age; or,

2. The recruitment, harboring, transportation, provision, or obtaining of a person for labor or services, through the use of force, fraud, or coercion for the purpose of subjection to involuntary servitude, peonage, debt bondage, or slavery.

By definition in the Palermo Protocol and the TVPA, in the case of a minor (under age 18 years), prostitution is a crime, whether or not there was consent.

The term *human trafficking* is not the same as smuggling where a person is willing to be transported to another location, usually across international borders, and has paid someone to take them there. In human trafficking, a person may be willing initially to be moved and may have paid something in advance. The deception, fraud, or coercion that evolves within that process, however, is the distinguishing hallmark.

The terms *country of origin, transit,* or *destination* are used to broadly classify countries and trafficking movement. A country can serve in all three roles, although some countries tend to be source countries, and others tend to be destination countries. For purposes of foiling investigators and law enforcement, traffickers may use some countries as places of transit. The use of fake passports and visas, coupled with cheap ticketing for transport and low-budget accommodations, aid in the covert nature of trafficking. Many people, even unknowingly, can be involved along the way, making it difficult to identify the head of the criminal activity. Yet they are all traffickers. In China, the lead traffickers are sometimes referred to as "snakeheads," signifying their leadership role and implying the venom they can inflict on those not cooperative with their evil intent and purposes.

Not all the terms used in trafficking are uniformly agreed upon. Some may choose to use the term *trafficked person*; others use the term *victim*. Although this latter term can appear stigmatizing, this term legally differentiates a victim from a criminal.

FORMS OF HUMAN TRAFFICKING

Human trafficking is categorized as either labor trafficking or sex trafficking. One category of trafficking does not preclude the other because some victims who are initially labor trafficked can also be sex trafficked. Children who were abducted or forcibly recruited to serve as combatants, cooks, messengers, or spies can also find themselves sexually abused by their troops.

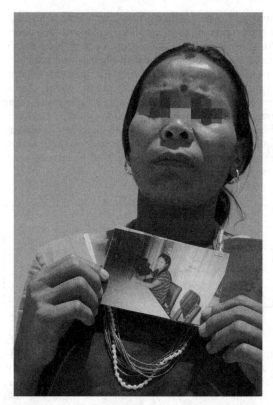

Figure 5-3. This desperate mother traveled from her village in Nepal to Mumbai, India, hoping to find and rescue her teenage daughter who was trafficked into an Indian brothel. Nepalese girls are prized for their fair skin and are lured with promises of a "good" job and the chance to improve their lives. "I will stay in Mumbai," said the mother, "until I find my daughter or die. I am not leaving here without her." (*Courtesy of Kay Chernush for the U.S. State Department. http://www.gtipphotos.state.gov.*)

For migrant workers, invalid contract terms and unsafe working conditions are setups for abuse; imposition of huge debts that they are required to work off may be the path of debt payment through sexual favors. Domestic servants in an informal workplace may be physically, socially, and/or culturally isolated. As a result, their employer may take advantage of them, forcing them to live in small quarters and/or coercing them to provide sexual services to the employer or his or her guests and family.

Labor Trafficking

Three forms of exploitative practices are found in labor trafficking: bonded labor, forced labor, and child labor.

Bonded labor, or debt bondage, is the least known but most widely used form of slavery. The victim's work is meant to be their means of repayment for a loan or service; however, no contractual terms exist to define the worth of their services as repayment, and their services do not liquidate their debt. In other words, their debt is always greater than the value of their services. Debt bondage can entrap not only individuals but whole families and even generations of people. Forced labor is a situation in which force, threat, or punishment mark the relationship between the so-called employer and worker. Freedom is restricted, and ownership of the person is exerted. Examples include sweatshops and domestic servitude, and they are found in some hotel and restaurant industry work, the garment industry, agriculture, and even street begging.

BOX 5-2.

55% of forced labor victims are women and children.

Many millions of children between 5 and 17 years of age are likely victims of labor trafficking. Child labor interferes with the physical, mental, spiritual, and social, educational, and moral development of children. It can be manifest in industries that require the nimbleness of children's fingers, such as carpet weaving, or their small size and weight, such as camel jockeying, or simple dull tasks such as breaking up stones into smaller pieces to make sidewalks or roads, or carrying clay bricks to kilns. Children who live in remote and rural areas can also be labor trafficked to help with fishing or plantation work, such as cocoa plantations in West Africa. Their remoteness makes them less visible to outsiders who might recognize that these children are not in schools. Many children do help with family businesses or informal employment as street vendors, but when such work predominates and drives their days, prohibiting a normal childhood of play and school, then it may be labor trafficking. Children can also be the mules for transport of illicit drugs or arms, or serve as child soldiers in countries where civil conflict requires conscription to increase the number of combatants, or to serve the troops, or both. Child soldiers may be sexually molested to threaten them into service. To desensitize them to the killing and horrors of war, they may be forced to kill a parent, a friend, or a stranger, as part of a gang initiation and as part of the message of "kill or be killed."

BOX 5-3.

"Migrant workers from Nepal and other countries are like cattle in Kuwait. Actually, cattle are probably more expensive than migrant workers there. No one cares whether we die or are killed. Our lives have no value." – Nepalese man trafficked to Kuwait, during an interview with Amnesty International.

Sex Trafficking

Sex trafficking may be a component of sex tourism, gang activity, high-end escort services, or simply as a means to make a profit by exploiting another human being. Runaway adolescents are vulnerable to being sex trafficked. Even if their initial conditions seem favorable and their new relationships seem trustworthy and generous, they are ultimately being groomed to be sold and brutally seasoned to sexually service multiple customers. Sex trafficking tends to receive more media coverage because of its sensational nature, but it is not as common as labor trafficking. It is estimated that several hundred thousand people are trafficked within the United States each year. Given stricter labor laws in the United States, sex trafficking may represent a higher percentage of all trafficking there compared with other countries.

BOX 5-4.

"I walk around and carry the physical scars of the torture you put me through. The cigarette burns, the knife carvings, the piercings. . . .how a human being can see humor in the torture, manipulation, and brainwashing of another human being is beyond comprehension. You have given me a life sentence." – Victim of trafficking in the United States, to her trafficker at his sentencing.

Organ Trafficking

Usually not considered as human trafficking, organ trafficking still entails the use or abuse of humans through the sale of body parts for transplantation.

The demand for organs such as kidneys exceeds the global supply. Desperately poor people may see the sale of one of their kidneys as a means to better themselves economically. Recruited by traffickers in urban slums, they are promised a free round-trip ticket to a second- or even first-world hospital where their organ will be skillfully removed and provided to someone else in need. The combination of apparent altruism for a needy recipient with an economic benefit to the donor can be attractive to a vulnerable person and may lend an air of legitimacy. The particulars of their postsurgical care, however, are lacking. Follow-up for surgical and medical complications, or compensation beyond the organ donation, are not part of the package by the organ trafficker. Costs of care to the donor once returned to their home country may well offset any initial gains. In some instances, children are sought and kidnapped for organs or body parts, not so much for transplantation but for perceived magical powers.

THE MAGNITUDE OF THE PROBLEM

In June 2012, the ILO released a new global estimate of 20.9 million forced labor victims.[6] The ILO notes that this is a conservative estimate for this largely hidden crime. The ILO's definition of forced labor includes sex trafficking (forced commercial sex). Women and girls represent an estimated 55% of forced labor victims; men and boys represent 45%. An estimated 74% of victims are adults (18 years and older); children make up the other 26%. The Asia-Pacific region has the largest number of forced laborers (56% of the global total), followed by Africa (18%), Latin America and the Caribbean (9%), the Developed Economies and European Union (7%), Central, Southeast, and Eastern Europe (non-EU) and the Commonwealth of Independent States (7%), and the Middle East (3%).

About 90% of all victims are exploited in the private economy, by individuals or enterprises. Of those exploited in the private economy, 22% are victims of sex trafficking; 68% are victims of labor trafficking. The remaining 10% of all victims are in state-imposed forms of forced labor, such as in prisons or in work imposed by the state military or rebel armed forces. Some 44% of the total number of forced labor victims have been moved internally or internationally; 56% are subjected to forced labor in their place of origin or residence.

THE PUBLIC HEALTH MODEL OF HUMAN TRAFFICKING

As in traditional public health models, especially for infectious diseases, one can also think about human trafficking in epidemiologic terms: the host, agent, environment, and vector. Using malaria as an example, the agent is the parasite *Plasmodium*, the vector is the *Anopheles* mosquito, the environment is the warm and stagnant water where the mosquito can breed and its larvae develop, and the host is the malaria-susceptible man, woman, or child. In a parallel fashion, trafficking has a host, agent, vector, and environment. The environment comprises, among other factors, poverty, socioeconomic pressures, deception, and greed. The vector is the trafficker or the chain of traffickers. The agent is the pimp, the john, and/or the sex tourist. The host is the vulnerable man, woman, or child. Nevertheless, when applied to human trafficking, such infectious disease models are simplistic and cannot fully explain the phenomenon of modern-day slavery, where there are relational dynamics, complexities, and nuances. In human trafficking, the laws of supply and demand are operative; the agents cannot be defined as one individual or a set of individuals. (The mosquito is hardly the only reason for malaria.) The signs and symptoms are not so neatly categorized as in a diseased organ system, and major and minor criteria do not define the problem as they do in traditional medicine. This is what makes the public health model both fascinating and frustrating.

To some extent, however, an infectious disease model can be applied further as we look later at the health implications of human trafficking and the appropriate interventions at various levels: individual, community, policymakers, media, and so on. As in the fight against malaria, which requires a multipronged approach to prevention, diagnosis, treatment, and prognosis, combating human trafficking similarly requires such approaches. These are described as the four "P's," elaborated in the section on the public health approach to human trafficking.

Like infectious disease cycles, human trafficking can also be considered a process or continuum, rather than isolated steps.[7] The first stage in the cycle is at the predeparture or recruitment stage. This is followed by the travel and destination/exploitation stages. Once out of the exploitation, either by escape or rescue, the person finds themselves in a reception/detention stage. Ultimately victims enter the integration/reintegration stage. Integration refers to placement at the destination; reintegration usually refers to family reunification or return to the home country. The cycle can be uneven; a person may stay in one stage for a long or short time. They may return to one stage before advancing to the next, or not advance at all. Because there are vulnerabilities at each stage, the health care professional or public health specialist should be sensitive to the complications and nuances of the trafficked person's life and struggles. Shame and self-blame, as well as difficulty with disclosure, lack of self-respect, and mistrust of those attempting to help the trafficked person, can be significant hurdles to overcome for the victim and the health worker, child protection services personnel, and law enforcement.

Such models, however, are imperfect representations of a real-world situation. The situation can quickly become more complex when other agents and environmental conditions are operative. This is the case when the victim has family members who may be at risk or threatened by the trafficker if the victim attempts to leave one stage for the other. In other situations, the victim develops a dependency and identification relationship with their trafficker, known as the Stockholm syndrome.[8] Victims may claim to, or actually be in love with their trafficker, and they may have children with him. They become dependent on their trafficker for shelter, food, and clothing and, ironically, for their relative safety. In the case of trafficked children, they may see their trafficker as a person to look up to, to trust, fear, and obey, regardless of the harm and abuse they are experiencing. In addition, trafficked persons may see themselves as responsible for their situation, or they may have normalized this abuse in their lives. Lastly, some victims "advance" from being a victim to working as a perpetrator. Having survived the abuse and learned the business, they turn to "the trade" for their own economic gain. They may recruit or manage newer victims and have a special relationship with the head trafficker.

Risk Factors

For any public health assessment, it is important to ask what characterizes an exposure and the risks of that exposure. Risk is the probability that an event will occur, and in some occasions that event is an unfavorable outcome.[9] An exposure is defined as (1) proximity and/or contact with a source of disease agent in such manner that effective transmission of the agent or harmful effects of the agent may occur, and (2) the amount of a factor to which a group or individual was exposed.[10] So what constitutes risk of exposure in the world of human trafficking? And what constitutes a risk group?

The International Program on the Elimination of Child Labor (IPEC) categorizes five kinds of risk factors: individual, family, external and institutional, community, and workplace.[11] These risks can occur during recruitment or while looking for work or a new life. In general, individual factors include age and sex (usually young girls); being a marginalized ethnic minority with little access to services: no birth registration and lack of proof of citizenship; being an orphan or runaway; lack of education and skills; low self-esteem; innocence and naiveté, lack of awareness; and negative peer pressure. In addition, in countries or places deemed as sources or sending areas,

difficulties in school leading to dropout, experience of family abuse or violence, feeling bored with village life or rural living, city attraction, and perception of a better life are also risk factors.

Family risk factors include being from a marginalized ethnic group or subservient caste; poor single parent family, or poor large family; death in a poor family; power relations within the household (usually within a patriarchal home); serious illness(e.g., human immunodeficiency virus/acquired immunodeficiency syndrome [HIV/AIDS]); domestic violence and sexual abuse; alcohol abuse and drugs in the family; past debt and bondage relations of the family; traditional attitudes and practices (sending a daughter to the extended family); and history of irregular migration and a migration network.

External and institutional risk factors include war and armed conflict; high youth unemployment; natural disasters such as floods, drought, and earthquakes; globalization and improved communication systems; strict migration controls that push movements underground; weak legal frameworks and law enforcement; corruption; weak education not relevant to labor markets; gender discrimination in education and labor; shifting social mores; and ambiguity in teen roles.

Community risk factors include location close to a border with a more prosperous country; long distance to secondary school and training centers; roads that facilitate access to large urban areas; poor quality of village leadership and community networks; lack of police, trained railway staff and border guards; lack of community entertainment; and history of migration.

Workplace risk factors include unsupervised hiring of workers, for example in border areas; poor labor protection and enforcement; unregulated informal economy and "3-D" jobs (i.e., dirty, dangerous, demanding) with poor working conditions; lack of law enforcement, labor inspection and protection; inability to change employer; sex tourism; undercover entertainment (e.g., hairdresser, massage); public tolerance of prostitution, begging, and sweatshops; and lack of organization and representation of workers.

There are also risks when in transition. Victims may travel alone rather than in a group. They may travel unprepared and uninformed and without money, or without destination address or job; they may be emotionally upset, drugged, threatened, and constrained. They may be traveling without any identification or registration, or traveling illegally. These at-risk persons may therefore be tempted to go through a nonregistered agency or smuggler or to travel at night. Once they are at their destination they may be isolated and without any social network or contact with family; they may be unable to speak the language and unable to understand the system in which they live and work; they may have illegal status; and they may be

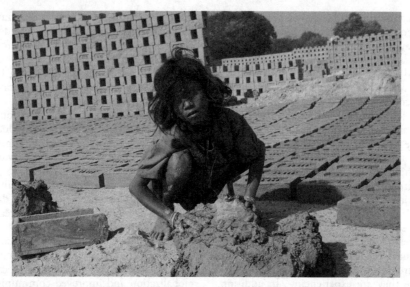

Figure 5-4. A 9-year-old girl toils under the hot sun, making bricks from morning to night, 7 days a week. She was trafficked with her entire family from Bihar, one of the poorest and most underdeveloped states in India, and sold to the owner of a brick making factory. With no means of escape, and unable to speak the local language, the family is isolated and lives in terrible conditions. (*Courtesy of Kay Chernush for the U.S. State Department. http://www. gtipphotos.state.gov.*)

dependent on drugs and alcohol. Many or all of these risk factors may result in working in terrible conditions, which potential victims may not recognize as situations ripe for exploitation or bondage.

However, it does not take the setting of a developing country or adverse economic conditions to put someone at risk. Some seek to better their lives or that of their family by seeking employment abroad. At some point, what seemed like an opportunity for advancement becomes a situation from which they cannot escape. Passports are confiscated, debts are incurred, earnings are insufficient to retire the debt, and communication with family or friends is forbidden or impossible.

CHARACTERISTICS OF TRAFFICKED PERSONS

Knowing these risk factors and exposures, how does the health care professional or public health specialist identify susceptible individuals or populations? One can conclude that many people around the world, as well as in your locale, are potential trafficking victims. Characteristically, these are adults (men and women) and children (boys and girls), runaway teens, so-called "throwaway kids," marginalized populations, the displaced, the stateless, and persons caught in

conflict-affected areas; and those caught in a cycle of poverty, poor education, and few vocational opportunities. The global mean age of entry into prostitution may be around 12 years of age.[12]

It is important to understand and appreciate the gender dimensions of trafficking. Although most think of sex trafficking when they hear the term *human trafficking* and therefore visualize the victim as a vulnerable woman or child, many men are trafficked victims. In studies by the International Organization of Migration (IOM) of migrant men in Belarus and Ukraine, men ages 18 to 44 years were trafficked into labor exploitation.[13] Some of these men cited the need to support families and children as their decision to migrate for work. The recruitment process mimicked the legal migration process, with agreements that appeared to be legally binding with legitimate companies. On arrival, however, working conditions were clearly substandard with unheated and unhygienic living space, poor quality food, crowding, and sometimes nonpayment of wages or abuses and threats. Some migrant workers left, but not all could exit freely. When rescued from their conditions, and offered assistance, some men were not inclined to receive that help. They did not see themselves as trafficked or exploited but regarded the situation as bad luck rather than a violation of their human rights.

Others saw their participation in the recruitment process as a disqualifier for assistance. Some viewed their situation as a better alternative to going home without any income at all; migration was a way to earn money, and they did not focus on the exploitative nature of the temporary work. The fact that some men either did not see themselves as trafficked victims, or even rejected that label, provides insights into providing assistance programs with gender sensitivities.

Disabilities play a role in trafficking as both a risk factor and an outcome of trafficking. Persons with disabilities are among the most at risk of being trafficked and more vulnerable to marginalization, stigmatization, and potential neglect and abuse. Health systems stretched to provide even basic services may not have the resources or advocates for care for the disabled. Disabilities include blindness, deafness, mental or physical challenges, developmental disabilities, and amputations. In some cultures, the disabled are seen as a burden on a family or community, and they risk being sold to a trafficker to unload the family of responsibility or burden. The disabled are more likely to be poorer, to be street children or beggars, or outcasts. The disabled may not be able to attend schools or are more likely to drop out, and thus they have less earning potential and fewer options, leading them to street begging, thievery, and forced prostitution. The disabled may also be more frequently perceived as virgins, less likely to be HIV positive (both conditions making them more attractive in high HIV-prevalent areas), and less likely to be able to fend off rapists or clients.

The disabled may also be disadvantaged because the loss of sight, speech, or hearing may compromise their ability to provide an understandable or credible witness and testimony against a trafficker in a court of law. Traffickers may take advantage of the disabled, thinking that the victim may be less successful in legal proceedings against them. Court systems may not be able to accommodate a disabled person in their testimony when sign language, interpreters, and physical access are not provided. Disabilities can also be the outcome of trafficking, as much as a risk. The exposure to trafficking can result in disabilities because physical and psychological abuse can be disabling. The disabilities thus engendered may cast them out of one form of trafficking and into another, continuing a vicious cycle of victimization, abuse, and helplessness.

A lesser known type of trafficked victim is the child bride. In some countries, for cultural reasons, young girls are promised to older men. Money is exchanged between the groom's family and the bride's family, in essence a sale of a young child or woman who may be forced to accept this new marital arrangement before the age of consent. She is not free to leave her husband and his family, may be required to work endless hours, provide sexual services to her husband, and may be resold to his friends if he has debts of his own. In Afghanistan, "opium brides"[14] are the girls sold by their farming fathers to Taliban who have advanced loans to the farmer to grow poppies and produce opium. When those poppy farms fail to produce or crops are destroyed, the only way to pay the debt may be to sell a daughter to the Taliban creditors.

CHARACTERISTICS OF PERPETRATORS

Anyone who participates in the recruitment, harboring, transportation, supply of provisions or helps to obtain a person through force, fraud, or coercion is considered a trafficker. Accordingly, someone who provides lodging, obtains travel tickets or visas, falsifies travel documents, books the flights, moves a person from one location to another, or helps along the trafficking route is considered a trafficker. There is typically a chain of services, with multiple people in that chain, to support trafficking. Physical transportation or direct contact is not necessary to define trafficking in persons.

The traffickers and perpetrators are not necessarily recognizable as overt criminals. They may be parents, relatives, boyfriends, neighbors, hotel owners, transportation agents, brothel owners, or managers of strip clubs or massage parlors. Pimps and johns may be middle-class citizens, married men, CEOs, town mayors and state governors, presidents of nations, well-regarded women, or they may be desperate people using trafficking as a means of income. Unfortunately, some law enforcement officials are also perpetrators, abusing their power and getting a cut in the earnings of the businesses they both protect and frequent as customers. They may be paid by the brothel owners and pimps to protect their space, thereby earning a salary greater than their official one. Where corruption reigns, court officials can be involved as well. Doctors and dentists can be hired by pimps and brothel owners to treat the medical/dental conditions of the trafficked victims, thereby eliminating the need for outside health consultations and avoiding raising suspicions when trafficked victims present with unusual conditions and injuries secondary to their abuse.

In some countries,[15] including the United States,[16] trucking routes and roadside rest stops can be prime places for human trafficking. In the earlier years of the HIV/AIDS epidemic, the spread of HIV was mapped to trucking routes because the stops along the way afforded casual and anonymous sex for men who had spent long hours on the road and were many miles from home. Brothels sprung up to support this business and offered small towns and villages a new form of income for their residents or for women brought into the area by pimps. These truck stops can also be the entry point for runaways and people escaping the law.

A common denominator for all traffickers is that they are all criminals; they have broken national and/ or international laws. Governments have the authority and responsibility to punish them and to provide legal recourse to survivors. Criminals need to be brought to justice, but punishment is not enough. Survivors need their rights and their health restored. Unfortunately, not all governments and authorities are able or willing to bring justice to bear.

THE RECRUITMENT PROCESS

In public health terms, how does exposure happen, given that some individuals are susceptible to being trafficked? In previous times, recruitment might happen by word of mouth or through seemingly legitimate announcements or ads placed in local papers. Nowadays, the Internet is becoming a means of recruitment, often in stepwise fashion, of the vulnerable and unsuspecting victim, and with increasing ease for the trafficker.

Mobile technology has become a vehicle for cyber seduction. Within the 21st century, the actors in human trafficking are no different than those predecessors of centuries before in terms of seeking out the vulnerable and looking to make a profit. However, the means of trafficking have changed. Perpetrators and their victims can be accessed through mobile technology and the Internet. Internet recruitment occurs in electronic chat rooms, on Web pages that offer escort services, in massage parlors, or jobs for the unsuspecting. For a while, Craig's List (used for individual advertising of items to buy or sell) also offered linkups for pimps and the human commodities they sold. Protests from anti-trafficking and anti-prostitution groups pressured Craig's List to remove this section. The Back Page of *The Village Voice*, however, continues to buy and sell sex services.

Recruitment can start when children and teens are surfing the Web, opening up Web pages and links that lead to sites that have secure "anonymizers" used by online predators. As the most common way to bypass Internet filters, anonymizers purport to be a Web site or a link or they link to another Web site once the Internet surfer has clicked on the site or Googled a term. Nearly 70% of parents are unaware that anonymizers exist.[17] Within chat rooms and e-mail and instant messaging, the predator may begin with questions that help him determine basics such as age, activities liked by that teen, and their living situation and then move on to a request for a photo or an inquiry about interest in older men, and so on. This initial probing is a risk assessment to see if the teen

is an easy target. The predators may introduce some ambiguous or sexually explicit conversation topics to assess whether the teen is willing to engage with him or her. At some point, the recruiter extends an invitation to meet in person. A blanket of secrecy is offered, a promise not to tell others, and then the bonding and "grooming" advance. Studies indicate that one in seven children is solicited online.[18] In those solicitations, 56% of kids are asked to send a photo; 27% of the photos are sexually oriented. In one study 44% of the solicitors were under the age of 18. Unfortunately, not all convicted sex offenders have to register on the offenders' U.S. registry. Of the 614,000 convicted sex offenders in the United States, more than 102,000 have been lost in the system.[19]

Child pornography, illegal in the United States, is the fastest growing online industry, and predators are on the cutting edge of technology. It has been said that home is the "virtual brothel" where the sex industry grows its clientele. Internet pornography is used by pimps to display photos of potential victims for buyers, and then a real meeting is arranged after a cash transfer.

Sexting on cell phones is done by a third of kids, most of whom think that it is okay.[20] To prevent such activity, parents can protect their kids by implementing "rules and tools" on all Internet-enabled devices such as desktop and laptop computers, cell phones, PDAs, and gaming devices. Such tools can filter dangerous content, dangerous contacts, and dangerous conduct.[21]

Not all recruitment is done online because vulnerable teens and runaways are unable to self-sustain on the street outside of home or protection. Statistics show that a runaway teenage girl will be on the street only 48 hours before her predator finds, grooms, and seasons her.[22] It may take a few months of special attention, clothes, food, jewelry and gifts before he demands or forces sexual favors from her for his friends or others. Money is exchanged, and she is now trafficked. A 2006 study of 13,000 U.S. youth revealed that 3.5% had exchanged sex for money or drugs.[23] Using census data, this percentage equates to 400,000 adolescents. Another study estimated that some 325,000 American youth were at risk for commercial sexual exploitation.[24]

The media play a role in promoting the acceptability of prostitution or condoning the maltreatment of women. Films such as *Pretty Woman* glamorize prostitution and can lead to the false conclusion that a john will be a kind and magnanimous rescuer, as was the protagonist in that film. Rap artists, fringe musicians, and lyricists have produced songs that reflect misogynist attitudes in keeping with pro-prostitution and human trafficking. In 2006, the Academy of Motion Picture Awards gave a music award to a group that glamorized the life of a pimp. Contemporary vocabulary includes the verb "to pimp," which means to make extravagant, as in "pimp my ride."

HEALTH IMPLICATIONS OF TRAFFICKING

Human trafficking has both individual and public health consequences. It is not the intent of this section to detail these medical aspects but rather to raise awareness of the issues and encourage you to seek out appropriate medical sources for diagnosis and treatment. Individual health problems have public health implications. The transport/migratory nature of some trafficking victims and contact with the public, particularly in sex trafficking and sex tourism, can have public health ramifications. Health care professionals need to be attuned to the fact that they may be the first responders to a trafficked person.

In the mid-2000s, semiquantitative studies on the physical and psychological health consequences of women and adolescents trafficked to Europe began to raise awareness of the health aspects of trafficking.[25] A five-country academic study on prostitution detailed the burden of physical and psychological trauma, as well as higher rates of sexually transmitted infections (STIs), hepatitis B, cervical cancer, and fertility complications.[26] The first study to document the health symptoms of trafficked women and adolescent girls quantitatively was conducted only recently. This study interviewed 192 women who had been trafficked and sexually exploited, and it evaluated their physical and mental health within 14 days of entering post-trafficking services.[27] Almost 95% reported physical or sexual violence while trafficked, and 59% had experienced pre-trafficking abuse.

The health consequences of labor and sex trafficking fall into several categories: reproductive and urogenital; neurologic and psychiatric (including substance use and abuse); infectious: constitutional (gastrointestinal, nutritional, musculoskeletal); occupational; and violence-related trauma (including dental and orofacial). The environments in which trafficked persons are forced to work contribute to the risks and exposures. Examples include crowded and unsanitary living conditions, poor nutrition, underventilated and overheated areas, noisy settings where sleep may not be possible, environments with social and cultural isolation, exposure to occupational environmental toxins, and lack of access to health care and prevention services. For the individual, predisposing and preexisting conditions may have also affected the health of the person before he or she was trafficked, especially if the person lived in a developing country or any setting where there was limited access to health services and health service disparities. Comorbidities add to the complexity of their health care and when coupled with exposure to clients whose health status is undetermined or not monitored, trafficked persons are further exposed to illness and disease.

Reproductive and Urogenital Disorders

Among those who are sex trafficked, problems of the reproductive tract are prominent and include STIs (e.g., HIV, chlamydia, gonorrhea, syphilis, hepatitis[28,29]), complications of pregnancy and abortions, urogenital complaints, and higher rates of cervical cancer. Sex trafficking has a direct cause and effect on the spread and mutation of HIV/AIDS in South Asia[30] and globally. Contributing factors include age, length of time in trafficking, number of sex partners, and lack of access to condoms and contraception. The physiologic and anatomic vulnerability of younger trafficked persons predisposes to higher risks of infections and trauma to internal and external genitalia. Studies of Nepali girls trafficked to India reveal a higher prevalence of HIV, particularly in girls younger than 16 years.[31] Young age has been a risk factor for HIV among female sex workers in India.[32] Furthermore, because menstruation is seen as an "interruption" for their work, victims and their traffickers may stuff the vagina with various materials to block obvious bleeding. These makeshift tampons can cause abnormal discharges, pain, and chronic infection including pelvic inflammatory disease.[33] Trafficked women also can have a number of urogenital symptoms including dysuria, pelvic and vaginal pain, vaginal discharge, and nonmenstrual vaginal bleeding.

Neurologic and Psychiatric Disorders

Neurologic complaints are also common and include headaches, blurred vision, dizziness and vertigo, memory problems, fainting, and back pain. Traumatic brain injuries, sustained during interactions with their pimps, employers, or clients, may lead to postconcussive syndromes, seizure disorders, or confusion. These conditions are further complicated when associated with alcohol and substance abuse. Neurologic problems can coexist with psychiatric conditions such as depression, anxiety, phobias, obsessive-compulsive behaviors, and posttraumatic stress disorders (PTSD), manifesting as hyperarousal and dissociative behaviors or frank psychoses. By far, mental health disorders predominate among those who have been trafficked: PTSDs, suicidal ideation, neuroses and psychoses, depression and anxiety, eating disorders, somatization, amnesias, vertigo and dizziness. The most common physical health symptoms reported by women included headaches

(81%), dizzy spells (71%), memory problems (63%), back pain (69%), and fatigue (82%).[34] In fact, trafficked persons are said to have more PTSD than soldiers in combat.[35] Flashbacks, hostility, and threats from coworkers and customers complicate the clinical picture.

Drugs and substance use/abuse play a role in the downward spiral of mental and physical health. Debate circles around the role and sequence of drug use in trafficked persons. Traffickers may drug their victims in the seasoning process to help them overcome resistance to forced sex; eventually the victims are addicted and prostitute themselves to support a drug habit. In other instances, victims may choose to use drugs to numb the physical and emotional pain of their abuse—whether sex or labor. This leads to a vicious cycle of needing money to pay for drugs and never having enough money to pay off debts.

Infectious Diseases

Seen in sex-trafficked persons are the previously mentioned STIs and viral hepatitides. Unhygienic working conditions and limited access to sanitation can lead to infestation by mites (scabies) and lice and infections of the skin caused by bacteria, viruses, and fungi. Vaccine-preventable diseases, malaria, tuberculosis, diarrheal diseases, and parasitic infestations may be related to the victim's place of origin. Prolonged transit in crowded, dirty conditions while moving from source to destination countries can also promote these diseases, and nutrition- or HIV-related immune suppression can exacerbate or reactivate diseases such as tuberculosis or opportunistic infections. Chronically poor nutrition may manifest as a low body mass index, anemia, gastrointestinal problems, or micronutrient deficiencies of essential vitamins and minerals.

Occupational Hazards

Long hours and hard labor, whether manual or sexual, can result in so-called occupational health effects such as fatigue, chronic headaches, gastrointestinal disorders, musculoskeletal disorders, and sleep disorders. Environmental toxins present in the agricultural and fishing industries may lead to respiratory, gastrointestinal, and dermatologic manifestations. Repetitive motion, such as carpet weaving or labor in garment factories, may present as carpal tunnel syndrome or other musculoskeletal disorders. Those who work with machinery or in the agricultural and fishing industries may present with back pain, dehydration, exposure to chemicals or pesticides, exposure to extremes of heat or cold, burns, lacerations, and amputation of fingers, hands, or feet. Malfunctioning equipment, lack of safety measures, lack of skills and training, pressures to meet production quotas, and understaffed factories or farms all can contribute to injury in the workplace. All these problems can be aggravated by sleep deprivation, psychological stressors, lack of proper nutrition, or preexisting health conditions that have not received care.

Violence-Related Trauma and Injuries

Violence is a fundamental component of trafficking. Violence takes many forms besides physical: verbal, sexual, emotional, cultural, and societal. Trafficked persons may be assaulted, beaten, or roughly handled during sexual and other encounters. Head, orofacial, and dental injuries are common and include orbital, temporal bone, mandibular and maxillary fractures, avulsed and missing teeth, and other dental trauma. Cigarette burns, attempted strangulation, and rope burns may be seen. Other injuries may include dislocations, major fractures, and traumatic brain injury. Lacerations, puncture wounds, bruising, and burns may be found in unusual places on the body. Pimps tend to make the injuries hidden, not wanting to turn away clients because obvious injuries may make a victim less marketable, and not wishing to raise suspicion if the trafficked person is allowed to seek medical care for other ailments. In very violent settings, homicide or suicide can be the ultimate outcome of trauma and violence.

Special Circumstances: Children of Trafficked Persons

Although not necessarily the direct victim of trafficking, children who have witnessed a parent being trafficked may have similar symptoms of PTSD, neuroses, attention deficits, and other cognitive, emotional, and behavioral disorders.[36] Such children may also suffer from lack of access to basic health services such as immunization programs, dental care, growth monitoring, and anticipatory guidance for developmental stages. These children may have vaccine-preventable diseases, be short statured due to malnutrition or endocrine reasons, and suffer from sleep deprivation because they sleep on the streets during the day, have no bed or place to sleep during the night while a parent is being prostituted, or may sleep under their parent's bed when the night's work is done. They may have physical disabilities secondary to road and traffic hazards as they dart between vehicles while begging at corners or "performing" for small change. Because of their small size and lack of personal agency, they are more subject to toxic environments, manipulation, and force. They may not be recognized as a secondary victim of trafficking, and they may have been separated from their parent for various reasons including pimp threats, forced and rapid evacuations, and frequent relocations for migrant work by the parent.

INITIAL ASSESSMENT OF TRAFFICKED PERSONS

The health care provider may be the first responder to a person who is being trafficked. Trafficked victims are more likely to seek care as a onetime visit in an emergency department, urgent care facility, or free community clinic. They may present with more advanced or more severe health problems. Control and surveillance by their unidentified trafficker or pimp may result in quiet deference during a clinic visit. They may be accompanied by someone who claims to be a relative or friend who may speak on behalf of the person. The latter may not speak the local language or be familiar with the neighborhood or environs. The health care provider will need to have a low threshold of suspicion when observing unusual trauma, fearfulness, or submissiveness. Because the trafficker is motivated to keep his victim working, he will eventually seek care for the victim, but this may not be until an injury or illness adversely affects performance. In some instances the trafficker may sell or even kill the trafficked person rather than deal with the health problems.

Interviewing of the patient should follow the guidelines for any suspected abuse; a safe and strictly confidential discussion must be assured, without the accompanying person present, and with informed consent at each step. Questions that may clue the health care provider in to abuse may include "Can you leave your job/work if you want? When not working, can you come and go as you please? Have you or your family been threatened with harm if you try to quit? What are your living and working conditions like? Where do you sleep and eat? Is there a lock on your door or windows so you cannot get out? Must you ask permission to eat, sleep, or go to the bathroom?" It is important to convey to the victim that their safety is the first priority.[37]

Because many victims have been exposed to violence and threats to them or to their family, they may be mistrustful or afraid to be exposed as a trafficked victim. Their loyalty and protectiveness of their trafficker is consistent with the Stockholm syndrome in which they identify or bond with their captor. They may fear punishment by their trafficker or, if they escape, fear deportation to their country of origin. A major limitation and reality is that the health care provider may have only one opportunity to see this patient without follow-up. Still, if the trafficked suspect is ready and willing to accept help, one can work with social services, child protective services, and law enforcement to take the next steps. It can be a long process to establish identities, guarantee witness protection, and meet short- and long-term needs.

A health care professional who is both trained and experienced/certified in sexual assault forensic examination (SAFE) is the person best equipped to perform the history and physical examination, although few facilities where trafficked persons present may have staff with these competencies. Using the list of physical findings and symptoms provided in the previous section, the health care provider should conduct a focused examination using a trauma-informed, patient-centered approach. Careful documentation of findings using the SAFE methodology will assess the victim's injuries and provide support to the investigation process led by law enforcement. The findings of the history and physical examination can provide key information in a court of law, allowing a judge or jury to make conclusions about the case brought forward by the victim against the suspected perpetrator. All involved must recognize that *the crime scene is a human body*. The health care provider is in a key position to collaborate with law enforcement to assess the severity and magnitude of injury to that body.

BOX 5-5.

The scene of the crime is the human body.

THE MULTI-DISCIPLINARY RESPONSE

Assistance to the trafficking victim is optimally offered through a multidisciplinary approach incorporating a team consisting of health care professionals, public health specialists, child protective services, sexual assault forensic experts, social workers, law enforcement, security staff, and legal experts. Protection and safety for the trafficked victim, the team, and the site of care are paramount. Skillful interaction and dialogue, informed consent, respect for patient autonomy, nondiscriminatory, trauma-informed, patient-centered and rights-based care, confidentiality, and linguistic and cultural competency all play roles in service provision.

The facility staff should be prepared to recognize and respond to both short- and long-term needs. They must know how to conduct and facilitate safe referrals to other health service providers and to higher-level care facilities. Staff should have updated, easily accessed lists of contact information for translation, domestic violence, child protection, security, and immigration services (including Customs and Border Protection, if in the United States), legal assistance, child labor specialists, and local law enforcement. They should have hotline numbers for suicide prevention, missing persons, and the National Human Trafficking Resource Center (NHTRC) hotline. These providers need to know the location and contact information for women's shelters, safe houses, migrant shelters, and faith-based organization shelters and established contacts with local networks, other providers, embassy and consular offices, and local government authorities.

The care and case management of the trafficked person are complex, and a detailed discussion is beyond the scope of this chapter. The IOM, among others, has developed manuals that lay out optimum direct assistance to the victim and guidelines for health care providers.

THE GLOBAL RESPONSE

Traditionally, criminal law framework has been used against the abusive practice of human trafficking. Criminal investigation and prosecution for perpetrators, or threats of sanctions for countries failing to take measures against human trafficking, have been the approach. For victims, the legal system has provided some means of protection and assistance. More recent legislative approaches have attempted to tackle root causes through prevention measures, but these remain the weakest and most difficult to implement and monitor.

Twenty-first century protocols and legislation have helped to formalize global and domestic efforts. One is the UN's Protocol to Prevent, Suppress, and Punish Trafficking in Persons, Especially Women and Children. Also known as the Palermo Protocol, this protocol supplements the UN's Convention Against Transnational Organized Crime and is accompanied by a protocol addressing smuggling. The Palermo Protocol defines the global approach to human trafficking as the "3 P's: prevention, protection, and prosecution. More recently a fourth "P," partnerships, has been added. This classification broadly categorizes the various means and entities working to counter human trafficking.

Historically, within the United Kingdom and United States, British parliamentarian William Wilberforce and President Abraham Lincoln, respectively, are prominent names in the abolition of slavery. However, many other individuals and organizations have worked and continue to work behind the scenes against trafficking in their neighborhoods, communities, and countries. During the Bush administration in the United States, the Trafficking Victims Protection Act (TVPA) of 2000 and its reauthorizations (TVPRA) in 2003, 2005, and 2008, helped to define punishment, authorize protection and victim assistance, and speak to prevention measures. The TVPA of 2000 also created within the U.S. Department of State (DOS) the Office to Monitor and Combat Trafficking in Persons (J/TIP), and required

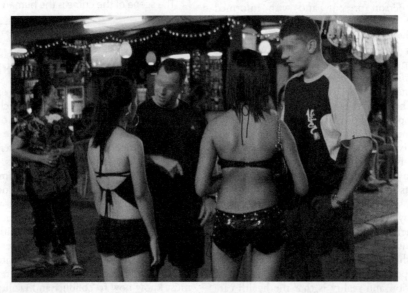

Figure 5-5. Customers/exploiters come from all over the world. Legalized or tolerated prostitution is a magnet for sex trafficking. The U.S. government considers prostitution to be "inherently demeaning and dehumanizing" and has opposed efforts to legalize it. The PROTECT Act makes it illegal for an American to sexually abuse a minor in another country. Perpetrators can receive up to 30 years in jail. (*Courtesy of Kay Chernush for the U.S. State Department. http://www.gtipphotos.state.gov.*)

from that office *The Trafficking in Persons Report*. The TVPA also increased penalties of 20 years to life for human trafficking, and created T- and U-visas to assist those victims who were willing and able to cooperate with the Department of Justice (DOJ) to prosecute the traffickers(s) involved in their cases. The T- and U-visas also provided temporary resident status as well as some tangible support benefits to the victims. Lastly, the TVPA of 2000 appropriated $60 million in resources to address human trafficking. In 2003, President George W. Bush signed a National Security Presidential Directive on Trafficking, the first of its kind. The directive called on all governmental agencies to create a strategic plan to advance the government's fight against human trafficking. The TVPRA of 2003 also created the President's Interagency Task Force on Human Trafficking, a cabinet-level inter-ministerial body.

Various nations have become more attuned to the level of the criminal activity of human trafficking within and across their borders. They have begun to work with legislators, law enforcement, the media, nongovernmental organizations (NGOs), and the general public to attempt to catalyze behavior change and decrease the incidence of human trafficking. The Swedish Parliament created legislative initiatives to shift emphasis from punitive measures for traffickers to addressing the demand for human trafficking. Some countries have tried to control and monitor human trafficking by legalizing prostitution, although with disappointing results. National and local travel and tourism offices have raised awareness of human trafficking in tourist spots, hotels, airports, train and bus stations, and other areas frequented by visitors. Film producers and directors have made visual and often graphic accounts of the crime of human trafficking, its victims, its perpetrators, and its heroes. Writers have catalogued in both books and journals the countless stories of desperate individuals who have been trafficked around the world.

U.S. federal agencies also play a role in countering human trafficking, both domestically and abroad. Their efforts are guided by the leadership at DOS/J/TIP and the DOJ. The U.S. Attorney General's office disseminates an annual report to Congress on the Assessment of U.S. Government Activities to Combat Trafficking in Persons. The U.S. Department of Health and Human Services (DHHS), through its Administration for Children and Families, conducts a program called "Rescue and Restore" that focuses on human trafficking. The Department of Homeland Security (DHS), the Federal Bureau of Investigation (FBI), Immigration and Customs Enforcement (ICE), Immigration and Naturalization Service (INS), Customs and Border Protection (CBP), and the Departments of Labor (DOL), Agriculture (DOA), Defense (DOD), and Education (DOE) are just some of the U.S. federal agencies that work on various aspects of human trafficking.

Within developing countries, the U.S. Agency for International Development (USAID) works closely with the DOS, U.S. embassies, other U.S. agencies, and host nation institutions to support anti-human trafficking programs in those countries that aim to prevent and protect individuals who are at risk of being trafficked or have been victims of human trafficking crimes. USAID is integrating counter trafficking activities into development programs across sectors. To prevent child trafficking on cocoa farms in Ghana, a "counter trafficking in persons" module was included in an agricultural program training cocoa farmers. USAID is committed to strengthening regional approaches to combat cross-border trafficking. In southern Eastern Europe, the agency supports a cross-border referral mechanism for trafficking victims in 10 countries. The referral guidelines and protocols help shape local laws including National Action Plans to Combat Trafficking. To raise awareness across Asia, USAID developed a multimedia trafficking awareness campaign through a partnership with MTV Exit. Impact assessments of the campaign suggest that people who have been reached are more aware of trafficking and its costs.

Various NGOs may focus on advocacy, communication, and social mobilization. End Child Prostitution and Trafficking (ECPAT) and National Center for Missing and Exploited Children (NCMEC) are just two of many examples. The latter's Innocence Lost Initiative disseminates information and photos of children missing in the United States and works with law enforcement to recover them. The U.S. DHHS funds Polaris, an organization based in Washington, DC, to run the Human Trafficking Resource Center's 24/7 hotline for information and reporting. They track and map the increasing number of phone calls that come from all over the United States and are making plans to develop a global center for hotline assistance.

Among the international and UN organizations, the UN Office on Drugs and Crime (UNODC), the UN Children's Fund (UNICEF), the IOM, the ILO, the International Program to Eliminate Child Labor (IPEC), and the Organization for Security and Co-Operation in Europe (OSCE) are some that have a major global reach and influence.

In partnership with many entities around the world, the U.S. DOS(J/TIP) compiles an annual report of the state of human trafficking in countries around the world.[38] This report is based on wide input from embassies, U.S. diplomatic posts, government officials, NGOs, international organizations, reports from journalists and academics, published reports, research trips to those countries and regions, as well as e-mail reports sent to J/TIP. The methodology consists of assessments under American law, with standards based in international law.

The U.S. DOS places every country in one of three tiers based on the extent to which its government works to combat human trafficking. The size of the problem in that country is an important factor, but key factors for tier placement include the government's action to enact laws to prevent human trafficking, to prosecute cases and prescribe criminal penalties, to fund victim protection efforts, and to partner with organizations that can help provide shelter, legal counsel, and other assistance. Although NGOs can be active within a country to combat human trafficking, it is the response of the government that forms the criteria for tier placement.

Tier 1 placement is for those countries whose governments comply fully with the TVPA's minimum standards; Tier 1 placement does not mean that a country has no trafficking problem however. Tier 2 countries do not fully comply with those standards but are making significant efforts to do so. Tier 2 Watch List countries have compliance problems (decreasing or no evidence of complicity and commitment to make changes) coupled with an absolute number of victims of severe trafficking, or a number that is significantly increasing. Tier 3 countries have neither commitment nor compliance. Countries that have been on the Tier 2 Watch List for two consecutive years are automatically downgraded to Tier 3. Other factors come into play for tier placement, including whether a country is a country of origin, transit, or destination for severe forms of trafficking. Penalties for Tier 3 placement include U.S. sanctions such as withholding or withdrawing nonhumanitarian and non–trade-related assistance as well as U.S. opposition to assistance from the World Bank and the International Monetary Fund. No tier ranking is permanent and the status is reviewed annually by the U.S. DOS.

THE PUBLIC HEALTH APPROACH TO HUMAN TRAFFICKING

The predominant means of combating human trafficking has largely been within the domain of criminal law and punishment. If one examines statistics on the number of prosecutions and convictions, those numbers pale in comparison to the estimated magnitude of human trafficking occurring worldwide. Clearly, the law-focused approach may have merit but cannot be the only solution to combating this crime. Public health approaches tackle problems from many levels, but the more successful interventions are those that deal with root causes. Drawing on the malaria example mentioned earlier in this chapter can drive home the point. Although using antimalarials for cases of malaria provides an individual needed relief and recovery, tackling environmental issues where

mosquitoes breed (residual spraying) and changing human behavior (use of insecticide-treated bed nets) have far reaching and more sustainable impact on the community, with resultant fewer cases of malaria. In a similar manner, immunization of children and adults can prevent diseases that otherwise would be known for their morbidity and mortality. Within immunization activities, we also know that herd immunity and community engagement lay the groundwork for decreased incidence of vaccine-preventable diseases and maybe eradication.

Some debate has surrounded whether human trafficking falls into the medical arena rather than public health because medicine deals with the health of individuals and human trafficking adversely affects the individual health of victims (and perpetrators). However, one can make a good case for human trafficking to be a public health issue, given its population dynamics and global nature, its magnitude with pervasive effects on large numbers of people, and the clear need for prevention interventions within the public arena.[39] Moreover, the fact that violence is seen as a public health issue is another reason for human trafficking to be seen in the light of public health concerns. The case is not whether it is primarily an issue for the practice of medicine or that of public health; it is both.

A moral imperative now exists for individuals and communities to act on knowledge of the harm of human trafficking, to engage in change to benefit both individuals and communities. One cannot become aware of human trafficking and not seek some level of involvement in combating this crime against humanity. That involvement can take many forms that range from policy development to hands-on activity. From the perspective of the public health specialist, prevention at the primary, secondary, and tertiary levels may be an effective way to frame that response. The following sections lay out some possible public health approaches—within the framework of the Palermo Protocol 4 P's—to combating human trafficking.

Prevention

Public health prevention occurs at one of three levels: primary, secondary, and tertiary. Primary prevention keeps a process from happening; secondary prevention interrupts the process before it becomes symptomatic or harmful; and tertiary prevention limits the physical and social consequences of the process. Prevention is more effective when it occurs in different forms and targets more than one population type or stakeholder. The Centers for Disease Control and Prevention (CDC) uses a four-level socio-ecological model in its work in violence prevention. Human trafficking can use a similar model.

Primary Prevention

Primary prevention can take the form of advocacy, communication, social mobilization, life skills training, mentoring, and counseling at the individual, family, and community levels, to name a few examples. Public education campaigns against trafficking can raise awareness about the definitions and drivers of TIP; it can include ways to recognize or suspect that TIP is occurring; and it can promote new behaviors or encourage the cessation of harmful behaviors. The media can play an active role in messaging about human trafficking, through public announcements, films, documentaries, social media such as Facebook and YouTube, as well as books, journal publications, music, concerts, and celebrity sponsorships. Given that some social media and music may promote forms of slavery and human trafficking, using the same mechanisms to combat abusive attitudes is appropriate. The tourism and travel industries also help to raise public awareness of trafficking. Travelers, whether on business or pleasure, or seeking new employment, are the targets for such public awareness about human trafficking. The NGO "Truckers Against Trafficking" spreads word among its own workforce and at truck stops to help identify trafficking victims and trafficking suspects (Figure 5-6). (Many NGOs perform excellent outreach and education, and cannot all be listed here.) Historically, the use of public awareness campaigns, social media, and other communication means have served public health purposes for smoking cessation, violence prevention, use of seat belts, and more recently obesity prevention or reduction. It is useful to study these examples to learn how public policy, mandates, and funding authorization occurred, what approaches were most effective, and how the impact was measured.

For the public health professional, primary prevention must be at the forefront. The old adage, "An ounce of prevention is worth a pound of cure" can be countered, however, in the world of anti-trafficking, with a newer saying: "An ounce of prevention is a pound of work." Primary prevention can be the most

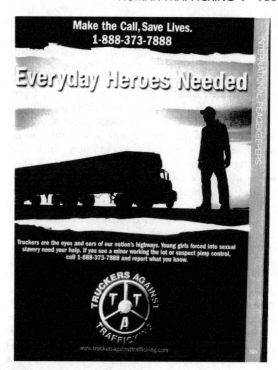

Figure 5-6. Truckers Against Trafficking poster. (*Courtesy of Kay Chernush for the U.S. State Department. http://www.gtipphotos.state.gov.*)

cost-effective but the hardest means to demonstrate positive impacts and sustainability within the TIP domain.

Prevention begins in many places but most deeply within the personal relationships that each person has within his or her family and community, no matter how those are defined. The definitions of roles, the place of respect for authority, the love and caring of parents, and the nurturing throughout the childhood years all contribute to a healthy sense of self. Where family relationships are fractured, or defined in abusive and exploitative ways, the risk of trafficking increases.

The challenges of prevention are no more acutely felt than during infancy and childhood and into the teen years, where the changing nature of relationships and the maturing definitions of self come into play. Studies have demonstrated that children who are abused are at higher risk of being abusers themselves or at risk for further abuse.[40] Although not all trafficked persons were abused as children, the child or adolescent who has experienced violence or cruelty in the home tends to be more vulnerable to repeat episodes of abuse later in life. Runaways, fleeing domestic turbulence or seeking to redefine their lives and self, are vulnerable to traffickers and opportunists. Data reveal that on the average it takes less than 48 hours for a trafficker or opportunist to spot and pick up a runaway on the street.[41] Teens whose sense of self is still forming or who are uncertain of their worth, gender, status among their peers, relationship to authority, or life direction are vulnerable to influence and suggestion from someone older, more persuasive, and appearing initially to be sympathetic to their plight. Traffickers have stated that they can intuit which child roaming the mall—or an Internet chat room—is likely to be susceptible to persuasion, deception, or a false offer of friendship. Lack of confidence, lonely habits, lack of belonging to a group, and/or inability to say no or to stay clear of strangers may be the first declining steps toward vulnerability. Therefore, it is the role of parents or guardians to develop, educate, and protect the child in healthy ways. Likewise, it is the role of the health care professional to provide anticipatory guidance and to inquire about family relationships, extended families, patterns of relating in the home, school performance, potential for abuse, violence, or substance use, and the chosen spiritual or moral compass. In addition the community and the place of worship can play an active role in guiding youth into right choices about their lives, relationships, health practices, and career paths, to name a few.

Prevention can also take broader forms, such as ensuring that each child and individual has a birth registration card and is included in the official registries. This problem is especially one of some developing countries, where vital records may be nonexistent, not a government priority, or not possible to implement for all its citizens. Birth registration helps to ensure access to health services, education, employment options, and official involvement in legal processes. Children lacking birth registration, undocumented workers, refugees, the marginalized, and the outcast may have none of these rights and privileges, making them more vulnerable to socio-economic pressures, illicit offers, deception, and fraud. The public health specialist or the health care provider can play a role in referring such individuals for social services and legal assistance.

Other ways of raising awareness about human trafficking include the use of the Internet and associated technology. An interactive Web-based tool called "The Slavery Footprint" takes the participant through a series of questions regarding lifestyle, possessions, work, and leisure. It then tallies up the likelihood of the participant's use of labor-trafficked goods.[42] The UNODC and the U.S. DHS have promoted the Blue Campaign, which also helps to raise awareness about global and domestic trafficking, respectively. The Administration for Children and Families within the DHHS has developed a series of webinars, posters, and educational material through its "Rescue and Restore" program. DHHS also funds Polaris, an NGO, to collect data on stateside human trafficking and to operate a trafficking hotline, where suspected trafficking can be reported and where further information about local law enforcement and other shelters can be requested.

Secondary Prevention

Secondary prevention for youth can come in the form of interventions and approaches for the individual who is found to be failing socially or academically, and who is at risk for dropping out from peer groups or school. Truancy from school, rebelliousness, and/or experimentation with drugs or sex may be gateways or early warning systems that the teen may be at higher risk. Secondary prevention can also take the form of Internet interventions in the home, such as computer chips and monitors to prevent those at home from accessing chat rooms and Web sites that can be venues for traffickers. The home is sometimes described as the "virtual brothel," the place where unsuspecting persons may be either enticed into pornography or recruited for in-person meetings where abuse, abduction, and exploitation can occur. Within the United States, various organizations, such as Enough is Enough, Covenant Eyes, Morality in Media, and Pure Hope, focus on Internet safety and prevention of pornography, and they have developed tools to alert parents to Internet-based risks.

Tertiary Prevention

Tertiary prevention occurs after the trafficking has occurred and attempts to mitigate the effects of harm.

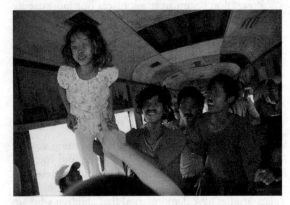

Figure 5-7. Members of the Cambodian NGO Phare Ponleu Selpak's prevention troupe perform on a train in Cambodia. The troupe uses a mixture of comedy, drama, acrobatics, and magic tricks to inform audiences about HIV/AIDS, land mines, drug addiction, and human trafficking. Credit: © 2006 Stephane Janin, Courtesy of Photoshare

The responses include rehabilitation programs, reintegration, and restoration/reunification with families, if that is desired by the trafficked person. This can include justice proceedings where the victim's rights may be restored. Many NGOs, including faith-based organizations, help trafficked victims regain their lives, through home group living, sheltered foster care, vocational training, life skill training, mentoring, and opportunities for starting up small businesses through micro-financing. USAID's Center of Excellence, within the Office for Democracy and Governance, has collected promising counter-trafficking practices that exemplify and chronicle ways in which international NGOs can help communities and trafficked individuals recover their lives and be reintegrated back into community life, whether it is the community of origin or a newly adopted one.

Protection

The second "P," protection, encompasses policy and legislation to support protection services and the establishment of networks, taskforces, and coalitions, physical protection such as safe havens, shelters, after-care facilities, and witness protection programs, and intangible victim assistance such as mental health counseling, legal assistance, social services, and chronic medical care. The needs of trafficked persons fall into short-term and long-term categories. Within the short term, victims need security, shelter, clothing, food, personal hygiene supplies, initial medical and mental health assessment, interpretation and translation services, and initial legal services. For the longer term, they need rehabilitation of physical and mental/emotional health disorders, housing, alternative employment (which includes assessment, training, and placement), legal services (especially immigration and criminal justice advocacy), and, in some instances, family reunification. If the trafficked person has children, they will likely need some of the services just described as well as birth documents, assistance with school registration, and updating of preventive services such as immunizations.

Within the United States, an additional aspect of protection is the availability of T-visas and U-visas. Victims who cooperate with law enforcement are able to obtain limited legal residence in the United States, as well as victim benefits such as the Supplemental Nutrition Assistance Program (formerly called food stamps), legal assistance, and help with housing.

Prosecution

Prosecution represents the means by which criminal justice is applied by law enforcement; it represents the courts' efforts to rectify the wrong done to the trafficked victim and an attempt to restore that person's human rights and dignity. The work of prosecution is supported by investigation involving law enforcement, border patrol personnel, bureaus of investigation, child protection officers, immigration officials, and other legal channels. Protection is often aided by expert witness by health care professionals, public health specialists, and forensic medical examiners, where appropriate. Obtaining informed consent during patient-provider procedures is critical for cases that may come to court. Issues of competency, capacity, and guardianship are also intricately entwined in trafficking cases, although far beyond the scope of this chapter. Various international organizations, including but not limited to the UN Office of the High Commissioner for Human Rights,[43] the World Health Organization (WHO),[44,45] the IOM,[46] Physicians for Human Rights,[47] and the Organization for Security and Co-operation in Europe (OSCE),[48] have resources on protection topics. Far fewer cases of human trafficking have been investigated and successfully prosecuted than occur. The DOS Trafficking in Persons Report for 2012 documents that for 42,291 victims identified, 7,909 cases were prosecuted of which only 3,969 led to convictions. These figures are out of an estimated 21 million trafficked persons worldwide. Reasons for this discrepancy reflect the shortcomings of a legal and law enforcement approach alone in stemming the tide of trafficking supply and demand. Reluctance of witnesses and victims to testify, lack of solid documentation, colluding law enforcement officers, and lack of legislation and judicial systems to bring traffickers to justice are just some of the reasons for this discrepancy.

Partnerships

Examples of partnerships include relationships between trafficking task force coalitions, NGOs, public-private partnerships, philanthropic groups, academic and community groups, survivor programs, street outreach, schools, local organizations, and businesses that strive for fair manufacturing and employment practices. These partnerships can be official or informal, secular or faith based. In 2004, End Child Prostitution, Child Pornography, and Trafficking of Children (ECPAT) launched a Code of Conduct to be implemented by the tourism industry. As of mid-2012, there were over 1,000 signatories on this document from over 42 countries. ECPAT-USA developed a Child Protection Tourism Code of Conduct that has now been extended to Brazil, Mexico, and Belize.

Various international entities such as the ILO, IOM, FAO, UN Global Initiative to Fight Trafficking (UNGIFT), UNODC, OSCE, USAID, USDOS, and others help develop policies and protocols, offer funding opportunities, and provide resource materials to catalyze partnerships. Much of the work of these partnerships is reflected in the prevention, protection, and prosecution activities previously described.

As mentioned earlier, as part of the U.S. government's global response effort, USAID works closely with U.S. embassies and its own missions in countries around the world to gather trafficking information, fund projects, and support other governments in fighting trafficking. These are usually countries of origin or transit. The United States is regarded as a desirable destination country.

DEMAND AND ITS REDUCTION

Although more attention is usually placed on the supply of victims of trafficking, one must consider the demand placed by a public that wants to buy another human for the purposes of sex and/or labor. As with drugs and arms for sale, the purchase of one human being equates to someone else's profit, profits whose margins are high and sheltered from regulation or taxation by their illicit and hidden nature. These profits are generated by service in the commercial sex industry or in labor industries such as garments, textiles, agricultural and produce sectors, and the fishing industry. Addressing and reducing the demand for trafficking must be part of the larger portfolio to abolish trafficking.

The foundation for the demand of trafficked victims is complex; however, disregard of basic human rights, attitudes and practices of female and male sexuality, and devaluation of men, women, and children are key underpinnings to this crime. Normalization of prostitution, zoning allowances for barrios and neighborhoods as so-called red light districts, turning a blind eye to sex tourism, or local law enforcement participation in prostitution all contribute to the demand.

It is ironic that within the countries where the value of women is great and where there are organized women's movements, relatively few local women are available for commercial sexual exploitation. Thus some of the brothels in first world countries are filled with women from the developing world, and countries like the United States, Germany, and the Netherlands have become desirable destination countries. More than 50% of prostitutes in Germany are not German but illegal immigrants, and more than 80% of Dutch prostitutes are not born in the Netherlands.[49] Movement is essential because of customer demand for "novelty." There are rings of networks that arrange for rotation of the trafficked persons to various cities so that the clientele have options, and so trafficked persons are kept from friends, families, and what is familiar to prevent escape.

When countries and laws have attempted to reduce sex trafficking and prostitution through legalization, the number of brothels and demand have increased.[50] Legalization brings in sex tourism and increases the demand by local men. When the supply of local women does not meet demand, women are trafficked in from outside the city or country.[51] These women are less expensive, more novel to the customer base, and easier to control by the pimps.

Laws that punish the john or pimp, rather than targeting the victim, have been shown to reduce demand. The experience of the Swedish government in combating trafficking demonstrates that legislative efforts and enforcement to identify and punish the trafficker significantly reduces the number of women in prostitution and the buyers of sex. In 1999, Sweden implemented a law that increased penalties and fines for traffickers, brothel owners, and pimps while removing the solicitation penalty for prostitutes. The government coupled this with a public awareness campaign about these changes in criminal law and penalties.[52] Two years after the new policy, there was a 50% decrease in women in prostitution, a 75% decrease in men buying sex, and trafficking decreased as well. Sex trafficking of eastern Europeans to Sweden decreased while neighboring countries saw a rise. The fear of prosecution plus the lowered demand discouraged further sex trafficking into Sweden.[53] Thus it appears that to reduce demand and to fight trafficking, prosecution of traffickers must be the focus of legislation and activism.

In the 2000 TVPA, demand was not mentioned; however, in subsequent reauthorizations addressing demand was included. In the 2005 TVPRA, addressing demand was mentioned as a way to prevent human trafficking, although it was not seen as having much impact. In contrast, the U.S. DoD, through a Presidential Order, took a zero tolerance approach to trafficking in 2005 by making the solicitation of prostitution a specific crime under the Uniform Code of Military Justice. The Wilberforce TVPRA of 2008 addressed demand reduction domestically and internationally and underscored the importance of DOJ reports on arrests in the Uniform Crime Reporting Systems.

More local examples point the way to possible success in demand reduction. The First Offender Prostitution Program in San Francisco is designed to educate men arrested for soliciting prostitutes about the negative consequences of prostitution. The program is a partnership between the local district attorney, police department, and a local nonprofit organization called, Standing Against Global Exploitation. Johns arrested are given a choice of prosecution or paying fines and taking classes, which are also known as "john schools." It is regarded as a cost-effective and transferable program to other states.[54] Other techniques such as use of billboards to show the face and name of a convicted trafficker, or impounding a trafficker's car, have demonstrated some anecdotal success.

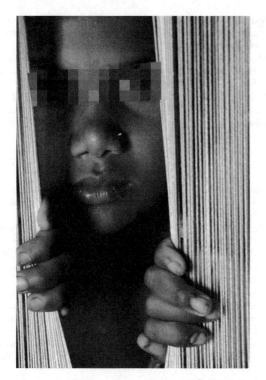

Figure 5-8. Children like this young girl are prized in the carpet industry for their small fast fingers. Defenseless, they do what they are told, toiling in cramped, dark, and airless village huts from sunrise until well into the night. (*Courtesy of Kay Chernush for the U.S. State Department. http://www.gtipphotos.state.gov.*)

Clearly, further research into the effectiveness and sustainability of demand reduction programs is needed before they can be rolled out and taken to scale.

MEASURES OF EFFECTIVENESS

Public health has had a strong tradition of monitoring and evaluation. Within the domain of anti-trafficking work, however, monitoring and evaluation are in a nascent stage. As management tools, monitoring allows for effective and efficient project implementation, and evaluation allows for objective ongoing periodic assessment or end-of-project assessment to determine if the intended goals and objectives of the intervention(s) were achieved. The IOM has produced a handbook on performance indicators for counter-trafficking.[55] The handbook is a resource and guide for project managers, developers, implementers, evaluators, and donors working in the field. It is not a comprehensive guide but suggests more objective measures of success in anti-trafficking work that anecdotal accounts or results do not translate into other project designs and plans. Indicators can reflect various stages of maturation of an anti-trafficking program. They can focus on input, process, output, outcome, or impact. They must be clearly defined, consensus driven, and SMART (specific, measurable, attainable, relevant, and trackable or timely). They should be developed at the project design stage and not as an afterthought. Besides their accountability functions, indicators of monitoring and evaluation can be used for advocacy purposes, project improvement, or course corrections.

In assessing the effectiveness of health services for trafficked victims, simple measures can include health providers' levels of knowledge or identification of suspected trafficked persons, the quality of medical treatment and care of trafficked victims, or the level of victim satisfaction with the medical services they receive. The IOM handbook details information on the project purpose, performance indicators, targets, and means of verification (data collection, data source).

RESEARCH NEEDS

The dearth of quantitative data on the health implications of human trafficking is a current limitation. There are seminal studies and researchers, but their numbers are small. This situation, therefore, calls for well-designed research and systematic collection of data that can form the evidence base for many purposes. Future studies can focus on prevention, protection, prosecution, and partnerships on health policy or health practice. Research data on services to trafficked persons should come from many sources including after-care facilities, urgent care and emergency department settings, community health centers, and free clinics. The lack of published data makes it difficult to advocate at both policy levels and local levels. Little data are available on the global burden of health issues, and there are few reports on trends or geographic patterns. Presently, data on health consequences of trafficking tend to be anecdotal or not generalizable to subpopulations because geographic, cultural practices, and local socioeconomic variables make data specific to a trafficked population. Further studies are needed on the characteristics of traffickers and victims, root causes and triggering events of trafficking, cost-effectiveness of models of aftercare and vocational training, and the impact of legislation on local trafficking activities. Researchers must investigate the socioeconomic, cultural, political, and legal factors that drive human trafficking. Such information can help to adapt messaging to vulnerable populations. Research data can provide compelling arguments for future funding. Collections of best or promising practices can serve to inform programs of more effective use of staff and funds.

```
┌─────────────────────────────────────┐
│                                     │
│             BOX 5-7.                │
│  - - - - - - - - - - - - - - - - -  │
│                                     │
│  National Human Trafficking Hotline: Call 1-888-373-│
│  7888 if you think someone is a victim of human     │
│  trafficking.                                       │
│                                     │
└─────────────────────────────────────┘
```

CONCLUSION

As a centuries-old practice, human trafficking continues to be a global problem. Clear estimates of its magnitude and impact are difficult to ascertain because of its illicit and criminal nature. However, we know that no country, culture, class, age, or gender is immune from trafficking. The health impact on individuals, communities, and countries is manifest in many ways, and for the unsuspecting health practitioner, the phenomenon may be hidden in plain sight. Data show that a law-centric approach is only part of the solution; a public health perspective on anti-trafficking can bring to light new ways of identifying and addressing this scourge. For the health care provider and the public health specialist, combating trafficking requires multipronged approaches in prevention, protection, prosecution, and partnership.

STUDY QUESTIONS

1. What are the common health consequences of human trafficking? Give examples of sex trafficking and labor trafficking. Are any of these more common in boys than girls or adults versus youth?

2. What measures do you think would be most effective in reducing demand for trafficking?

3. Study the list of tiered countries from the Department of State *Trafficking in Persons Report* for 2013. Do you see any patterns, trends, or reasons why some countries may be more likely to be on watchlists or tier 3 lists?

4. What could you do to engage in the fight against human trafficking? Provide examples of activities within each of the four P's.

5. Identify two key areas of research where data could be applied to more effective anti-trafficking work and to leverage funding.

SELECTED RESOURCES

Bales, K. *Disposable People: New Slavery in the Global Economy.* Berkeley: University of California Press, 2004.

Bales K. *Ending Slavery: How We Free Today's Slaves.* Berkeley: University of California Press, 2007.

Bales K, Soodalter R. *The Slave Next Door: Human Trafficking and Slavery in America Today.* Berkeley and Los Angeles: University of California Press, 2009.

Blunt R. *Crossed Lives—Crossed Purposes: Why Thomas Jefferson Failed and William Wilberforce Persisted in Leading an End to Slavery.* Searcy, AR: Resource Publications, 2012.

Cadet JR, Cadet CN. *Restavek. From Haitian Slave to Middle-Class American.* Austin: University of Texas Press, 1988.

Farley M, ed. *Prostitution, Trafficking, and Traumatic Stress.* New York: Haworth Press, 2003.

Grant B, Hudlin CL, eds. *Hands That Heal: International Curriculum to Train Caregivers of Trafficking Survivors.* Baltimore, MD: FAAST (Faith Alliance Against Sex Trafficking), 2007.

Haugen G, Hunter G. *Terrify No More: Young Girls Held Captive and the Daring Undercover Operation to Win Their Freedom.* Nashville, TN: Thomas Nelson, 2005.

Hochschild A. *Bury the Chains: Prophets and Rebels in the Fight to Free an Empire's Slaves.* Boston: Houghton Mifflin Harcourt, 2006.

International Organization for Migration. *Caring for Trafficked Persons: Guidance for Health Providers.* Geneva: IOM, 2009.

International Organization for Migration. *Listening to Victims: Experiences of identification, Return and Assistance in South-Eastern Europe.* Geneva: International Center for Migration Policy Development, 2007.

International Organization for Migration. *The IOM Handbook on Direct Assistance for Victims of Trafficking.* Geneva: IOM, 2007.

Kristof ND, WuDunn S. *Half the Sky: Turning Oppression into Opportunity for Women Worldwide.* New York: Vintage Books, 2010.

Lloyd R. *Girls Like Us: Fighting for a World Where Girls Are Not for Sale: A Memoir.* New York: Harper Perennial, 2011.

U.S. Department of State, Office to Monitor and Counter Trafficking in Persons. *Trafficking in Persons Report* 2012 and prior years. http://www.state.gov/j/tip/rls/tiprpt/2012/.

Zimmerman C, Hossain M, Yun K, et al. *Stolen Smiles: A Summary Report on the Physical and Psychological Health Consequences of Women and Adolescents Trafficked to Europe.* London: The London School of Hygiene and Tropical Medicine, 2006.

REFERENCES

1. Actual cases (names changed) from the U.S. Department of State, Office to Monitor and Combat Trafficking in Persons, 2012.

2. Teen Girls' Stories of Sex Trafficking in the US, *ABC News*, February 9, 2006. http://abcnews.go.com/Primetime/story?id=1596778&page=1.

3. Bales K. *Ending Slavery: How We Free Today's Slaves.* Berkeley: University of California Press, 2007.

4. International Labor Organization, June 2012. http://www.ilo.org/global/lang–en/index.htm.

5. Bales, K. *Disposable People: New Slavery in the Global Economy.* Berkeley: University of California Press, 2004.

6. To learn more about the new estimate, go to: http://www.ilo.org/global/about-the-ilo/press-and-media-centre/news/WCMS_181961/lang–en/index.htm.

7. Zimmerman C, Yun K, Shvab I, et al. *The Health Risks and Consequences of Trafficking in Women and Adolescents: Findings*

from a European Study. London: London School of Hygiene and Tropical Medicine, 2003.

8. Strenz T. The Stockholm Syndrome: law enforcement policy and ego defenses of the hostage. *Ann N Y Acad Sci* 1980;347: 137–150.

9. Last John. *A Dictionary of Epidemiology,* 2nd ed. Oxford, UK: Oxford University Press, 1988:115.

10. Ibid., 46.

11. International Programme on the Elimination of Child Labour Trafficking: The ILO's response through IPEC. Geneva, 2007. http://www.ilocarib.org.tt/index.php?option=com_content&view=article&id=9 15:world-day-against-child-labour-2007-to-focus-on-the-elimination-of-child-labour-in-agriculture&catid=204:2007-news&Itemid=1210.

12. Shared Hope International. Vancouver, WA. www.sharedhope.org.

13. IOM. 2008 CTM database and CTM thematic research series. Geneva. http://www.iom.int/jahia/webdav/shared/shared/mainsite/activities/ct/iom_ctm_database.pdf.

14. Yousafzia S, Moreau R, Bourreau M. The opium brides of Afghanistan. *Newsweek,* April 7, 2008.

15. Sex trafficking of young people in Poland. ECPAT International-http://ecpat.net/EI/Publications/Trafficking/Factsheet_Poland.pdf.

16. Stratford D, Ellerbrook T, Akins J, et al. Highway cowboys, old hands, and Christian truckers: risk behavior for human immunodeficiency virus infection among long-haul truckers in Florida. *Soc Sci Med* 2000;50:737, 746.

17. Internet Safety 101, Enough is enough, 2009. http://www.internetsafety101.org/.

18. Wolak J, Finkelhor D, Mitchell K. *Online Victimization of Youth: Five Years Later.* Durham, NH: National Center for Missing and Exploited Children, 2006. http://www.unh.edu/ccrc/pdf/CV138.pdf.

19. State or Territory Sex Offenders Registries—States and Puerto Rico. U.S. Census Bureau, July 2006; and U.S. Department of Justice Statistics, 2008; Internet Safety Workbook, p. 55. http://www.nsopw.gov/Core/PublicRegistrySites.aspx.

20. Enough is Enough, www.enough.org.

21. *Internet Safety 101 Workbook: Rule and Tools.* Reston, VA: Enough Is Enough, 2009:95–132.

22. National Center for Missing and Exploited Children. www.missingkids.com.

23. Edwards J, Iritani B, Hallifors D. Prevalence and correlates of exchanging sex for drugs or money among adolescents in the United States. *Sex Transm Infect* 2006;82:354–358.

24. Estes RJ, Weiner NA. *The Commercial Sexual Exploitation of Children in the US, Canada, and Mexico.* Philadelphia, PA: University of Pennsylvania, 2001. http://www.sp2.upenn.edu/~restes/CSEC_Files/Complete_CSEC_020220.pdf.

25. Zimmerman C, Hossain M, Yun K, et al. *Stolen Smiles: The Physical and Psychological Health Consequences of Women and Adolescents Trafficked to Europe.* London: London School of Hygiene and Tropical Medicine, 2006.

26. Raymond J. *A Comparative Study of Women Trafficked in the Migration Process.* New York: Ford Foundation, 2002.

27. Zimmerman C, Hossain M, Yun K, et al. The health of trafficked women: a survey of women entering post-trafficking services in Europe. *Am J Public Health* 2008;98(1):55–59.

28. Silverman JG, Decker MR, Gupta J, et al. Syphilis and hepatitis B co-infection among HIV infected sex trafficked women and girls, Nepal. *Emerg Inf Dis* 2008;14(6): 932–934.

29. Chacham AS, Diniz SG, Maia MB, et al. Sexual and reproductive health needs of sex workers: two feminist projects in Brazil. *Reprod Health Matters* 2007;15(29):108–118.

30. Huda S. Sex trafficking in South Asia. *Int J Gynaecol Obstet* 2006;94(3):374–381.

31. Silverman J, Decker M, Gupta J. HIV prevalence and predicators of infection in sex-trafficked Nepalese girls and women. *JAMA* 2007;298(5):536–542.

32. Sarkar K, Bal B, Mukherjee R, et al. Young age is a risk factor for HIV among female sex workers—an experience from India. *J Infection* 2006;53(4):255–259.

33. Dovydaitis T. Human trafficking: the role of the health care provider. *J Midwifery Womens Health* 2010;55(5):462–467.

34. Farley M. *Prostitution, Trafficking and Traumatic Stress.* New York: Haworth Press, 2003.

35. Farley M. Prostitution and trafficking in nine countries: an update on the violence and post-traumatic stress disorder. *J Trauma Pract* 2003;2(3–4):33–74.

36. Willis BM, Levy BS. Child prostitution: global health burden, research needs, and interventions. *Lancet* 2002;359:1417–1422.

37. World Health Organization. *Ethical and Safety Recommendations for Interviewing Trafficked Women.* Geneva: WHO, 2003.

38. Department of State. J/TIP link to annual TIP reports. http://www.state.gov/j/tip/rls/tiprprt/index.htm.

39. Todres J. Moving upstream: the merits of a public health approach to human trafficking. *Georgia State Law, 89 NCL Rev 447 2011.* Social Science Research Network Electronic Paper Collection. http://ssrn.com/abstract=1742953.

40. American Academy of Child and Adolescent Psychiatry Fact Sheet #9. Child Sexual Abuse. http://www.aacap.org/cs/root/facts_for_families/child_sexual_abuse.

41. National Center for Missing and Exploited Children. www.ncmec.org.

42. Slavery Footprint. How Many Slaves Work for You? www.slaveryfootprint.org

43. UNHCR. *Recommended Principles and Guidelines on Human Rights and Human Trafficking, Report of the United Nations High Commissioner for Human Rights to the Economic and Social Council (E/2002/68/Add.1).* New York: United Nations Economic and Social Council, May 20, 2002.

44. World Health Organization. *Resource Book on Mental Health, Human Rights, and Legislation.* Geneva: WHO, 2005.

45. World Health Organization. *Guidelines for Medico-Legal Care for Victims of Sexual Violence.* Geneva: WHO, 2003.

46. International Organization for Migration. *The IOM Handbook on Direct Assistance for Victims of Trafficking.* Geneva: IOM, 2007.

47. Physicians for Human Rights. *Examining Asylum Seekers: A Health Professional's Guide to Medical and Psychological Evaluation of Torture.* Cambridge, MA: Physicians for Human Rights, 2001.

48. Organization for Security and Cooperation in Europe. *National Referral Mechanisms Joining Efforts to Protect the Rights of Trafficked Persons: a Practical Handbook.* Warsaw: OSCE, 2004.

49. Leidholdt D, Executive Director. *Demand and the Debate.* Coalition Against Trafficking in Women, 2003. http://www.catwinternational.org/.

50. Malarek V. *The Natashas: Inside the New Global Sex Trade.* New York: Arcade, 2004.

51. Hughes D. *Foreign Government Complicity in Human Trafficking: A Review of the State Department's 2002 Trafficking in Persons Report.* Testimony before the U.S. House Committee on International Relations. Washington, DC, June 19, 2002.

52. Swedish Ministry of Industry. *Employment and Communications. 2004 Fact Sheet*: Prostitution and Trafficking in Women.

53. Ekberg GS. Prostitution and trafficking: the legal situation in Sweden. Paper presented at Journeésde formation sur la mondialization de la prostitution et du traffic sexuel. Association Québécoise des organisms de cooperation international. Montreal, Quebec, Canada.

54. Shively M, Jalbert SK, Kling R, et al. Final report on the evaluation of the first offender prostitution program. National Institute of Justice/National Criminal Justice Reference Service, March 2008.

55. International Organization for Migration. *Handbook on Performance Indicators for Counter-Trafficking Projects*. Geneva: IOM, 2008.

Environmental Health in the Global Context

6

Jeffrey K. Griffiths and Edward Winant

LEARNING OBJECTIVES

- *Understand the major ways in which environmental pollutants such as industrial chemicals make their way into humans*
- *Learn appropriate methods of personal drinking water treatment and sanitation for traveling and living in the developing world*
- *Learn to recognize health problems caused by contaminated drinking water or inadequate wastewater treatment and the benefits enjoyed by populations with good drinking water and sanitation*
- *Gain a basic understanding of appropriate methods of treating community drinking water and wastewater in the developing world*
- *Understand the magnitude of, health effects associated with, air pollution*

Environmental factors profoundly influence human health. A 2006 report by the World Health Organization (WHO) estimated that 24% of the world's burden of disease, and about a third of the burden in children, is due to preventable environmental factors.[1] By *preventable,* it is meant that these risks can be altered or mitigated. This burden of avoidable disease is disproportionately felt by the residents of poor countries, with attributable disease burdens often 10-fold higher or more than that seen in wealthier nations.[2] Reasons for the disproportionate effects felt in developing countries include a lack of modern technology, weak protective environmental laws and regulations, a lack of awareness, and poverty.[3] Nonetheless, residents of wealthy countries are also

affected by air pollution, poorly designed urban environments, flooding, and lead poisoning, among other risks, and thus environmental health is truly of global concern.

Unclean water and poor sanitation remain the most potent environmental causes of illness worldwide. Industrial chemical contaminants affect health everywhere. Of the more than 30,000 chemicals commonly used today, fewer than 1% have been studied in detail as to their health effects and toxicity,[4] and our understanding of the effects of simultaneous low-level exposure to hundreds or thousands of chemicals is rudimentary at best. Air pollution has been found to be a top-ranked problem in nearly every country undergoing economic transition. This chapter outlines a number of the global environmental challenges to health.

BIOLOGIC, PHYSICAL, AND CHEMICAL ENVIRONMENTAL RISKS AND THEIR AVOIDANCE

Environmental hazards include biologic, physical, and chemical ones, along with the human behaviors that promote or allow exposure. Some environmental contaminants are difficult to avoid (the breathing of polluted air, the drinking of chemically contaminated public drinking water, noise in open public spaces); in these circumstances, exposure is largely involuntary. Amelioration or elimination of these factors may require societal action, such as public awareness and public health measures. In many countries, the fact that some environmental hazards are difficult to avoid at the individual level is felt to be more morally egregious than those hazards that can be avoided. Having no choice but to drink water contaminated with very high levels of arsenic, as is the situation in Bangladesh, or being forced to passively inhale tobacco smoke in restaurants, outrages people more than the personal choice of whether an individual smokes tobacco. These factors are important when one considers how change (risk reduction) happens.

It should be noted that environmental health hazards often affect political elites as well as the poor in many countries. Although there are usually higher risks for the poor than the rich, principally because the rich enjoy improved disinfection of drinking water and sanitation, other hazards, such as air pollution or chemical and heavy metal contamination of foodstuffs, can affect all sectors of society, assisting in the development of a political consensus for change.

Some environmental hazards are associated with specific individual human behaviors, which in principle can be changed. In the absence of clean water and sanitation, simple handwashing with soap has been shown to dramatically decrease the rates of infectious diseases such as diarrhea, pneumonia, and impetigo.[5] Occupational exposures to pesticides, fertilizers, and microbial pathogens can be minimized by the use of protective gear, careful application techniques, and the provision of water and soap for decontamination. Irrigation not only improves crop production but also provides a conducive environment for the expansion and transmission of waterborne diseases such as schistosomiasis. In this case, reducing body contact with water will decrease rates of disease.

The handling of environmental hazards to human health must be tailored to the contaminant(s) and to the associated behaviors. It usually involves an assessment of the health burden, the routes of exposure, and identification of the stakeholders. Economic factors are often critical. Because the burden of disease may fall on people who do not share in the economic or social benefits of an environmental hazard, community action or political negotiations are often involved in the amelioration of environmental risks.

Biologic Hazards

The term *biologic hazards* usually refers to diseases caused by pathogens such as viruses, bacteria, prions, fungi, and parasites. It should be noted that the product of an infection can cause disease as well as the live pathogen. For example, in Ghana and other countries where foodstuffs may be stored in a damp state, fungal infections of tubers or maize (corn) produce aflatoxins, proteins that are potent carcinogens that especially affect the liver.

An astounding 94% of the disability-adjusted life years (DALYs) of disease burden due to diarrhea, principally caused by viruses and bacteria, is environmental in origin.[1] Approximately 1.5 million deaths a year, mostly in young children, are caused by poor sanitation, contaminated water, and lack of hygiene (a complex behavioral and socioeconomic component).

When feces and urine are not disposed of carefully, and when hygiene (the ability to wash hands with soap) is absent, human pathogens contaminate food, surface and groundwater, and hands. Lifespan in the United States increased in the period from 1900 to 2000 by more than 3 decades, and a good two thirds of this increase has been attributed to clean water, clean food, and sanitation.[6] One reason that some countries with limited budgets for health, such as Cuba and Costa Rica, have recently achieved major increases in lifespan and major decreases in childhood mortality and adult morbidity is that they have focused on water and sanitation risks.[7] If you take a single point away from this chapter, it is the crucial importance of keeping human and animal feces out of water and food.

Pathogens found in human feces are exquisitely adapted to causing human disease, and it should be obvious that breaking the cycle of transmission through basic sanitation and the provision of clean water should be an extraordinarily high societal priority.[8] The major pathogens causing illness and death through these transmission pathways include rotavirus, enteroviruses (a group that includes polio), *Salmonella, Shigella, Escherichia coli, Cryptosporidium, Campylobacter,* and hepatitis A and E viruses. Some of these are shared with domestic or peridomestic animals of economic importance, such as *Salmonella, Campylobacter, E. coli,* and *Cryptosporidium.* Typhoid (*Salmonella typhi*), in contrast to most of these pathogens, is a disease only of humans, and one way to judge the adequacy of water treatment and sanitation is to look at decreases in typhoid incidence.

Water Supply

The issues of water supply and sanitation in the developing world are of great importance. As the saying goes, "An ounce of prevention is worth a pound of cure." More to the point is the fact that public health engineers have saved many more lives than doctors over the course of human history. Safe, clean drinking water and adequate sanitation are critical needs for the developing world. However, projects to improve these conditions must include appropriate technology, cultural sensitivity, and long-term management procedures or they will quickly fail.

Water supply starts at the source, either surface water or groundwater. Surface water (i.e., streams, lakes, rivers, or ponds) is easily found and used. Large rivers and lakes provide year-round sources of water, whereas small streams and ponds may fail in dry seasons. Impoundments (dams) may be used to store stream flow from the wet season to supply community needs during the dry season. However, all surface water sources are unprotected. That is, they are very susceptible to pollution and should not be used without treatment.

Groundwater falls into two sources, shallow and deep. Shallow groundwater comes from water infiltrating the soil and trickling down until it is caught on top of the bedrock. This upper aquifer, or water table, fluctuates in depth depending on the season, dropping in dry seasons and rising in wet weather. Although the soil can filter out many pollutants, shallow groundwater is susceptible to pollution and should be used with care.

Shallow groundwater is tapped through wells or springs. Shallow wells are typically hand dug down to the water table and use a hand pump or bucket to bring water up. Springs are natural points where the water table meets the ground surface and water seeps out. Typically these occur at the toes of slopes or on hillsides.

Shallow wells and springs are very common water sources for developing countries. Although they are not pristine sources of water, the method of getting water from them can add considerable pollution to the water, and the solutions are usually easy and inexpensive to use. For wells, a small wall around the top of the well made of stone, brick, or concrete serves to keep animals and small children from falling in and diverts rainwater runoff from entering the well. A cover also serves to protect the well from trash and pollution; providing a bucket and rope, with a windlass to gather the rope when out of use, solely for the well helps keep these items clean and keeps dirt out of the well (Figure 6-1).

Hand pumps provide the best protection for a shallow well because the well remains covered while the water is withdrawn. Further, using a bucket and rope will introduce some contamination because buckets are frequently set on the ground, and ropes pass through the unwashed hands of the users. Many types of hand pumps are available in developing countries, and their use is limited only by cost. They typically cost more than submersible electric pumps in the United States but have the advantage of working without power (Figure 6-2).

If an event occurs to contaminate a well, perhaps an animal drowning in the bottom, it is possible to "shock" the well to cleanse it. This will remove the existing pollution but will not guard against recontamination. The procedure is to add chlorine, typically in the form of bleach, to the well and then draw out all of the chlorinated water and dispose of it. This prevents people from drinking overchlorinated, and dangerous water, and removes the source of contamination. The bleach should be added to a bucket of water, mixed well, and then lowered into the well to mix with all of the water at the bottom. It is necessary to get an idea of how much water is in the bottom of the well so that the proper amount can be withdrawn. Without too much math, the volume is the area of

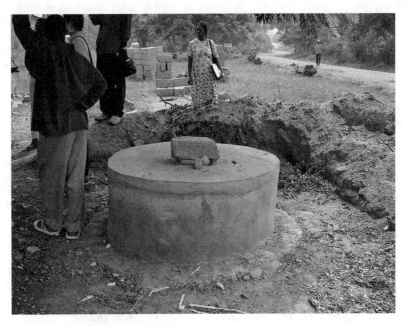

Figure 6-1. Protected well. (*Photo by Edward H. Winant.*)

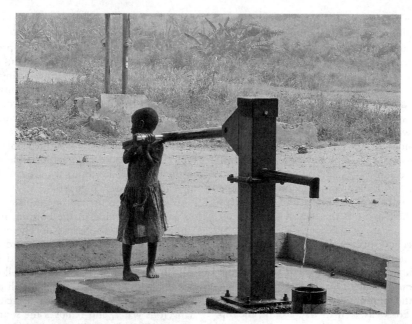

Figure 6-2. Hand pump. (*Photo by Edward H. Winant.*)

the well times the water depth. A typical circular well, 1 meter in diameter (3.28 feet) with a water depth of 2 meters (6.56 feet), holds

$h \times (\pi\ d^{2/4})$
$2 \times (3.14 \times 1^{2/4}) = 1.6$ cubic meters or 1,600 liters (410 gallons)

For a spring, a spring box or house helps gather the water from the ground and stores it in a protected place until needed. Typically, a pipe drains the box and allows users to fill their buckets under the pipe, keeping buckets and dirt out of the spring. Also, washing and bathing activities then take place downstream of the spring and do not affect the water quality at the source.

Deep wells, or boreholes, tap a water source (aquifer) that is much deeper and more protected than shallow wells. These deeper aquifers are contained in water-bearing rock layers under layers of impermeable rock. Thus their waters are safe from most forms of pollution but are also more of a finite resource because they are so hard to recharge.

Reaching these deep aquifers can be quite a challenge. They need to be drilled or bored into the rock with specialized machinery. Further, the hole has to be cased through the upper soil levels to keep potentially dirty waters out of the well. Finally, an electric submersible pump is extended into the hole to access the deep waters, thus requiring modern machinery and electricity for use.

A final source of drinking water is collecting rainwater. This is most commonly done on the roofs of houses, with gutters to collect and carry the rain to a storage basin, the prototypical American rain barrel. Gutters are fairly easy to install, but sizing the storage basin can be a problem. Ideally, it would be large enough to store all the water needed by the inhabitants of the building from one rainfall until the next. The difficulty arises because so many locations on earth have wet seasons and dry seasons, and the time between rainfalls may last weeks or even months. Storing enough rainfall from a rainy season to last through a dry season requires large and expensive storage tanks (Figure 6-3).

The other aspect of rainwater collection is that roofs are typically quite dirty, with leaves, sticks, and bird droppings. There are two solutions to the problem of a dirty roof: foul flush tanks and filters. The foul flush tank diverts and stores the initial rainfall, which is assumed to rinse the roof clean. After a short time, the rest of the rain is collected in the main storage tank. Filters are usually sand columns placed on top of the storage tank to remove contamination. Filtration is discussed in more detail later in the chapter.

Water Delivery

Once the water source has been identified and developed, some thought must be given to getting it to the users. The most common and low-tech method is to have users come to the water source and carry their

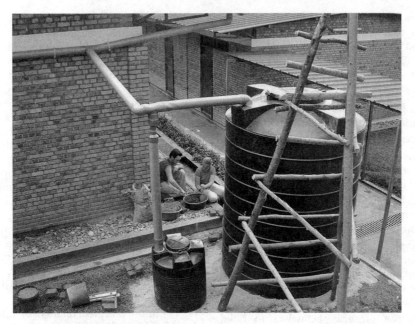

Figure 6-3. Rain water. (*Photo by Edward H. Winant.*)

daily supply home in buckets or jars. This requires a lot of human effort and also serves to reduce daily consumption. People are not inclined to take long baths or to waste water when they have to tote it a long way. In these cases, water use is usually restricted to cooking, cleaning, drinking, and occasionally bathing. Washing clothes and bathing may take place nearer to the source. This reduces the need for transporting water but usually leads to further contamination of the source water unless protective steps are taken as outlined previously.

Another method of water delivery is the commercial water cart. Here, larger supplies of water are brought to homes by cart, and the water is sold to the homeowner. Carts can vary from small pushcarts carrying 50 gallons or so to animal-drawn carts with a few hundred gallons, or to tanker trucks capable of delivering thousands of gallons.

The "modern," or preferred, method of water delivery is through pipes. Laying pipes in the ground is an expensive investment in community infrastructure, which is the main drawback to its universal adoption. When using pipes, it is also necessary to provide pressure to force the water through them. This is typically done by pumps, which require a power source. Water towers are usually included in the system because the demand for water varies through the day and can exceed the pumping rate. Thus towers store water at night, when demand is low, and assist the pumps in the morning and evening, when demand is highest.

In some places pressure may be provided by gravity, if the water source is sufficiently elevated above the users. When relying on gravity, storage tanks are sometimes required to maintain a sufficient supply of water.

A commonly adopted system is to pipe water into a community center from a remote source and then require users to carry their daily supply from the tap to their homes. This reduces individual treks to find water from miles of walking to more reasonable distances, but it also saves money on laying pipes throughout the community to every home.

Water Quantity

What options exist for poor rural people in the developing world? It must be recognized that in many places, an adequate *quantity* of water is more important than *quality*. Water may have to be carried, sometimes for miles, which consumes a huge amount of time, principally for women and children. In developed countries, the basic assumption is that each person uses 50 to 70 gallons per day (195 to 275 liters per day). Of course, this covers various uses such as watering the lawn, washing cars, laundry, automatic dishwashers, and teenagers taking long showers. The WHO suggests that the minimum amount in the developing world, where people must carry their own water, is 2.5 gallons per day (10 liters per day). An adult in the setting of drought needs at least 5 liters of water per day for basic food and hydration needs, without even considering the needs for basic hygiene (washing hands, etc.).[9] Actual use will fall somewhere in this range and will tend to increase if water is piped directly into each house. Thus efforts to decrease the environmental risks of unclean water must often address both quantity and quality.

- Feces should be kept out of water supplies with the use of basic or improved pit latrines.
- Water can be boiled if there is sufficient fuel in the area.
- Simple filtration (e.g., through cloth, such as a sari) will remove some pathogens, as has been amply demonstrated in Bangladesh and India.[10]
- It is being increasingly recognized that simply letting water settle after collection will carry many pathogens down with the sediment.
- Relatively simple methods for treatment at the household point of use—such as chlorinating water with the use of household bleach, or storing water in translucent or transparent vessels that allow ultraviolet (sunlight) sterilization to occur—are being tested.
- Communities can organize themselves to build simple water distribution systems, using PVC or similar pipes, where the source water is upstream of the community and therefore unlikely to be fecally contaminated.

Water Quality

With water provided to homes, the next thought is treating it to improve the water quality and reduce incidents of sickness. Treatment may occur on many levels, from small doses for the individual, to a household system for all occupants, to communitywide treatment systems. However, the basic steps and methods of treatment are similar at all levels.

Water treatment consists of three basic steps, although not every method includes all the steps.

1. Primary, or physical, treatment consists of settling out particles in the water.
2. Secondary, or biologic, treatment involves filtering the water through a benign biologic layer to reduce organic contamination. The biologic layer is typically fixed or suspended in some type of filter medium, such as sand. Modern plants in the developed world sometimes use plastic shapes or grids for the same purpose.
3. Tertiary, or chemical, treatment (also known as disinfection) is aimed at killing and removing harmful pathogens in the water. The most common chemical for disinfection is chlorine.

Personal water treatment, mostly used in travel situations, consists of either portable filters (backpacking water filters) or chemical tablets. Backpacking filters use a hand pump to force water through extremely small pores in a filter medium and remove particles, organic materials, and possibly pathogens, depending on the pore size. Tablets, either chlorine or iodine, disinfect the water, killing pathogens but not removing any silt, particles, or organic material. These tablets will not remove color or existing bad taste from the water.

Household treatment accounts for daily water use for several people. The simplest method is to store water in large covered barrels. This form of primary treatment will settle out particles in the water that lead to bad taste and color. Secondary treatment, or filtration, can be achieved with a range of commercially bought units that use porcelain candles or fabric bags to strain out contaminants. In general, the pore sizes on these filters are not small enough to remove pathogens, so a disinfection step is also required. Forcing water through a pore size small enough to remove pathogens requires pressure, and this complication would make most home-sized filters too complex (Figure 6-4).

The most accepted method of disinfection for a household is boiling. Water temperatures higher than

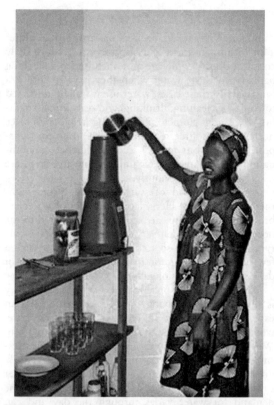

Figure 6-4. Home water. (*Photo from "Water in Africa" U.S. Peace Corps Photograph Archive. http://www.peacecorps. gov/wws/educators/enrichment/africa/index.html.*)

140°F (60°C) will kill pathogens. Of course, without a thermometer it is hard to judge 140°F, so bringing the water to boiling temperature is a nice visual indication of the proper amount of heat. Some authorities recommend boiling water for 30 minutes to ensure complete disinfection. This can be quite wasteful of fuel, however, and simply bringing the water to a rolling boil at sea level is sufficient. At higher elevations, boiling water for 5 minutes or less will typically give good results. The water should be boiled in a covered pot for protection and be allowed to cool. When sufficiently cool, it may be poured into the filter or other storage container.

Household filters can also be constructed using local materials. Typically the container is an oil drum or other large barrel. Gravel is placed at the bottom around the outlet pipe, which needs to be punched through the barrel wall. The gravel should be small enough, such as pea gravel, so that the sand does not settle into the pore spaces. Over the gravel, at least 24 inches (0.60 m) of sand should be placed. This should leave enough room at the top of the barrel for water to stay while it filters through the sand. The outlet pipe should also be equipped with a tap, so that water may be withdrawn without problem. Of course, this means the filter needs to be raised enough to get a container under the tap.

Another good household disinfection method is using clay filters treated with colloidal silver, such as those made by Potters for Peace.[11] These filters, which can be made locally in almost any village, are inexpensive and do a fair job of destroying pathogens. The silver impregnation lasts for about a year of normal use before replacement is needed.

Of all these household treatment methods, the single most important is boiling because this does an effective job of removing pathogens, and every household has a way of heating water. Thus teaching villagers to boil water is the single most effective way of getting them to improve their water quality. It can be difficult to convince them of the need, however, because the fuel cost of boiling all drinking water can be excessive. However, this simple step can reduce the incidence of sickness dramatically, especially for infants, young children, and the aged.

Community water treatment is generally an extension of the procedures just mentioned. Settling basins are used to remove solid particles suspended in the water. Filters are then used to further purify the water, and then it is disinfected and stored.

Historically, the first community filters were slow sand filters. These were large beds of sand through which water slowly percolated. The slow rate of application kept the sand from getting clogged too often. When the sand had trapped enough contamination to clog the filter and reduce the percolation, the filter

was cleaned by manually raking the sand and removing the top layer. As demand for water in cities grew, these slow filters soon became too large, and rapid sand filters were introduced. As the name implies, the water is applied much more quickly to a rapid sand filter, and the filter tends to clog much sooner. The cleaning method is to apply a backwash periodically to the filter. Backwashing means forcing water through the filter in the reverse direction, which expands the sand, cleans out the clogging material, and readies the filter for continued operation. In developing countries with available land, especially for small communities, slow sand filters are preferred for their low cost and easily understood maintenance. Where land is not available, rapid sand filters should be considered.

For disinfection, the most commonly used chemical is chlorine. It comes in three forms: gas, liquid, and solid tablet. The gas form can be somewhat tricky, so for small systems, a liquid drip is the preferred method. This drip is introduced by a small feed pump into the water line so that the concentration of chlorine in the water is roughly constant. Chlorine is a dangerous chemical, both for the operator and for the end user if the concentration is too high. However, it is well understood, relatively inexpensive, and leaves a residual in the water line that continues to protect the quality of the water throughout transmission.

People living in the developed world as well as the developing world have the need to maintain rigorous water treatment and sanitation practices. The methods used for water treatment—halogenation, usually with chlorine or chloramines, and then filtration—were devised over a century ago, and although effective when optimally implemented, they suffer the deficiencies of old technology. Chlorination is highly effective against bacterial and viral infections, and when first instituted it uniformly leads to major decreases in the burden of disease due to these infections. However, it is ineffective against a number of emerging pathogens that are chlorine resistant. Many of these resistant pathogens are most active where especially susceptible populations exist, such as people with acquired immunodeficiency syndrome (AIDS) or pregnant women.

An epidemic of waterborne toxoplasmosis was detected in Vancouver, Canada, stemming from the use of water from a reservoir that was chlorinated but not filtered. Astute clinicians noted an increase in the number of cases of in utero (congenital) *Toxoplasma* infections, as well as retinal disease in the general population. An epidemiologic investigation revealed that cougar feces in the watershed contained *Toxoplasma* oocysts. Presumably, the infectious oocysts were washed by rainfall into the reservoir and (unaffected by the chlorination) then directly entered the drinking water supply.[12] To globalize this incident, one only needs to reflect on the absence of filtration in many countries where basic chlorination is provided. Estimates from Central America and Africa suggest that most cases of toxoplasmosis are the result of infection with the oocyst form of the parasite, which is only excreted by felines. In the United States and Europe, most toxoplasmosis is the result of eating undercooked meat that contains *Toxoplasma* cysts.[13] The addition of filtration to water treatment, even simple sand filtration, is believed to decrease the risk of infection from pathogens such as *Giardia, Cryptosporidium* (and, one supposes, *Toxoplasma*) by about 100-fold.[14]

Filtration is not a perfect defense, even though it may remove the vast majority of pathogens (99.00% to 99.99% of pathogens is typical for modern conventional treatment plants).[14] Unfortunately, the infectious dose needed to infect 50% of people for *Cryptosporidium* is under 10 oocysts for some strains,[15] suggesting that even the rare organism that slips through the filtration system can cause illness. The largest outbreak of waterborne disease in the history of the United States occurred in Milwaukee in 1993 when more than 400,000 people became clinically ill with cryptosporidiosis when one of the two filtration plants in Milwaukee failed.[16] Of note, infection rates in households with tap water filters were approximately 80% lower than in households without them. In 1994, an epidemic of cryptosporidiosis in Las Vegas in people with AIDS was epidemiologically linked to the municipal water supply, even though it met all relevant chlorination and filtration standards.[17] It must be emphasized that the two major causes of persistent diarrhea in people with HIV/AIDS in the developing world are cryptosporidiosis and microsporidiosis.[18] These pathogens cause chronic diarrhea and malabsorption with wasting. Neither of these diseases has reliably effective drug treatment, and thus prevention (through paired drinking water treatment and sanitation) is the only real option against these scourges.

The use of halogens in treating water introduces variable levels of these elements into water. Halogens have been linked (at higher levels) to bladder cancer, fetal congenital defects, and miscarriages.[19] The balance between a halogen level sufficient to kill pathogens and low enough to minimize other risks is a delicate but necessary one.[20] Failures of chlorination have led to outbreaks of dysentery and diarrhea in Canada[21] and typhoid in Central Asia,[22] proving the point that water treatment systems cannot be allowed to fail, no matter the location. One of the ironies of water treatment practices is that source water protection (e.g., not letting fecal material enter source water for drinking purposes) has been ignored in many communities, under the assumption that water treatment will invariably render the water completely safe.

A safer, although somewhat more expensive, method of disinfection is ultraviolet (UV) light. This involves passing the water past UV light bulbs, where the radiation kills off the pathogens. UV disinfection requires relatively "clean" water, meaning that most of the suspended solids have been removed.

Of course, the application of water treatment depends heavily on the source water available. Surface waters, being unprotected, are usually suspected of being highly contaminated with organic material and pathogens. Further, many rivers and streams carry a high silt load, so settling basins (primary treatment) are almost always required when treating surface waters. Springs and shallow wells may be contaminated, depending on what is "upstream" of them in a groundwater sense. Mountaintop springs, which basically are fed by pure rainwater, can be of very high quality. Springs situated below farms or houses are likely to be quite contaminated. Still, groundwater does not carry the silt loads that surface waters do, so in many cases disinfection is all that is required of spring or well water. Deep wells, if properly constructed and drawing from a quality source, may not require any treatment to be safe for drinking.

Sanitation

Sanitation deals with treating the waste products of human society and making them safe for the environment and for public health. This section discusses human waste (feces and urine) and solid waste (garbage).

As with water treatment, wastewater treatment falls into the same three levels: primary (physical), secondary (biologic), and tertiary (disinfection and polishing). Further, these apply to all wastewater treatment, from individual house systems up to the largest municipal plants.

Sanitation provides benefits beyond those of decreasing diarrheal disease. For example, intestinal nematode infections from *Ascaris, Trichuris,* and hookworm are all transmitted after fecal contamination of soil. The first two nematodes are ingested (either in soil or in contaminated uncooked food), and hookworm larvae penetrate the skin of people without shoes. All three of these cause diseases that contribute to malnutrition and to anemia but can be completely prevented by the implementation of adequate disposal of feces. In the United States, rural poor farmers residing in the southern areas of the country were once regarded as lazy, before it was understood that most of them were severely anemic from hookworm infections. After World War I, the Rockefeller Foundation devoted enormous resources to convincing people to spend scarce resources on shoes and sanitation facilities.[23] Schistosomiasis, a trematode infection, affects hundreds of millions of people, and the infectious eggs are all excreted in urine or feces. Again, simple sanitation would abolish this disease over time in affected regions.

The most common form of sanitation in developing countries is the latrine or outhouse. Latrines may be provided for individual houses or combined into a community facility. The latrine is a simple pit, covered with a durable slab, where users go to relieve themselves. Concrete slabs, at least 6 inches (15 cm) thick and reinforced with iron bars, make the best latrine floors. They are easy to clean, last a long time, and are very sturdy. A less expensive floor may make use of wooden planks or even logs.

Because no water is used to transport the waste, there is no need for wastewater treatment. The pit holds the solids, allowing for some biologic degradation, but in general serves only for storage. Eventually the pit will reach capacity, leading to removal of the solids or digging a new pit. Ash or lime is sometimes added to the pit to help control odors.

The pit is usually left unlined if it is dug in a stable soil such as clay. Where sandy soils predominate, some reinforcement of the pit may be required. Although there is no effluent to treat, the urine will seep out the pit floor and walls into the surrounding soil. This is normal, even beneficial, but some care must be taken to separate the pit from the surrounding groundwater.

Two feet (0.61 m) of soil separation is sufficient to protect the groundwater. Thus the pit should not be dug deeper than 2 feet above the water table. The water table may be determined roughly by the water depth of nearby shallow wells. Remember, however, that the water table will fluctuate according to wet and dry seasons; the latrine should be sited using the wet season water levels. If the groundwater level reaches the bottom of the pit, it will become contaminated and threaten nearby shallow wells and springs.

Where there are high groundwater tables, it may be necessary to construct vault latrines. This variation includes a lining for the pit of concrete, brick, or stonework to prevent groundwater contamination. Obviously, this method is more expensive, and so it is used only when absolutely required to protect the groundwater (Figure 6-5).

An implementation that many groups prefer is the ventilated, improved pit latrine (VIP latrine). This involves building solid walls that do not allow light through, a tight roof covering, and a screened ventilation pipe running to the top of the roof. The doorway must be set away from the prevailing winds, so that the wind draws air out of the latrine rather than forcing it in. Further, with no light in the latrine, the only light available to the pit comes from the pipe, which draws the flies up to the screen. Unable to escape, they die (Figure 6-6).

Culturally, VIPs are unacceptable to some people. Because they are so used to latrines, they consider it improper to relieve oneself inside. Adding a roof to a latrine makes it a building, and thus not suitable. Many latrines are thus simple affairs with walls of

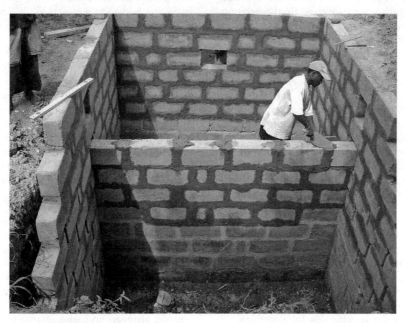

Figure 6-5. Vault latrine. (*Photo by Edward H. Winant.*)

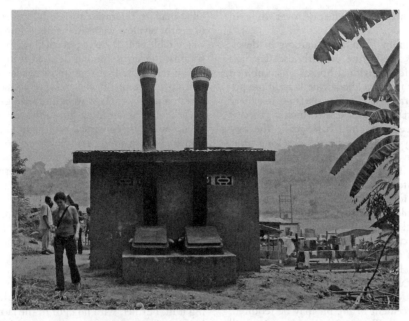

Figure 6-6. VIP latrine. (*Photo by Edward H. Winant.*)

plaited leaves or sheet metal for privacy, or situated so they are screened naturally by trees.

Another improvement on the common latrine is the composting latrine. This involves improvements to the pit so that air and heat are available to promote the composting process. Additionally, access is needed because the pile needs to be turned. This is usually done manually with a pitchfork to stir the accumulated waste. A carbon source is also needed and can be provided by sprinkling sawdust or throwing paper waste down the latrine hole after every use.

Once water is provided to individual homes, flush toilets can be installed, at which point wastewater becomes a much larger problem. The first step toward treatment is usually to pipe wastewater to the latrine pit, thus making it into a cesspool. However, this pit now has to deal with a great quantity of polluted water in addition to the solids it was storing. The water will leach out the sides of the pit; given the amounts of water used and the organic contamination, this will eventually clog the soil around the pit and back up into the house.

Septic systems, in which the solids settle into a tank and the effluent passes to a field of perforated pipes to soak into the ground, are much more effective in the long term. They require additional investment and a larger area for application, however. In areas of low housing density, they are undoubtedly the best method for wastewater treatment.

For areas of greater housing density, sewers are the preferred method. These large pipes, laid so gravity will convey the sewage, collect wastewater and convey it to a central treatment location. This treatment plant usually consists of settling tanks (primary treatment); biologic treatment, such as filters or aeration tanks (secondary treatment); perhaps some polishing or additional filtration, and then disinfection (tertiary treatment). The treated effluent is then discharged to a nearby surface water body; the removed solids, now called sludge, will be deposited in a land fill, incinerated, or used as a soil amendment or crop fertilizer.

Biologic treatment for community wastewater may be in several forms. The least technological is lagoons, or sewage ponds, where the sewage is contained for long periods of time to allow proper treatment. Lagoons do occupy large areas of land, but they do not require much maintenance. Sand filters are also frequently used to treat wastewater, as are aerobic tanks and wetlands. Aerobic tanks introduce air into the sewage to promote the growth of aerobic bacteria, which are very efficient at consuming organic waste. Filters work much the same as for water treatment, supporting a layer of bacteria that consume the organic waste, as well as physically straining the water to remove solids.

Constructed wetlands combine both methods of treatment. Here, the effluent flows through a gravel bed, which performs the tasks of a filter. Water-loving plants, such as reeds or cattails, grow in the gravel, and their roots provide oxygen for treatment, take up some of the effluent for their water needs, and also remove nitrogen and phosphorus from the waste as plant nutrients.

Proper sanitation also includes solid waste, or garbage. Sadly, this is commonly overlooked, and many villages have no way of dealing with their accumulating garbage. It is frequently piled in heaps or scattered about carelessly. Both conditions are unsightly, smelly, and can support rodents, insects, and other disease vectors.

When garbage is collected in central locations around the community, it is common to periodically set fire to the collected waste and burn off the combustibles. Although incineration is certainly an accepted method of reducing the volume of solid waste, it is helpful to attempt it in controlled conditions. Certain materials, notably plastics and tires, give off noxious fumes when burned. In general, the smoke from trash fires can be hazardous and is certainly annoying to nearby residents. Finally, some materials will not burn and will remain after the attempted incineration.

Another method of solid waste treatment is land filling. This requires a suitable area of land set aside to receive the solid waste, preferably away from most residents. It also requires soil to be placed over layers of garbage to contain the odors and disease vectors. The soil cover, with accompanying ditches and landscaping to control runoff, is important to keep water contaminated by the waste (termed *leachate*) away from other sources of water that serve the community. If possible, the floor of the landfill should be a heavy clay soil, compacted by machinery to further contain the leachate.

Given that landfills and dumps should not be too close to communities, a garbage collection and transport method should be established. Although it is certainly possible for each resident to make a trip to the town dump, it is more convenient to have local community collection points throughout the town and have the garbage picked up and taken to the landfill using community resources.

Recreational Water Exposure

Recreational water exposure has also been recognized as a potent source of fecal-oral contamination. Indeed, the U.S. Centers for Disease Control and Prevention defined swimming in pools and other recreational waters as "communal bathing" and has published studies on the average mass of feces carried by swimmers into pools. In the United States, epidemics of disease caused by *Giardia, Shigella,* and *Cryptosporidium* occur every year because of fecal contamination of recreational swimming sites such as pools, lakes, rivers, and beaches.[24] Recreational waters in some countries are contaminated not only by diarrheal fecal pathogens but also by parasitic pathogens such as schistosomes and by viruses such as polio, other enteroviruses, and hepatitis A. Historically, polio was frequently waterborne in the now-developed world, and swimming in rivers, ponds, or lakes (which are obviously not chlorinated) was a recognized risk for the disease.

Management of Water and Sanitation Systems

Use of community resources brings up an important point: management. In many cases, it is not the technology or even the resources that are a barrier to project implementation; it is the continued management of the project that causes failure. Any village in the world can dig latrines and shallow wells and provide for trash collection. What is lacking is the community management needed to marshal the community resources to accomplish these tasks and see to their continued operation and maintenance.

For instance, tales of broken and unrepaired pumps, caved-in wells, or dilapidated spring boxes are common throughout the developing world. Many of these projects are installed by well-meaning and dedicated volunteers and nonprofit organizations. The projects work well and are much appreciated for several years. But something eventually breaks, and there is no money to fix it. The impressive and helpful project goes to waste, and the residents return to their previous ways of getting water or eliminating waste.

It is important to involve local residents in project planning and implementation. This means more than just asking the opinions of the village elders. In many cases the elders, usually men, want a project that will bring prestige or honor to their village. However, the women and children who must make use of the new infrastructure have other ideas. For instance, when it is the children's job to get water, it is no good installing a hand pump that requires great strength to use. It is also sometimes the case that women who walk a good way to gather water at a remote spring cherish the communal time they have together and resent the piping of this spring into the village to relieve them of some of their hard work.

Thus project planning should involve representatives of all groups in a community. It should also deal with requirements for upkeep and use of the installed equipment. The minimum level of management should be the creation of a community committee charged with overseeing and maintaining the project. This committee should have a maintenance budget and a way to collect money from the users. For example, a hand pump costing $1,500 and expected to last 20 years should have $75 collected each year in a replacement fund ($6.25 each month). If this pump serves 25 homes, then each family would be expected to contribute $0.25 each month.

What happens, in many cases, is that some people do not pay, even when they have the best of intentions. Perhaps the harvest failed, or a child was sick and they needed the money for medicine. If they fail to pay and yet can still use the community resource (pump or spring box or latrine), they have less incentive to pay in the future. Neighbors, seeing this, are also less inclined to pay. Sadly, it is very common for no one to pay into community repair funds. Then, 15 or 20 years down the road, when the pump breaks or the latrine is full, there is no money to fix it.

It is helpful, therefore, to have some enforcement capacity for the committee. At the very least, peer pressure can be exerted on noncontributing families to encourage their participation. The most effective management, of course, is the utility model, where users pay for the amount of water or sanitation services that they use and can be cut off for nonpayment. This provides an enforcement action to ensure continued participation.

Disturbance of the Natural Environment and Risks for Infectious Diseases

Some ecosystems support *Anopheles, Culex,* or *Aedes* mosquitoes, which transmit diseases such as malaria, filariasis, dengue, and yellow fever. Brackish water, as found in coastal mangrove swamps, is a reservoir for *Vibrio cholerae,* the agent of cholera. Perhaps by convention or out of reverence for the natural environment, we do not usually consider a pristine swamp an environmental hazard. However, it is clear that our forebears did, for they industriously drained swamps to provide more arable land and to decrease the risks of diseases such as malaria. One of the greatest accomplishments of the fascist Italian dictator Mussolini was the drainage of the swamps near Rome and the eradication of malaria from the region. When the Tennessee Valley Authority in the United States built dams in the 1930s and 1940s to provide electricity to Appalachian areas, studious care was taken to alter the water levels periodically in dams and rivers to disrupt the hatching of mosquito eggs. This had, at times, devastating effects on the aquatic habitat of the affected rivers, but the incidence of malaria was dampened by these tactics.

A counterexample demonstrating the importance of intact ecosystems to human health is that of the Naivasha Lake region in the Rift Valley of Kenya. The town of Naivasha does not treat its sewage, which flows into a lake that is used for both drinking water purposes and fishing. Fortunately, the Kenya Wildlife Service maintains a game preserve where the contaminated water from the town flows into wetlands. The wetlands detoxify and decontaminate the wastes before they enter the lake. Indeed, the use of artificial wetlands in tropical countries is being promoted globally as a way to treat wastewater without the capital expense of a modern treatment plant.[25]

There is substantial evidence that the destruction of ecosystems increases the hazards of infectious diseases. Malaria epidemics often follow the construction of roads and houses in forested areas because new water pools (breeding sites for mosquitoes) are unintentionally left without adequate drainage near the construction. Indeed, deforestation of tropical forests, and the concomitant construction of crude logging roads to remove the trees, results in predictable increases in mosquito-borne infections. As an example, yellow fever is maintained in a high forest canopy (sylvan) cycle between primates and mosquitoes in South America that does not involve humans. When trees are felled by loggers, however, the yellow fever–infected mosquitoes then bite the workers, who carry the infection to cities, where the cycle is maintained in humans via *Aedes aegypti* mosquitoes (the urban cycle).

Other examples are plentiful. The damming of the Nile River at Aswan in Egypt led to an explosion in the incidence of schistosomiasis, as did the damming of the Volta River in Ghana. Schistosomes have difficulty penetrating the skin of human hosts in rapidly flowing waters, but the damming led to placid waters and greatly increased transmission. The introduction of irrigation in Puerto Rico for sugarcane production led to extremely high rates of schistosomiasis at the turn of the last century.[26] The several decades long increase in the incidence of Lyme disease in the densely populated northeastern United States is considered by most biologists to be the result of an exploding deer population (after elimination of their natural predators) and the desire of humans to live in suburban or semirural areas. Both of these factors increase the likelihood of exposure to the tick vector, which normally feeds on deer and mice. Thus environmental risks for acquiring infectious diseases often are linked to both disturbed or changed ecosystems and increasing human presence in the involved area.

As delineated by the WHO, three approaches to the environmental management of mosquito-borne diseases such as malaria, Japanese encephalitis, and dengue are as follows[1]:

1. Modification of the environment to reduce vector habitats
2. Manipulation of the environment on some periodic basis
3. Modification of human behavior or habitation

Draining swamps, leveling land, filling in pools, modifying river boundaries, lining irrigation canals to prevent water loss, and avoiding stagnant waters are examples of the first approach. In urban environments, these methods include the construction of drains, improving house design so that water does not pool in gutters, and providing wastewater and sanitation facilities to remove mosquito breeding sites.

The second approach is represented by efforts such as changing the levels of reservoirs. The third includes simple methods such as fine screens in household windows to decrease contact with mosquitoes, and the use of bednets. Bednets are an interesting tool because they incorporate both an environmental barrier between the vector and humans, and, if insecticide treated, a chemical defense as well. Treated bednets have been found to reduce overall mortality in children younger than 5 living in malaria-endemic regions by as much as 40%.[27]

Climate, the Environment, and Human Health

The linkage between climate, alterations in the environment, and specific diseases is regarded as well founded. The incidence of cholera in western South America and of diseases such as Oroya fever in the Andes has been linked to the sea temperature of the Humboldt Current, especially during El Niño phenomena.[28] The details and mechanistic explanations for these relationships are still being delineated, but it is not hard to imagine that sea temperature affects land conditions, which in turn affect vegetation and humidity, and in turn the density of insect vectors of disease. By way of example, my colleagues and I have shown that cases of *Salmonella* and *Campylobacter* infection reported to the Massachusetts Department of Public Health are tightly linked to the ambient temperature, whereas reported cases of *Cryptosporidium, Shigella,* and *Giardia* infections peak some weeks after the peak in summer temperature.[29] *Salmonella* and *Campylobacter* are known to reproduce in foodstuffs, and the coinciding peaks of temperature and infection with these two bacterial pathogens probably represent the product of maximal bacterial growth during the hottest days of the year. In contrast, it can be argued that the triad of *Cryptosporidium, Shigella,* and *Giardia* infections in Massachusetts represents transmission via recreational water exposure. Surface waters used for recreational purposes (ponds, rivers, outdoor pools) achieve their highest temperatures some weeks after ambient air temperatures peak, explaining the lag period, because people are most likely to swim when the water is warmest.

Environmental factors also include rainfall. In many cities and towns in the United States, surface water runoff is drained into the sewage treatment system because separate runoff and sewage treatment systems are more expensive than a combined system. However, heavy rainfall can overwhelm the capacity of sewage systems, leading to the discharge of untreated sewage into rivers or lakes. Indeed, Curriero and colleagues have shown that waterborne disease epidemics in the United States tend to follow periods of very heavy rainfall.[30] In the developing world, it has been noted that epidemics of diseases such as cryptosporidiosis tend to occur at the beginning of the rainy season when rainfall is likely to sweep human and animal wastes into waters eventually used for drinking and cleaning.[31]

Infectious disease is also the final mechanism by which other physical environmental factors cause human disease. For example, air pollution both decreases lung function and increases the risk of pneumonia.

Physical Hazards

Physical environmental hazards include not only catastrophic events such as hurricanes, drought, earthquakes, cyclones, and floods, but also the hazards of the human-constructed, or human-altered, environment. One way the constructed environment interacts with catastrophic environmental events is the building of towns in floodplains. Another way is extensive deforestation above towns, which promotes increased flash flooding and mudslides after heavy rains. The rainwater is no longer retained in the sponge of forest vegetation. In addition to the risk of catastrophic loss of life and property, even periodic minor flooding can be dangerous. It has been shown in Brazil that periodic flooding of lower-lying neighborhoods is strongly associated with hemorrhagic fever due to leptospirosis.[32]

Global warming is another physical hazard. Scientific consensus concludes that higher overall global temperatures have led to both higher and lower rainfall for different areas, higher sea levels, and at times drastic changes in climate and vegetation. Whereas climate determines the geographic range of infectious diseases, extreme weather related to climate variability (and manifested in our physical environment through rain, heat, cold, etc.) affects the timing and intensity of infectious disease outbreaks.[33]

The linkage between a changing climate, the environment, and human health may prove dramatic or subtle. Drought, which can be the result of both climate change and of deforestation, can lead to such severe economic shocks that the risk of civil war increases.[34] Catastrophic environmental events often lead to displaced populations and refugee communities. These catastrophes can be rapid (a flood, a drought) or slow (desertification near the Sahel, slow sea-level rises) but are, in either case, severe. For example, should the sea level rise by a meter in the next 50 years, a substantial minority of the population of Bangladesh will lose their low-lying land. How will they survive? Will they die of starvation as they lose their subsistence farmland, or will they attempt to emigrate into neighboring countries that are unlikely to welcome them (e.g., India, Myanmar)? Some Pacific island nations may become submerged. One can argue that this form of slowly advancing catastrophe is no less profound than a dramatic, immediate one.

The Built Environment

There is a growing recognition that the *built environment* (of towns, cities, and roads) can contribute to, or be deleterious to, health. Urban environments often provide social, economic, and cultural opportunities that more rural areas do not, and in so doing, they provide a mixture of environmental benefits and risks. For example, water treatment systems and sewerage (with their major benefits) are often more available in urban environments than in rural ones because cities have the ability to raise the capital for water and sewerage projects. Other aspects of urban life are negative: for example, some wealthy towns have eliminated sidewalks in residential areas and isolated commercial areas so they can only be reached by automobiles. This practice promotes the use of (polluting) automobiles even for minor errands and, through discouraging exercise, indirectly promotes obesity, diabetes, and cardiovascular disease.[35,36] High levels of noise are common in urban areas and in some occupations. It has been estimated that 16% of all deafness can be attributed to such occupational exposures.[1,37]

Pedestrian and traffic deaths are also a major concern. In northern Europe, roadway designs have been developed over the past 50 years that minimize pedestrian deaths from traffic accidents. Traffic speed is limited by "traffic calming" through roadway bumps, one-way streets, road narrowing, traffic circles, and other measures that decrease speed and increase the likelihood of pedestrian survival. These intelligent designs are uncommon; thus increased deaths from traffic accidents (as well as air pollution) commonly accompany urbanization. In many parts of the world, improvements in roadways are not accompanied by segregated bicycle lanes, parallel walking paths with roadside barriers, or designated pedestrian crossways. Pedestrian deaths then occur when people walk on roadways. Other contributing factors include a lack of street lighting and signage, narrow roads, and poor road maintenance. Traffic accident death rates in many countries are an order of magnitude higher than they are in developed countries such as the United States.[38] (Unbelievably, most motor vehicles imported into India are not currently equipped with seat belts as a so-called cost-saving measure.) Traffic accidents are believed to account for 2.6% of DALYs worldwide.[1] The leading cause of tourist death is traffic accidents, not infectious diseases.

Chemical Hazards

Naturally Occurring Chemical Risks

The natural physical environment can be a source of naturally occurring chemical and radiologic risks, such as heavy metals (arsenic) or radionuclides (uranium, radium, thorium, actinium, radon, etc.). For example, the U.S. Environmental Protection Agency (EPA) estimated that approximately 420,000 and 620,000 United States residents are potentially exposed to elevated levels of radium-228 and uranium, respectively, from drinking water.[39] Radon is the decay product of radium, which in turn is the decay product of uranium. It is a risk factor for lung cancer and usually present as a dissolved gas in groundwater. It is released into household basements from the surrounding ground or when groundwater with dissolved radon is aerosolized (e.g., in the shower). The EPA estimates that approximately 1 in 15 households in the United States is at risk of exposure to elevated levels of radon. The global burden of risk is unknown.[40] Uranium miners are at a very increased risk of cancer because of their occupational exposures to this potent carcinogen. In Europe this risk was recognized as early as 1879, yet little protection was afforded to miners in the United States before 1962, again demonstrating the need for adequate health regulations and standards for environmental exposures.[41]

Heavy metals exposure is common. Lead is ubiquitous: it is used in batteries and in industrial processes, added to paint and gasoline, and found in water distribution pipes and fittings. Lead exposure leads to mental retardation, anemia, and hypertension, among other conditions. Acutely high lead levels lead to anemia and seizures, but even chronically low levels are a cause for concern. In 2002, the WHO estimated that lead-associated mental retardation represented about 0.75% of all DALYs.[37] These risks existed even in ancient times; for example, the Romans ate and drank from lead cups and plates, and they added lead to foodstuffs. This practice is thought to have led to an epidemic of infertility. Leaded gasoline is still frequently used globally, and lead poisoning is common where its use in paint and gasoline has not been banned. The extent of this burden has been poorly studied.

Globally, more than 100 million people are believed to be exposed to high levels of arsenic from drinking water.[42] The digging of deep tube wells to provide potable water in Bangladesh has sharply decreased deaths due to fecally contaminated water but has sharply increased the incidence of skin disease, renal impairment, hypertension, and cancer because of arsenic contamination of the groundwater.[43] Estimates exist that a third of the Bangladeshi population is drinking water with an unacceptably high level of arsenic. In one study from the Matlab region of Bangladesh, 54% of people consumed water containing more than 50 µg/L of arsenic.[44] The U.S. National Academy of Sciences has concluded that there is no safe level of arsenic in water.[45] In contrast to the situation in Bangladesh, arsenic exposure in other areas is secondary to industrial processes or mining.

For example, exposure to high levels of arsenic (via water contamination) in the western United States is usually due to abandoned mine wastes (tailings) entering the water supply. In the eastern United States, high levels of arsenic are naturally found in some groundwater or in waters contaminated by industry over the past 150 years.[46]

Occupations such as sandblasting, place workers at risk of the scarring lung disease known as silicosis. Occupational exposures to hazardous physical environments are common and a major opportunity for decreasing the human disease burden. Occupational risks can include exposure to industrial chemicals and solvents, including carcinogens such as benzene as well as heavy metals such as mercury. Mercury is used to isolate gold from ore; in informal gold mines in South America, mercury poisoning affects not only the miners but also their families because they bring contaminated clothing home. In the rivers where the mercurial wastes are dumped, the mercury is concentrated in fish, which are then consumed by the population, further distributing the ill effects of mercury.[47] As described later in this chapter in the section on air pollution, the combustion of coal for power generation is another significant source of mercury exposure.

Synthetic Chemicals

As the world has industrialized, risks from nonnatural synthetic chemicals associated with manufacturing and agriculture have risen sharply. The manifestations of exposure to these chemicals depend on the class of chemical. Suffice it to say these manifestations may include damage to fetuses; malignancies; damage to specific organs such as the nervous system, kidneys, or liver; metabolic syndromes; and damage to fertility. Exposure to these chemicals can occur occupationally; through contamination of food, water, or air; and through dermal contact. It is not possible in the space of this chapter to review all of these, and indeed the global burden of disease from synthetic chemicals is unknown.

Pesticides and herbicides have achieved a level of notoriety related to their overuse and application without safety precautions. Many examples exist of neurologic effects due to acute exposures.[48] Chronic exposures to these agents can lead to unexpected results. For example, the pesticide 1, 2-dibromo-3-chloropropane (DBCP) was developed in the 1950s to kill banana root nematode parasites. In the mid-1970s, a group of 35 workers in California were found to be sterile after applying DBCP, and its use was banned in 1979. However, it continued to be exported and used in countries such as Ecuador, Guatemala, Nicaragua, Honduras, the Philippines, and Costa Rica. It is believed that many thousands of workers became sterile after using DBCP without proper equipment. Pesticides and other noxious chemicals that are otherwise useful may be casually stored at the household level in unmarked leaky containers. These containers can be opened by children, allowing accidental poisonings and exposures. Better packaging and storage could eliminate these frequent events.[49] Ingestion of a pesticide is also a frequently used method of suicide.[50]

Air Pollution

Studies over the past 30 years have identified air pollution as one of the most, if not the most, important environmental hazards to humans. Air pollution has been linked to respiratory disease (infections, asthma, and chronic obstructive pulmonary disease); cardiovascular diseases, including myocardial infarction; cancer; impaired lung development in adolescents; and intrauterine growth retardation and congenital anomalies.[51-55] Rapidly growing societies, such as modern China, are characterized by severe air pollution in nearly all major cities. The principal causes of outdoor air pollution include exhaust products of internal combustion engines and power generation, as well as industrial releases. Air pollutants are a complex mixture of gases (carbon monoxide, nitrogenous compounds, ozone, etc.) and particulates, which vary in size. The gases may have effects in isolation but also undergo chemical reactions once produced, resulting in smog that may contain sulfuric acid and other respiratory irritants. Particulates (soot) can act as inanimate vectors that deliver carcinogenic polyaromatic hydrocarbons into the lungs when inhaled.

Buses and trucks in some cities are the major sources of air pollution, and reducing air pollution may require mandatory modifications to their engines. Interestingly, in studies done in the Andean countries of South America, the modifications made to reduce pollutants usually led to increased engine energy efficiency, decreased costs for fuel, and a net increase in profits for the operators of the buses and trucks.[56] This point is made to remind you that the benefits of remediating environmental risks may easily outweigh the costs when fully examined. Cost-benefit analyses in the United States and the European Union have strongly suggested that the control of air pollution leads to major improvements in human health.

Air pollution can occur very locally, such as in the household from heating or cooking, or across a large swath of land. Power-generating plants and incineration facilities tend to release pollutants from high chimney stacks, and thus the pollutants are dispersed much higher in the atmosphere than those from houses or automobiles. In the United States, approximately 48 tons of mercury are released into the environment every year from coal-burning plants. This amount is about 40% of the annual release of around

120 tons of mercury. Half of this amount is deposited locally, and the other half distantly.[57] The global burden of mercury release has been estimated to be between 4,400 and 7,500 tons per year.

Indoor air pollution, from the use of biofuels such as wood and from tobacco smoke exposure, is now understood to be a major contributor to respiratory infections. Lower respiratory infection (LRI), especially pneumonia, remains the leading cause of death in children younger than 5 years, and 36% of all LRIs have been attributed to the use of biofuels for cooking and heating.[58,59] This percentage translates into approximately 1 million deaths a year in children younger than 5. Environmental exposure to tobacco smoke leads to recurrent otitis media in children[60,61] and to lung cancer and chronic obstructive lung disease, even in people who are not active smokers.[62,63] Fuels such as natural gas and propane gas burn more cleanly and efficiently than biofuels, and their use reduces household pollution levels. Innovative cooking stoves that use biofuels are being devised that are both more fuel efficient and ventilate outside the household, so that indoor pollution levels are minimized. Volatile organic compounds, nitrogen dioxide, carbon monoxide, and biologic allergens are other forms of indoor air pollution. These contribute to a total of perhaps 1.5 to 2.0 million deaths yearly from indoor air pollution.[64]

Increased rates of tuberculosis have been linked to both indoor air pollution and environmental tobacco smoke, but the degree of this association is not well understood.[1]

SUMMARY

This brief overview has used a definition of environmental health that tries to encompass the biologic, physical, and chemical risks to humans that are mediated through the environment. Major improvements to human health could be accomplished by increased attention to these risks because they represent a large proportion of the total global disease burden. It is important to emphasize that this burden of disease disproportionately falls upon developing and transitional countries. Indeed, it is difficult to see how progress toward meeting the Millennium Development Goals[65,66] can be achieved without attention to these factors. Reducing child mortality and improving maternal health (goals 4 and 5), combating the major infectious and noncommunicable diseases (goal 6), ensuring environmental sustainability (goal 7), and promoting responsible development (goal 8) all require addressing environmental issues. Even the developed richer countries are by no means immune to environmental risks, given the increased use of chemicals in agriculture and industry, heavy reliance on road transportation, and air pollution.

Despite the enormity of the challenge, there is room for hope. Environmental issues are being addressed, and many of the risks are well understood and easily avoided. Complex technology is not needed to remove lead from the environment, clean water and sanitation are not new processes, and there are now many examples of the successful control of air pollution. In addition, many societies have now successfully tackled these problems and improved the lives of their citizens. From the global perspective, these instances of success should be models for others.

STUDY QUESTIONS

1. Name three leading pollutants that influence human health and describe their health consequences, delineating both their magnitude and how these health effects can be prevented.

2. The three levels of water treatment are physical, biologic, and chemical. What are the effects of each type of treatment? Are they always necessary? How can they be combined or avoided?

3. In a situation in which raw sewage disposal is contaminating a water supply, what problem should be addressed first, treating the sewage or the drinking water? What are the advantages or disadvantages to doing one project before the other?

SELECTED BIBLIOGRAPHY ON WATER AND SANITATION

Brush RE. *Wells Construction: Hand Dug and Hand Drilled.* Washington, DC: Peace Corps, 1979. Information Collection and Exchange Manual M-9.

Cairncross S, Feachem R. *Small Water Supplies.* London: Ross Institute of Tropical Hygiene, 1986.

Elder JR. *Manual of Small Public Water Supply Systems.* Washington, DC: US Environmental Protection Agency, 1991.

Hutton LG. *Field Testing of Water in Developing Countries.* Marlow, UK: Water Research Center, 1983.

Manja KS, Maurya MS, Rao KM. A simple field test for the detection of faecal pollution in drinking water. *Bull World Health Organ* 1982;60(5):797–901.

Mara D. *Sewage Treatment in Hot Climates.* New York: John Wiley and Sons, 1976.

Pickford J, et al. *The Worth of Water: Technical Briefs on Health, Water and Sanitation.* London: Intermediate Technology Publications, 1991.

Ross Institute of Tropical Hygiene. *The Preservation of Personal Health in Warm Climates.* London: Ross Institute of Tropical Hygiene, 1985.

Talbert DE. *Water/Sanitation Case Studies and Analysis.* Washington, DC: Peace Corps, 1984.

U.S. Environmental Protection Agency. *Onsite Wastewater Treatment Systems Manual.* Washington, DC: US Environmental Protection Agency, 2002. EPA/625/R-00/008.

Viessman W, Hammer MJ. *Water Supply and Pollution Control.* 4th ed. New York: Harper & Row, 1985.

Wilkie W. *Jordan's Tropical Hygiene and Sanitation.* London: Bailliere, Tindall and Cox, 1965.

Winblad U, Kilama W. *Sanitation Without Water.* London: Macmillan, 1985.

USEFUL INTERNET SITES

American Waterworks Association: http://www.awwa.org.

London School of Hygiene and Tropical Medicine, University of London, United Kingdom: http://www.lshtm.ac.uk

National Small Flows Clearinghouse and National Drinking Water Clearinghouse, West Virginia University: http://www.nesc.wvu.edu.

U.S. Army Corps of Engineers Institute for Water Resources: http://www.iwr.usace.army.mil/.

Water Engineering and Development Centre (WEDC), Loughborough University, United Kingdom: http://wedc.lboro.ac.uk/.

REFERENCES

1. Prüss-Üstün A, Corvalán C. *Preventing Disease Through Healthy Environments. Towards an Estimate of the Environmental Burden of Disease.* Geneva: World Health Organization, 2006.

2. Ezzati M, Lopez AD, Rodgers A, et al. Selected major risk factors and global and regional burden of disease. *Lancet* 2002;360:1347–1360.

3. Briggs D. Environmental pollution and the global burden of disease. *Br Med Bull* 2003;68:1–24.

4. Royal Commission on Environmental Pollution. *Chemicals in Products: Safeguarding the Environment and Human Health.* London: Royal Commission on Environmental Health, 2003.

5. Luby SP, Agboatwalla M, Feikin DR, et al. Effect of handwashing on child health: a randomised controlled trial. *Lancet* 2005;366(9491):185–187.

6. Esrey SA, Habicht JP. Epidemiologic evidence for health benefits from improved water and sanitation in developing countries. *Epidemiol Rev* 1986;8:117–128.

7. World Health Organization. *Evaluation of the Costs and Benefits of Water and Sanitation Improvements at the Global Level.* Geneva: WHO, 2004.

8. World Health Organization and UNICEF. *Water for Life: Making It Happen.* Geneva: WHO, 2005.

9. Howard G, Bartram J. *Domestic Water Quantity, Service Level and Health.* Geneva: World Health Organization, 2003. http://www.who.int/water_sanitation_health/diseases/WSH03.02.pdf.

10. Huo A, Xu B, Chowdhury MA, et al. A simple filtration method to remove plankton-associated *Vibrio cholerae* in raw water supplies in developing countries. *Appl Environ Microbiol* 1996;62:2508–2512.

11. Potters for Peace. Filters. http://www.pottersforpeace.org/.

12. Bowie WR, King AS, Werker DH, et al. Outbreak of toxoplasmosis associated with municipal drinking water. *Lancet* 1997;350:173–177.

13. Griffiths JK. Exotic and trendy cuisine. In: Schlossberg D, ed. *Infections of Leisure.* Washington, DC: American Society for Microbiology Press, 2004.

14. U.S. Environmental Protection Agency. National primary drinking water regulations: long term 2 enhanced surface water treatment rule. *Federal Register* 2006;71:653–702.

15. Teunis PF, Chappell CL, Okhuysen PC. *Cryptosporidium* dose response studies: variation between isolates. *Risk Anal* 2002; 22:175–183.

16. MacKenzie WR, Hoxie NJ, Proctor ME, et al. A massive outbreak in Milwaukee of *Cryptosporidium* infection transmitted through the public water supply. *N Engl J Med* 1994;331(3):161–167.

17. Goldstein ST, Juranek DD, Ravenholt O, et al. Cryptosporidiosis: an outbreak associated with drinking water despite state-of-the-art water treatment. *Ann Intern Med* 1996;124(5):459–468.

18. Franzen C, Muller A. Cryptosporidia and microsporidia-waterborne diseases in the immunocompromised host. *Diagn Microbiol Infect Dis* 1999;34(3):245–262.

19. U.S. Environmental Protection Agency. National primary drinking water regulations: long term enhanced surface water treatment rule. Final rule. *Federal Register* 2002;67(9):1811–1844.

20. Nieuwenhuijsen MJ, Toledano MB, Eaton NE, Fawell J, Elliott P. Chlorination disinfection byproducts in water and their association with adverse reproductive outcomes: a review. *Occup Environ Med* 2000;57(2):73–85.

21. Ellis A. Waterborne outbreak of gastroenteritis associated with a contaminated municipal water supply, Walkerton, Ontario, May–June 2000. *Can Commun Dis Rep* 2000;26(20):170–173.

22. Mermin JH, Villar R, Carpenter J, et al. A massive epidemic of multidrug-resistant typhoid fever in Tajikistan associated with consumption of municipal water [see comment]. *J Infect Dis* 1999;179(6):1416–1422.

23. Ettling J. *The Germ of Laziness: Rockefeller Philanthropy and Public Health in the New South.* Cambridge, MA: Harvard University Press, 1981.

24. Dziuban EJ, Liang JL, Craun GF, et al. Surveillance for waterborne disease and outbreaks associated with recreational water—United States, 2003–2004. *MMWR CDC Surveill Summ* 2006;55(12):1–30.

25. Stottmeister U, Wiessner A, Kuschk P, et al. Effects of plants and microorganisms in constructed wetlands for wastewater treatment. *Biotechnol Adv* 2003;22(1–2):93–117.

26. Hillyer GV. The rise and fall of Bilharzia in Puerto Rico: its centennial 1904–2004. *P R Health Sci J* 2005;24(3):225–235.

27. D'Alessandro U, Olaleye BO, McGuire W, et al. Mortality and morbidity from malaria in Gambian children after introduction of an impregnated bednet programme. *Lancet* 1995;345(8948): 479–483.

28. Chinga-Alayo E, Huarcaya E, Nasarre C, del Aguila R, Llanos-Cuentas A. The influence of climate on the epidemiology of bartonellosis in Ancash, Peru. *Trans R Soc Trop Med Hyg* 2004; 98(2):116–124.

29. Naumova EN, Jagai JS, Matyas B, et al. Seasonality in six enterically transmitted diseases and ambient temperature. *Epidemiol Infect* 2007;135(2):281–292.

30. Curriero FC, Patz JA, Rose JB, Lele S. The association between extreme precipitation and waterborne disease outbreaks in the United States, 1948-1994. *Am J Public Health* 2001;91(8):1194–1199.

31. Gatei W, Wamae CN, Mbae C, et al. 2006. Cryptosporidiosis: prevalence, genotype analysis, and symptoms associated with infections in children in Kenya. *Am J Trop Med Hyg* 2006;75(1):78–82.

32. McBride AJ, Athanazio DA, Reis MG, Ko AI. Leptospirosis. *Curr Opin Infect Dis* 2005;18(5):376–386.

33. Epstein PR. Climate change and emerging infectious diseases. *Microbes Infect* 2001;3(9):747–754.

34. Miguel E, Satyanath S, Sergenti E. Economic shocks and civil conflict: an instrumental variables approach. *J Political Economy* 2004;112:725–753.

35. Frank L, Andresen M, Schmid T. Obesity relationships with community design, physical activity, and time spent in cars. *Am J Prevent Med* 2004;27:87–96.

36. Ewing R. Can the physical environment determine physical activity levels? *Exerc Sports Sci Rev* 2005;33:69–75.

37. World Health Organization. *World Health Report 2002: Reducing Risks, Promoting Healthy Life.* Geneva: WHO, 2002.

38. Nordberg E. Injuries as a public health problem in sub-Saharan Africa: epidemiology and prospects for control. *East Afr Med J* 2000;77(Suppl 12):S1–S43.

39. U.S. Environmental Protection Agency. National primary drinking water regulations; radionuclides; final rule. *Fed Reg* 2000;65(236):76708–76753.

40. U.S. Environmental Protection Agency. Radon information. http://www.epa.gov/radiation/radionuclides/radon.html.

41. Brugge D, Goble R. The history of uranium mining and the Navajo people. *Am J Public Health* 2002;92:1410–1419.

42. Alaerts G, Khouri N, Kabir B. Strategies to mitigate arsenic contamination of water supply. In: *Arsenic in Drinking Water. United Nations Synthesis Report on Arsenic in Drinking Water.* 2001. http://www.who.int/water_sanitation_health/dwq/arsenicun8.pdf.

43. Rahman MM, Chowdhury UK, Mukherjee SC, et al. Chronic arsenic toxicity in Bangladesh and West Bengal, India—a review and commentary. *J Toxicol Clin Toxicol* 2001;39(7):683–700.

44. Parvez F, Chen Y, Argos M, et al. Prevalence of arsenic exposure from drinking water and awareness of its health risks in a Bangladeshi population: results from a large population based study. *Environ Health Perspect* 2006;114:355–359.

45. National Research Council. *Arsenic in Drinking Water: 2001 Update.* Washington, DC: National Academies Press, 2001.

46. Durant JL, Ivushkina T, MacLaughlin K, et al. Elevated levels of arsenic in the sediments of an urban pond: sources, distribution and water quality impacts. *Water Res* 2004;38(13): 2989–3000.

47. Tarras-Wahlberg NH, Flachier A, Lane SN, Sangfors O. Environmental impacts and metal exposure of aquatic ecosystems in rivers contaminated by small scale gold mining: the Puyango River basin, southern Ecuador. *Sci Total Environ* 2001;278(1–3): 239–261.

48. Jamal GA. Neurological syndromes of organophosphorus compounds. *Adverse Drug React Toxicol Rev* 1997;16(3):133–170.

49. McGuigan MA. Common culprits in childhood poisoning: epidemiology, treatment and parental advice for prevention. *Paediatr Drugs* 1999;1(4):313–324.

50. Gunnell D, Eddleston M. Suicide by ingestion of pesticides: a continuing tragedy in developing countries. *Int J Epidemiol* 2003;32:902–909.

51. Pope CA III, Burnett RT, Thun MJ, et al. Lung cancer, cardiopulmonary mortality, and long-term exposure to fine particle air pollution. *JAMA* 2002;287:1132–1141.

52. Kaur S, Cohen A, Dolor R, Coffman CJ, Bastian LA. The impact of environmental tobacco smoke on women's risk of dying from heart disease: a meta-analysis. *J Womens Health* 2004;13:888–897.

53. Gauderman WJ, Avol E, Gilliland F, et al. The effect of air pollution on lung development from 10 to 18 years of age. *N Engl J Med* 2004;351:1057–1067.

54. Ritz B, Yu F. The effect of ambient carbon monoxide on low birth weight among children born in southern California between 1989 and 1993. *Environ Health Perspect* 1999;107(1): 17–25.

55. Ritz B, Yu F, Fruin S, Chapa G, Shaw GM, Harris JA. Ambient air pollution and risk of birth defects in Southern California. *Am J Epidemiol* 2002;155(1):17–25.

56. Environment and Sustainable Development Project. Enhancing competitiveness while protecting the environment. Center for International Development, Harvard University. http://www.cid.harvard.edu/sd/.

57. Stockstad E. Toxic air pollutants. Inspector general blasts EPA mercury analysis. *Science* 2005;307:829–830.

58. Smith KR, Smet JM, Romieu I, Bruce N. Indoor air pollution in developing countries and acute lower respiratory infections in children. *Thorax* 2000;55(6):518–532.

59. Smith KR, Mehta S, Maeusezahl-Feuz M. Indoor air pollution from solid household fuels. In: Ezzati M, Lopez AD, Rodgers A, Murray CJL, eds. *Comparative Quantification of Health Risks.* Geneva: World Health Organization, 2004.

60. Sternstrom R, Bernard PA, Ben-Simhon H. Exposure to environmental tobacco smoke as a risk factor for recurrent acute otitis media in children under the age of five years. *Int J Pediatr Otorhinolaryngol* 1993;27(2):127–136.

61. Etzel RA, Pattishall EN, Haley NJ, Fletcher RH, Henderson FW. Passive smoking and middle ear effusion among children in day care. *Pediatrics* 1992;90(2 Pt 1):228–232.

62. Taylor R, Cumming R, Woodward A, Black M. Passive smoking and lung cancer: a cumulative meta-analysis. *Austr N Z J Public Health* 2001;25(3):203–211.

63. Vineis P, Airoldi L, Veglia P, et al. Environmental tobacco smoke and risk of respiratory cancer and chronic obstructive pulmonary disease in former smoker and never smokers in the EPIC prospective study. *BMJ* 2005;330(7486):265–266.

64. Viegi G, Simoni M, Scognamiglio A, et al. Indoor air pollution and airway disease. *Int J Tuberc Lung Dis* 2004;8: 1401–1415.

65. United Nations. UN Millennium Development Goals. http://www.un.org/millenniumgoals/.

66. United Nations. *The Millennium Development Goals Report 2006.* New York: United Nations. http://mdgs.un.org/unsd/mdg/Resources/Static/Products/Progress2006/MDGReport2006.pdf.

Nutrition

Clydette Powell and John R. Butterly

LEARNING OBJECTIVES

- *Describe nutrition problems around the world: their extent, causes, and manifestations*
- *Identify the signs and symptoms of micronutrient deficiencies and understand approaches to addressing these deficiencies*
- *Describe key interventions for malnutrition in various settings: in developing countries, during complex humanitarian emergencies, and in the context of HIV/AIDS and tuberculosis*
- *Identify some tools for measuring malnutrition and distinguish between growth monitoring and rapid emergency assessment*
- *Describe how national and international policies can shape nutrition strategies and approaches. Give examples of potential beneficial and adverse effects of such policies*

INTRODUCTION

During the past few decades we have become increasingly aware of the central role that nutrition plays in all aspects of population health. We have recognized that access to adequate nutrition is a human right since the promulgation of the Universal Declaration of Human Rights in 1948, as stated in Article 25: "Everyone has the right to a standard of living adequate for the health and well-being of himself and of his family, *including food*" [emphasis added]. Although it may seem intuitively obvious that such access is also a basic human need, there is value in reviewing the biologic factors that inform our understanding of this. We will come back to a more detailed discussion of these concepts later in this chapter, but keep these two fundamental truths in mind while reading

the following pages. In addition, we wish to introduce another concept for you to consider while reading this chapter; all of the major causes of death of the people of this globe, be they living in high-income, middle-income, or low-income countries, are inextricably linked to the nutritional environment in which they find themselves.

THE GLOBAL CONTEXT

Undernutrition

In a century characterized by modern approaches to identifying and solving global health problems, undernutrition prevails in the world's children, contributing to a third of all deaths in children under 5 years of age.[1] An estimated 195 million children under 5 years in developing countries are stunted in growth (height-for-age), and some 120 million are wasted (weight-for-height).[2] Overall, 80% of the world's undernourished children live in just 20 countries around the world, according to the World Health Organization (WHO).[3] In addition, a third of the developing world suffers from micronutrient deficiencies—deficiencies that accompany poor nutrition and are silent until their effects are advanced and, in some instances, irreversible. In these settings, infections, such as human immunodeficiency virus (HIV), tuberculosis (TB), and parasites, intensify the impact of undernutrition, and vice versa.

We can define direct causes of undernutrition as primary undernutrition, caused by inadequate food intake, or secondary undernutrition, caused by underlying diseases such as TB or HIV/AIDS. In addition, there are many indirect causes of undernutrition: poverty, the low status of women, unsanitary health conditions, wars and conflict, low national income growth, as well as poor governance and corruption. Factors underlying poor health services are human, economic, and organizational resources and their control. This is one reason that undernutrition can be seen in conflict-affected areas or in areas where a local governing authority does not have the will, the commitment, or the effectiveness to carry out services for a population. Political ideologies, ethnic discrimination, and marginalization of the poor can create pockets of undernutrition in countries where abundant nutritional sources are inequitably allocated. However, not all undernutrition is seen in developing countries or in complex humanitarian emergencies. Consider inner cities, where food may not be accessible (the "food deserts" seen in disadvantaged neighborhoods), not affordable due to poverty, or where lack of knowledge about (and unavailability of) good nutritional choices leads to poor selection of foods and poor eating habits. At the time of this writing, it is conservatively estimated that 14% of the population of the United States, in isolated rural areas as well as disadvantaged urban areas, is either chronically or intermittently food insecure if not actually malnourished.[4] The U.S. Department of Agriculture (USDA) Supplemental Nutrition Assistant Program (SNAP), commonly referred to as the food stamp program, supplies food purchasing support to 46 million people each month (14.6% of the total population as of 2012),[5] and various state food banks report serving between 12% and 14% of the population within their respective states.[6] A somewhat disturbing set of statistics applies to the elderly population in the United States. According to one study, 18% of elderly patients living in long-term facilities were severely undernourished, with 27.5% mildly to moderately undernourished.[7] Prevalence in the hospitalized population is even more alarming, varying between 40% and 60% depending on the study cited.[8]

Respected leaders throughout history have pointed out that one of the most meaningful measures of a society is reflected by how they treat their most vulnerable members. We should keep this in mind as we learn more about the statistics of preventable morbidity and mortality as they relate to our children and senior citizens.

Where in the developing world does undernutrition remain a problem for 21st-century populations? The countries of South Asia (India, Bangladesh, Afghanistan, and Pakistan) have both high numbers and high rates of undernourished children, with India leading the list. In fact, although undernutrition is decreasing in Asia overall, the prevalence of undernutrition in South Asia (41% to 43%) is much higher than that in sub-Saharan Africa (SSA; 25%) (Figure 7-1).[9] In SSA, undernutrition is a major contributing factor in over 60% of deaths of children under the age of 5 years, with pneumonia and diarrhea accounting for the highest percentage, closely followed by perinatal causes. Other infections, specifically TB, HIV/AIDS, and malaria, account for the rest.[10] For Africa, it is estimated that 25% of children 5 years or younger are underweight (moderate to severe), and some 34% are stunted.[11]

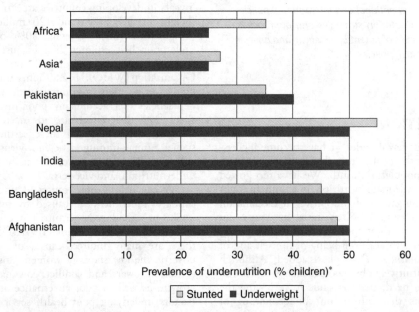

Figure 7-1. The prevalence of undernutrition in South Asian countries is much higher than in Africa. From World Bank. *Repositioning Nutrition as Central to Development: A Strategy for Large-Scale Action.* Washington, DC: World Bank, 2006. *(Reproduced with permission.)*
*Estimates are based on WHO regions.

Populations, and children in particular, do not die of undernutrition per se, but of infectious diseases that would generally not be fatal to well-nourished individuals. They are vulnerable to these infections because of the direct effects undernutrition has in weakening the natural defenses of the immune system (they are compromised hosts), as well as the indirect effects of having poor access to health services, poor sanitation, unsafe water supplies, and ignorance of basic health care practices. Poverty and lack of education exacerbate and prolong undernutrition. Although poverty is the ultimate underlying problem, the resultant undernutrition leads to possibly irreversible loss of each individual's potential due to damage to physical and intellectual capacity, and the lack of education adds to this synergistically, resulting in a severe loss of the development of human capital. Thus a vicious cycle is created. Poor feeding practices and lack of adequate nutrition result in poorly nourished children; if they survive to be of reproductive age, they are likely to be poorly nourished parents. Stunted mothers can give birth to low-birth-weight babies. Undernutrition in the mother can result in major damage to a child's health and well-being, much of which is irreversible, manifesting as less physical capacity, lowered intelligence, and more frequent illnesses. Those factors may result in irregular school attendance or diminished ability to learn, and ultimately in lower likelihood of employment, lowered productivity, and inability to meet the daily economic demands of life. Because this can be a generational phenomenon in households and communities, it is a difficult cycle to break. These children and adolescents rarely escape the cycle of poverty and despair into which they are born.

It is this inability of people suffering from chronic food insecurity and undernutrition that is fundamental to the loss of human capital that defines the so-called poverty trap. Jeffrey Sachs, in his book *The End of Poverty,*[12] notes that extreme poverty occurs when there is a lack of six types of capital, starting with human capital. It is for this reason that we suggest, if indeed a poverty trap exists, chronic hunger and undernutrition are the locks on that trap. Stated another way, acknowledging that the ultimate problem underlying inequities in global health today is that of poverty, hunger is surely its cruelest manifestation.

Graphs of undernutrition (weight-for-age by region) show that undernutrition happens early in life (Figure 7-2).[13] Studies demonstrate that for younger

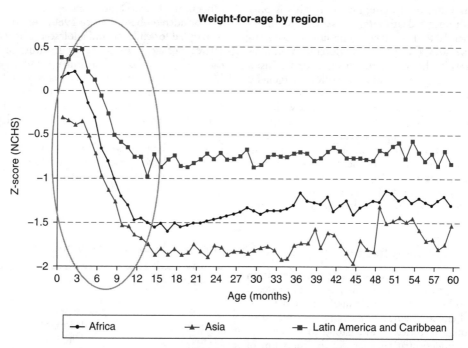

Figure 7-2. Malnutrition happens early. From Shrimpton R, Cesar G, et al. The worldwide timing of growth failure; implications for nutritional interventions. *Pediatrics* 2001;107(5):e75. NCHS, National Center for Health Statistics. Circled area represents a window of opportunity. (*Reproduced with permission.*)

children, the risk of dying increases exponentially with degree of undernutrition.[14] As children get older, however, the degree of undernutrition drops off in part because younger undernourished children have died and in part due to the fact that older children are better able to fend for themselves in an environment of scarce resources. In other words, younger children are more represented in the data showing undernutrition.

Although there is some debate in the nutrition literature as to the temporal and causative relationship between undernutrition and mortality in any specific population, there is general agreement that this relationship is an exponential one. That is, as the severity of undernutrition increases, mortality rates increase exponentially rather than linearly, explaining the alarming increases in mortality we see as food insecurity evolves into overt famine. Where low rates of undernutrition exist, high mortality rates in children of refugee populations can be explained by acute illnesses such as acute diarrhea and dehydration when access to adequate infrastructure is lacking. In populations where public health services and stable home environments are able to support the necessary infrastructure, higher rates of undernutrition can be weathered when severe food insecurity and famine occur. High mortality rates can mask deteriorating nutrition status because they can occur for reasons other than undernutrition. This is only true when under-5 death rates are very high—more than 10 per 10,000 per day. Some nongovernmental organizations (NGOs) have developed models to characterize whether a situation is a food crisis, a health crisis, or a combination of both (emergencies out of control).

One solution to undernutrition begins with preventing and treating undernutrition in pregnant women and in children up to 2 years of age. Providing health and nutrition education along with micronutrient fortification and supplementation is also very important. Contrary to popular perception, school feeding programs do not intervene soon enough, although they may draw children into school and keep them there.[15]

Overnutrition and Obesity

In the introduction to this chapter we made mention of the concept that all of the major causes of death of the world's population are causally related to the nutritional environment, and that the term *malnutrition,* although historically understood to be synonymous with undernutrition, includes the spectrum of physiologic deviations from the norm caused by overnutrition. When we incorporate this insight into the calculus of our policy decisions and widen the scope

of concern in a global sense, we recognize that malnutrition is not limited to developing countries. Its presence, as the recognized biometrics of overweight, obesity, and morbid obesity, has become epidemic in developed nations, most readily apparent in poor urban slums and underserved rural areas. Sedentary lifestyle, dietary excesses, high-fat content in food, and consumption of the empty calories in processed and fast foods lead to overnutrition and obesity. These diets can also be marginal in certain nutrients; stunted growth coupled with excess body fat can be the result. The increasing stress levels of modern life have also resulted in rising morbidity and mortality. Data from the Centers for Disease Control and Prevention (CDC) indicate that nearly two thirds of the U.S. population is either overweight or frankly obese.[16] To put this into perspective, consider the fact that in 1990 obesity prevalence rates in the United States for adults varied from less than 10% to 14%. In the year 2000, those numbers had increased to 15% to 25%, and in 2010, the numbers had increased to between 20% to over 30% depending on the registry we examined.[17]

Obesity is defined using body mass index (BMI) as a metric for maladaptive fat storage. BMI is calculated as body weight in kilograms divided by height in meters squared. Acceptable BMI varies by age and gender (Table 7-1). Some 17% of children and adolescents in the United States between 2 and 19 years old are considered obese.[18] Since 1980, obesity prevalence has tripled for children and adolescents between 2 and 19 years of age.[19] In 2005, the Institute of Medicine called these trends a "harmful upward trajectory."[20] Many factors are strong predictors of childhood obesity: genetics (having overweight parents), childhood characteristics (having been overweight in middle childhood), psychosocial factors (such as depression), and behavior (such as eating while watching TV and lack of regular exercise). Of specific interest, a number of studies have demonstrated a clear link between childhood obesity and the presence of a television in the child's bedroom.[21]

Table 7-1. Body mass index and medical status.

Body mass index	Medical status
≥30.0	Obese
25–29.9	Overweight
18.5–24.9	Normal
17–18.4	Mild PEM
16–16.9	Moderate PEM
<16	Severe PEM

PEM, protein-energy malnutrition.

The marked increase in the prevalence of obesity just noted is accompanied by parallel increases in deaths due to noncommunicable chronic disease, such as cardiovascular disease, diabetes, stroke, and cancer, all of which are linked to excess calories, saturated fat, salt (sodium), cholesterol, and sugars, along with inadequate fiber intake. Dietary factors also are linked to higher risks for hypertension, dental and renal disease, and osteoporosis.

Diseases of Infrastructure and Diseases of Affluence

We have developed our understanding that there is a difference between the specific diseases that cause the morbidity and mortality due to undernutrition or overnutrition. We can now give consideration to a distinction between diseases of infrastructure and diseases of affluence. What do we mean by this?

Most of this chapter deals with the physiologic consequences of undernutrition, and as we have discussed, undernutrition weakens a person's ability to fight off infectious diseases that would, under normal circumstances, be reasonably well tolerated (i.e., the person becomes a compromised host). Coupled with this poor access to adequate nutrition in impoverished regions we see overcrowding due to inadequate living quarters and a lack of access to safe water supplies and adequate sanitation facilities. This creates what we might think of as a "perfect storm"; not only is the population compromised in their ability to fight off infection, but also people are more likely to encounter pathogenic organisms through exposure to contaminated water supplies and/or contact with infected individuals. Because of this association between undernutrition, on the one hand, and these communicable diseases related to inadequate public health facilities, on the other, we can consider these diseases to be diseases of infrastructure. (The proximate examples of infrastructure given here are, of course, only a part of a more complex infrastructure including issues of economic development and governance.)

At the other end of the spectrum of nutritionally related diseases, we have seen the exponential growth of the prevalence of obesity in middle- and high-income nations, with its associated chronic metabolic diseases. All of these are major risk factors for the development of coronary artery disease, explaining why coronary artery disease is the major cause of death in both men and women in developed nations. Due to this association of higher rates of obesity-related metabolic diseases and higher levels of income, we can refer to these diseases as diseases of affluence.

Paradoxically, overnourished populations have the greatest access to information and approaches that would increase their health and well-being, suggesting that populations in developed nations are as at much risk of suffering the ill effects of unhealthy nutrition due to poor choices as are populations in developing nations due to poor access. To counter food advertising and the convenience of fast foods, public health messages promote awareness of better food choices and lifestyle. Package labeling, media campaigns, and social marketing have led to some increased nutrition awareness among the public as well as among health care providers. However, food availability and affordability, ethnic preferences, and levels of education and income still negatively influence these choices.

The Nutritional Transition

Many low- and middle-income countries are caught in a situation referred to as *nutritional transition*. These countries face simultaneous public health challenges: undernutrition in some populations and obesity in others, along with diet-related noncommunicable diseases, such as cardiovascular disease, cancer, and diabetes. This phenomenon can be very costly for countries because it presents competing priorities for limited health budgets and health personnel, who may still be grappling with programs to combat traditional communicable diseases.[9] The prevalence of obesity tends to follow a bimodal distribution in these countries, becoming evident at first in the more well-to-do members of the population, but invariably having a greater prevalence in the poor.[22]

Over- and undernutrition can coexist not only in the same country but also in the same household. In Mauritania, more than 40% of mothers are overweight while at the same time more than 30% of children are underweight. As many as 60% of households with an overweight person also had an underweight person.[9]

In the introduction to this chapter we presented the argument that access to adequate nutrition is a human right and a basic human need. If we accept Article 25 of the Universal Declaration of Human Rights (and subsequent contemporary documents such as the Millennium Development Project [MDP]) as our moral authority for stating that access to adequate nutrition is a human right, to what authority do we turn to assert that access to adequate nutrition is a human need?

In 1943, Abraham Maslow, considered the father of humanistic psychology, published his seminal article on his theory of human motivation.[23] Commonly known as Maslow's hierarchy of needs, he pointed out that there were five levels of human development, starting with physiologic needs, and then advancing through issues of safety, love and belonging, self-esteem, and self-actualization. Although there is significant detail to be learned about each of these levels of individual growth, a critical point to be understood about this concept is that one cannot advance to the next level of personal development until the needs of the level below are met. In other words, if the basic needs of the physiologic level are not met, and this includes access to adequate nutrition, one can never advance along the continuum of personal growth, and therefore never realize one's full potential. To quote Maslow, "For the man who is extremely and dangerously hungry, no other interests exist but food. He dreams food, he remembers food, he thinks about food, he emotes only about food, he perceives only food and he wants only food. (This) allow(s) us to speak . . . of pure hunger drive and behavior, with the one unqualified aim of relief." In the following sections we discuss the physiologic consequences of inadequate intake of calories, protein, and certain micronutrients, but we should always consider these issues in the context of the physical and psychological suffering associated with chronic hunger.

PROTEIN-ENERGY MALNUTRITION

In an introduction to any discussion of an unhealthy diet, it is important to say a few words on what is considered to be a healthy diet. Basic caloric needs depend on age, gender, body size, and activity level, but calories alone are not sufficient. A proper balance of calories from the macronutrient carbohydrates, fats, and proteins is critically important in growth and maintenance, as is the intake of sufficient amounts of the micronutrient vitamins and minerals. The first publicly published accounts of what would be considered a balanced diet appeared in 1974 in Sweden as a food pyramid, with most of the calories (55% to 75%) being supplied by unrefined carbohydrates, 15% to 30% being supplied by fats, and 10% to 15% supplied by protein. A similar food pyramid for the United States was published in 1992. More recently, the USDA has replaced the food pyramid with My Plate, a divided plate that not only offers suggestions as to a balance of macro and micronutrients, but also offers advice on what would be considered healthy choices (e.g., whole grains and fresh fruits and vegetables, lean meats for proteins, and fat-free or low-fat calcium-rich dairy products.) In this section we describe the effects of undernutrition of these food groups and certain micronutrients, with the reminder that overnutrition (especially too much intake of calorically dense fats and oils) can be just as damaging to one's health, albeit for different reasons.

Throughout this chapter we have been using the terms *undernutrition* and *overnutrition,* as we have become increasingly aware of the fact that overnutrition is as costly a form of malnutrition as undernutrition in terms of health outcomes. Traditionally, however, malnutrition has been understood to mean undernutrition, and very specifically undernutrition due to inadequate intake of the macronutrients carbohydrates, fats, and protein. For this reason, undernutrition has been referred to as protein-energy malnutrition (PEM). When the body's basic maintenance needs for the caloric energy found in carbohydrates or fats, or the basic building blocks (amino acids) found in protein, exceeds its dietary intake of them, undernutrition is the result. People develop PEM for many reasons, such as inadequate food intake, poor composition of the diet, and unclean environments (poor hygiene), diarrhea, and infections. Children are especially vulnerable due to their increased needs during periods of growth and development as well as their dependence on others to help them meet those needs.

To understand the pathophysiology of the different forms of PEM, we need very briefly to review the basics of nutrition. The energy we need to grow and maintain our own bodies, and to perform the functions of life, are obtained through the ingestion of calories. (A calorie is defined as the amount of energy required to raise the temperature of 1 cubic centimeter of water 1 degree Centigrade. When we refer to dietary calories, we are actually talking about a kilocalorie, or 1,000 calories. This is usually written as Calorie, although conventional usage tends to omit the capital "C.") Most of our caloric needs is met by the ingestion of carbohydrates (sugars and starches), which supply 4 calories per gram, and fats (mostly triglycerides), which supply 9 calories per gram. Proteins are a special case. They also supply 4 calories per gram, but because humans can only synthesize 10 of the 20 naturally occurring amino acids needed to make our own internal proteins, we normally use only about 25% of ingested protein for energy. The remaining 75% is recycled. We use the amino acids in ingested proteins that we cannot synthesize (the *essential amino acids*) to synthesize our own protein in order to preserve the integrity of our internal environment. When diets are lacking in adequate high-quality protein (that containing adequate amounts of the essential amino acids), a particularly pernicious form of undernutrition occurs (see later). This explains why we have referred to undernutrition as protein-energy undernutrition.

Classically, three types of PEM have been described: marasmus, kwashiorkor, and marasmic kwashiorkor.

Marasmus (the term comes from the Greek word for "withering") is due to prolonged caloric deprivation or frank starvation. It is characterized by severe wasting of fat and muscle, which results in an old-person skin-and-bones appearance (Figure 7-3). This is the most common form of PEM seen in nutritional emergencies where food shortages are severe. In contrast to the relative anorexia seen in children with

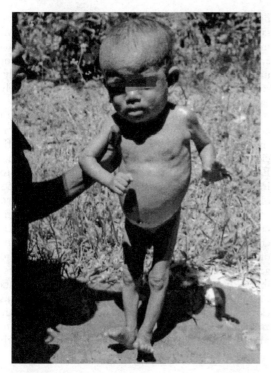

Figure 7-3. Cambodian child with marasmus. (*Photo credit: Debra Coats, FNP.*)

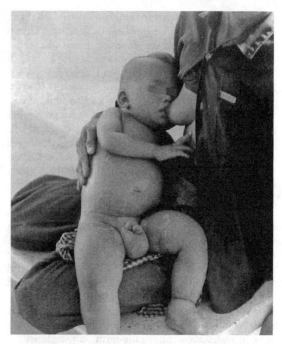

Figure 7-4. Cambodian child with kwashiorkor. (*Photo credit: Debra Coats, FNP.*)

kwashiorkor (who may be getting enough calories but not enough protein), children with marasmus are hungry. Marasmus may also be the result of chronic or recurring infections with decreased food intake.

Kwashiorkor comes from the Ghanaian term meaning "the sickness that the older child gets when the next baby is born"; the older child is displaced from breastfeeding by the newborn, who is offered the breast first. The older child is left to forage from the family table or may be given complementary foods for which he or she is not yet ready. Because breast milk is frequently the only source of high-quality protein available in these settings, the child quickly becomes protein deficient and unable to synthesize his or her own internal proteins for normal body function. One of these proteins is the albumin found in blood plasma. Due to the resultant hypoalbuminemia, kwashiorkor is accompanied by edema, mostly in the feet and legs, along with flaky skin, sparse light-colored (even red) hair, apathy or irritability, and poor appetite. Because of the edema, children may look "fat" and appear to be well fed to the untrained observer or to the parent who is not aware of the silent effects of undernutrition in their child. Children with severe kwashiorkor may have hair that falls out easily and skin that looks burned or ulcerated

and peels easily (Figure 7-4). In addition, they may have cardiac, renal, and gastrointestinal failure due to their inability to adequately maintain the protein in their internal organs. The third form of PEM, marasmic kwashiorkor, has both wasting and edema.

Chronic PEM has both short-term effects, such as lowered resistance to infections, and long-term effects, such as growth retardation, reduced intellectual development, and increased death rates, especially among children 1 to 5 years old, who are more vulnerable to respiratory infection and diarrhea. These children are also more vulnerable to TB, which is highly prevalent in many developing countries. Undernutrition is closely associated with TB in developing countries and often is considered a clinical sign of TB because TB has an increased metabolic demand (as do many chronic diseases such as AIDS and cancer). Undernutrition can lead to immune compromise, which then sets the stage for an opportunistic infection. To quantify the degree of undernutrition, public health specialists and health care providers speak of wasting and stunting in terms of muscle mass (weight) and height, respectively. In children 6 to 59 months old, *wasting* (low weight-for-height [WFH]) is defined as more than 2 standard deviations (SDs), or Z scores, below the reference values set by the WHO or the National Center for Health Statistics (NCHS); the term excludes edema. Almost 25% of children younger than 5 years in developing nations suffer from wasting. This puts them at great risk for death or severe growth impairment and delayed psychological development. Populations in which 10% to 14.9% of children are wasted are said to have a high (serious) risk of death. Usually the crude mortality rates (CMRs) in those populations are 2 to 4.9 deaths per 10,000 per day. Populations that are considered critical have wasting percentages of 15% or higher; CMRs tend to be more than 5 deaths per 10,000 per day. The prevalence of wasting in any population is considered a good measure of acute undernutrition.

Stunting (low height-for-age) occurs when children fail to reach their linear growth potential. As with wasting, stunting is associated with poverty, poor feeding practices, and risk of illnesses. Its prevalence varies widely, from less than 5% (United States and Chile, for example) to 59% (Afghanistan), around the world. India alone has an estimated 61 million stunted children, accounting for 30% of all the stunted children under 5 years in the world. Stunting is a manifestation and long-term consequence of chronic undernutrition. Stunted children may never reach their full growth potential, even when nutritional interventions are introduced. The prevalence of stunting in any population is considered a good measure of chronic or past undernutrition.

MICRONUTRIENT DEFICIENCIES

Micronutrients are vitamins and minerals required in very small quantities (micrograms or milligrams per day) for good health. For example, the average person requires only about one teaspoon of iodine during his or her entire lifetime. Because the human body does not produce most of these micronutrients, they have to be obtained from foods in the daily diet, as supplements added to food (i.e., food fortification), or in the form of capsules, powders, tablets, or injections. Although these micronutrients are only required in small amounts, the absence of any one of them will lead to severe disability and eventual death because they are important either as building blocks to grow and maintain our anatomy, or as critical cofactors in the basic biochemical reactions necessary for our physiology. Among the many micronutrients, the ones of greatest interest and importance are iron, iodine, and vitamin A, followed by zinc, vitamin D, and folic acid. Although deficiency of vitamin C (scurvy), vitamin B_1 (beriberi), and vitamin B_3 (pellagra) have in the past caused substantial morbidity and mortality in affected populations, they are relatively uncommon today (although not unheard of). Micronutrient deficiencies have several causes:

poverty, poor diet, lack of clean water and adequate sanitation, illness, and malabsorption. Unlike PEM, micronutrient deficiencies may not be readily apparent. In fact, micronutrient deficiencies may be silent until major signs and symptoms appear. Fortunately, solutions to micronutrient deficiencies are relatively easy, inexpensive, available, and politically feasible.

Of the billions of people in the world, WHO and UNICEF estimate that some 2 billion are at risk for iron deficiency, 1.6 billion for iodine deficiency, and 0.8 billion for vitamin A deficiency. Each day some 300 mothers die in childbirth due to iron deficiency, 4,000 children die from the effects of vitamin A deficiency, and 50,000 infants are born with reduced mental capacity due to iodine deficiency.[24] Correction of readily apparent macronutrient deficiency without recognition (and correction) of concurrent micronutrient deficiency can lead to acute syndromes of disabling, potentially irreversible morbidity, and mortality. Country-specific data on micronutrients as well as overall nutritional status can be found in Macro International's Demographic and Health Surveys that collect and analyze data to monitor and evaluate populations, health, and nutrition programs.[25]

Iron

Iron deficiency is the most common micronutrient deficiency in the developing world and usually manifest by anemia. Anemia can also be seen in inflammatory processes, inherited disorders of hemoglobin, and deficiencies of vitamins A, B_{12}, and folate. However, at least 50% of cases of anemia are due to iron deficiency. Iron deficiency can be caused by inadequate dietary intake, insufficient iron absorption, or periodic bleeding, as in menstruation. Anemia in women of childbearing age is defined as a hemoglobin concentration less than 12 g/dl (at sea level). The diagnosis of iron deficiency anemia is usually established by measuring the concentration of serum ferritin, iron, transferrin, or total iron-binding capacity.

Often the cause is poor nutritional intake and lack of adequate iron sources in the diet, although chronic occult blood loss due to intestinal parasites can contribute significantly as well. Early childhood and the childbearing years in women (due to monthly blood loss and sequential pregnancies) are the two most vulnerable periods in life for iron deficiency. Iron depletion in the full-term infant occurs by about 6 months of age and may be marked by age 1 year when anemia is apparent. The consequences of iron deficiency may be anemia, lowered immunity to fight infection, adverse pregnancy outcomes, reduction in work capacity or school performance, and behavioral and learning difficulties in the child.

Correction of iron deficiency can be a targeted intervention in which vulnerable populations are screened and then provided iron supplements, or it can be a universal approach in which everyone is given iron supplements in areas where iron deficiency anemia is prevalent. Routine iron supplementation for pregnant women is a standard practice in most of the world. Hookworm infection can account for a large portion of iron deficiency. In these instances periodic deworming programs, coupled with sanitation and hygiene practices, can decrease the worm burden in the local population. When nutrition education is added to such programs, including at the time of growth monitoring, better food choices and feeding practices can help communities to be self-vigilant and self-monitoring and less reliant on rescue micronutrients from outside providers. Promotion of exclusive breastfeeding, delayed introduction of tea water given to infants, and iron fortification of commonly consumed foods (e.g., flour, cereals) can make a difference in lowering the incidence of iron deficiency in the community.

When the prevalence of anemia among non-pregnant women of reproductive age is equal to or greater than 20%, WHO recommends a weekly regimen of 60 mg of elemental iron along with 2,800 micrograms (2.8 mg) of folic acid for all menstruating women. This weekly regimen should be taken for 3 months, followed by 3 months off treatment, in an alternating pattern.[26] When the woman is anemic, she should take 120 mg elemental iron daily along with 400 micrograms (0.4 mg) of folic acid daily until her hemoglobin returns to normal. Then she should resume the intermittent regimen as described.[26] Preschool children living in areas where the prevalence of anemia is equal to or greater than 20% should receive weekly 25 mg of elemental iron; school-age children should take 45 mg of elemental iron each week. If they are anemic, they should take elemental iron daily until their hemoglobin reaches normal levels. Where hookworm infection is higher than 20%, it is best to combine iron supplementation with antihelminthics in children older than 5 years. At least annual universal antihelminthic treatment should be administered, irrespective of infection status.[27]

Iodine

Lack of iodine in the diet of a pregnant mother has several adverse effects on the growing fetus: it may result in stillbirth or infant death or may manifest as mild mental retardation or even cretinism, which includes severe brain damage, deafness, and dwarfism. Iodine deficiency reduces intelligence, education potential, and productivity. The average reduction in IQ is 13.5 points with iodine deficiency; in cretinism, this reduction is far greater.[28]

Iodine deficiency is the greatest cause of preventable brain damage in fetuses and infants, with over 130 countries and 2 billion people affected worldwide. If the allocation of iodine deficiency were visualized as a pyramid, it would show 2 billion people at risk at the bottom of the pyramid, 655 million with goiter, 26 million with brain damage, and 6 million with cretinism.

Iodine deficiency must be corrected before conception. This can be accomplished through food fortification, such as salt iodization. Major advances have been made over the last 15 years.[29] In 1990, only 46 countries had iodized salt programs, whereas in 2007, 120 countries had such programs and 54 countries still had problems with iodine deficiency.[30] Universal iodization of salt is a known safe way to control iodine deficiency for most of the world. The public health challenge is in getting the job done. Fortification also reduces the short-term effects on children and adults, such as lethargy and motor and mental impairment. Additional economic and social benefits include improved health and work capacity, improved efficiency of education, reduced health care expenditure, and improved quality of life.

Vitamin A

Vitamin A deficiency affects about 19 million pregnant women and 190 million preschool-age children in over 90 countries, but mostly from the WHO regions of Africa and Southeast Asia.[31] Some 40% of preschool children are estimated to be vitamin A deficient. Infants and children have increased vitamin A requirements to support rapid growth and to help them combat infections. Inadequate intake of vitamin A can result in vitamin A deficiency, which can be manifest as night blindness as the earliest sign, to increased morbidity and mortality from measles, diarrhea, and respiratory infections. Overall, 6% and 8% of deaths in children under 5 in Africa and Asia, respectively, are solely due to vitamin A deficiency. When vitamin A deficiency is combined with undernutrition, iron and zinc deficiencies, and inadequate breastfeeding, this combination accounts for 7% of under-5 deaths.

Vitamin A deficiency is the leading cause of preventable blindness in young children and increasingly recognized as a contributor to maternal mortality. Up to half a million children become blind each year due to vitamin A deficiency. Of those who develop blindness, half die within 1 year, in part because of their impaired ability to combat infection, particularly measles. Of the 190 million children with vitamin A deficiency, 13.5 million have night blindness, 3.1 million have xerophthalmia, and nearly half a million are blind.[32] Clinically, there is dryness of the cornea and conjunctiva (xerophthalmia), with scars and ulceration, Bitot's spots (keratinization), and ultimately keratomalacia. This is because vitamin A is used to regenerate epithelial cells including the retina.

Vitamin A deficiency is usually seen in community clusters, meaning that cases of xerophthalmia are surrounded by groups of affected mothers and young children. This phenomenon reflects community dietary practices and shared risks of undernutrition and infection. As children grow older, their tastes change, they are able to search more widely for food on their own, and they are less likely to have vitamin A lacking in their diet. Vitamin A deficiency may also be seasonal when dietary need is mostly supplied through vegetable sources, as availability may be high during harvest time but essentially absent during the months that just precede harvest.

Diarrhea, liver disease (hepatitis, cirrhosis), and intestinal infections with worms decrease the body's ability to absorb vitamin A. The infection-undernutrition cycle is the downward spiral of decreased food intake, decreased nutrients, and decreased ability to fight infection. This is sometimes seen in cases of measles. Metabolic needs for vitamin A are higher during growth, infection, and pregnancy. Any kind of corneal ulceration, especially when associated with measles, is an indication to provide vitamin A immediately, on the presumption that vitamin A deficiency exists.

Treatment is urgent and not expensive. In the mid-1980s, research in Indonesia—the Aceh trial—demonstrated that 2 cents' worth of vitamin A decreased child mortality by 34% (Figure 7-5).[33] Studies between 1986 and 1992 from India, Nepal, and Africa confirmed that preschool mortality could be reduced by 25% to 30%. The Nepal Nutrition Intervention Project studied 44,000 rural women, half of whom were pregnant. Results showed that a weekly dietary supplement of vitamin A or beta-carotene could reduce maternal mortality by 40%.[34] Public health surveys for night blindness and other manifestations of eye problems are one way of determining the prevalence of vitamin A deficiency in populations at risk. Trained interviewers and observers and large samples of children are necessary for such surveys. Among children younger than 5 years in SSA, about two fifths are at risk for vitamin A deficiency, and adequate vitamin A programs could avert 645,000 deaths each year. Vitamin A supplements can decrease infant mortality by 25%; reduce HIV-related morbidity, measles, and kwashiorkor mortality in children; and decrease maternal mortality by 40%. Vitamin A is often distributed at the time of immunization campaigns called national immunization days, as well as with other child survival interventions, such as deworming and nutrition education. Recent meta-analyses show that vitamin A does not alter seroconversion (antibody response) to measles vaccination, an important point because vitamin A is often co-administered at the time of measles vaccination.[35] One way to prevent vitamin A deficiency is breastfeeding because breast milk is a rich source of vitamin A. Exclusive breastfeeding for the first 6 months is strongly recommended. Dietary counseling is important for mothers of children who are beyond the breastfeeding years.

Vitamin A occurs naturally in animal products (dairy, egg yolks, liver) as well as vegetable sources (palm oil, dark green leafy vegetables) and colored fruit (such as papayas and mangos) that are rich in

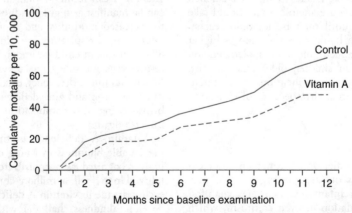

Figure 7-5. Mortality of 1- to 5-year-old children in vitamin A–supplemented versus control villages in Aceh, Indonesia, 1982–1984. From Sommer A, TarwotJo I, Djunaedi E, et al. Impact of vitamin A supplementation on childhood mortality: a randomized controlled community trial. *Lancet* 1986;1:1169. (*Reproduced with permission.*)

carotenoids and beta-carotene. Vegetable sources of vitamin A are less bioavailable than animal sources, partly because the plant sources are provitamins that must be metabolically converted to the active form, but also because diets that are lacking in animal sources tend to have very little fat, and fat is necessary in the diet to facilitate absorption of this fat-soluble vitamin. Foods such as sugar, cooking oil, and flour can also be fortified with vitamin A. Children and women after childbirth can be given supplements for 6 months: 200,000 IU for children and 300,000 IU for the mother 4 to 8 weeks postpartum. Finally, dietary diversification can help guarantee that vitamin A is consumed in adequate amounts. UNICEF now supplies between 600 and 800 million 2-cent vitamin A capsules to more than 75 countries around the world, essentially covering some 300 to 400 million children each year.

High-dose vitamin A supplementation is recommended in infants and children 6 to 59 months of age in settings where vitamin A deficiency is a public health problem,[36] and especially where night blindness prevalence is equal to or greater than 1%. Children 6 to 11 months old, including those who are HIV positive, should receive 100,000 IU once; children 12 to 59 months should be given 200,000 IU every 4 to 6 months.

In three settings vitamin A supplementation is not recommended by WHO: for newborns, for infants 1 to 5 months of age, and for HIV-positive pregnant women. Neonatal vitamin A supplementation and supplementation in infants 1 to 5 months of age is not recommended as a public health intervention to reduce infant morbidity and mortality.[37,38] The quality of the available evidence for mortality-related outcomes was found to be moderate. Mothers should continue to be encouraged to exclusively breastfeed infants for the first 6 months to achieve optimal growth, development, and health. Vitamin A supplementation in HIV-positive pregnant women is not recommended as a public health intervention for the prevention of mother-to-child transmission of HIV, nor is it recommended for postpartum or pregnant women.[39] It should be noted that concerns have been raised regarding increased progression to death for HIV-positive mothers and infants because of universal maternal or neonatal vitamin A supplementation in HIV-endemic areas.[40]

Zinc

Zinc is an essential element for growth, in both humans and plants, and for proper immune function and mucosal integrity. Lack of zinc in the human diet increases risk for diarrhea, respiratory infection, and developmental delays. In its severe form, zinc

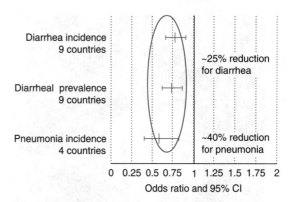

Figure 7-6. Effects of daily zinc supplement use on diarrhea and pneumonia in preschoolers. From Zinc Investigators' Collaborative Group. Prevention of diarrhea and pneumonia by zinc supplementation in children in developing countries: pooled analysis of randomized controlled trials. *J Pediatr* 1999;135:689–697. (*Reproduced with permission.*)

deficiency is characterized by acrodermatitis, gastrointestinal discomfort, diarrhea, and slow growth.

Many studies have demonstrated scientifically that daily zinc supplements reduce diarrhea and pneumonia in preschoolers (Figure 7-6).[41] In addition, zinc supplementation (taken as 20-mg tablets) decreases the frequency and the volume output of diarrhea and shortens the time to recovery. The effervescent tablets can be dissolved in breast milk or oral rehydration solution. Zinc supplementation for 10 to 14 days has a preventive effect on childhood illnesses in the 2 to 3 months after treatment.

Zinc is found in breast milk, meats, and crustaceans. It is generally low in most vegetables, grains, and fish. Years of over cultivation of the soil and mismanagement of land can deplete zinc in the soil, leading to low zinc levels in plants, crop yields, and seeds, contributing to the deficiency cycle.

Vitamin D

Vitamin D is needed for bone growth. Bone softening and ultimately rickets are the result of defective mineralization of growing bone—an imbalance of calcium and phosphorus. Nutritional rickets typically affects children younger than 2 years, during the period of rapid growth when demands for calcium and phosphorus are high. Vitamin D–deficient children will fail to thrive, be short in stature, be developmentally delayed, and have gait abnormalities (Figure 7-7).

Vitamin D deficiency can be prevented in all breast-fed babies by the daily administration of 400 IU of

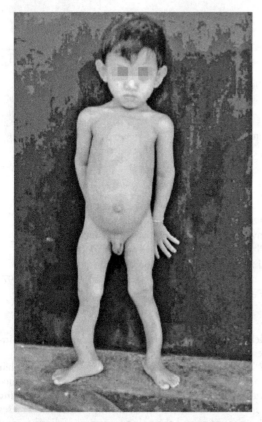

Figure 7-7. Cambodian child with rickets. (*Photo credit: Debra Coats, FNP.*)

vitamin D for the first 2 months of life. All formulas have at least 400 IU/L. A multivitamin tablet that contains that amount should be given if the formula intake is less than 500 ml per day or if the child does not get regular sunlight exposure (30 to 60 minutes each week). In nutritional rickets caused by vitamin D deficiency, calcium supplementation is essential. Daily oral administration of 2,000 to 5,000 IU vitamin D for 3 to 6 months or 300,000 to 600,000 IU intramuscularly every 3 to 6 months is the standard of care. It takes about 3 to 6 months for the physical changes to resolve, and some deformities may still require orthopedic correction.

Natural sources of vitamin D include fish liver oils, egg yolks, and fatty fish. Vitamin D precursors are converted in the skin by exposure to sunlight. Living in places where the weather is constantly cloudy, wearing clothing all the time, and residing mostly indoors will diminish exposure to sunlight and therefore can lead to vitamin D deficiency.

The mineral calcium plays a critical role with vitamin D. Vitamin D stimulates calcium absorption from the intestines and deposition in the bones. Calcium-deficient rickets, in contrast to vitamin D–deficient rickets, is seen during the toddler and childhood years, and it can occur even with sunshine exposure. Vitamin D–deficient rickets may present in the first year of life with hypocalcemic tetany or bowing of the legs. Daily oral calcium supplements of 1,000 mg elemental calcium (2.5 g of calcium carbonate) can meet the need. Therefore, when one encounters a case of rickets, it is important to consider deficiencies of either vitamin D, calcium, or both as the causes and treat accordingly.[42,43]

Folic Acid

Folic acid, also known as folate or vitamin B_9, is required for the production of DNA and is needed for the development of tissues and organs early and throughout pregnancy.[44] It prevents neural tube defects (NTDs), as well as other birth defects, such as in the lip/palate, the heart, and the limbs. NTDs are serious birth defects of the spine and brain that are the result of incomplete formation or closure of the neural tube. NTDs are the leading cause of infantile paralysis in the United States, with spina bifida as the most frequently occurring permanently disabling birth defect.

The WHO and the U.S. Public Health Service recommend that all women capable of becoming pregnant should consume 400 micrograms (0.4 mg) of folic acid daily to reduce their risk of a pregnancy resulting in neonatal spina bifida or other NTDs. Research in 1998 demonstrated that the incidence of NTDs in the United States had declined by almost 20% since folic acid fortification began.[45] Data from Chile show a decline by 31% in NTDs in 2000–2001 following wheat fortification. This implies that fortification with folic acid is effective in preventing NTDs and should be given due consideration in flour fortification programs.[46] The dietary approach to increase consumption of folic acid/folate is to improve overall dietary habits, take a daily folic acid supplement, and consume fortified foods.

Dietary folate is found in fresh green vegetables and some fruit. Intestinal malabsorption, such as chronic diarrhea, diminishes the uptake of folate. This results in anemia and failure to thrive, nonspecific signs and symptoms that should prompt the health care provider to include the diagnosis of folic acid deficiency in the differential.

When the prevalence of anemia among nonpregnant women of reproductive age is equal to or greater than 20%, WHO recommends a weekly regimen of 60 mg of elemental iron along with 2,800 micrograms (2.8 mg) of folic acid for all menstruating women.

This weekly regimen should be taken for 3 months at a time, alternating with 3 months off.[26] When the woman is anemic, she should take daily 120 mg elemental iron along with 400 micrograms (0.4 mg) of folic acid until her hemoglobin returns to normal. Then she should resume the intermittent regimen as described here.[26]

Other Potentially Significant Vitamin Deficiencies

Vitamin C

Vitamin C is found in fresh fruits (especially citrus) and vegetables, including leafy greens, potatoes, and sprouted beans. It is also found in the breast milk of humans, as well as in the milk of goats, camels, and cows. It is easily lost in cooking and boiling, which may be done for sterilization. Famine-affected and drought-affected populations are particularly prone to scurvy when fresh fruits and vegetables are in short supply. Signs and symptoms of scurvy are bleeding and swelling of the gums, easy bruisability, bone pain, and anemia.[47,48] Pain may lead to contractures and unusual positions for more comfort. Prevention of scurvy is accomplished by the daily consumption of 10 mg vitamin C, or such items as a quarter of an orange, a small tomato, a guava, or 20 grams of leafy green vegetables.

Vitamin B₁ (Thiamine)

Found in whole-grain cereals, unmilled rice, dried beans, ground nuts, red meat, dairy products, and some vegetables, vitamin B_1 can easily be deficient in populations where the main staple is polished white rice, cassava (manioc), and carbohydrates. B_1 deficiency, also known as beriberi, can be manifest as "wet" beriberi or "dry" beriberi. The wet form is due to high output acute cardiac failure, in which shortness of breath, swelling (edema), and an enlarged heart are the primary findings. It occurs more commonly in infants from 2 to 5 months of age and can be preceded by an infection. The infant first becomes listless, uninterested in feeding, has a weak cry, then becomes agitated, and finally cyanotic with poor peripheral perfusion. Death can occur abruptly within the following 24 hours.

The dry form is a more chronic condition in which the signs and symptoms are predominantly neurologic: initially weakness and peripheral sensory deficits, followed by ascending paralysis and areflexia. Beriberi may also resemble other neurologic disorders that have central nervous system findings, such as convulsions and coma, as well as spasms of the facial muscles. Among chronic alcoholics, thiamine deficiency can manifest as Wernicke's encephalopathy.

Apart from adequate dietary sources, prevention of beriberi can be achieved with the daily administration of 1 mg of thiamine. Mothers who are pregnant or lactating can be given 50 mg daily of thiamine to prevent beriberi in their children. The diagnosis of beriberi in an infant should lead the health care provider to consider the same condition in the mother. For management of acute medical conditions, treatment guidelines should be consulted.

Niacin

Niacin (B₃) is found in dried beans, nuts, lightly milled cereals, liver, fish, milk, meat, eggs, and cheese. Its deficiency can be seen in populations where the dietary staples are maize (corn) and sorghum, and generally where undernutrition is prevalent. Usually niacin deficiency (pellagra) causes severe diarrhea and mental deterioration. Classically, the deficiency is recognized as "the four D's": diarrhea, dermatitis, dementia, and death. The rash is typically in sun-exposed areas of the body. The tongue can become red and painfully swollen, making eating all the more difficult. Treatment of pellagra with thrice-daily 50 to 100 mg of nicotinamide (rather than niacin) can result in dramatic improvements within a few days.

Other Micronutrient Deficiencies

Cobalamin (B₁₂) and selenium deficiencies are less frequently found, but they may be seen, respectively, in strict vegetarians and in some parts of China, Scandinavia, and central Africa.[49] Cobalamin deficiency can present as macrocytic anemia and diarrhea, with failure to thrive. Selenium deficiency may be complicated by cardiomyopathy, osteoarthropathy, and myxedematous cretinism. Riboflavin (B₂) deficiencies are seen in children with very restricted diets because it is widely available in animal protein and green vegetables. These children have angular stomatitis, glossitis, and keratitis.

You can consult medical references for the daily allowances for the most important micronutrients and preventive and curative treatments for their deficiencies.

Food Fortification

Home fortification of foods with multiple micronutrient powders is strongly recommended by WHO to improve iron status and reduce anemia among infants and children 6 to 23 months of age.[50] However there is no available evidence on the harms or benefits of multiple micronutrient powders for pregnant women for improving maternal and health outcomes as an alternative to iron and folate supplementation.

In an attempt to reach large populations without behavior change strategies, some countries have chosen to fortify foods with micronutrients such as iron, iodine, or vitamin A. Food fortification strategies have included fortification of condiments (soy and fish sauce), milk, sugar, cooking oils, rice, wheat and maize flour, processed foods (biscuits), water, and salt.[51]

The success of food fortification depends on a number of factors, ranging from governments to private sector to the public sector. First of all, food fortification plans must take into account at least three points: (1) the food quantity eaten by the target population; (2) the likeliness of acceptability in terms of taste, color, and other characteristics; and (3) the price of the fortified product. These three factors can drive the plan to success or lead to failure. Food fortification plans require technical experts and industries to work together to identify scientifically sound approaches to adding vitamins and minerals to enhance the nutritional content of food. In addition, it calls for governments to encourage industries to envision benefits of investment in large-scale production of fortified foods. Governments also need to support the establishment and enforcement of national standards and quality processes. Moreover, communication and public education are necessary to create market demand. This requires strategic and informed use of the media coupled with effective public and private partnerships.

Large-scale use of iodized salt has been shown to reduce goiter by 19% to 64%. Water iodization studies show goiter reduction to range from 51% to 89%. Studies from Mexico and India of food fortified with iron and zinc showed reduced rates of anemia in Mexican toddlers and decreased incidence and duration of diarrhea and respiratory illnesses among Indian children. Some organizations in Mongolia have used Sprinkles, a home-based fortification sachet that includes iron and vitamin D. Fortification of monosodium glutamate with vitamin A showed that mortality in children ages 6 to 49 months was reduced by 30%.[52]

NUTRITION SURVEILLANCE AND MONITORING PROGRESS

The collection and analysis of nutrition data provides information that can be useful in various settings. For example, as a routine part of maternal and child health programs, nutrition surveillance can monitor population trends in nutrition status. During an emergency situation, the rapid assessment of nutrition status can determine the extent and severity of undernutrition and thereby predict change or the threat of deterioration. Nutrition surveillance can guide public health programs and assist governments and NGOs in project monitoring and evaluation. These data can indicate

the effectiveness of an intervention and track overall trends for preparedness reasons. Donor organizations often require such benchmarks for assessment of the delivery and performance of humanitarian assistance. Demographic and health surveys collect nutrition information on a 5-year basis in developing countries. UNICEF makes use of multi-indicator cluster surveys.

Global efforts at collecting and analyzing nutrition data during complex humanitarian emergencies began in 1993 as the Refugee Nutrition Information System (RNIS). RNIS evolved to become a Geneva-based system called the Nutritional Information in Crisis Situations (NICS). The NICS is the only system that considers all causes of undernutrition, key constraints in delivering humanitarian assistance, and the prevalence of acute undernutrition. Deriving its information from a wide range of voluntary UN and NGO sources, it issues quarterly reports that judge risks and threats to a population's nutrition status. As a warning system, NICS considers a prevalence of 5% to 8% undernutrition to be a concern and 10% to be a serious situation. NICS reports are meant to raise awareness and advocacy for interventions when action or donor responses are insufficient. However, delays in reporting sometimes result in the lack of timely intervention by donors and key stakeholders.

In the United States, the National Health and Nutrition Examination Surveys collect data from dietary interviews, physical examinations, and biochemical tests on samples of the U.S. population, including minority populations and elderly Americans. In addition, the NCHS collects and analyzes data, including nutrition status of the U.S. population, and publishes data briefs for public review and education. These sources of information provide trends in the health of the U.S. population and thereby allow other federal and state agencies as well as local health authorities to promote information on health practices and nutrition choices that would benefit their population.

RAPID ASSESSMENT IN EMERGENCY CONTEXTS

The SPHERE Project guidelines, developed by a large consortium of humanitarian NGOs, emphasize the importance of investigating the possible causes of undernutrition before attempting an anthropometric survey.[53] Information on the extent of undernutrition and its underlying causes can help to shape interventions. For humanitarian relief needs, it is important to identify the most affected populations and at-risk geographic areas and then to prioritize them for nutritional interventions. Assessments allow more effective use of limited resources as well as the monitoring of the effectiveness of local aid, in terms of both coordination and the impact on at-risk populations or individuals already affected. Many studies in the literature illustrate the approach to assessing undernutrition in developing countries.[54,55]

Survey assessments may be conducted for different purposes. An organization that delivers food rations in bulk metric tons will have different objectives and population-based indicators compared with an organization that sets up therapeutic feeding programs for affected individuals. Another organization may focus on identification of the underlying causes of undernutrition, with a plan for targeted interventions. Whereas one set of surveys may be for assessing food stores (food security), market activity, land use, livestock, and livelihoods, another may be for conducting anthropometric surveys in targeted populations. A challenge occasionally encountered is that nutrition surveys may not conveniently overlap with surveys of food security and livelihood assessments. Data may be specific to the area surveyed and not readily extrapolated. Broader surveys may miss the smaller remote pockets of poverty, undernutrition, or mortality.

Surveys also measure the extent of coverage of populations by interventions. Therefore, they have a place in both relief and development settings, that is, in measuring progress toward objectives that are either implicitly or explicitly stated and required by donor agencies or international organizations. Many of the standards for humanitarian assistance have been agreed on within the international community through the Sphere Humanitarian Charter and Minimum Standards in Disaster Response Project and Standardized Monitoring and Assessment of Relief and Transitions (SMART) (see Chapter 15).[56] Data in emergency settings are sometimes collected by a standard two-stage cluster-sampled survey to estimate the prevalence of acute undernutrition in program areas.[57] Cluster-sampling methodology selects 30 clusters (e.g., villages) and then surveys 30 units (e.g., households) in those 30 villages. Such an approach, although appearing straightforward, can be limited by difficulties in identifying the sampling frame for targeted populations. This limitation is especially seen in settings where refugee communities are closely integrated into host communities, making them hard to disaggregate for study purposes; where populations are highly mobile (nomadic or migrating); and where population density is sparse or households are small. As a result, such surveys can be resource intensive in terms of time, personnel, and costs. Alternative survey methodologies use a stratified design, defining strata from a central systematic area sample method.[58] Before a new survey is planned, it is useful to see if population-based data already exist, for example, trends in the

health of children seen in primary health care clinics or data from recent surveys. If an assessment still needs to be done, it can be achieved fairly quickly by measuring middle upper arm circumference (MUAC) among affected children or by sampling high-risk populations and measuring WFH.

MUAC measurement is both easy to teach and do and therefore gaining in popularity and use. It can be applied to rapid triage settings, especially where quick assessment of children (6 months to 59 months old) is needed. MUAC measurement uses a tricolored band around the middle upper arm (Figure 7-8). Position and placement are critical so that proper correlation can be made with the protein composition and lean tissue mass.

MUAC is more closely correlated with mortality than is WFH, thereby making MUAC a more reliable measure for planning emergency nutrition interventions and predicting mortality rates. Some international organizations also recommend that this measure be used as a criterion for admission to an outpatient therapeutic feeding center.

COMMUNITY-BASED GROWTH MONITORING AND PROMOTION

In contrast to rapid assessment of nutrition status in populations for emergency and food distribution purposes, growth monitoring serves as an ongoing public health activity in nonemergent settings in both developed and developing countries. *Anthropometry* is the scientific term used to describe this process of weighing and measuring. Anthropometry provides both the prevalence and incidence of undernourished children in a community. Moreover, it can serve as an early warning system in both acute and nonurgent settings. In situations where there is a massive influx of refugees or internally displaced persons, anthropometry can serve as a quick triage tool, rapidly identifying those who need acute nutrition interventions. Anthropometry can also serve to monitor ongoing programs where food distribution or onsite preparation and feeding are occurring.

Measurement of a child's weight and height is accompanied by recording those data points in a child's health record, commonly known in developing countries as a "road-to-health" chart. Such measurement can result in a significant interaction between a health care provider and the child's caretaker, where both look to see if the child's weight and height are progressing on the road to health.

Although this activity may be done privately in a health center, in developing countries it is more often performed in the outdoors or in a public place. Salter scales for weighing an infant or young child

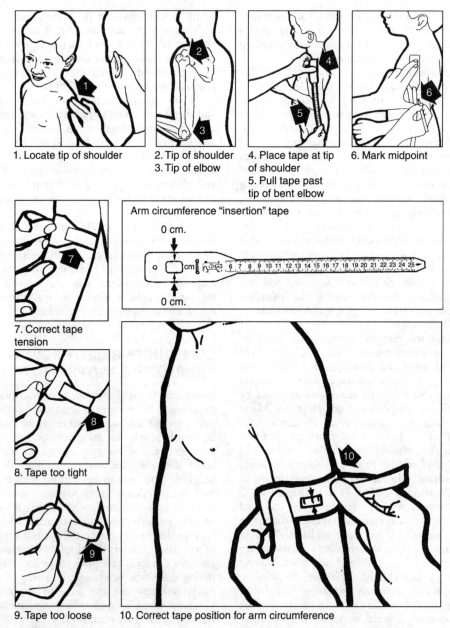

1. Locate tip of shoulder

2. Tip of shoulder
3. Tip of elbow

4. Place tape at tip of shoulder
5. Pull tape past tip of bent elbow

6. Mark midpoint

Arm circumference "insertion" tape

0 cm.

0 cm.

7. Correct tape tension

8. Tape too tight

9. Tape too loose

10. Correct tape position for arm circumference

Figure 7-8. Child middle-upper arm circumference measurement. From Coghill B. *Anthropometric Indicators Measurement Guide*. Washington, DC: Food and Nutrition Technical Assistance Project, Academy for Educational Development, 2001. (*Reproduced with permission.*)

hang from a tree in the outdoor setting (Figure 7-9). Mothers gather around to see the measurement of their own child as well as that of the children of their neighbors. Much talk and laughter can accompany this process. The measurement activity also benefits the bystanders who gather to watch the process. The experienced health care provider takes timely advantage of these sessions for community instruction about good nutrition, proper food choices, breastfeeding practices, and even broad health and

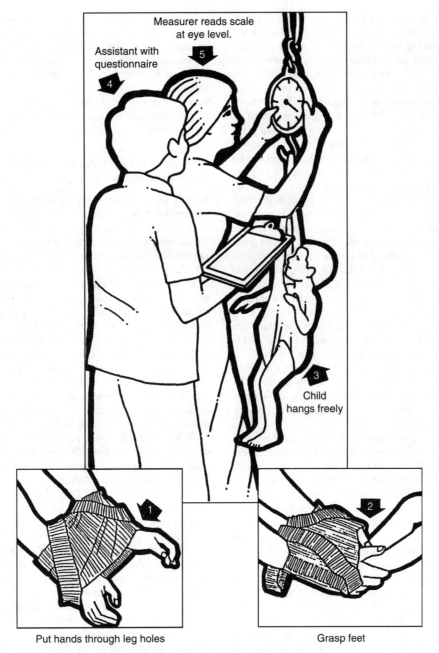

Measurer reads scale
at eye level.

Assistant with
questionnaire

Child
hangs freely

Put hands through leg holes

Grasp feet

Figure 7-9. Child measurement using Salter scale. From Coghill B. *Anthropometric Indicators Measurement Guide.* Washington, DC: Food and Nutrition Technical Assistance Project, Academy for Educational Development, 2001. (*Reproduced with permission.*)

hygiene messages. He or she can reinforce the importance of good nutrition and can publicly acknowledge mothers who made the appropriate nutrition and feeding choices for their children. Other mothers may learn the reasons for undernutrition or lack of growth in their own offspring. In addition, this activity can be coupled with immunization activities, supplementary feeding activities, family planning discussions, and general monitoring of family health and health needs.

Because anthropometry is easy and simple to apply, relatively untrained staff can effectively assist in the activities. Training should start with careful selection and qualification of community workers who have an interest in the process and are willing to receive instruction. Although they do not necessarily need to be literate or previously trained as health workers, they must be capable of being objective, comfortable with children, and able to work in a team. Role playing often helps to reinforce key teaching points as well as to identify strengths and weaknesses of the candidate trainees. It is useful to have them work in pairs because this will be the requirement in the field. Trial runs can highlight the steps in the process of child selection, measurement, and recording. It is essential to have a separate session on writing numbers on the records and charts because the number 7 can look like 1, and sixes, zeros, and eights can be confused. When both height and weight are being measured, height should be done first. Use a separate team for age assessment to keep the teams focused on specific tasks in the growth monitoring process.

Because it may be difficult to know the exact age of a child, WFH rather than weight-for-age (WFA) is often used. In instances where a child's age is needed, age sometimes can be determined by asking questions that relate physical, historical, or seasonal events to the birth of the child: for example, was the child born during the rainy season, when the president came to power, or when the tsunami struck?

Although relatively easy and simple, anthropometry data can be subject to unintentional errors. Errors of weight include those of taring the scales, movement by the child being measured, the degree of undress or cooperation, the presence of edema, parasite and stool load, dehydration status, and reading errors by those not adequately trained to read and record numbers. Health care workers performing the measurements should be sure that the child is not holding onto the scale or onto an anxious parent or caregiver.

Height can be more difficult to measure. An approved height/length board should be used (Figure 7-10). Ideally, the measurement requires three people: one to hold the child's head, one to straighten the knees, and a third to record the measurement called out by the assistants. It is important to ascertain that the child is standing straight, looking straight ahead, not slouching or wearing shoes, nor manifesting clubfoot or other deformities of the spine or legs. Hairdos can sometimes interfere with an accurate measurement and should be noted on the chart. For those children who are unable to stand or are too young to cooperate, length is measured instead of height (Figure 7-11).

Other measures of nutrition status include measurement of the thickness of fat folds (triceps and subscapular). However, fatfolds are usually not measured in developing country settings, and they exist primarily for academic purposes. In addition, fat fold measurements do not have good international references, and fat folds stabilize after 1 year, making this measurement less useful in anthropometry of children younger than 5 years. Some training and consistency of application of the calipers are also required to measure fat folds.

Interpreting Weight and Height Measurements

Results are commonly expressed in Z scores, for ease in interpreting anthropometric measurements. The Z score is an SD score, which is reflective of an individual measurement in relation to a standard reference population (the expected value). The Z score is derived by taking the difference between the observed value of a measurement and the median value in the reference population and dividing that difference by the SD value for the reference population. The Z scores can be for height-for-age, WFA, and WFH.

WFH is preferred because it has two objective measurements and it is often not possible to know the exact age of a child. Cut-off points for moderate undernutrition are defined as 2 SDs below the median of the reference population, or 80% of the median of the reference population. For severe undernutrition, this is 3 SDs, or 70% of the median.

When WFA is used, percentages of the standard expected WFA are used. Ninety percent of the standard is roughly at or above the 15th percentile on a standard growth curve (specific for age and gender), 80% is at the 3rd percentile of that growth curve, and 60% is about 3 SDs below the mean. Therefore, for kwashiorkor, the WFH is 60% to 80% of the expected; for marasmus, this is less than 60%; and for nutritional dwarfism, this is also less than 60%. Gender, age, the presence of edema, and sometimes measles immunization status are noted as part of the data collection to assist in the interpretation.

International reference standards are generated by the WHO,[59] the CDC, and the NCHS. In 2006, the WHO announced growth standards that more closely parallel growth trends in developing countries.[60] It will take some time for these growth standards to be disseminated and utilized around the world and to be accepted by the ministries of health responsible for dissemination of the standards.

In contrast to individual measurements, surveys for prevalence of undernutrition in populations use percentages of sampled populations that are below 2 SD for moderate undernutrition and below 3 Z scores for severe undernutrition. This is somewhat akin to the interpretation of individual measurements. Frequency distributions in tables or charts serve to profile the population.

Data need to be interpreted within their context. The public health provider or the researcher must ask several questions to derive a rational perspective.

What might be the causes of undernutrition? Is there food insecurity, a lack of adequate health care for a population, or is there an external factor (drought, natural disaster) that has led to poor harvests, displacement of populations, and other adverse conditions?

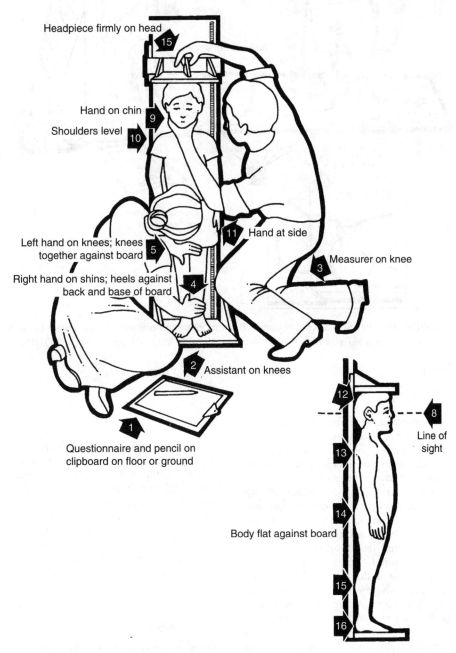

Figure 7-10. Correct position for child height measurement. From Coghill B. *Anthropometric Indicators Measurement Guide.* Washington, DC: Food and Nutrition Technical Assistance Project, Academy for Educational Development, 2001. (*Reproduced with permission.*)

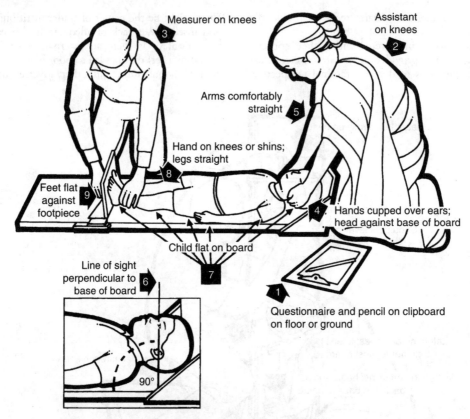

Figure 7-11. Child length measurement. From Coghill B. *Anthropometric Indicators Measurement Guide.* Washington, DC: Food and Nutrition Technical Assistance Project, Academy for Educational Development, 2001. (*Reproduced with permission.*)

Seasonal trends should be taken into consideration. Some countries experience droughts every 7 to 10 years. Populations can suffer from poor harvests, dying livestock (such as food sources), debilitation, and death of those who already have marginal health.

Infectious diseases may lay the groundwork for subsequent undernutrition; conversely, undernutrition can predispose an individual to infectious disease, as well as increase the risk of dying from that cause. When interpreting undernutrition data, it is important to keep in mind that undernutrition can be mimicked by infectious disease, notably TB and HIV/AIDS. Children who are chronically malnourished and do not respond to feeding supplementation are frequently assumed to have active TB. Although this is not a good diagnostic criterion on which to make the diagnosis of childhood TB, it is often the approach in settings where TB prevalence is high in the community and good diagnostic means are lacking.

PREVENTION

Several components make up the package of essential preventive actions against undernutrition: breastfeeding, complementary feeding, maternal nutrition, food fortification (vitamin A and iodine), integrated management of childhood illness (IMCI), and hygiene and sanitation as well as food safety, and lastly education about healthy habits and food preferences. Moreover, larger community issues such as food security and food safety must also be considered in preventing undernutrition among the most vulnerable.

Breastfeeding

Strong evidence supports the advantages of breastfeeding over the use of breast milk substitutes (formula) or early addition of foods. The benefits of exclusive breastfeeding for the first 6 months of life are particularly strong.[61] Practices vary widely over time, and recommendations continue to change as experts learn more about breast milk, population behavior, and individual preferences. The nutrient content of breast milk is regarded as the best source of protein (including immunoglobulins), carbohydrates, lipids, minerals, and vitamins (except iron and vitamins K and D) for newborns, including premature babies, and infants. Protective immunoglobulins in breast milk reduce the risk of diarrhea, respiratory illness, and otitis media (Figure 7-12). Moreover, for premature babies, breastfeeding reduces the incidence of necrotizing enterocolitis and may enhance their neurocognitive development. In addition to these nutritional benefits, breast milk is contamination free, a key distinction in areas where water can be a source of disease. In addition to providing immunoglobulin-rich colostrum, suckling stimulates oxytocin release in the mother that assists in uterine contractions, delivery of the placenta, and reduces postpartum blood loss. It is important to note that lactating women have higher caloric and other nutrient needs, which means that breastfeeding is not cost free.

Neurobehavioral (bonding) and maternal (faster recovery postpartum) benefits also accrue with breastfeeding. Other benefits include economic benefits, which are especially important to those with limited household income. There is no need to purchase formula, bottle-feeding equipment, or have accessible the sanitary conditions needed to mix it, and breastfed infants tend to have fewer medical illnesses and lower infant and childhood mortality.

The nutrient content of breast milk remains fairly constant and independent of the mother's dietary intake until her own bodily stores are severely depleted.[62] The caloric density of breast milk averages about 21 kcal/30 cc (range: 14 to 35 kcal/30 cc), depending on its fat content, which is not directly related to the mother's diet. Original concerns that breastfed infants did not gain as much weight as formula-fed infants were based on comparisons with infant growth curves of formula-fed white babies. The curves have been considered inappropriate for human milk–fed infants, and some newer WHO growth standards reflect better sampling frames (breastfed babies from numerous countries). The growth of breastfed infants should be considered the norm.

With regard to the practice of breastfeeding, it is essential to instruct new mothers that the colostrum (first milk) should be offered to the newborn by putting the baby to the breast right after birth. This should be exclusive of any other administered fluids or other foods, which is the case in some cultures (prelacteal feeding). Breast milk is the only food an infant needs for the first 6 months of life. There are some instances, because of particular maternal health problems and some medications, for example, when breastfeeding may be contraindicated; however, these are rare exceptions that require consultation with medical and nursing experts. Each feeding contains two types of milk: foremilk and hind milk. Foremilk is more watery and meant to address the child's thirst and encourage sucking. As the child continues to feed, the fat content of the milk rises. This hind milk is meant to satiate the baby's appetite. Both milks contain nutrients and are beneficial and required for proper growth.

The WHO and UNICEF support exclusive breastfeeding of infants in the first 6 months of life, particularly as part of the Baby Friendly Hospital Initiative. The American Academy of Pediatrics (AAP) reaffirmed its recommendations of exclusive breastfeeding for about 6 months, followed by continued breastfeeding after introduction of complementary food for 1 year or longer as mutually desired by mother and infant.[63] In addition, the AAP endorses the WHO/UNICEF "Ten Steps to Successful Breastfeeding." Although rates of breastfeeding initiation continue to rise in the United States, not all demographic groups have increased breastfeeding practices. Ethnicity, education, employment, age, and multiparity can influence breastfeeding choices. Support and promotion of breastfeeding by many groups, including the Special Supplemental Nutrition Program for Women, Infants, and Children

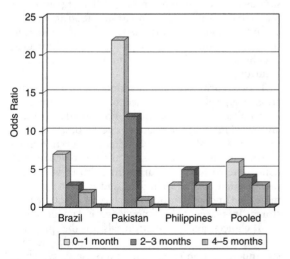

Figure 7-12. Infant mortality due to infectious diseases associated with not breastfeeding, by country and age group. From Hill Z, Kirkwood B, Edmond K. Family and Community Practices That Promote Child Survival, Growth and Development: A Review of the Evidence. Geneva: World Health Organization, 2004:21–26.

(commonly referred to as WIC), have helped raise awareness and lower barriers to breastfeeding among eligible populations. In addition, the Healthy People 2020 goals focus on breastfeeding initiation and maintenance and on the elimination of health disparities, including racial and ethnic, as they pertain to breastfeeding.[64]

Newborn and infant feeding recommendations in the context of HIV were recently updated in the WHO Prevention of Mother-to-Child Transmission (PMTCT) and Breastfeeding Guidelines 2010.[65] The advent of antiretrovirals (ARVs), along with their greater availability and acceptability, have changed the incidence of postnatal transmission of HIV through breastfeeding and thereby have shaped guidance about breastfeeding and replacement feeding after weaning. All women presenting for antenatal care should be HIV tested and, if positive, they should be enrolled in a HIV PMTCT program. Approximately 80% of all MTCT occurs in mothers whose CD4 count is less than 350 and thus eligible for lifelong antiretroviral treatment (ART). With ART, MTCT rates are typically lowered from greater than 35% to less than 5%, even with extended breastfeeding. Among the approximately 60% of HIV-positive mothers who choose to breastfeed and are not eligible for ART (CD4 greater than 350), there are two recommended prophylaxis regimens involving primarily ARV dosing to the infant (option A) or maternal triple-ARV dosing (option B) for the duration of breastfeeding, both with MTCT rates of less than 5%. A number of countries have adopted a modification of option B—Option B+—initiating all HIV-positive women on lifelong ART in pregnancy, even if their CD4 is greater than 350.

Breastfeeding should be exclusive in the first 6 months and extended to at least 12 months with adequate complementary feeding, and the infant should only be weaned if the mother can provide a safe and adequate replacement diet. Weaning should be gradual (about 1 month), and ARV prophylaxis should continue for 1 week beyond any breastfeeding. For mothers who choose to replacement feed from birth or wean early, commercial infant formula should be used exclusively in the first 6 months.

Further, the 2010 WHO PMTCT Guidelines call on countries to establish as a national policy whether they will primarily promote breastfeeding or replacement feeding for all HIV-positive mothers. Mothers may opt out and choose an infant feeding option not aligned with the national policy without ostracism or sacrifice of counseling and support from health services. It is also recognized that ARVs are not yet universally available, and guidance from maternal and child health services will need to take that into consideration. The design of breastfeeding promotion interventions should consider these recommendations in the context of the local prevalence of HIV, ARV services, and the balance of risks between MTCT associated with breastfeeding and mortality associated with replacement feeding from birth or early weaning. Multiple studies showed no benefit to HIV-free survival with formula feeding from birth or early weaning and replacement feeding versus extended breastfeeding, even prior to the advent of postnatal ART or ARV prophylaxis among breastfeeding mothers, which should now dramatically shift the balance of risks in favor of breastfeeding as long as there is good ARV adherence.

Food Security

Food security can be defined as those conditions in which people have both physical access to affordable food and the economic means to obtain it. Food should be available in sufficient quality and quantity to meet nutritional needs and to allow for a healthy and productive life. When poverty, policies, forced migration due to conflict or war, environmental factors (drought, floods), or other natural disasters disrupt this access and availability of food for prolonged periods of time, global acute malnutrition (GAM) and severe acute malnutrition (SAM) can ensue. SAM and GAM are often used as health indicators of food insecurity. Médecins Sans Frontières (MSF) uses four stages to describe progressively worsening conditions: food insecurity, food crisis, serious food crisis, and famine. Other organizations may refer to suffering from chronic food insecurity, extended food crisis, prevalence of acute undernutrition, mortality, access to food, coping strategies, livelihood assets, probability of hazards, and civil security.

Food security is usually descriptive of a macro situation (e.g., a district, province, or nation). However, it can also apply to individual households. Cultural and religious practices, knowledge of best nutrition practices for infants and children, or even limited varieties of food and lack of dietary diversity can contribute to food insecurity. In cultures where the men are fed first and children and women last, one might see undernutrition in the face of adequate food stores. In places where knowledge is lacking about food choices and nutrient needs in the pregnant women or in the growing infant or child, one may see undernutrition in the face of food security. There may also be adequate caloric intake but inadequate micronutrient intake.

Food security assessments tend to be qualitative and can be based on rainfall data, crop production, and market prices. Famine Early Warning Systems Network (FEWSNET), which is supported by the

U.S. Agency for International Development (USAID), publishes regional monthly or bimonthly reports to track these and other parameters. FEWSNET and other assessments take into account food production, market prices, coping strategies, and population migration. This information may be derived from a variety of local sources. Some surveys are supplemented by dietary diversity information, such as number of types of food available, weekly consumption of selected foods, and main sources of food used by a household. Although these data do not reveal the whole picture, they do reflect local conditions where populations are at increased risk due to ethnic and political marginalization, conflict and violence, or natural disasters such as drought. Demographic and health surveys also complement this information and provide valuable trends assessments.

On a more focused basis, local market surveys and household surveys can complement nutrition assessments. A market survey will indicate whether meats or fish can be bought, for what price, and in what quality or quantity. It is helpful to see if alternate sources of protein are available in the form of legumes and nuts and beans. Much can be learned by visual inspection of a household: the cooking and eating areas, food preparation utensils, food storage areas, hygiene conditions, number of family members eating in one household, gender and ages of those members, sick relatives who are bedridden, and the presence of rats, dogs, and cats, as well as other basic health measures, such as bednets, water storage pots (covered or not), and latrines.

Sometimes in the rush to address food insecurity and to provide emergency food supplies, the "food-first" approach by donor agencies and their implementing partners predominates. Such an approach may fail to consider underlying causes of undernutrition that could be tackled directly. In the culture of donors, however, it is easier to quantify and fund food commodities. Such aspects of the humanitarian relief effort carry more visibility, goodwill, and political impact. Nevertheless, food interventions per se do not address the root causes of undernutrition in maternal and child populations, those populations living with HIV/AIDS, or the elderly who are chronically malnourished.

Food Safety, Hygiene, and Sanitation

Food safety—the proper handling of food and its preparation—plays an indirect role in nutrition problems. Although a thorough discussion of food safety is not the purview of this chapter, acute food poisoning as well as periodic contamination of food due to unclean food handling and preparation can have a significant public health impact. Pesticides can also contaminate food and provoke serious reactions when ingested. Chronic undernutrition can occur when bacteria, parasites, and even viruses are found regularly in food sources.

Foodborne outbreaks can be attributed to poor personal hygiene, improper storage temperatures, contaminated equipment, inadequate cooking, and food from unsafe sources. Primary symptoms are usually gastrointestinal (nausea, abdominal cramps, vomiting, diarrhea), as well as neurologic and systemic manifestations in some instances.

Classically, food handling and preparation by those who have not washed their hands or who have not washed or cleaned the food can lead to illness in any susceptible person. Typical organisms and illnesses such as typhoid, *Salmonella, Shigella,* staphylococcal toxins, botulinum toxins, hepatitis A, cholera, *Escherichia coli, Yersinia, Clostridium perfringens, Bacillus cereus, Giardia,* and amebiasis plague many locals and visitors alike. Parasites, such as tapeworms (in beef, pork, and fish), *Cryptosporidium,* and *Cyclospora,* and toxins in shellfish and bottom-feeders (e.g., paralytic shellfish poisoning) can be prevalent. It is worth inquiring what pathogens and illnesses predominate in the area. Of interest is that in some communities, the most common cause of epilepsy is neurocysticercosis from the pork tapeworm. Tuberculosis of the gut can be traced back to consumption of unpasteurized cow's milk.

Health Education

Underlying all these factors is that individuals need to be taught healthy practices that prevent undernutrition: exclusive breastfeeding for infants in the first 6 months; healthy dietary intake and variety of food choices during pregnancy, infancy, and childhood; iron and folate supplementation for women of childbearing age; safe food-handling practices; oral rehydration and zinc for diarrhea; vaccination for rotavirus (where available); and promotion of good handwashing practice, to name a few. These health education lessons are not taught separately but should be incorporated into other health encounters, into community activities, such as health fairs, or special visitor events. Infant and child growth monitoring, for example, is a good time to reinforce health messages or to introduce new ones. Moreover, antenatal and family planning sessions, immunizations, and IMCI services are opportune times. For persons with chronic illnesses, such as diabetes, tuberculosis, HIV/AIDS, and epilepsy, the nutrition component of their care must not be overlooked; nutrition is as much a part of their clinical management as the glycemic control, the anti-TB drugs, the ARVs, or the anticonvulsants. Persons must understand the critical nature of early feeding strategies to prevent stunting as much as to avoid wasting. They must understand the nutrition link to psychosocial development, cognitive skills, academic achievement, and better employment options later in life.

INTERVENTIONS

From time to time, when undernutrition is widespread in a community, the question arises as to whether health providers should start community-based or camp-based nutrition programs. WHO's framework states that undernutrition rates under 10% (10% of children 6 to 59 months old who are either below 2 SDs of the reference median WFH or 80% of the reference WFH) do not require population interventions.[66] Instead, individuals may need attention through regular community services. MUACs can also be used as eligibility criteria for selective feeding programs. MUACs less than 11 cm indicate severe undernutrition, and those between 11.0 and 12.49 cm reflect moderate undernutrition.[67]

For undernutrition rates between 10% and 14%, the WHO recommends starting targeted supplementary feeding programs (SFPs) and therapeutic feeding programs (TFPs) for those who are severely malnourished. With undernutrition rates of 15% or more, the WHO recommends the distribution of general rations, plus SFP for all members of vulnerable groups (Table 7-2),

Table 7-2. Supplementary food types.

Blended food[a]
Corn-soya blend (CSB)
Wheat-soya blend (WSB)
Corn-soya-milk (CSM)
Wheat-soya-milk (WSM)
Locally produced mixes
1. Base: Cereal
Rice
Maize
Sorghum
2. High-protein source
Beans
Groundnuts
Lentils
Soya beans
Dried skim milk
Oil seeds
3. High-energy source
Vegetable oil
Oil seeds
Butter oil
Groundnuts
Sugar

[a]Blended foods may be available through the World Food Programme or directly from donors. They are nutritionally valuable (fortified with vitamins and minerals), easy to transport and store, and can be very useful to initiate a supplementary feeding program when appropriate local foods are lacking. From Médicins Sans Frontières. *Nutrition Guidelines.* 1st ed. Paris: Médicins Sans Frontières, 1995.

particularly children and pregnant/lactating mothers, and TFP. These recommendations can be modified when other deteriorating circumstances so indicate—for example, general food rations below the mean energy requirement; CMRs above 1 per 10,000 per day; epidemics of measles or pertussis; severe cold and inadequate shelter; high prevalence of respiratory and diarrheal disease; and severe public health hazards.

The treatment of malnourished children,[68] although beyond the scope of this chapter, includes key steps: the prevention or treatment of hypoglycemia, hypothermia, and dehydration; correction of electrolyte imbalance and micronutrient deficiencies; gradual initiation of feeding; rebuilding of wasted tissues (catch-up growth); provision of stimulation, play, and loving care; and preparation for follow-up after discharge.

Premature termination of treatment increases the risk of recurrence of undernutrition. Children should reach the expected weight for their height before discharge from a feeding program. Some children will always remain underweight because they are on the low end of the normal distribution curves of WFH. If they demonstrate continued growth rates and no functional impairments, they can be discharged after 1 month of adequate food intake and weight gain. The parents or caregivers should be instructed in the causes of PEM, the proper use of foods (quality and quantity), personal and environmental hygiene, immunizations, and early management of diarrhea and respiratory infections.

Community-Based Therapeutic Care

First implemented in Ethiopia in 2000, community-based therapeutic care (CTC) is a community-based approach for managing large numbers of acutely malnourished people as a viable alternative to therapeutic feeding centers.[69,70] Although it was primarily designed to meet the needs of children younger than 5 years, it is being considered for treatment of severe and acute undernutrition among adults, particularly those with HIV/AIDS. It can be used in emergency situations or in development settings.[71] CTC uses people's homes, not hospitals, so the focus of assistance is on villages rather than health centers. It works through local people wherever possible rather than through imported experts. It considers the social, economic, and cultural aspects of undernutrition in addition to the medical ones.

Home-based treatment accommodates the fact that women should not spend prolonged periods of time away from their homes. Although undernutrition often is recurrent in households that are chronically vulnerable, the risk of acquiring infection at home is less than at a facility where other sick people are located. This risk would argue for home-based treatment rather than hospitalization for undernutrition.

BOX 7-1. COMMUNITY-BASED THERAPEUTIC CARE: MANAGEMENT OF ACUTE MALNUTRITION. IMCI, INTEGRATED MANAGEMENT OF CHILDHOOD ILLNESSES; WHO, WORLD HEALTH ORGANIZATION. (DATA FROM CTC RESEARCH AND DEVELOPMENT PROGRAMME. COMMUNITY-BASED THERAPEUTIC CARE (CTC): A FIELD MANUAL. OXFORD, UK: VALID INTERNATIONAL, 2006.)

Management of Acute Malnutrition

If complications are present
Malnutrition is severe and IMCI/WHO protocols are instituted

If no complications, but malnutrition is still severe
Institute an Outpatient Therapeutic program

If no complications and malnutrition is moderate
Institute a Supplementary Feeding Program

Protocols for CTC (Box 7-1) are different from those used by the WHO for managing SAM in facilities. CTC has four components: community mobilization and participation, SFPs, outpatient therapeutic care, and stabilization centers.[72]

Most experts recommend that MUAC should be the key criterion for who should participate in CTC activities.[73] MUAC is more closely correlated with muscle mass than WFH, is a better measure of nutritional status than WFH, and tends to predict the risk of death better than WFH. Because MUAC increases with age, a fixed cut-off point will preferentially select younger children, who have a higher risk of death. The choice of MUAC or WFH by agencies will depend on whether it is more important to identify the risk for death or the response to treatment because the latter is better gauged by WFH.

CTC relies on the availability of ready-to-use therapeutic foods (RUTFs),[74] such as Plumpy'nut (Nutriset). RUTFs are a mix of cereals, legumes, oil, water and sugar, vitamins, and minerals, providing a protein source and an energy source. RUTFs often have a peanut base, but not all countries grow peanuts. RUTF can be made at home, does not have to be cooked (no firewood), is easy to store, and can be a vehicle for additives. Plumpy'nut comes as a 92-gram bar that provides 500 calories.

RUTF is easier to prepare than the water-based F100 (a fortified dried milk formula) and does not require high volumes of intake to meet energy requirements, unlike F100. Access to safe water may be limited in disaster and crisis settings. Newer RUTFs do not use milk powder and use only locally produced crops. RUTF can also be considered for replacement feeding of non-breastfed children older than 6 months because it is less expensive than infant formula. Because HIV stigma can be associated with the use of infant formula, RUTF may be more acceptable. Some experts think that RUTF should be included in the essential drugs list. Such inclusion would simplify logistics because RUTF would then be part of the normal package of drugs.

On an emergency scale, RUTFs are imported, regardless of costs, to meet acute needs. As time goes on, it is desirable to encourage local production with locally available ingredients because the cost of RUTF is tied to the sustainability and success of CTC. CTC provides a market for RUTF; conversely, RUTF is needed for the success of CTC. Other factors that play into the success of CTC are the availability of community volunteers, their motivation, the ability to train and retain them, the availability of training materials, the possibility that volunteers from other development programs could be employed, and whether CTC can be combined with the IMCI strategy.

Two types of indicators can be used to determine whether a nutritional intervention, such as a feeding program, is performing effectively: process indicators, such as the number of staff working at a feeding center; and outcome indicators, such as the percentage of children recovered. The relief and development community debates about other indicators, such as weight gained or length of stay at a facility. Although donors tend not to use these indicators, international and nongovernmental organizations may use them for internal monitoring. SFPs use indicators such as recovery rate, death rate, and defaulting rate. TFPs use these three indicators plus weight gain, coverage, and mean length of stay. Organizations such as the World Food Programme, the UN High Commission for Refugees, MSF, and Save the Children have different thresholds at which "alarming" percentages set into motion other responses.

SPECIAL CIRCUMSTANCES: HIV/AIDS

Over the last 25 years, the story of undernutrition has been made more complicated by HIV. Undernutrition and HIV/AIDS have a mutually adverse relationship. By decreasing the natural immune defenses, undernutrition increases susceptibility to HIV and may also contribute to lowered effectiveness of ARVs. HIV/AIDS can be accompanied by gastrointestinal disorders that diminish the body's ability to absorb food and essential micronutrients, further jeopardizing nutritional status. In addition, opportunistic infections, such as TB, increase the body's metabolic demands and burn vital calories, worsening the degree of undernutrition.

PEM negatively affects all aspects of the immune system: cell-mediated immunity, antibody production, acute phase response, and protection of the integument. HIV diminishes the immune system and T-cell function. The lack of micronutrients, such as vitamins A, B, C, and E, as well as iron, zinc, and selenium, also affects the immune system, making the body more susceptible to infection. Consequently, PEM and HIV together can be significantly destructive.

HIV-positive women are more likely to deliver low-birth-weight babies, who are more likely to experience slower growth and be at higher risk for undernutrition. Along with the previously mentioned rationale and recommendations regarding exclusive breastfeeding and early cessation, periodic vitamin A supplementation lowers morbidity and mortality and improves growth in HIV-positive children. Malnourished HIV-positive adults are known to have an increased risk of opportunistic infections, a shorter survival, and a higher risk of death.

Nutritional needs for people living with HIV/AIDS are different from the noninfected person or child.[75] Moreover, the synergism between infectious disease and undernutrition compounds the problem of morbidity and mortality, especially in low-resource settings.[76] HIV increases resting energy expenditure, reduces food intake, and can be accompanied by malabsorption or loss of key nutrients. Asymptomatic HIV-positive individuals require 10% more energy calories; symptomatic HIV-positive individuals require 20% to 30% more.[77] For HIV-positive children with weight loss, energy requirements increase by 50% to 100%. Given that it would be impossible for children to consume large volumes of food to make up that need, early detection of weight loss and encouragement of feeding is especially important.[78]

The overlap between SAM and HIV/AIDS is considerable. The association of inadequate food intake, malabsorption and diarrhea, and altered metabolism and nutrient storage leads to nutritional deficiencies. These are exacerbated by increased oxidative stress and immune suppression, which in turn allow for more HIV replication, faster disease progression, and increased morbidity and mortality. Special nutritional interventions, therefore, need to be integrated into the medical management of HIV.[79]

The interactions among HIV, livelihood, and food security are complex. People may stay at home to care for sick and dying family members, making them less available for community activities, including food

crop production and food sales in the marketplace. This downward spiral further decreases income available for health care and treatment.

The use of home-based care for HIV/AIDS patients shares a number of features with CTC, which can be modified to meet the nutritional needs of people living with HIV/AIDS.[80] CTC can potentially reduce hospitalization rates. It is also seen as a point of entry for voluntary counseling and testing as well as a means for facilitating adherence to ART. Trust, proximity to home for easier referrals, and the credibility of the CTC work may all increase voluntary counseling and testing in the local population. Just as DOTS (directly observed treatment, short course) programs for TB are enhanced by the supply of food to TB patients to facilitate case management, so too may CTC help with antiretroviral therapy.

Nutritional interventions have a wide range of activities, from good nutrition counseling for positive living, to counseling on special food and nutrition needs in conjunction with treatment for opportunistic infections and the use of ARVs, including instances in which ARVs should or should not be taken with food. ARVs can aggravate nutritional problems and cause metabolic derangements of glucose, fat stores, lipid and cholesterol, and pancreatic enzymes needed for digestion. Good nutrition is essential for response to treatment. Children, pregnant and lactating mothers, and those who lose weight or do not respond to medication may need supplementary feeding; in the case of severe undernutrition, they need therapeutic feeding. Children who are vulnerable or orphaned by parents who died of HIV/AIDS will need special nutrition assistance as well. Palliative care and assistance with coping mechanisms are also important interventions for those doubly affected by undernutrition and HIV/AIDS.

Micronutrients are especially important for people living with HIV/AIDS. Clinical trials have shown that supplementation improves many clinical and laboratory parameters, such as increasing survival times, preventing adverse birth outcomes, and reducing mother-to-child transmission of HIV in nutritionally vulnerable women with advanced disease.

THE GLOBAL POLICY RESPONSE

Economists and others recognize that undernutrition negatively affects a country's economic growth, perpetuates poverty, and results in increased health costs. On a larger scale, where larger proportions of a country's population are affected, the gross national product reflects the result of a long cascade beginning with undernutrition.

To bring global attention and pressure to bear on this situation, the first MDG is to halve poverty and hunger in target populations where individual income

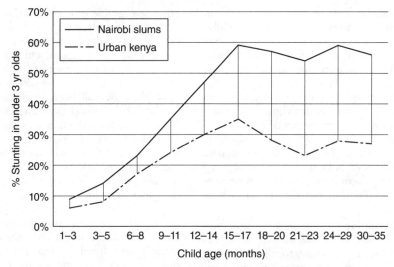

Figure 7-13. Stunting prevalence among children under 3 years old: comparing the Nairobi slums with overall urban Kenya. Data from Source: Urbanization, Poverty and Health Dynamics—Maternal and Child Health data (2006–2009); African Population and Health Research Center; and Kenya DHS (2008–2009).

is less than US$1 per day and where large proportions of children younger than 5 are underweight. MDGs are just a part of the response. It is well known that better incomes and food security are part of the route to solving undernutrition. Yet these alone are not the answer. Inappropriate feeding and care practices in the face of food-secure environments result in underweight or stunted children. Moreover, poor access to health services, poor sanitation, and ignorance of basic health care exacerbate the problem.

That first MDG includes a target to halve between 1990 and 2015 the proportion of people who suffer from hunger.[81] The MDG report for 2012 indicated that hunger may have spiked in 2009, as a consequence of the global food and financial crisis, and that progress to end hunger has been stymied in most regions. Moreover, it indicated that one in four children in the developing world is still underweight and that children in rural areas are nearly twice as likely to be underweight as those in urban areas. This is also reflected in the UNICEF Report on the State of the World's Children 2012 (see the end-of-chapter Resources section). The association with poverty and undernutrition shows that, in some regions, the prevalence of underweight children is dramatically higher among the poor. Underlying all this is that over 42 million people have been uprooted by conflict or persecution.

In fact, the UNICEF report for 2012 indicates that for children the locus of poverty and undernutrition has been shifting from rural to urban areas, thereby closing the gap between rural and urban areas. The urban poor child is likely to be undernourished, and if chronically deprived of adequate caloric and micronutrient intake, to be stunted as well. This was borne out in a study of Indian children in eight cities, in which the National Family Health Survey from 2005 to 2006 found at least 25% of urban children under 5 years were stunted. For the poorest quartile of urban dwellers, over 50% of the children were stunted and 47% were underweight.[82] Not limited to Asian children, stunting in children younger than 3 years is also documented in prevalence surveys in Nairobi's slum area Kibera (Figure 7-13).

Therefore one must ask, "What are the key actions that countries must undertake to reverse these figures of high prevalence of undernutrition and stunting in children, particularly those in urban slums?"

1. Ensuring that nutrition is on the list of national priorities, and keeping it there. This means there must be an official nutrition policy and implementation plan, along with a line item in the national and subnational budget to address this. However, unclear perspectives about what should be done occasionally lead policymakers to see the root of undernutrition as a poverty issue that should be addressed through poverty alleviation programs.[83] The voices of educated, motivated, and influentially placed champions can help motivate decision makers who are challenged by competing priorities in their health and population strategies.[84]

2. Applying evidence-based interventions, such as promotion of breastfeeding, complementary feeding for children 6 to 9 months of age, vitamin A

supplementation, iron fortification, iron and folate supplementation for women of child-bearing age, universal salt iodization, and zinc in the management of diarrhea, as well as good handwashing techniques and use of adequate sanitation facilities. On a broader scale, national investments in agriculture (such as irrigation schemes), better roads, health clinics, and community markets are improvements in infrastructure that may help diminish food insecurity.[85] In addition, encouragement to farmers to raise crops, which have been bred for disease resistance and may have greater micronutrient content, will contribute to better nutrition in local populations.

3. Not implementing activities that have not proven to be effective. This includes food-for-work, microcredit programs, growth monitoring (without a link to nutrition counseling and referrals), preschool feeding programs targeting children over 24 months of age, and school feeding programs targeting children older than 5 years.[52]

Other key points include acting at scale, by identifying promising practices and seeing them piloted and then quickly scaled up—that is, large-scale effectiveness assessments, targeting those most in need in situations where socioeconomic inequities and politics might prevent reaching those most in need, investigating the proper role of the private sector, and strengthening strategic and operational capacity within the national government and its health workforce to manage a national nutrition agenda.

What about international food aid? This is a major resource, often used more visibly in times of natural disasters or conflict. Around two thirds of all food aid, both emergency and development, is handled by the World Food Program (WFP). The WFP reports in 2012 its work in 73 countries, for 90 million beneficiaries, delivering 3.7 million tons of food, with projected resource needs of over US$5 billion.[86] Food aid is best if it is linked to and leverages other interventions in health, water, and sanitation. When it becomes a stand-alone activity for food distribution, it can divert human resources and logistics. Private sector projects, such as the Global Alliance for Improved Nutrition, also help indirectly with food aid, such as investment in new equipment for food fortification, micronutrient premix, quality assurance systems, and marketing infrastructure.[87]

On an international scale, the Scaling Up Nutrition (SUN) movement was launched by the UN in 2010 to stimulate leaders to focus on nutrition and to commit to effective national policies. It has a broad range of stakeholders from many sectors and was endorsed by more than 100 governments plus civil society, academic, and business organizations. These stakeholders developed a "road map" for advancing the SUN Framework that targets the "1,000-day window of opportunity" to improve the nutrition of pregnant and breastfeeding mothers and children under the age of 2 years. The SUN movement is not an initiative, institution, or fund.

Within the collaborative global effort to address hunger, chronic food insecurity, and undernutrition, Feed the Future is the U.S. government's contribution to a process that supports country-owned processes and plans and that works with other global development partners and stakeholders. The government has pledged $3.5 billion to help countries transform their own agricultural sectors for sustainable production to feed their nations. Feed the Future draws on the expertise of other governmental agencies, the private sector, and research institutions to facilitate sustainable agricultural development in partner countries that are particularly affected by undernutrition. Feed the Future, led by USAID, leverages the strengths of agencies across the government including the State Department, Peace Corps, Millennium Challenge Corporation, the Treasury Department, U.S. Trade Representative, the Overseas Private Investment Corporation, the U.S. African Development Foundation, and the USDA. Feed the Future "aims for economic growth by improving linkages along the entire value chain—from farm to market—by improving connections to local, regional, and global markets, promoting sustainable intensification, and supporting an enabling environment for agricultural trade to minimize the impact of food price hikes."[88]

If we look at the example of Africa, we can see why an initiative like Feed the Future is needed. According to the UN, only 3.5 % of African cropland is irrigated, compared with 39% in South Asia. In addition, Africa uses a twentieth of the fertilizer that Asia uses, and it has not developed new lines of crops to withstand drought cycles and other agricultural challenges. Moreover, the International Food Policy Research Institute states that yields in Africa account for just a third of global yields, coupled with a drop in Africa's agricultural trade to a low 3%.[89]

As we consider the economics and policies affecting agriculture in the developing world, it is also important to consider the advances in agricultural science (and the related policies) that can have a significant effect on a developing country's ability to feed its own population. We can refer to the progress made during the 4 decades from the 1940s to the 1970s, termed the "Green Revolution" by USAID director William Gaud in 1968. This collaboration between agricultural science, on the one hand, and governmental policymaking, on the other, began in 1943 in Mexico through the efforts of Norman Borlaug (considered the father of the Green Revolution). The success of his efforts in Mexico led the Rockefeller Foundation to work to spread these new techniques to other parts of the world, including India, other parts of Asia, the Philippines, and Africa (where it met with less success). Although the Green Revolution has been criticized more recently for the effects on the environment due to the use of petroleum-based fertilizers and insecticides, there is a general consensus that billions of people were spared the suffering and early mortality of starvation due to its successes. Borlaug was awarded the Nobel Peace Prize in 1970 for his work in increasing the world's food supply. We are now faced with the opportunity of a second Green Revolution, in the form of genetically modified organisms (GMOs). The term *GMO* is applied to any organism (in this case plants or animals purposefully altered for use as food) in which the genetic code has been altered by sophisticated techniques in a laboratory setting (as opposed to the genetic alteration we have been practicing for millennia through selective breeding and artificial selection). These genetic modifications are used to increase agricultural yields and decrease susceptibility to insect infestation (and thereby decrease the amount of insecticide needed) among other things. Controversy around the ultimate safety of these techniques has led some governments to ban the use of such methods as well as the importation of GMO foods. A full discussion of the pros and cons of GMOs is beyond the scope of this chapter, but you may refer to the excellent book on the subject by Pinstrup-Andersen and Shioler, *Seeds of Contention* (see Resources section).

The international community knows that solutions do not simply lie in investing more money in struggling countries. In addition, other health interventions and poverty reduction strategies will be undercut if the basic problems of hunger and undernutrition are not addressed. Beyond policy analysis, there must be strong linkages between policies and nutrition actions, commitments to forging new partnerships and equipping actors to manage nutrition programs, and the engagement of the business, private, and corporate sectors to act responsibly when it comes to nutrition messaging, food choices, and new markets and products. In the perspective of the World Bank and others, tackling undernutrition is seen as an excellent economic investment.[9] In fact, in May 2004 a consensus of eminent economists (including several Nobel laureates) concluded that the returns on investing in micronutrient programs are second only to the returns on fighting HIV/AIDS among a lengthy list of ways to meet the world's development challenges.[9,90]

Governments will need to show commitment to nutrition programs on a wide scale. This will lay a foundation for the broader agenda of poverty reduction

and sustainable growth. Otherwise, undernutrition—the world's largest public health problem and the leading contributor to child mortality—will continue to undermine other worthy public health responses in both the developed and developing world.

CONCLUSION

Undernutrition prevails in the world's children and contributes a third of all child deaths. We know that undernutrition happens early in life, and its multisystem consequences track children into their adolescent and adult years. Many reasons exist for undernutrition, yet there are many solutions, including the prevention and treatment of undernutrition in pregnant women and children younger than 2 years. The developed world faces problems with overnutrition. Nearly two thirds of the population in the United States is either overweight or frankly obese. Countries in between these extremes are undergoing nutritional transition, where the traditional health morbidities and mortalities, usually communicable diseases, are now being replaced with diet-related noncommunicable diseases. Addressing the challenges of global nutrition requires evidence-based research, policy changes, creative partnerships, and keeping nutrition as a national and global priority.

STUDY QUESTIONS

1. What factors predispose to undernutrition? How are these different for countries? Communities? Individuals?

2. What are the advantages of community-based therapeutic care?

3. What are the special considerations for nutrition in HIV-affected and HIV-infected populations?

4. What micronutrient deficiencies require immediate attention? Can you think of why it might be dangerous to correct caloric deficiency but fail to recognize concurrent protein deficiency or micronutrient deficiency?

5. Would you use MUAC or WFH in assessing severe acute malnutrition (SAM)? Why? What are the advantages and disadvantages of each?

6. What is the cycle of poverty and its link with undernutrition? How does chronic undernutrition perpetuate this cycle?

7. What areas of research would help inform nutrition interventions for vulnerable populations?

8. How are the nutrition problems different in developing countries versus in the developed world? What diseases are associated with each?

9. What is the role of policy formation in influencing ministries of health, the donor community, and nongovernmental organizations in addressing global undernutrition?

10. How might the thoughtful introduction of GMOs help in alleviating world hunger? What are possible pitfalls?

ACKNOWLEDGMENTS

We would like to acknowledge the editorial assistance of Tammie Henderson, as well as the technical input on breastfeeding from Anne Peniston, Jessica Tilahun, and Timothy Quick.

RESOURCES

Books

Butterly J, Shepherd J. *Hunger: The Biology & Politics of Starvation.* Hanover, NH: Dartmouth Press, 2010.

Pinstrup-Andersen P, Shioler E. *Seeds of Contention: World Hunger and the Global Controversy over GM Crops.* Baltimore, MD: International Food Policy Research Institute, 2001.

Pollan M. *The Omnivore's Dilemma: A Natural History of Four Meals.* New York: Penguin Press, 2007.

Sachs, J. *The End of Poverty: Economic Possibilities for Our Time.* New York: Penguin Press. 2006.

Documents

The Lancet Series on Maternal and Child Undernutrition, Black RE, Allen LH, et al. Maternal and Child Undernutrition. Lancet 2008;371(9608):243–260.

UNICEF. The State of the World's Children 2012: Children in an Urban World http://www.unicef.org/publications/index_61789.html.

World Health Organization and Food and Agriculture Organization of the United Nations. Nutritional Care and Support for People Living with HIV/AIDS. Training manual for participants and facilitator's guide. Geneva: WHO, 2009. http://www.who.int/nutrition/publications/hivaids/9789241591898/en/index.html.

A Scaling Up Nutrition: Progress Report from countries and their partners in the Movement to Scale Up Nutrition (SUN). United Nations High Level Meeting on Nutrition, September 20, 2011. First edition http://www.scalingupnutrition.org/wp-content/uploads/2011/05/summmary-note.pdf.

World Health Organization. Indicators for assessing infant and young child feeding practices, Part 2: Measurement. Geneva: WHO, 2010. http://whqlibdoc.who.int/publications/2010/9789241599290_eng.pdf.

Nutrition Advisory Service. Addressing undernutrition in external assistance: an integrated approach through sectors and aid modalities, Tools and Methods series, Reference document No. 13, European Commission, September 2011. http://capacity4dev.ec.europa.eu/t-and-m-series/blog/reference-document-nr-13-%E2%80%93-addressing-undernutrition-external-assistance-%E2%80%93-integrated-approach.

Epi Info. EpiNut software (for anthropometric data entry and analysis).

Prudhon C, Briend A, et al. *WHO, UNICEF, and SCN Informal Consultation on Community-Based Management of Severe Malnutrition in Children.* Food and Nutrition Bull 2006:27(3) Tokyo: United Nations University Press, 2006. SCN Nutrition Policy Paper 21. http://www.unscn.org/layout/modules/resources/files/Policy_paper_No_21.pdf.

World Food Programme. Vulnerability Assessment and Mapping team reports. http://wfp.org/operations/vam/vam_docustore/index.asp.

Web Sites

Emergency Nutrition Network (ENN): http://www.ennonline.net.

ENN Online, Infant Feeding in Emergencies: http://www.ennonline.net/ife/orientation

Famine Early Warning Systems Network: http://www.fews.net/.

Food and Nutrition Technical Assistance: http://www.fantaproject.org/

The Sphere Project: http://www.sphereproject.org/.

Standardized Monitoring and Assessment of Relief and Transitions: http://www.smartindicators.org/.

United Nations System Standing Committee on Nutrition: http://www.unscn.org/.

Allen L, deBenoist B, Dary O, Hurrell R. Guidelines on food fortification with micronutrients. WHO, 2006. http://www.who.int/nutrition/publications/guide_food_fortification_micronutrients.pdf.

REFERENCES

1. UNICEF. State of the World's Children, 2012. http://www.unicef.org/publications/index_61789.html.
2. UNICEF. Tracking Progress on Child and Maternal Nutrition: A survival and development priority, 2009. http://www.unicef.org/publications/index_51656.html.
3. Black R, Allen L, Bhutta Z, et al. Maternal and child undernutrition: global and regional exposures and health consequences. *Lancet* 2008;371:5–22.
4. USDA. Food Security in the US. 2012. http://www.ers.usda.gov/topics/food-nutrition-assistance/food-security-in-the-us.aspx.
5. USDA. Supplemental Nutrition Assistance Program. 2012. http://www.fns.usda.gov/snap/.
6. Feeding America. Hunger in America. 2012. http://feedingamerica.org/hunger-in-america/hunger-facts/hunger-and-poverty-statistics.aspx.
7. Keller HH. Malnutrition in institutionalized elderly: how and why? *J Am Geriatr Soc* 1993;41(11):1212–1218.
8. Thorsdottir I, Jonsson PV, Asgeirsdottir AE, Hjaltadottir I, Bjornsson S, Ramel A. Fast and simple screening for nutritional status in hospitalized, elderly people. *J Hum Nutr Diet* 2005; 18(1):53–60.
9. World Bank. *Repositioning Nutrition as Central to Development: A Strategy for Large-Scale Action.* Washington, DC: World Bank, 2006.
10. Black R, Morris S, Bryce J. Child Survival I. *Lancet* 2003;361: 2226–2234.

11. UNICEF. *Tracking Progress on Child and Maternal Nutrition: A Survival and Development Priority.* New York: UNICEF, 2009.

12. Sachs J. *The End of Poverty: Economic Possibilities for Our Time.* New York: Penguin, 2006.

13. Shrimpton R, Victoria CG, de Onis M, Lima RC, Blössner M, Clugston G. Worldwide timing of growth faltering: implications for nutritional interventions. *Pediatrics* 2001; 107(5):E75.

14. Pelletier DL. The relationship between child anthropometry and mortality in developing countries: implications for policy, programs and future research. *J Nutr* 1994;124(Suppl): 2074S–2081S.

15. World Food Program. School Meals, 2012. http://www.wfp .org/school-meals.

16. Ogden C, Carroll M, Kit B, et al. Prevalence of obesity in the United States, 2009–2010. *NCHS Data Brief No. 82*, CDC, January 2012.

17. Centers for Disease Control and Prevention. Behavioral Risk Factor Surveillance System, CDC. http://www.cdc.gov/obesity/ data/adult.html.

18. Ogden CL, Carroll MD, Curtin LR, Lamb MM, Flegal KM. Prevalence of high body mass index in U.S. children and adolescents, 2007–2008. *JAMA* 2010;303(3):242–249.

19. Ogden C, Caroll M. Prevalence of obesity among children and adolescents: United States, Trends 1963–1965 through 2007–2008. Division of Health and Nutrition Examination Surveys, CDC, 2010. http://www.cdc.gov/nchs/data/hestat/ obesity_child_07_08/obesity_child_07_08.htm.

20. Institute of Medicine, Committee on Prevention of Obesity in Children and Youth. *Preventing Childhood Obesity: Health in the Balance.* Washington, DC: National Academies Press, 2005.

21. Adachi-Mejia AM, Longacre MR, Gibson JJ, Beach ML, Titus-Ernstoff LT, Dalton MA. Children with a TV in their bedroom at higher risk for being overweight. *Int J Obes* 2007;31:644–651.

22. Caballero B. Global Health: A Nutrition Paradox-Underweight and Obesity in Developing Countries. *N Engl J Med* 2005; 352(15):1514–1516.

23. Maslow A. Theory of human motivation. *Psychol Rev* 1943;50: 370-396.

24. World Health Organization. *World Health Report 2011.* Geneva: WHO, 2011.

25. Nutrition Update (2010) and Micronutrient Update (2007), MEASURE DHS, Macro International, Calverton, MD.

26. World Health Organization. *Guidelines: Intermittent iron and folic acid supplementation in menstruating women.* Geneva: WHO 2011.

27. World Health Organization. *Guidelines: Intermittent Iron Supplementation in Pre-School and School-Age Children.* Geneva: WHO, 2011.

28. Bleichrodt N, Born M. A meta-analysis of research on iodine and its relationship to cognitive development. In: Stanbury J, ed. *The Damaged Brain of Iodine Deficiency: Cognitive, Behavioral, Neuromotor and Educative Aspects.* Elmsford, NY: Cognizant Communication Corporation, 1994.

29. Andersson M, Takkouche B, Egli I, Allen HE, De Benoist B. Current global iodine status and progress over the last decade towards the elimination of iodine deficiency. *Bull World Health Organ* 2005;83(7):518–525.

30. De Benoist B, McLean E, Andersson M, et al. Iodine deficiency in 2007: global progress since 2003. *Food Nutr Bull* 2008;29(3):195–202.

31. World Health Organization. Vitamin and Mineral Nutrition Information System. Geneva: WHO. http://www.who.int/vmnis/en/.

32. Micronutrient Initiative and UNICEF. *Vitamin and Mineral Deficiency: A Global Progress Report.* Ottawa: Micronutrient Initiative, 2004.

33. Sommer A, Tarwotjo I, Djunaedi E, et al. Impact of vitamin A supplementation on childhood mortality: a randomized controlled community trial. *Lancet* 1986;1:1169.

34. West K, Katz J, Khatry S, et al. Double blind, cluster randomized trial of low dose supplementation of vitamin A or beta-carotene on mortality related to pregnancy in Nepal. *BMJ* 1999;318:570–575.

35. Savy M, Edmond K, Fine PE, et al. Landscape analysis of interactions between nutrition and vaccine responses in children. *J Nutr* 2009;139:2154S–2218S.

36. World Health Organization. *Guidelines: Vitamin A supplementation in infants and children 6–59 months of age.* Geneva: WHO, 2011.

37. World Health Organization. *Guidelines: Vitamin A supplementation for newborns.* Geneva: WHO, 2011.

38. World Health Organization. *Guidelines: Vitamin A supplementation in infants 1–5 months of age.* Geneva: WHO, 2011.

39. World Health Organization. *Guidelines: Vitamin A supplementation in pregnancy for reducing the risk of mother-to-child transmission of HIV.* Geneva: WHO, 2011.

40. Humphrey J, Illif P, et al. Effects of a single large dose of vitamin A, given during the post-partum period to HIV-positive women and their infants, on child HIV infection, HIV-free survival, and mortality. *J Infect Dis* 2006;193:860–871.

41. Zinc Investigators' Collaborative Group. Prevention of diarrhea and pneumonia by zinc supplementation in children in developing countries: pooled analysis of randomized controlled trials. *J Pediatr* 1999;135:689–697.

42. Fischer PR. Thatcher TD, Pettifor JM. Pediatric vitamin D and calcium nutrition in developing countries. *Rev Endocr Metab Disord* 2008;9:181–192.

43. Thatcher TD, Fischer PR, Strand MA, Pettifor JM. Nutritional rickets around the world: causes and future directions. *Ann Trop Paediatr* 2006;26:1–16.

44. Scholl TO, Hediger ML, Shall JI, Khoo CS, Fischer RL. Dietary and serum folate: their influence on the outcome of pregnancy. *Am J Clin Nutr* 1996;63:520–525.

45. Green NS. Folic acid supplementation and prevention of birth defects. *J Nutr* 2002;132(8 Suppl):2356S–2360S.

46. Castilla E, Orioli IM, Lopez-Camelo JS, et al. Preliminary data on changes in neural tube defect prevalence rates after folic acid fortification in South America. *Am J Med Genet* 2003;123A(2):123–128.

47. Heymann WR. Scurvy in children. *J Am Acad Dermatol* 2007;57:358–359.

48. Olmedo JM, Yiannis JA, Windgassen EB, Gornet MK. Scurvy: a disease almost forgotten. *Int J Dermatol* 2006;45:909–913.

49. Zou K, Liu G, Wu T, Du L. Selenium for preventing Kashin-Beck osteoarthropathy in children: a meta-analysis. *Osteoarthritis Cartilage* 2009;17:144–151.

50. World Health Organization. *Guideline: Use of Multiple Micronutrient Powders for Home Fortification of Foods Consumed by Infants and Children 6–23 Months of Age.* Geneva: WHO, 2011.

51. http://www.unitedcalltoaction.org/documents/Investing_in_the_future.pdf: Investing in the Future: A united call to action on vitamin and mineral deficiencies. Global Report, 2009.

52. Butta ZA, Ahmed T, Black RE, et al. What works: interventions for maternal and child undernutrition and survival. *Lancet* 2008;371(9610):417–440.

53. Sphere Project. *The Sphere Humanitarian Charter and Minimum Standards in Disaster Response.* 2004 revised edition. Oxford, UK: Oxfam, 2011. http://www.sphereproject.org/handbook/index.htm.

54. Salama P, Spiegel P, Talley L, Waldman R. Lessons learned from complex emergencies over past decade. *Lancet* 2004;364(9447): 1801–1813.

55. Spiegel P. Quality of malnutrition assessment surveys conducted during famine in Ethiopia. *JAMA* 2004;292:613–618.

56. SMART 2005. *Measuring mortality: nutritional status and food security in crisis situations—the SMART protocol. Version 1.* Final draft, January 2005. http://www.smartindicators.org/SMART_Protocol_01-27-05.pdf.

57. Salama P, Assefa F, Talley L, Spiegel P, van Der Veen A, Gotway CA. Malnutrition, measles, mortality, and the humanitarian response during a famine in Ethiopia. *JAMA* 2001;286:563–571.

58. Myatt M, Feleke T, Sadler K, Collins S. A field trial of a survey method for estimating the coverage of selective feeding programmes. *Bull World Health Org* 2005;83(1):20–26.

59. World Health Organization. The WHO child growth standards. Geneva: WHO, 2006. http://www.who.int/childgrowth/standards/en/.

60. United Nations Standing Committee on Nutrition. SCN endorses the new WHO growth standards for infants and young children. April 27, 2006. http://www.unsystem.org/scn/publications/html/who_growth_standards.htm.

61. Hill Z, Kirkwood B, Edmond K. *Family and Community Practices That Promote Child Survival, Growth and Development: A Review of the Evidence.* Geneva: World Health Organization, 2004:21–26.

62. Picciano MF. Nutrient composition of human milk. *Pediatr Clin North Am* 2001;48:53–67.

63. AAP. Breastfeeding and the Use of Human Milk. Policy Statement. *Pediatrics* 2012;129(3):e827–e841.

64. U.S. Department of Health and Human Services. *Healthy People 2010.* 2nd ed. With *Understanding and Improving Health and Objectives for Improving Health.* 2 vols. Washington, DC: U.S. Government Printing Office, 2000.

65. World Health Organization. *Guidelines on HIV and Infant Feeding: Principles and Recommendations for Infant Feeding in the Context of HIV and a Summary of the Evidence.* Geneva: WHO, 2010.

66. World Health Organization. *The Management of Nutrition in Major Emergencies.* Geneva: WHO, United Nations High Commissioner for Refugees, International Federation of the Red Cross and Red Crescent Societies, and World Food Programme, 2000.

67. World Health Organization. *Child Growth Standards and the Identification of Severe Acute Malnutrition in Infants and Children.* Geneva: A Joint Statement by the World Health Organization and the United Nations Children's Fund, 2009.

68. Collins S, Dent N, Binns P, et al. Management of severe acute malnutrition in children. *Lancet* 2006;368(9551):1992–2000.

69. CTC Research and Development Programme. *Community-Based Therapeutic Care (CTC): A Field Manual.* Oxford, UK: Valid International, 2006.

70. Collins S. *Community-Based Therapeutic Care—A New Paradigm for Selective Feeding in Nutritional Crises.* London: Overseas Development Institute, 2004. Humanitarian Policy Network paper 48.

71. Emergency Nutrition Network. *Operational Challenges of Implementing Community Therapeutic Care: ENN Report on an Inter-Agency Workshop, Washington DC, February 28–March 2, 2005.* Oxford, UK: Emergency Nutrition Network, 2005:6.

72. Guerrero S, Mollison S. Engaging communities in emergency response: the CTC experience in Western Darfur. In: Humanitarian Policy Network, eds. *Humanitarian Exchange.* London: Overseas Development Institute, 2005:20–22.

73. Myatt M, Khara T, Collins S. A review of methods to detect cases of severely malnourished children in the community for their admission into community-based therapeutic care programs. *Food Nutr Bull* 2006;27(Suppl):S7–S23.

74. Ashworth A. Efficacy and effectiveness of community-based treatment of severe malnutrition. *Food Nutr Bull* 2006; 27(Suppl):S24–S48.

75. World Health Organization. *Guidelines for an Integrated Approach to the Nutritional Care of HIV-Infected Children (6 Months to 14 Years).* Geneva: WHO, 2009.

76. Duggan C, Fawzi W. Micronutrients and child health: studies in international nutrition and HIV infection. *Nutr Rev* 2001;59: 358–369.

77. World Health Organization. *Nutrient Requirements for People Living with HIV/AIDS: Report of a Technical Consultation.* Geneva: WHO, 2003.

78. World Health Organization. *HIV and Infant Feeding: A Guide for Health Care Managers and Supervisors.* Geneva: WHO, 2003.

79. Irlam JH, Visser ME, Rollins N, Siegfried N. Micronutrient supplementation in children and adults with HIV infection. *Cochrane Database Syst Rev* 2010:CD003650. http://onlinelibrary.wiley.com/o/cochrane/clsysrev/articles/CD003650/pdf_fs.html.

80. Guerrero S, Bahwere P, Sadler K, Collins S. Integrating CTC and HIV/AIDS support in Malawi. *Field Exchange* 2005;25: 8–10.

81. United Nations. Millennium Development Goals, 2012. http://www.un.org/millenniumgoals/.

82. Agarwal S. The state of urban health in India: comparing the poorest quartile to the rest of the urban population in selected states and cities. *Environment and Urbanization* 2011; 23:(1):13–28.

83. Morris S, Cogill B, Uauy R, for the Maternal and Child Undernutrition Study Group. Effective international action against undernutrition: why has it proven so difficult and what can be done to accelerate progress? *Lancet* 2008;371: 608–621.

84. Shiffman J. Generating political priority for maternal mortality reduction in 5 developing countries. *Am J Public Health* 2007; 97:796–803.

85. Pinstrup-Andersen P, Shimokawa S. Rural infrastructure and agricultural development. Tokyo, 2006. http://siteresources.world bank.org/INTDECABCTOK2006/Resources/Per_Pinstrup_Andersen_Rural_Infrastructure.pdf.

86. World Food Program. Overview of Operations in 2012. http://documents.wfp.org/stellent/groups/public/documents/op_reports/wfp242503-1.pdf.

87. Global Alliance for Improved Nutrition, 2012. http://www.gainhealth.org/.

88. Feed the Future, US Government's Global Hunger and Food Security Initiative, 2012. http://www.feedthefuture.gov/.

89. International Food Policy Research Institute, Washington DC. http://www.ifpri.org/.

90. Bhagwati J, Fogel R, Frey B, et al. Ranking the opportunities. In: Lomberg B, ed. *Global Crises, Global Solutions*. Cambridge, UK: Cambridge University Press, 2004.

Primary Care In Global Health

8

Jeffrey F. Markuns and Alain J. Montegut

 LEARNING OBJECTIVES

- *Understand the definitions of primary care and primary health care*
- *Understand the development of primary care historically and its global importance today*
- *Understand the role of primary care in health systems and how countries with inadequate primary health care are adversely affected*
- *Be able to compare and contrast four countries with different health policies, priorities, and resources*

INTRODUCTION

Primary health care is a phrase introduced to our lexicon in the 1970s. It is, however, an approach to health care that in fact has been present for centuries. It is important for us to understand the roots of primary health care in general practice as well as its current practice to fully understand its role in society and health. It is also important to distinguish between *primary health care,* as a comprehensive strategy for health promotion, and *primary care,* typically representing the element of clinical service delivery in that broader strategy toward health.[1]

Health care has become a major issue for many countries in the 21st century. Health care includes economic, social, political, and technical issues. The questions that surround national debates regarding health care around the globe are similar. How do we best promote health and treat disease? Who should provide this care? How should the system be organized? What is the right balance and mix of health providers, and how should they be distributed? What health services should be provided for all, and who should pay? How much should health care cost?

For individuals and families, the core question can be synthesized as follows: How do I attain the highest possible level of health, and how do I best access health services in times of need?

This chapter focuses on primary health care and how it is organized and practiced around the globe. It offers a definition of primary care and looks at how it is delivered in the context of a comprehensive primary health care strategy among different health care systems. It explains how primary care can have an impact on disease and on health indicators. It looks at what some goals could be for improving health systems through advocacy for primary care education and delivery and discusses health workforce issues as they relate to models for training of primary care physicians and other members of primary care teams. The chapter focuses on primary care physicians because of the limitation of space; however, we recognize there are many other health professionals who often compose the primary care team.

Additionally, the chapter explores how four countries with vastly different political and socioeconomic conditions have tried to improve health in their countries—some through the advent of strong primary health care delivery systems, others through systems traditionally based on specialist care, and others who have selected primary health care as the central theme for health care reform and are in the early years of implementation. It is hoped that you will gain an appreciation for the complex challenges involved in improving opportunities for health for all.

THE HISTORY OF PRIMARY CARE

Healing has been practiced for centuries around the globe. In fact, in the premodern era it was practiced in broadly similar ways. The healer was often an elder of the community who over time had gained respect and knowledge. Disease was believed to come from both natural and supernatural causes. Often the causes were felt to be spiritual, involving the entry or exit of spirits to or from the body. Primary care has its roots in the premodern era when healers had strong ties within communities and used this status to improve the health of the members of the community. Over time some of these healers became known as *physicians,* the person who "heals or exerts a healing influence."[2] Others became nurses, midwives, pharmacists, and allied health professionals, among others. Traditional healers continue to provide health advice and treatment worldwide as well.

Over time, the art of healing was joined with the science of prevention. The Yellow Emperor, the first sovereign of civilized China, wrote the *Neijing* roughly 2,000 years ago, which has come to be known as *The Yellow Emperor's Classic of Medicine.*

> In the good old days the sages treated disease by preventing illness before it began, just as the good government of emperor was able to take the necessary steps to avert war. Treating illness after it has begun is like suppressing revolt after it has broken out.
>
> A superior doctor arrests disease at the skin level and dispels it before it penetrates deeper. An inferior doctor treats illness after it passes the skin.
>
> A good healer cannot depend on skill alone. He must also have the correct attitude, sincerity, compassion, and a sense of responsibility.[3]

Hippocrates later articulated the importance of a holistic approach to health. In Plato's *Phaedrus* we learn that "Hippocrates the Asclepiad says that the nature even of the body can only be understood as a whole,"[4] and "it is more important to know what sort of person has a disease than to know what sort of disease a person has."[5]

The Renaissance brought the beginning of modern medicine in 1543 with the publication of the first complete textbook of human anatomy, *De Humanis Corporis Fabrica* by Andreas Vesalius. Vesalius was a classicist by education. He knew Greek and Latin and had studied the ancient writings and extolled them. He was considered a true humanist; in his teachings, he was able to blend the approach to the whole person with his science. The evolution of the physician as scientist and humanist continued.[6]

The ensuing three centuries brought many changes in the science of medicine. Alongside progress in medical science most of the world continued to use traditional healers. In countries that were becoming industrialized through the 19th and early 20th century, however, physicians and nurses assumed the primary responsibility for patient care. Before the political changes of 1917 in the Soviet Union, there was a rich tradition of general practice. The Zemstvo physicians combined traditional medical care with the humanitarianism and reformism of the contemporary

populist movement. These physicians believed that if medical care was to be effective, it had to be given in tandem with improvements in the sanitation, nutrition, and living standards of the time.[7]

In the United States, the generalist was also the primary physician. This was advocated by William Osler in an article entitled "Internal Medicine as a Vocation" published in the *Medical News* in 1897: "By all means, if possible, let [the young physician] be a pluralist, and—as he values his future life—let him not get early entangled in the meshes of specialism."[8]

The end of the 19th and early part of the 20th centuries brought with them desires for reform in medical education. The Medical Act of 1858 in Great Britain[9] and the 1910 report entitled *Medical Education in the United States and Canada: A Report to the Carnegie Foundation for the Advancement of Teaching,*[10] authored by Abraham Flexner, offered recommendations that would change the face of medical education in these countries and then the world. The activities generated by these reports developed standards for the accreditation of medical schools and policies related to the qualifications of physicians. Although these reforms raised the quality of medical education, they concurrently caused a disproportionate reduction in the number of physicians serving disadvantaged communities.[11]

The role of the generalist physician continued to evolve during this period. There was a progressive separation of the role of community-based general practitioners from physicians and surgeons who specialized and held hospital appointments. In this division the general practitioner became the doctor of first contact working in the community, whereas consultant physicians and surgeons controlled the hospitals with their scientific and technical facilities. Patients who needed these additional services were referred by their general practitioners.

As medical education reforms evolved through the early part of the 20th century, so did the need for good generalist physicians. In his book, *A Time to Heal,* Flexner wrote, "The small town needs the best and not the worst doctor procurable. For the country doctor has only himself to rely on: he cannot in every pinch hail specialist, expert, and nurse. On his own skill, knowledge, and resourcefulness, the welfare of his patient altogether depends. The rural district is therefore entitled to the best trained physician that can be induced to go there."[11]

In nonindustrialized parts of the world, the value of the generalist health care provider of first contact was also recognized. *Barefoot doctors* were farmers who obtained basic medical training and worked in rural villages in China to bring health care to areas where urban-trained doctors would not settle. There had been scattered experiments with this concept before 1965, but with Mao's famous 1965 speech about health care,[12] it became institutionalized as part of the Cultural Revolution, which radically diminished the influence of the Weishengbu, China's health ministry, dominated by Western-trained doctors. In Vietnam, a national Commune Health Center system was created in the 1950s; it was staffed by health care workers initially but then began to receive staffing by generalist physicians in the late 1960s and 1970s.[13]

Health care professionals of first contact have evolved and become more stratified in response to advances in medical sciences and therapies. Health care services are often organized into four overlapping levels of care: primary care, which is the focus of this chapter; secondary medical care, which includes consultations by specialists for patients with more unusual problems; tertiary care, which is care for patients with disorders that are so uncommon in a population that the primary care physician would not be expected to maintain skills in caring for them; and emergency care, which is initial care for urgent problems or trauma.[14]

THE DEFINITION OF PRIMARY CARE

In 1978, the World Health Organization (WHO) convened a conference in Alma Ata, the capital of the Soviet Republic of Kazakhstan. It was attended by 3,000 participants from 134 governments and 67 international organizations. The purpose of the conference was to look for ways to improve health. Ideas about primary health care had been discussed in many countries and across many organizations. The outcome of this conference was a declaration regarding health and primary health care. The group declared health to be a fundamental human right, called for an attainment of a minimum level of health by the year 2000, and identified primary health care as key to achieving this goal. The declaration provided a framework for the definition of primary health care as essential, practical, affordable, scientifically sound, and the main focus of overall social and economic development. The group recognized needs fulfilled by primary health care will vary depending on the location, burden of illness, demographics, and socioeconomic circumstances of the community.[15]

In the 21st century, although there has been great progress in various arenas of health, it is now also clear that the goal of Alma Ata remains too distant, with many countries still struggling to adequately meet the health care needs of all people. A variety of issues contribute to this continued health deficit, but it is also recognized that there remains a wide range of commitment to, and subsequent implementation of, primary health care across nations. As a result, in 2008, the WHO renewed the call for development

of high-quality primary care throughout the world in their report "Primary Health Care—Now More Than Ever."[16]

Traditionally, the terms *primary health care* and *primary care* were often used interchangeably, intended mainly to indicate any health improvement effort that principally takes place in the community, as distinct from secondary or tertiary care provided in hospitals. Over the years since Alma Ata, however, the definitions of *primary health care* and *primary care* have become more distinct. In today's lexicon, *primary health care* typically refers to a broad approach to improving health at both the individual and community level. Primary health care may include public health elements such as nutrition, clean water and sanitation, maternal and child health, family planning, immunizations, mental health services and provision, and essential drugs, as well as community-based individual clinical services.[17]

In the lexicon of this expansive definition, the meaning of *primary care* has evolved to refer primarily to the specific element of clinical service delivery such as preventive and curative services for individuals and families provided within the broader context of primary health care. The unique quality of primary care is that it does not focus specifically on the diagnosis and treatment of specific disease processes, but rather it aims for the broader goal of quality health through the provision of health services utilizing principles of care founded in the primary health care approach.

Even with this refined meaning of primary care, the role and specific elements of what constitutes high-quality primary care remains far reaching. In their 2008 report, the WHO outlined that primary care:

- Provides a place where people can bring a wide range of health problems
- Is a hub through which patients are guided through the health system
- Facilitates ongoing relationships between patients and clinicians
- Builds bridges between personal health care and patients' families and communities
- Opens opportunities for disease prevention, health promotion, and early detection of disease
- Utilizes teams of health professionals with specific and sophisticated biomedical and social skills
- Requires adequate resources and investment but provides better value for money than its alternatives[16]

Primary care may be provided by public or private practitioners and includes efforts to coordinate services across sectors. In economically developed countries, primary care professionals include family doctors, nurses, pharmacists, and a variety of allied health professionals. In less economically developed countries, primary care may be delivered by health workers who have received shorter courses of training, such as barefoot doctors in China or Aboriginal health workers in Australia, as part of a national strategy to provide improved primary health care. These health workers are often community members and therefore knowledgeable about the communities they serve; they provide a vital link to other health care providers.

Primary Care and Its Relationship to Disease

As countries work to provide the highest possible level of health care services at the lowest cost, researchers have analyzed how the organization and composition of health services affect health outcomes. There are many determinants of health for individuals and for populations. The basic determinant, of course, is the gene pool, but this is "heavily modified by the social and physical environment, by behaviors

that are culturally or socially determined, and by the nature of the health care provided."[18] Across all countries, evidence shows us that health outcomes are often adversely affected by poverty both within and between countries.

Although health care services is one of the wide range of determinants of health outlined at Alma Ata, greater spending on health care does not necessarily improve health outcomes. Very strong evidence exists that access to comprehensive primary health care improves health outcomes. Increasing the ratio of primary care physicians to specialists improves health outcomes even more.[19]

The benefits of primary health care become apparent by reviewing the relationship between primary care orientation and the health indicators of the population. A review of life expectancy reveals general trends in health outcomes across the world, recognizing life expectancy is greatly impacted by infant and child mortality (Figure 8-1).

These data reveal clusters of countries with similar rankings on a logarithmic scale.[20] Although efforts

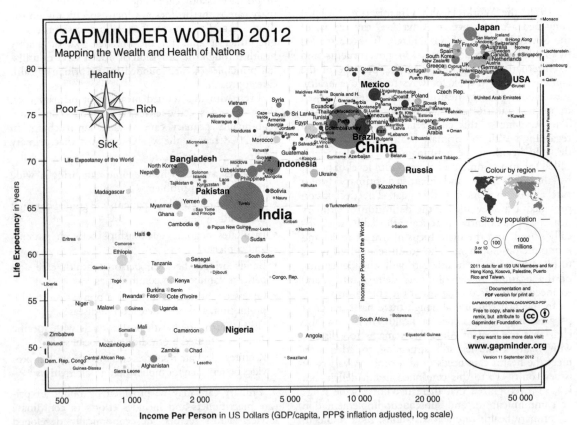

Figure 8-1. Life expectancy compared with per capita income.

toward accomplishing the Millennium Development Goals have resulted in significant improvements over recent years, large disparities remain. Much of Africa, ravaged by the human immunodeficiency virus (HIV) epidemic, remains with very low life expectancy and continues to struggle with high child mortality, despite a broad range of income. In Asia, we can see important variations, such as Vietnam's higher life expectancy compared with China, despite China's substantially greater income. Among high-income countries, we see the United States sits below its peers in life expectancy despite generally higher income. Economic factors play a significant role in determining health outcomes, but evidence is mounting that development and access to primary health care services play an important role as well.

Data have been analyzed from Western industrialized countries, looking at the strength of primary care as evaluated based on nine characteristics of health systems' infrastructure (Table 8-1) and six practice characteristics of the patients' experiences in receiving care (Table 8-2). A scoring system was developed to assign a relative value to the countries studied based on their level of primary care. The countries with higher rankings in primary care were found to have had better health indicators. Additionally, those countries that had weak primary care infrastructures had higher costs and poorer outcomes.[14,21]

A correlation also exists between primary care and age-standardized mortality. With a 20% increase in the number of primary care physicians, there is an associated 5% decrease in mortality (40 fewer deaths per 100,000). Most important, the effect is greatest if the increase is in family physicians. One more family physician per 10,000 people (an estimated

Table 8-1. Health system characteristics.

Extent to which the system regulates the distribution of resources throughout the country
Mode of financing of primary care services
Modal type of primary care practitioner
Percentage of active physicians involved in primary care versus those in conventional specialty care
Ratio of average professional earnings of primary care physicians compared with other specialists
Requirement for cost sharing by patients
Requirement for patient lists to identify the community served by practices
Twenty-four-hour access arrangements
Strength of academic departments of primary care or general practice

From Starfield B, Shi L. Policy relevant determinants of health: an international perspective. *Health Policy* 2002; 60:201–218. (*Reproduced with permission.*)

Table 8-2. Practice characteristics.

First-contact care
Longitudinality
Comprehensiveness
Coordination
Family-centeredness
Community orientation

From Starfield B, Shi L. Policy relevant determinants of health: an international perspective. *Health Policy* 2002; 60:201–218. (*Reproduced with permission.*)

33% increase) is associated with 70 fewer deaths per 100,000 (an estimated 9% decrease). In contrast, an estimated 8% increase in the number of specialist physicians is associated with a 2% increase in mortality.[22] An association also exists between primary care and infant outcomes. The greater the supply of primary care physicians, the lower the infant mortality and percentage of low-birth-weight infants. An increase of one primary care physician per 10,000 has been associated with a 2.5% reduction in infant mortality and a 3.2% reduction in low birth weight.[23]

Numerous studies have demonstrated that earlier detection of diseases such as breast cancer,[24] melanoma,[25] colon cancer,[26,27] and cervical cancer[28] improves with greater access to primary care. A decrease in total mortality and the mortality for colon cancer, heart disease, and stroke is also correlated with increased access to primary care.[29] Increased access to primary care results in better health outcomes and lower costs.[30,31]

Almost all of the evidence concerning the benefits of primary care systems comes from industrialized countries. There remains little data from developing countries. A study in Indonesia that looked at primary health care and infant mortality rates showed that as the government shifted spending away from primary care and toward the hospital and technological sector, there was a worsening of infant mortality.[32]

PRINCIPLES OF PRIMARY CARE

Essential to delivery of quality primary care services is sufficient training in the core principles of primary care:

- Access or first contact care
- Comprehensiveness
- Continuity
- Coordination
- Prevention
- Family- and community orientation
- Patient-centeredness

Although many of these principles have been taken for granted since evidence to support them was first outlined decades ago, many developing countries lack experience with the implementation of these principles in their health systems and thus require explicit training programs in these principles.

Maximizing the effectiveness of human resources for health also requires more than training. In developed countries and in the wake of the increasing evidence to suggest high-quality primary care offers an opportunity for improved individual and population health at lower costs, there is a renewed interest in health system concepts related to high-quality primary care. It is now being recognized that even in those countries where dedicated training programs in core principles of primary care have been ongoing for some time, broad health system supports are needed to promote practical and uniform implementation of these principles. Standardized evidence-based approaches are being piloted on a wide scale, such as patient-centered medical home initiatives.[33-35] As a result, interest in primary care development now goes well beyond training to explore what overall system supports can be implemented at the governmental, societal, and institutional level to promote clinical service delivery that adheres to these core principles of primary care. Although there may need to be a shift in emphasis of specific principles depending on local health system needs, each principle plays an important role in the delivery of primary health care.

Access or First-Contact Care

Access to health care is increased when primary care services are provided at the community level, usually through primary care team members. Access is determined by availability, convenience, proximity, affordability, and acceptability.[18] Of course, barriers to each of these exist in most settings to some degree, and countries may face greater barriers in some aspects than others.

Under ideal circumstances, a usual source of care is identified by the patient representing the point of first contact with the health care system for most health issues. This point of first contact should offer patients continuous access to health care services through coverage arrangements, along with referrals for patients who require services that are not available at the local level. When patients can readily access primary care services in the community, they are less likely to seek hospital services, which are often less convenient and more expensive.[36]

Comprehensiveness

The principle of comprehensiveness focuses on the concept that the capacity for addressing a wide range of issues is necessary at the point of first-contact care. Patients who typically present to sources of first-contact care are undifferentiated and unfiltered by their very nature, and so a broad range of medical problems may face providers at the grassroots level.[18] Providers need to be trained to handle the most common medical problems encountered at their local level, and also be sufficiently skilled in recognizing, managing, and referring more complicated or unusual problems.

Insufficient training in a broad range of problems can quickly lead to dissatisfaction among providers' ability to provide quality care and result in increased turnover at the primary care level. In addition, the site of first contact needs to have adequate supplies to deal with this broader range of medical issues.

Continuity

Continuity of care can be present on three levels: informational, longitudinal, and personal.[37] Informational continuity refers to the maintenance and communication of medical information about a patient. Core to this concept is the creation and maintenance of a personal medical record that may be kept by the patient, stored at the point of first contact, or maintained electronically. Continuity of information may occur over time from visit to visit, among providers within a single health care facility, and between independent facilities such as the point of first contact and a hospital.

Longitudinal continuity involves health care that is provided over time at a single facility or with a specific health care team. Continuity is expedited when patients can identify a usual source of care, sometimes referred to as a *medical home*. In response, care is enhanced when a team of providers assumes primary responsibility for promoting the health of a specific group of patients.

Personal continuity involves an ongoing personal relationship between an individual patient and a personal physician or other primary care provider; alternatively, this relationship might include a few select team members in an effort to maintain longitudinal continuity when the personal provider is not available. In this interpersonal relationship, the patient knows the physician by name and develops a basis for trust.[37]

Continuity is enhanced when patients can identify and readily access their own primary health care providers, but the various barriers to access cited earlier can also negatively impact the various levels of continuity. Furthermore, efforts to overcome these same barriers and provide enhanced access may also at times unintentionally reduce continuity, such as in an effort to offer more convenient and timely care but that occurs when the patient's personal provider is not available.[38,39]

Coordination

Coordination is perhaps one of the most important and universal aspects of primary care. This can mean collaboration among team members, between a range of specialty providers, or simply with the patient and their family. At its essence, coordination of care involves the responsible provider collecting and interpreting all the relevant information and placing it in the context of a specific patient, and then assisting the patient in all aspects of his or her health. This assistance might range from prescribing a medication to provision of relevant immunizations to communication with a specialist or group of specialists focused on a single but more complicated aspect of the patient's health. Coordination of care is known to improve patient outcomes, making it an effective tool for management and treatment of illness, especially chronic disease.[40,41]

Coordination can also refer to health management skills, and the need to coordinate a primary health care team. In some primary care systems, doctors may supervise the care provided by nurses, physician assistants, community health workers, and other health team members to ensure continuity of care for a greater number of patients.[42] In these situations, doctors typically focus their direct service delivery efforts on the care of patients with more complex conditions while nurses and other health professionals provide preventive services, manage less complex patient problems, and pursue more time-intensive case management activities in chronic disease care.

Prevention

Prevention is often situated at the intersection between public health and primary care. It is an essential element of primary health care and often responsible for the greatest quantitative improvements in health outcomes.

Primary care is uniquely situated to promote public health–based preventive services at the individual patient level. Primary care can leverage the enhanced access, repeated clinical encounters over time, as well as the interpersonal relationship with a health care provider to encourage adherence to a variety of preventive measures. In many settings, the point of first-contact care is the most logical and effective place to dedicate resources toward disease prevention.[43]

Family and Community Orientation

The orientation of primary care to include family and community is an important principle for maximizing the effectiveness of health care. The focus on family acknowledges the crucial role family members play in health and illness. Engaging family members can help individual patients achieve lifestyle modifications and improved adherence to therapies. Understanding the family situation can put an individual's medical problems into a more holistic context and identify potential caregivers for assistance when needed.

Community-oriented primary care provides an opportunity for the primary care provider to apply the experiences from their daily clinical service delivery to the public health context.[18] It is important for the primary care provider to recognize the influence of the greater community—including social, environmental, and economic impacts—on both the scope of medical problems presenting to their clinic and the approach to health for individual patients. Conversely, through regular interaction with the local population seeking first-contact care, the primary care provider is provided with a vital window on the overall health of the community. The daily diagnoses presenting to the provider can act as a barometer of the overall health of the community. For health systems to take full advantage of this feature of primary care, providers need to be equipped with the skills and procedures to act effectively on their health observations.

Patient-Centeredness

In the rush toward improved health outcomes, the need for patient-centeredness can easily be forgotten. Disease-based approaches to improved health are often seen as more likely to provide scientifically proven and statistically significant quantitative improvements in focused health outcome measures. The increased focus on these approaches is compounded when such outcomes need to be demonstrated over a very limited period of time, a common demand of funders in global health improvement efforts. Although the desire for proven improvements in specific health indicators over short funding periods is certainly understandable, these disease-based approaches fail to take into consideration the specific health of individuals. Each individual represents a complex system in itself, typically impacted by an interaction of influences from family, community, and a variety of individual health problems, commingled with an individual patient's personal life and health goals. A provider equipped to understand the complicated interactions of these determinants of health and identify the most relevant interventions has the potential to bring together a variety of health improvement strategies in a powerful and synergistic way.

Primary care utilizes the principles just outlined to accomplish this synergy and aid patients in achieving their desired level of health. The well-trained primary care provider uses all of these principles to identify the problems and concerns of a patient, build a body of evidence relevant to the patient to support specific diagnoses or management plans, elicit the influencing factors surrounding the patient, and then counsel the patient in a shared decision-making venture toward the patient's personal goals. In this setting, patient satisfaction enters the equation as both an important health determinant and health indicator.

At times, a patient's personal goals may not include a maximum level of health—and thus can be at odds with government or funder goals, running contrary to a usual public health approach. It stands to reason that a patient that is not motivated toward maximal health is likely to act as a drag on a variety of population health indicators. By developing health systems that support primary care providers in focusing on the core principles of primary care, however, the grassroots provider has an opportunity to bring a variety of powerful tools to bear on improving every individual's health to a maximal achievable level. Systems that fail to account for the interaction of individuals' many health determinants miss an opportunity to maximize effectiveness at best and can unintentionally negatively impact overall patient health at worst.[44] In primary care, improved health is achieved while respecting the individual's specific needs in the context of a health system's overall goals.

HUMAN RESOURCES FOR HEALTH

People are at the heart of all effective health systems. Health professionals and their support staff, or human resources for health, organize and provide services and health education and assess outcomes. A wide array of skills is required for the effective delivery of comprehensive primary care services; these services may be delivered by a variety of personnel.

Ample evidence exists that the number, quality, and distribution of health personnel strongly affect health outcomes. For example, birth outcomes are strongly associated with the presence of a skilled birth attendant at deliveries.[45] A minimal density of health workers is needed to ensure that all women will have access to a skilled attendant.

The WHO estimates that there are 59.2 million full-time health workers worldwide. Approximately two thirds of these workers are health services providers; the other third are health management and support workers.[46]

Individual health professionals are usually integrated into teams to deliver primary health care services. Primary care physicians, nurses, and outreach workers are of particular importance to well-functioning primary health care teams. They are called on to assess and treat a wide range of patients at the community level including those with urgent or complex disorders. They function to bridge the gaps between patients and health resources, between individual and public health, and between communities and secondary and tertiary care services.[17]

A primary health care team is composed of people who contribute to delivering health services. Each team is unique: local conditions determine the members, relationships, and responsibilities of the team; regional and national conditions influence the resources and contexts in which the teams operate. Enormous diversity exists in the composition of primary health care teams. They often consist of physicians, nurses, medical assistants, midwives, social workers, community health workers, and others who provide direct patient care. Supportive members of the team may include receptionists; administrative professionals and administrators; health educators; and laboratory, pharmacy, and radiology personnel. Consultative members of the team may include those who provide specialized health services or those with expertise in community health.[47,48]

Flexibility in the makeup of primary health care teams is necessary for dealing with the unique circumstances and resources of a particular community. For instance, not all of the personnel just described may be available, in which case others may assume essential roles. Achieving a sustainable and balanced health workforce requires the coordination of many sectors of society: educational institutions, policymaking bodies, communities, and financiers (Figure 8-2).

Achieving the right distribution of health workers is challenging within and between countries. Health professionals tend to congregate in urban areas, resulting in rural shortages in most nations. Additionally, there are absolute shortages of health workers in many areas of the world, most notably in the sub-Saharan African Region, where it is estimated that there is a shortage of a million health workers to meet even the minimal standards for delivery of essential health care services (Figure 8-3).

Ensuring there is an adequate supply of local health workers to provide sufficient access to services is a key factor in promoting health. Quantity, however, is not the only factor in human resources for health. The supply of health workers needs to be adequately trained in primary care, along with sufficient resources and system supports, so that the accessible services represent the vision of health care outlined at Alma Ata and in the 2008 WHO report. Dedicated training programs in primary care are necessary to offer an adequate quality of services that can realistically meet population needs.

Health professional education requires eligible students, intact educational institutions, sufficient faculty, and years of investment. Health professionals are likely to practice in environments to which they have been exposed in training. If students do not see primary care as attractive, they are unlikely to pursue

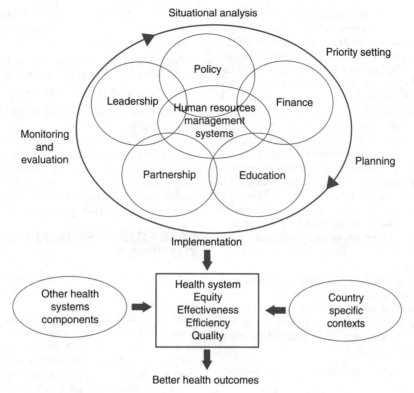

Figure 8-2. Human resources for health technical framework: achieving a sustainable health workforce.

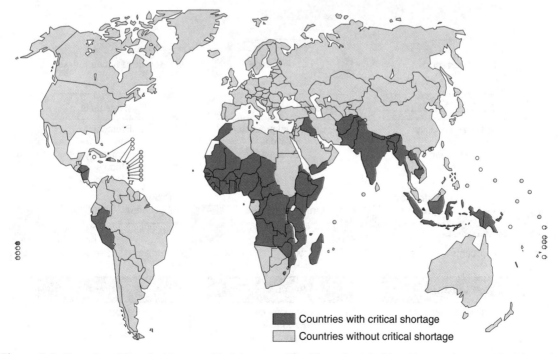

Figure 8-3. Countries with and without a critical shortage of health service providers (doctors, nurses, and midwives).

primary care careers. Therefore, much of the education of the primary health care workforce should be in well-supported primary care and community settings.

Train, sustain, and retain refers to the steps necessary to prepare, deploy, and support health professionals where they are needed. To be satisfied, health professionals need to feel sufficiently prepared and competent to work in their specific practice setting. Health professionals do not work in a vacuum, and thus they also require a system that encourages and supports their efforts and provides adequate facilities with good working conditions. If workers are unprepared, salaries are too low, or facilities are inadequate, it is difficult to recruit or retain workers where they are needed (Figure 8-4). There is an ongoing relationship between education, labor and health services markets, and the human resources considered necessary in each sector. (See Chapter 20 for more information on this topic.)

International comparisons of primary health care outcomes in economically developed countries suggest that the greatest differences in health between countries are associated with the degree to which the following principles have been implemented in their health services delivery system[18]:

- Equitable distribution and financing of health care services
- Similar level of professional earnings for primary care physicians and specialists

- Comprehensiveness of primary health care services
- Absent, or very low, requirements for copayments for primary health care services
- Primary care physicians providing first-contact care and entry into the health delivery system
- Person-focused longitudinal care

Globalization has resulted in the flow of ideas, goods, and people around the world. Powerful economic forces lure many health professionals to greener pastures and better facilities. Strong global, national, and local alliances are needed to ensure that health professionals are not only trained to meet the needs of communities but also that they are retained to practice in areas where they are needed (Figure 8-5).

CASE STUDIES FROM AROUND THE WORLD

The cost of health care has been rising across the globe, and many countries are now facing an aging population and seeing a shift from infectious diseases to chronic disease. As a result, countries have been trying to reorganize the delivery of health care in many ways. The evidence that provision of primary care and the existence of a sound primary health care infrastructure lead to improved health has led many countries to choose this model on which to base reform. Other countries have continued to base their systems on a disproportionate share of secondary

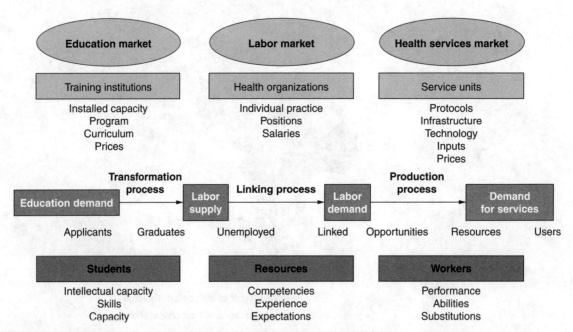

Figure 8-4. Relationship of education, labor, and health services markets with human resources.

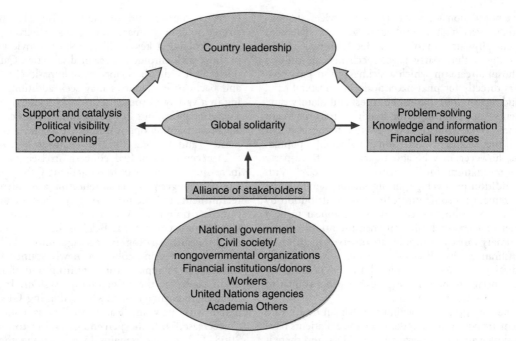

Figure 8-5. Global stakeholder alliance.

and tertiary care. One can consider a variety of health systems to be designed along such a continuum.

This section discusses four countries to illustrate disparities in health care delivery systems around the globe. These examples were chosen specifically to demonstrate inequalities and disparities in health. They demonstrate that wealth is not an isolated indicator for improved health for all and that creative solutions to provide primary care are important for all countries.

Belgium

The Kingdom of Belgium is located in Western Europe, with the capital city of Brussels having the distinction of acting as headquarters for the European Union (EU). Belgium is largely urban and legally bilingual with three official languages and a population of almost 11 million with 99% literacy, of which approximately 60% speak Dutch, 40% speak French, and less than 1% speak German. Belgium functions as a parliamentary democracy under a constitutional monarchy, with a complicated political system including federal, regional, and linguistic levels of government. Life expectancy for the population in 2012 was 79.7 years, ranking 38th in the world, and Belgium generally experiences very low infant, child, and maternal mortality.[49]

Responsibility for health policy is shared between the federal authorities and federated entities (regions and communities). The federal authorities regulate and finance compulsory health insurance, manage the hospital system including accreditation criteria and hospital financing, register pharmaceuticals and prices, and oversee professional qualifications. The regions and communities are largely responsible for primary health care including health promotion and prevention, maternal and child health care and social services, community-based care, accreditation standards, and financing hospital investment. Belgian health care is influenced by a number of professional and trade organizations, as well as patient associations. Communities are responsible for coordinating outpatient care policy including initiatives in primary health care, home care services, and palliative care.[44,49]

Belgium offers near universal public health insurance with a broad benefits package covering over 8,000 services, financed by a combination of proportional social security contributions from taxable income and progressive direct taxation. Health care expenditure in 2009 represented 11.8% of the gross domestic product (GDP), ranking 12th in the world and third among EU member states. There are 6.6 hospital beds per 1,000 population and almost 3 physicians per 1,000, with a near even split in physicians between general practitioners (GPs) and specialists.[50]

Initially, health insurance coverage primarily covered hospital services, but it has now been expanded to include outpatient care. Over a 3-year period, 95%

of the population accesses outpatient services, demonstrating a very high level of access to care.[49] Payment is generally structured on a fee-for-service basis. Typically, a third-party payer mechanism is utilized for hospital care, in which a sickness fund pays providers directly for pharmaceuticals and hospital care, excluding any copayments. For most ambulatory care, patients are responsible for making direct payment to the provider and then obtaining a reimbursement from the sickness fund. Some vulnerable populations, however, may be able to access the third-party payer mechanisms for ambulatory care as well.[50] With the addition of coverage for ambulatory services, the requirement for some direct financial contribution by patients to health care costs does not appear to be a barrier to accessing health care because no differences in primary care consumption are observed by category of insurance. Overall costs for patients with chronic medical problems can be high however, because the total amount of personal expenses is proportional to the amount of care required.[51]

The core principles behind the Belgian health care system are equity and freedom of choice. Patients have free choice among primary care providers, and there is no gatekeeper function, so referrals are not required to consult with a specialist physician. For their part, physicians have freedom in diagnostic and therapeutic decision making and may choose to participate or not in the national health insurance scheme. Just as autonomy for patients is paramount, there is an equal respect for the autonomy of care providers and their diagnostic and therapeutic decisions.[49] Doctors are also free to choose their practice location, although government incentives exist to promote primary care practice in underserved areas.

There is a long tradition of primary care training for physicians in Belgium, known as GPs. Medical training in Belgium is a 6-year undergraduate university course right after high school, and further postgraduate training is required to obtain a license to practice. Postgraduate specialty training programs range from 3 to 6 years in length, with General Practice training programs requiring 3 years. GPs do not need to be accredited, but financial incentives encourage accreditation through certification by fulfilling criteria in the four domains of medical practice, continuing medical education (CME), medical practice evaluation, and rational prescribing. Physicians are required to maintain medical records on patients, complete 20 credits of CME, and have at least 1,250 patient encounters per year.[49]

Physicians primarily work in solo practice, with about a quarter in group practices, and they often work without other medical staff. Less than 1% of physicians in clinical practice are salaried. Although GP offices are typically only staffed with a medical secretary, nurses and physiotherapists also have a strong role in primary care service delivery, with nurses playing a key ancillary role in providing care to those with chronic disease or disabilities. Qualified nurses have either bachelor- or diploma-level training, and bachelor-level nurses may seek additional training in a variety of specialty fields. Nurses may obtain special qualifications in wound and diabetes care, and advanced training opportunities are available through master's and doctoral (PhD) programs in nursing.

A recently identified concern in Belgium is an increasing percentage of nonpracticing GPs, especially among younger physicians, reflecting a problem with recruitment and retention of physicians in primary care after training.[50] Although there has been suggestion in some corners that Belgium has an oversupply of physicians, a rising average age among GPs suggests the decreasing cohort of newly trained GPs is insufficient to replace those retiring and thus may begin to strain the primary care system. In addition, the percentage of newly graduating GPs compared with new medical specialists is continuing to decrease, with the percentage falling to 30% in 2008. GP income remains lowest among the various specialties, but capitation grants have begun to enhance GP income, bringing the average significantly closer to that of other specialties.[50] In addition, a variety of programs offering grants, loans, and administrative assistance to new GPs have been instituted in recent years to incentivize primary care as an attractive career option.

Although there is overall good coverage and accessibility to GPs, because there is no required referral system in Belgium some patients still see specialists as their point of first-contact care. The population is highly satisfied with GPs, however, and prefers contact with their GP. Only 10% of GP contacts result in a patient referral to a specialist, but 95% of patients who had an outpatient contact with a physician consulted a GP. Despite low barriers to accessing the specialist system, very few patients consult only a specialist. It is quite common, however, especially in older age groups, for combined consultation with a GP and specialist.[49]

In general, although there is robust primary care coverage by GPs throughout Belgium, GPs have recognized a need for greater collaboration and coordination. There have been a number of initiatives to try to promote and strengthen the primary care system.

A medical record system was established to improve informational continuity and promote the establishment of a usual source of care. An individual GP is charged with maintaining the record and can charge health insurance for maintenance of the record. A corresponding incentive is offered to patients, who have copayments reduced by 30% for consultations to the GP who holds their medical record. There is no strict gatekeeper function in Belgium, but an additional incentive to utilize the primary care physician is increased reimbursement for a patient's first visit to a specialist if they are referred by a GP. Emergency department visits are also discouraged as a first-contact access point through reduced copayments if referred by a primary care physician.[52]

In 2003, GP cooperatives (GPCs) were established for the organization of out-of-hours medical care and have been a positive development in structuring primary care. The GPCs are designed for improved longitudinal continuity, offering out-of-hours coverage by a group of affiliated providers for a designated area. GPCs offer a centralized location for out-of-hours primary care and organize available physicians to offer home visits. There is a long tradition of home visits in Belgium as part of primary care service delivery, but only in recent years with the development of the GPCs has telephone consultation and triage been made widely available. The establishment of the GPCs has been associated with a shift in the type of primary care contact, with the total number of home visits remaining relatively stable but also decreasing as a proportion of total encounters when compared with in-office consultations.[50] This is consistent with a general trend in recent years of decreasing home visits and increasing office consultations seen in encounters during normal working hours. Although emergency department use has not been shown to decrease with establishment of the GPCs, the overall GP caseload and number of encounters has increased with this improved access.[51]

A study on implementation of the chronic care model in Belgium noted most general practitioners had no support staff in place, and primary care providers lack opportunities to take up full responsibility for chronic care.[50] Nonetheless, nearly all chronic patients see a GP yearly, with over 10 contacts per year on average.[49] In recent years, there have been efforts to strengthen the role of the general practitioner including incentives to both patients and physicians for patients to register with a primary care provider. In 2009, system supports for primary care management of chronic diseases were implemented, including the development of care pathways and financial incentives to both physicians and patients for participation. In addition, local multidisciplinary networks were established to assist in chronic disease care.[53]

One longtime coordinated function of GPs over the last 30 years in Belgium has been their integration with the public health system through a network of sentinel general practitioners, designed to provide periodic and standardized reports on epidemiologic characteristics of the population as experienced in the primary care system.[53] Efforts are underway to increase extraction of this information from electronic health records, and there is now an increasing computerization among GPs as a result of an information technology bonus, with uptake greatest among younger physicians.

Lesotho

The Kingdom of Lesotho is a land-locked country in sub-Saharan Africa, completely surrounded by South Africa. Designated as a least developed country (LDC) by the United Nations, Lesotho struggles under the burden of the world's third highest HIV prevalence rate. About 24% of Lesotho's population of almost 2 million people lives primarily in rural villages with a temperate climate that thankfully allows it to be free of many tropical diseases that plague other developing nations. Many families rely on subsistence farming and migrant labor, with many men working in mines in South Africa. Lesotho is bilingual with primary official languages of Sesotho and English and a single primary ethnic group, the Basotho. Both languages are taught in school, and Lesotho boasts a literacy rate of about 90%, one of the highest in all of Africa.

Lesotho has a stable political system consisting of a parliamentary constitutional monarchy, one that recognizes the HIV epidemic as the single greatest threat to the nation's viability. Health indicators are quite poor overall, with a life expectancy of 51.9 years, ranking 213 as one of the very lowest in the world. Maternal mortality is very high at 620/100,000 and has increased over the last decade; infant and child mortality are also quite high.[44] Malnutrition is another common health problem, with 16.6% of children under the age of 5 reported as underweight.[54]

Government health services in Lesotho are organized into vertical, largely disease-based systems, superimposed on an overall clinical delivery system. The total system is overseen by a Ministry of Health with the support of the parliament. The vertical system consists of various programs and taskforces of the ministry, including programs in HIV/AIDS control, tuberculosis control, mental health, primary health care, and environmental and occupational health programs.

The clinical delivery system consists of health service areas representing geographic divisions containing roughly 40,000 people. Each health service area is served by a district hospital with approximately 100 to 250 beds, with a national average of 1.3 hospital beds/1,000 population as of 2006.[44] The district hospital is also responsible for supervising all the health centers and clinics in the area. At the grassroots level, health centers and clinics typically serve between 6,000 and 10,000 people and are intended to be geographically accessible by foot.[55] Overall, the clinical delivery system consists of 72 health centers, 9 district hospitals, a national referral hospital, a mental hospital and leprosarium. In addition to the governmental systems, the Christian Health Association of Lesotho operates another 73 health centers and 7 district hospitals with substantial financial support from the government of Lesotho. Seriously ill patients or others requiring tertiary care are referred to South Africa for further management.[56]

As an LDC, Lesotho is challenged with inadequate funding for the health system, despite the Ministry of Health representing the third largest government expenditure and despite receiving additional financial support from international agencies and governmental organizations.[55] At 13.2% of GDP, Lesotho has the fifth highest health expenditure as a percentage of GDP in the world.[44] An effective health insurance scheme is not yet in place, with the government charging fees intended to recover 15% to 20% of expenditures, and higher fees approximating 20% to 50% recovery from the Christian Health Association of Lesotho. Although the fees are quite low compared with developed countries, they remain out of reach for many families with subsistence living.

The government has adopted the principles and objectives of the Alma Ata declaration, recognizing primary health care as a key approach to implementing health for all, even if both financing and implementation remain a challenge.[55] Overall, the government has tried to implement the best primary health care system possible in the face of extremely limited financial and human resources. The Lesotho health system depends heavily on nursing, with only approximately 5 physicians per 100,000 population. Lesotho's primary care system depends primarily on nurses and nursing assistants for grassroots clinical service delivery at the health centers and clinics.[57] Traditional birth attendants also work at the grassroots level to assist with deliveries.

Despite four nursing schools in the country, the total supply of skilled health workers is still inadequate. The number of nurses for the population falls far short of the WHO recommended minimum.[58] Many health workers migrate to South Africa for better economic opportunities, and the HIV/AIDS epidemic has devastated the workforce in all sectors. For training of physicians, there is no medical school in the country. Most Basotho medical students obtain their education in South Africa with financial support from the government of Lesotho, but then without postgraduate programs in Lesotho, many remain in South Africa to obtain postgraduate training and never return to practice in Lesotho. In this setting where training options remain limited, recruitment takes its place and policy efforts to sustain and retain health workers take on a much greater significance.

A variety of efforts have been attempted to improve the human resource situation in primary care and primary health care in general in partnership with a variety of nongovernmental organizations. Patients are provided with medical records known as *bukanas* on first consultation to help with informational continuity. As with many newly implemented health system improvements however, surveys of bukanas are showing that very little and inconsistent patient information is written in the record.[59] Grassroots training programs have developed for primary care nursing skills, and the first postgraduate training program in the country has been developed in the specialty of family medicine.[60]

Family medicine was identified as a critically needed specialty in Lesotho, although with a different emphasis than might be seen in a more developed nation. In Lesotho, because of the extreme shortage of health care personnel, it is unlikely a physician could be spared to work full time only in the ambulatory setting, and so first-contact care in the community is provided by the primary care nursing staff. As a result, although physicians may still play an important role in first-contact care at the hospital level, physicians as a precious resource may not have the same emphasis on continuity of care. In such a low-resource setting, a greater emphasis is placed on postgraduate training in comprehensive care so that a physician provider is prepared for the widest scope of practice possible at the first-contact level, and capable of performing and managing illness at the highest level possible when no other specialist is readily available for referral.

In the setting of an overwhelming burden of specific diseases and extremely low human resources, Lesotho is challenged to maintain a broad-based and person-centered approach to primary health care. Disease-based public health interventions play an incredibly important role in combating the disease burden, even while some programs may unintentionally neglect or inhibit core principles of primary care. Although the government intention remains to offer an equitable and broad-based health system approach founded in primary care, existing plans of the government and supporting organizations continue to focus primarily on disease-based approaches. In recent years these approaches have begun to broaden in recognition of the continued and essential need for comprehensive primary health care and include specific elements targeted at overall health system strengthening, albeit in the context of disease-focused health care programs.[61,62]

Vietnam

The Socialist Republic of Vietnam, a country with more than 90 million people and a distribution of 70% of the population in its rural areas, does better than many other developing countries in its region on some health indicators, but not all. The infant mortality rate of 20/1,000, life expectancy at birth of 72.4 years, and under-5 mortality rate of 23/1,000 are comparable with those in some of the more developed countries in the region. Since 1985, with the inception of the government policy of *Doi Moi* (change and newness), Vietnam has been moving toward a market-oriented socialized economy. The resulting rapid economic growth appears to have fueled quite significant improvements in typical health indicators, although in many ways these are better than expected when compared with other countries of similar GDP per capita. The policy of Doi Moi has allowed for the development of health care delivery on a private fee-for-service basis and the early advent of purchased health insurance products in the belief that a planned public and private health care mix can maximize access and efficiency to promote the rational growth of health care.[13]

Although Vietnam has made good progress over the last 20 years toward the Millennium Development Goals, the prevalence of malnutrition and communicable disease is still quite high.[63] The leading causes of death have changed little over the last decade, with head injury and other injuries leading this category. Even though the total expenditure on health has slowly been increasing to now 6.9% of GDP, with public health expenditures only a minority portion (37.5%) of this,[54] this communist state has maintained a strong political commitment to provide health care to all in Vietnam consistent with its socialist philosophy of governance.

In the 1950s, this commitment to health care for all led to the development of a remarkable medical network of commune health centers across the country that now number over 10,000. Although this network provides outstanding geographic access for patients, other components of a high-quality primary care system were lacking. The Ministry of Health (MoH) trained a cadre of health care workers for each of these health centers early on. Although there have been attempts since that time to introduce generalist physicians into these health centers, this has met with limited success. Many of the barriers experienced by other countries around the world to bringing physicians to rural areas exist in Vietnam as well. As a result, midwives, nurses, and assistant physicians have primarily staffed the commune health centers. In the 1990s, only 15% of the commune health centers were staffed with physicians. There has been increasing success since that time and now most commune health centers, both urban and rural, have general doctors; however, these doctors do not have a postgraduate medical education and are perceived as poorly trained.[64]

There are eight institutions currently training physicians in Vietnam: two medical universities under the direction of the MoH and six medical colleges under the direction of the Ministry of Education. Vietnam's current system of training physicians is based on the French system of medical education.[65] Candidates are eligible to enter 6 years of medical school directly after completion of high school. Medical training consists of classroom academics, with the basic sciences taught in the first 2 years, the medical sciences in the next 2 years, and then clinical rotations within the hospitals during the final 2 years. Very little time is spent in outpatient centers outside the hospital system, and there is little to no training in the core principles of primary care. At the end of this undergraduate medical education, the physicians are called "general doctors." They are immediately faced with compulsory service in outpatient services in urban areas or in village community care centers according to the needs outlined for the distribution of labor by the provincial health directors.[66] Many graduates either oppose relocating to a rural commune or simply feel unprepared for primary care practice at the commune level, and therefore they elect to decline the service. These graduates then become unemployed or pursue alternative nonclinical employment.

Following a minimum of 3 years of work in the community, physicians may then take a competitive examination specific to a desired specialty. Two to 6 years of postgraduate training is required for specialties such as internal medicine, pediatrics, obstetrics, and surgery. Until 2001, there were no postgraduate or continuing medical education requirements for general practice physicians (Figure 8-6). Postgraduate specialty training begins with a 2-year program, at the end of which the graduate is classified as a first-degree specialist in that discipline. That physician may then practice in that discipline or continue with additional training to obtain the second-degree certification. Physicians may also pursue research and academic tracks within the disciplines by pursuing master's- and PhD-level training. There is an emerging "residency" that allows physicians to obtain a master's degree in a clinical specialty that is offered to encourage community-based practice with the credentials reserved in the past for academic physicians.

The health care delivery system in Vietnam is hierarchical (Figure 8-7). The expectation is that medical care will be entered at the commune health center level and that referrals will then be made to the next level of care. There is no significant gatekeeper function however, and because of the perceived poor quality of the general doctor and most grassroots facilities, many patients choose to bypass the commune health centers and present directly to district or provincial hospitals. With the advent of the private sector, the

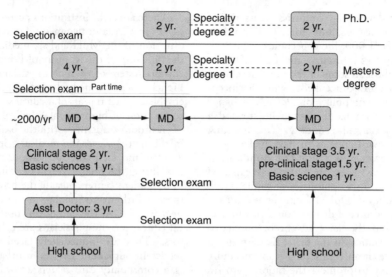

Figure 8-6. Medical education system in Vietnam.

expectations of patients regarding the quality of their medical care have increased, and they are less likely to follow the traditional avenues of health care delivery. In a 1991 survey in Cu Chi Province, only 10% of the population sought services from the commune health centers, 15% to 20% sought services directly from the hospitals, 40% sought services in the private sector, and the rest sought services at the district health level. In the urban areas, a more affluent family can go to a private physician or to a hospital clinic, where there is a 90% chance of being seen by a physician.[67]

In a more recent study examining the utilization of commune-level primary care services in Thai Nguyen Province, perceived quality care was noted to enhance community health center (CHC) utilization. When quality of care was perceived to be low, even subsidized services were insufficient to entice patients not to seek care elsewhere.

In 1996, a report entitled *Strategic Orientation for People's Health Care and Protection from Now to the Years 2000 and 2020* was published from the proceedings of the VIIIth Congress of the Communist

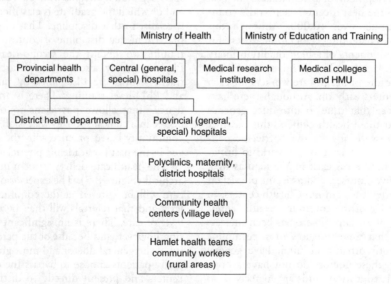

Figure 8-7. Health care delivery system, Vietnam.

Party of Vietnam.[68] The report set out new goals for the health care delivery system. These included goals for the continued improvement of the health care indicators and policies by which these goals should be reached. In particular, these new policies included streamlining the organizational structure, developing a national health care network to provide quality health care to all, and improving training programs with criteria for new and annual retraining. Provisions were made for the development of training networks. The report spelled out that in the "training of community health doctors, [the] commune doctor should be [trained] different[ly] from . . . doctors who . . . work in hospitals. To do this a training environment should be created so that trainees will acquaint themselves with the environment where they will work in the future."[68]

This document also promoted increased investment in health-related activities. The MoH of Vietnam, acknowledging the difficulties it was having meeting the people's needs for primary health care services, also began to investigate alternative approaches to meet this need in 1995. As a result it commissioned a needs assessment to investigate the current status of the primary health care system and to make recommendations for change in the Vietnamese health care system.[69] The request highlighted the special interest by the ministry on focusing on primary health care delivery at the rural community level.

The consultation spanned 4 years and included site visits to multiple areas of the country and discussions with many stakeholders. By the end of the needs assessment, it became clear that the MoH was seeking to develop a primary care physician with a patient-centered, family-focused, and community-oriented model of training. The criteria for a primary care physician as described by the MoH included comprehensiveness and continuity of care. The stakeholders in the needs assessment recommended to the MoH that its objective should be "to create educational programs that will lead to a specialty that will be the cornerstone for the delivery of primary health care to the people of Vietnam." This report was accepted by the MoH in March 2001 and created the specialty of family medicine.

Since 2001, with support from international colleagues, six of the eight medical schools have initiated training of family physicians. Programs have focused on retraining of general doctors already in practice to the level of first-degree specialists as the usual postgraduate training model. In this model, a physician, after having served in the community in a general practice, may take an entrance examination and then enter a 2-year program that, when completed, results in the awarding of a first degree specialist in family medicine. This model was successful in various

pilots, but it was recognized that urban university-based training programs would never be sufficient for retraining of the entire general doctor workforce, and such a model runs a high risk of diverting physicians away from their rural commune health centers after graduation. As a result, a modular retraining program was developed and implemented at the rural district level to engage the current rural general practice workforce in enhancing their knowledge and skills at a location closer to their commune.

In this model, university faculty travel to the rural district hospital to deliver the didactic component, and local hospital faculty are provided with faculty development so they might provide on-site practical clinical training between didactic modules. This program allows training general doctors to return to their communes on weekends and between training sessions so they might continue to maintain their existing clinical practice and access to care for their community.

Since the inception of the first degree specialist in family medicine training programs in 2001, over 500 first-degree specialist family physicians have been trained. Overall, there has been a high retention rate of these physicians at the commune level, and they report increased satisfaction with their work. Surveys of graduates have indicated statistically significant increases in clinical knowledge and confidence in multiple clinical topics compared with untrained peers, and early assessments have shown increased satisfaction of patients with their retrained commune physicians. Observational assessments have also shown that primary care practiced by graduates at the commune level has expanded the quality and scope of local health care.

Perhaps most importantly, local provincial health authorities have found the new trainees to be an important upgrade in the quality of local primary care delivery. To maximize the recognized benefit of their investment in these newly trained family doctors and provide improved primary care system supports, one provincial health authority worked with international partners to establish and pilot a primary care referral system integrated with the local district hospital, as well as develop a curriculum for teams training nurses and assistant physicians in family medicine. In addition, this provincial health authority sought authorization for an expanded medication formulary in communes with specialty-trained family medicine physicians.

To date, the bulk of training is being done by specialty physicians with a commitment to improving primary care in their country, who have been trained from 1 month to 1 year in faculty development fellowships in U.S. family medicine residencies and who have received ongoing support through training of trainer workshops by U.S. consultants in Vietnam. In addition, there is also a cohort of faculty trained with master's degrees in family medicine through south-south institutional partnerships and a small cadre of faculty enrolled in PhD programs in family medicine through south-north partnerships. More recently, the Hanoi Medical University, with outside support, has received approval for and developed a master's degree in family medicine, providing an important mechanism for the sustainability of primary care faculty training.

As a result of the success of the program, the government has now begun to seriously explore both financial and policy mechanisms to dramatically expand the family medicine program as part of a national effort to build a strong primary care foundation for the health system, with a goal of staffing 80% of commune health centers in key provinces with specialty-trained family doctors. The government recently approved the inclusion of a core module on family medicine in the undergraduate curriculum as part of an effort to expose more students to primary care. This inclusion in the undergraduate curriculum now also results in a mandate for all medical schools to develop and maintain formal departments of family medicine. In addition, the MoH has recommended the prime minister adopt expansion of the National Family Medicine program, including substantial government investment in the program, as an essential component of a comprehensive plan to reduce hospital overcrowding. A national steering committee has been formed to consider how primary care might be more fully integrated with universal health insurance and how to develop nationwide referral guidelines from the primary care commune systems through the national health care delivery system. New pilot programs are also being developed to adopt the successful pilot in Khanh Hoa Province as the foundation for utilizing a continuing medical education-based approach to upgrading general doctors across the country to the level of a family medicine specialist.

United States

The United States, a country of over 300 million people, spends a greater share of its GDP on health than almost every other nation at 16.2%. Despite the amount of money spent, the United States ranks far from number one for health outcomes as compared with countries that spend much lower percentages of their GDP on health. In fact, with the exception of the average length of life left for those who have already attained 80 years of age, the United States ranks last or near last on most rankings of the major health indicators for industrialized nations. Lower life expectancy among high-income countries was previously shown in Figure 8-1.[70]

In spite of this significant health care expenditure, increasing numbers of Americans have been without health insurance or adequate access to care, and medical bankruptcy has become an increasingly common problem for families. Until recently, the United States was the only industrialized nation lacking a government program to ensure financial access to health care services for all. A patchwork of both public- and private-sector safety nets left well over 40 million adults between 18 and 65 years old (or 18.5%) without health insurance and many more with only sporadic coverage.[71]

In response to this crisis of access, as well as skyrocketing costs to the economy, the Affordable Care Act was signed into law in 2010, with a multi-year rollout of various elements of the law. Although the law is far reaching with many different components, perhaps the core feature of the law is a requirement for all individuals to purchase health insurance, coupled with government mechanisms to ensure access to affordable coverage for lower income people.

As noted in the introduction to this chapter, it is important to distinguish between a primary health care system and "primary care," or the place of first contact for health. The United States ranks poorly in the strength of its primary care orientation; there is currently no overarching system of physicians, nurse practitioners, and physician assistants who serve as the point of first contact for all patients in the United States.[21]

The medical system in the United States is rooted in specialization. In fact, the term *primary care* was not a part of the medical lexicon until the mid-1960s. The American Board of Medical Specialties currently recognizes more than 70 specialties and subspecialties. The first of these, ophthalmology, was established in 1908; the boards of pediatrics and general internal medicine were established in 1935 and 1936, respectively. The American Board of Family Practice, not established until 1969, preceded only five other currently recognized specialty boards: thoracic surgery (1970), nuclear medicine (1971), allergy and immunology (1971), emergency medicine (1979), and medical genetics (1991).

The medical specialties presumed to provide first-contact care in the United States are known as generalists. The type of physicians who fall into this category is somewhat controversial; some statistical sources have included "general obstetric/gynecology" under this rubric in the past. For the purposes of this chapter, this specialty is not included as primary care and has been excluded from the following statistical citations. According to the Bureau of Health Professions, approximately 34% of all practicing physicians in the

United States in 2009 were "generalists." Of these, 12% were in family or general practice, 15% general internists, and 7% were pediatric providers.[72] Although there were more "generalists" (i.e., physicians without residency training) practicing prior to 1950, the current percentages have remained stable for the past 30 years.

By contrast, specialist providers represent more than 60% of the physician workforce, and their numbers continue to increase in spite of government efforts to encourage medical graduates to enter primary care. According to the *Dartmouth Atlas of Health Care*, there were almost 72 primary care providers and 127.8 specialists per 100,000 residents in 2006. The distribution of primary care physicians varies regionally, however, with a range from 46/100,000 residents in Owensboro, Kentucky, to 117/100,000 in San Francisco, California (Figure 8-8).[73]

The Affordable Care Act, in addition to developing a mechanism to finance and mandate health care for all, also includes several mechanisms to try to promote improved primary care. As is evident from the distribution of both primary care and specialist physicians, access to primary care depends, in part, on its geographic availability. In an effort to address the needs of medically underserved areas, the federal government created the community health center program in 1965. These not-for-profit health centers provide care in federally designated medically underserved areas and/or underserved population groups. Federally qualified health centers (FQHCs) can be CHCs, health care for the homeless, school-based health programs, migrant health centers, and health care for public housing. There are currently over 3,000 FQHC clinics in the United States, and they have been shown to provide high-quality care at

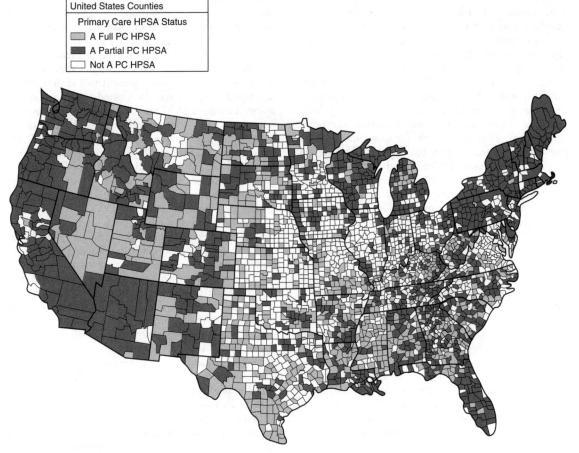

United States Counties

Primary Care HPSA Status

- A Full PC HPSA
- A Partial PC HPSA
- Not A PC HPSA

Figure 8-8. Primary care physician distribution in the United States. PC HPSA, primary care health personnel shortage area.[51]

lower cost.[74] Although they form a partial safety net, these centers serve only 25% of people living below the poverty line and only an eighth of all uninsured Americans.[75] The Affordable Care Act now includes a dramatic increase in funding for CHCs in an effort to further expand the program.

Several other mechanisms have also been included in the Affordable Care Act to promote primary care. The act includes a modest but significant increase in reimbursement to primary care providers. The act calls for the development of pilot programs to explore improvements in quality and efficiency, many of which are expected to focus on the development of patient-centered medical homes designed to standardize the implementation of many primary principles in health care delivery. The act includes additional incentives for primary care practice through the National Health Service Corps, and scholarship and loan repayment programs.

Although perhaps not fundamentally changing the core payment mechanism for health care, the act calls for the development of accountable care organizations, a mechanism intended to align incentives between hospitals and primary care in an effort to increase quality of care while lowering costs. Accountable care organizations will be groups of hospitals and providers responsible for caring for a specific group of patients. Through the Medicare program, the organizations would be rewarded with shared savings in the event they are able to provide high-quality low-cost care. These same organizations would also be at risk of being held accountable for losses should they provide low-quality care at too high an expense. By joining primary care physicians and hospitals in this shared benefit and risk, it provides new incentives for both sides to find new ways to enhance primary care and reduce unnecessary hospitalizations and high-cost low-benefit medical interventions.

As reflected in the ratios of specialist to generalist physicians noted previously, the distribution of health providers in the United States is out of balance. Taken together, the data in several population-based investigations of health outcomes and quality indicators in U.S. counties suggest that optimal health outcomes occur when 40% to 50% of the physician workforce is made up of family physicians, general internists, and general pediatricians.[76] Because, as previously noted, only 32% of the physician workforce are currently primary care physicians, there is a need for more generalists. The remedy for this imbalance, however, will not soon be fulfilled. The number of medical students choosing to enter general pediatrics, general internal medicine, or family medicine has been declining since its peak in 1998. Currently, only 28.7% of all physicians who began residency training in 2008 were expected to ultimately practice primary

care, and projections suggest a continued downward trend. When one considers that only a smaller percentage of those entering residencies in family medicine (91%), pediatric (44%), and internal medicine (10% to 20%) will be likely to have substantial outpatient primary care practices, it is anticipated that only 16% to 18% of medical students who matched into National Resident Matching Program residencies in 2010 are likely to practice primary care. Some of the primary care need is also filled, however, by additional osteopathic physicians, as well as nurse practitioners and physician assistants.[77] In the residency program selection process of 2012, the proportions of positions filled by U.S. graduates were 70% for pediatrics, 56% for internal medicine, and 48% for family medicine.[78]

COMPARING CASES: POLITICAL WILL AND PRIMARY CARE

We have defined primary health care as an integrated system based in the community that provides first-contact, continuous, comprehensive, and coordinated care. The four country cases illustrate a variety of primary care systems in practice and provide examples of the spectrum of governmental commitment to ensuring adequate primary health care for their populations. The four countries represent two each from the developed (Belgium and the United States) and developing (Lesotho and Vietnam) worlds. They represent some extremes—for example, the U.S. per capita spending on health care or Lesotho's HIV/AIDS disease burden. Although they do so on widely different scales and with huge variation in available resources, all four countries confront challenges of developing adequate workforce to support the primary care needs of their populations.

There is a striking difference in each country's commitment and strategy to providing health for all. In some cases, the desire to provide such care is explicit. Recall Vietnam's government report declaring its commitment to "developing a national health care network to provide quality health care to all" or Lesotho's political declaration toward the goals of Alma Ata. More indirectly, we can discern a commitment to primary health care for all in Belgium by the existence of a national universal health insurance scheme, and a new governmental commitment to such access in the United States, where 18.5% of adults under 65 are without any health insurance.[79]

The lack of health insurance has consequences for access to primary care. In an article comparing primary care in five developed countries, Schoen and her colleagues noted the outlying characteristics of the United States, where about 1 in 10 adults had no usual person or place where they sought first contact care and nearly 1 in 5 could not report a usual doctor.[80] This contrasts with Belgium, where 95% of adults access primary care. Of note, adults with lower incomes in all five countries were particularly affected by cost of care; this was especially striking in the United States, where 57% of respondents who were below the median income reported either not seeing a doctor when sick, not getting recommended tests or follow-up care, or not getting prescription medications because of costs in the past year. By comparison, in the United Kingdom, only 12% of adult respondents with below-median income did not seek needed care.

The late Dr. Barbara Starfield developed a method of ranking countries on primary health care.[18] Based on average scores on 11 essential features of primary care, she ranked countries in the developed world on a scale from 0 to 12 (Figure 8-9). Using this ranking, we can see that the United States is worst in primary care rank and also worst in the average of health care outcomes. Belgium fares somewhat better in both categories.

Starfield also ranks these countries for their primary health care score as compared with their per capita health expenditures. This comparison illustrates the high-expenditure yet inferior primary care score of the United States compared with Belgium (Figure 8-10).

Such primary health care rankings are not available for Lesotho and Vietnam. However, by comparing health outcomes and expenditures for the four countries (Tables 8-3 and 8-4), we can compare and contrast several salient issues. Each of the four countries makes a disparate financial commitment to health. Note that although the United States spends well over 15% of its GDP on health, more than half of that expenditure is from private sources. Compare this with Belgium, where the national universal health insurance system funds the vast majority of health care costs. Vietnam and Lesotho have much more limited resources, each spending much lower amounts per capita on health, with a range of expenditures as represented by percentage of GDP. In spite of the low expenditure, Vietnam does relatively well on health outcomes, with a life expectancy at birth of 72 years and a low under-5 mortality rate compared with Lesotho.

It is perhaps most striking to see the difference in political will of countries such as Belgium and Vietnam, where systems are deliberately designed to provide primary health care to the entire population, in comparison with the United States, where the need for a delivery system that ensures a source of good primary care and minimizes inappropriate services remains controversial.[81]

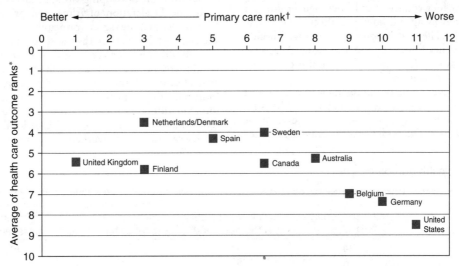

*The average health care outcome rank is an average of ranks for the following outcome measures: patient satisfaction, expenditures per person, 14 health indicators, and medications per person.

†Primary care rank is a rank of primary scores. The primary score is derived form the average of scores on 11 features of primary care. (See Starfield B. Primary care: concept, evaluation, and policy. New York: Oxford University Press, 1992)

Figure 8-9. Primary care rank versus average of health care outcome ranks. (*Adapted with permission from Starfield B. Is primary care essential? Lancet 1994;344:1129–1133.*)

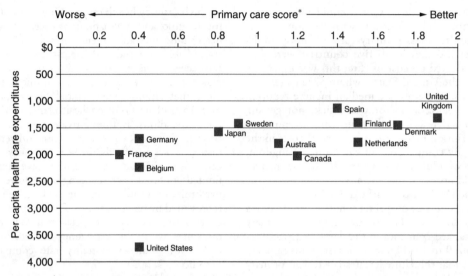

*The primary score is derived form the average scores on 11 features of primary care. (See Starfield B. Primary care: concept, evaluation, and policy. New York: Oxford University Press, 1992).

Figure 8-10. Per capita health care expenditures versus primary care score. (*Adapted with permission from Starfield B. Policy relevant determinants of health: an international perspective.* Health Policy 2002;60:201–221.)

CONCLUSIONS

This chapter tries to answer the questions posed at the outset, which health care policymakers are asking. It looked at four countries and how their health care policies are evolving and how they affect the health of their people. The goal is common: improved health. The approaches found around the globe to achieve this goal through the structuring of health care delivery systems are dissimilar.

The evidence from the industrialized countries is clear: where primary care is the fundamental basis for access to health care systems, the costs are less and the outcomes better. The evidence is yet to be determined in the developing world. To date, however, there is no correlation between government spending on health care and the health of the population. Will the outcomes from the developing world be any different?

In the Declaration of Alma Ata, primary health care is defined by seven principles. These can be summarized by stating that a solid system of primary health care "reflects and evolves from the economic conditions and sociocultural and political characteristics of the country and its communities"; "addresses the main health problems in the community, providing promotive, preventive, curative and rehabilitative services"; and "relies, at local and referral levels, on health workers, including physicians,

Table 8-3. Health outcomes.

	Life expectancy at birth, years[a]	Under-5 mortality ratio, per 1,000[b]	Children receiving measles vaccine by age 2, %[c]	Births attended by skilled personnel, %[d]
Belgium	80	4	94	>99
Lesotho	48	85	85	62
United States	79	8	92	99
Vietnam	65	23	98	84

[a]Data from 2009.
[b]Data from 2010.
[c]Data from 2011.
[d]Latest available data since 2005.
Adapted from World Health Organization, *World Health Statistics 2012.* Geneva: WHO, 2012.

Table 8-4. Health expenditure.

Year 2003	Total expenditure on health as % of GDP	Gov't expenditure on health as % of total health expenditure	Private expenditure on health as % of total health expenditure	Gov't expenditure on health as % of total gov't spending	Per capita gov't expenditure on health at average exchange rate (US$)	Out-of-pocket expenditure as % of private expenditure on health
Belgium	10.8	75.1	24.9	15.1	3,567	19.1
Lesotho	9.4	74.3	25.7	10.3	56	69.0
United States	17.6	47.7	52.3	19.6	3,795	23.4
Vietnam	6.9	37.5	62.5	7.8	29	92.7

GDP, gross domestic product; gov't, government.
Adapted from World Health Organization, *World Health Statistics 2012.* Geneva: WHO, 2012.

nurses, midwives, auxiliaries, . . . community health workers, [and] traditional practitioners."[15] The four countries used in this chapter's case studies have followed these principles, with different outcomes.

Perhaps the soundest principle is that we know that "health for all" can be achieved by providing health care access that is first-contact, continuous, comprehensive, and coordinated and provided to populations undifferentiated by gender, disease, or organ system—that is, through primary care.

ACKNOWLEDGEMENTS

We would like to acknowledge the contributions of Cynthia Haq, Debra Rothenberg, and Leon Piterman to the original version and core concepts of this chapter. We would also like to thank Anselme Derese and Jan De Maeseneer for their assistance with the description of primary care in Belgium, as well as Brian Penti and Amber Steorts for their help with the description of Lesotho.

STUDY QUESTIONS

1. Define primary health care and describe the various components and health personnel requirements.
2. Compare the primary care systems of Belgium and the United States and relate their systems to health outcomes.
3. How can countries use limited resources to most efficiently improve the health of their populations?

REFERENCES

1. Jurberg C. Flawed but fair: Brazil's health system reaches out to the poor. *Bull World Health Organ* 2008;8:241–320.
2. Answers.com. Physician. http://www.answers.com/topic/physician.
3. Ni M. *The Yellow Emperor's Classic of Medicine.* Boston: Shambhala, 1995.
4. Greek Medicine: Hippocrates and the rise of rational medicine. U.S. National Library of Medicine, History of Medicine Division, 2002. http://www.nlm.nih.gov/hmd/greek/greek_rationality.html.
5. Brainy Quote. *Hippocrates quotes.* http://www.brainyquote.com/quotes/authors/h/hippocrates.html.
6. Vesalius the humanist. http://www.hsl.virginia.edu/historical/artifacts/antiqua/vesalius.cfm.
7. Weber S. Soviet health delivery. *Health Soc Work* 1977;2(1):7–25.
8. Bowman RC. Osler and rural practice. http://www.ruralmedicaleducation.org/osler.htm.
9. Crowther A, Dupree M. The invisible general practitioner: the careers of Scottish medical students in the late nineteenth century. *Bull History Med* 1996;70(3):387–413.
10. Flexner A. *Medical Education in the United States and Canada.* New York: Carnegie Foundation for the Advancement of Teaching, 1910.
11. Bowman RC. Flexner's impact on American medicine. http://www.ruralmedicaleducation.org/flexner.htm.
12. Wang S. China's health system: from crisis to opportunity. *Yale-China Health J* 2004;3:5–50.
13. Dung PH. The political process and the private health sector's role in Vietnam. *Int J Health Plann Manage* 1996;11(3): 217–230.
14. Starfield B. Is primary care essential? *Lancet* 1994;344(8930): 1129–1133.
15. World Health Organization. *Primary Health Care: Report of the International Conference on Primary Health Care, Alma Ata, USSR.* Geneva: WHO, 1978: 25.
16. *Primary Health Care: Now More Than Ever.* Geneva: World Health Organization, 2008.
17. Boelen C. *Improving Health Systems: The Contributions of Family Medicine. A Guidebook.* Singapore: WONCA, 2002.
18. Starfield B. *Primary Care: Balancing Health Needs, Services, and Technology.* Rev. ed. New York: Oxford University Press, 1998.
19. Starfield B, Shi L, Grover A, Macinko J. The effects of specialist supply on populations' health: assessing the evidence. *Health Aff (Millwood)* 2005;(Suppl): Web Exclusives:W5-97–W95-107.

20. GapMinder 2012. *Mapping the wealth and health of nations*, 2012. www.gapminder.org/downloads/world-pdf/.

21. Starfield B, Shi L. Policy relevant determinants of health: an international perspective. *Health Policy* 2002;60(3):201–218.

22. Shi L, Macinko J, Starfield B, Wulu J, Regan J, Politzer R. The relationship between primary care, income inequality, and mortality in US States, 1980–1995. *J Am Board Fam Pract* 2003;16(5):412–422.

23. Shi L, Macinko J, Starfield B, et al. Primary care, infant mortality, and low birth weight in the states of the USA. *J Epidemiol Community Health* 2004;58(5):374–380.

24. Ferrante JM, Gonzalez EC, Pal N, Roetzheim RG. Effects of physician supply on early detection of breast cancer. *J Am Board Fam Pract* 2000;13(6):408–414.

25. Roetzheim RG, Pal N, van Durme DJ, et al. Increasing supplies of dermatologists and family physicians are associated with earlier stage of melanoma detection. *J Am Acad Dermatol* 2000;43(2 Pt 1):211–218.

26. Ferrante JM, McCarthy EP, Gonzalez EC, et al. Primary care utilization and colorectal cancer outcomes among Medicare beneficiaries. *Arch Intern Med* 2011;171(19):1747–1757.

27. Roetzheim RG, Pal N, Gonzalez EC, et al. The effects of physician supply on the early detection of colorectal cancer. *J Fam Pract* 1999;48(11):850–858.

28. Campbell RJ, Ramirez AM, Perez K, Roetzheim RG. Cervical cancer rates and the supply of primary care physicians in Florida. *Fam Med* 2003;35(1):60–64.

29. Shi L, Macinko J, Starfield B, Xu J, Politzer R. Primary care, income inequality, and stroke mortality in the United States: a longitudinal analysis, 1985–1995. *Stroke* 2003;34(8):1958–1964.

30. Lee J, Park S, Choi K, Kwon SM. The association between the supply of primary care physicians and population health outcomes in Korea. *Fam Med* 2010;42(9):628–635.

31. Franks P, Fiscella K. Primary care physicians and specialists as personal physicians. Health care expenditures and mortality experience. *J Fam Pract* 1998;47(2):105–109.

32. Simms C, Rowson M. Reassessment of health effects of the Indonesian economic crisis: donors versus the data. *Lancet* 2003;361(9366):1382–1385.

33. Malouin RA, Starfield B, Sepulveda MJ. Evaluating the tools used to assess the medical home. *Manag Care* 2009;18(6):44–48.

34. Backer LA. The medical home: an idea whose time has come . . . again. *Family Pract Manag* 2007;14(8):38–41.

35. Sia C, Tonniges TF, Osterhus E, Taba S. History of the medical home concept. *Pediatrics* 2004;113(5 Suppl):1473–1478.

36. Duong DV, Binns CW, Lee AH. Utilization of delivery services at the primary health care level in rural Vietnam. *Soc Sci Med* 2004;59(12):2585–2595.

37. Saultz JW. Defining and measuring interpersonal continuity of care. *Ann Fam Med* 2003;1(3):134–143.

38. Phan K, Brown SR. Decreased continuity in a residency clinic: a consequence of open access scheduling. *Fam Med* 2009; 41(1):46–50.

39. Bennett KJ, Baxley EG. The effect of a carve-out advanced access scheduling system on no-show rates. *Fam Med* 2009;41(1): 51–56.

40. Powell Davies G, Williams AM, Larsen K, Perkins D, Roland M, Harris MF. Coordinating primary health care: an analysis of the outcomes of a systematic review. *Med J Aust* 2008;188 (8 Suppl): S65–S68.

41. Stille CJ, Jerant A, Bell D, Meltzer D, Elmore JG. Coordinating care across diseases, settings, and clinicians: a key role for the generalist in practice. *Ann Intern Med* 2005;142(8):700–708.

42. De Maeseneer J, van Weel C, Roberts R. Family medicine's commitment to the MDGs. *Lancet* 2010;375(9726): 1588–1589.

43. Iliffe S, Lenihan P. Integrating primary care and public health: learning from the community-oriented primary care model. *Int J Health Serv* 2003;33(1):85–98.

44. Central Intelligence Agency. *The World Factbook, 2012*. Agency USCI, ed. https://www.cia.gov/library/publications/the-world-factbook/.

45. Wilson A, Gallos ID, Plana N, et al. Effectiveness of strategies incorporating training and support of traditional birth attendants on perinatal and maternal mortality: meta-analysis. *BMJ* 2011;343:d7102.

46. World Health Organization. *The World Health Report 2006: Working Together for Health*. Geneva: WHO, 2006.

47. Kark SL. *The Practice of Community-Oriented Primary Health Care*. New York: Appleton-Century-Crofts, 1981.

48. Pritchard P. *Manual of Primary Health Care: Its Nature and Organization*. 2nd ed. Oxford, UK: Oxford Medical Publications, 1981.

49. Gerkens S, Merkur S. Belgium: health system review. *Health Syst Transit* 2010;12(5):1 266. http://www.euro.who.int/__data/assets/pdf_file/0014/120425/E94245.pdf.

50. Meeus P, Van Aubel X. *Performance of General Medicine in Belgium, a Check-Up*. Brussels: National Institute for Health and Disease Insurance (NIHDI), 2012.

51. Sunaert P, Bastiaens H, Feyen L, et al. Implementation of a program for type 2 diabetes based on the Chronic Care Model in a hospital-centered health care system: "the Belgian experience." *BMC Health Serv Res* 2009;9:152.

52. Philips H, Remmen R, Van Royen P, et al. What's the effect of the implementation of general practitioner cooperatives on case load? Prospective intervention study on primary and secondary care. *BMC Health Serv Res* 2010;10:222.

53. Boffin N, Bossuyt N, Vanthomme K, Van Casteren V. Readiness of the Belgian network of sentinel general practitioners to deliver electronic health record data for surveillance purposes: results of survey study. *BMC Fam Pract* 2010;11(1):50.

54. *World Health Statistics*. Geneva: World Health Organization, 2012. www.who.int/gho/publications/world_health_statistics/EN_WHS2012_Full.pdf.

55. Shonubi AM, Odusan O, Oloruntoba DO, Agbahowe SA, Siddique MA. "Health for all" in a least-developed country. *J Natl Med Assoc* 2005;97(7):1020–1026.

56. Babich LP, Bicknell WJ, Culpepper L, Jack BW. Social responsibility, international development, and institutional commitment: lessons from the Boston University experience. *Acad Med* 2008;83(2):143–147.

57. Veidis AN, Nkholongo E, Steorts A. *Strengthening community health in a nurse driven system*, 2012. http://www.bu.edu/lesotho/files/2009/10/Izumi-Program-Summary-Sept-2010.pdf.

58. Médicines Sans Frontières. *Help wanted: Confronting the health care worker crisis to expand access to HIV/AIDS treatment: MSF experience in Southern Africa*, 2007. https://www.doctorswithoutborders.org/publications/reports/2007/healthcare_worker_report_05-2007.pdf.

59. Steorts A. Personal communication, 2012.

60. Nkabane-Nkholongo EL, Jack B. *The Family Medicine Specialty Training Program: A Program of the Ministry of Health and Social Welfare and the Lesotho Boston Health Alliance: Progress Report to PEPFAR, October 2010 to June 2012*, 2012.

61. *National HIV and AIDS Strategic Plan 2006 - 2011*: National AIDS Commission, The Government of Lesotho, revised 2009. http://www.ilo.org/wcmsp5/groups/public/—ed_protect/—protrav/—ilo_aids/documents/legaldocument/wcms_126751.pdf.

62. *Lesotho Strategy*. U.S. Government Global Health Initiative, 2011. http://www.ghi.gov/documents/organization/178898.pdf.

63. World Health Organization. *Viet Nam: Health Profile*. Geneva: WHO, 2012. http://www.who.int/countries/vnm/en/.

64. Montegut AJ, Schirmer J, Cartwright C, et al. Creation of postgraduate training programs for family medicine in Vietnam. *Fam Med* 2007;39(9):634–638.

65. Singer I. Editorial: The medical education project in Vietnam: an obituary. *JAMA* 1975;234(13):1405–1406.

66. Project of Vietnam-Netherland. *Strengthening in teaching epidemiology and primary healthcare in 8 medical faculties in Vietnam: survey to evaluate the knowledge, attitude and skills of medical curriculum in 8 medical faculties*, 2000–2001.

67. Gellert GA. The influence of market economics on primary health care in Vietnam. *JAMA* 1995;273(19):1498–1502.

68. Socialist Republic of Vietnam Ministry of Health. *Strategic Orientation for People's Health Care and Protection in the Period of 1996–2000 and Vietnam's National Drug Policy*. Hanoi: Socialist Republic of Vietnam Ministry of Health, 1996.

69. Montegut AJ, Cartwright CA, Schirmer JM, Cummings S. An international consultation: the development of family medicine in Vietnam. *Fam Med* 2004;36(5):352–356.

70. Starfield B. The importance of primary care to health. *Medical Reporter*, 1999.

71. Kaiser Commission on Medicaid and the Uninsured. *The Uninsured: A Primer. Key Facts About Americans Without Health Insurance*. Washington, DC: Kaiser Family Foundation, 2006.

72. *Health, United States, 2011: with special feature on socioeconomic status and health*. Hyattsville, MD: National Center for Health Statistics, 2012.

73. Dartmouth Atlas of Health Care: The Dartmouth Institute for Health Policy and Clinical Practice; 2012. http://www.dartmouthatlas.org/.

74. Proser M. Deserving the spotlight: health centers provide high-quality and cost-effective care. *J Ambul Care Manage* 2005;28(4):321–330.

75. Starfield B, Shi L, Macinko J. Contribution of primary care to health systems and health. *Milbank Q* 2005;83(3):457–502.

76. Kruse J; Association of Departments of Family Medicine. Family medicine legislative advocacy: our powerful message. *Ann Fam Med* 2005;3(5):468–469.

77. COGME. *Advancing Primary Care: COGME 20th Report*. Washington, DC: Council on Graduate Medical Education, 2010. http://www.hrsa.gov/advisorycommittees/bhpradvisory/cogme/Reports/twentiethreport.pdf

78. *National Resident Matching Program. Results and Data: 2012 Main Residency Match*. Washington, DC: National Resident Matching Program, 2012.

79. Phillips RL, Jr., Starfield B. Why does a U.S. primary care physician workforce crisis matter? *Am Fam Physician* 2004;70(3):440–446.

80. Schoen C, Osborn R, Huynh PT, et al. Primary care and health system performance: adults' experiences in five countries. *Health Aff (Millwood)* 2004;(Suppl Web Exclusives): W4-487–W4-503.

81. Starfield B. Insurance and the U.S. health care system. *N Engl J Med* 2005;353(4):418–419.

Malaria

9

Paul R. Larson and Mark W. Meyer

LEARNING OBJECTIVES

- *Describe the current global burden of malarial disease*
- *Incorporate knowledge of clinical syndromes associated with malarial disease into diagnosis and initial management*
- *List medications that may be used in both acute therapy and prevention of malaria with consideration for local resistance patterns*
- *Outline the social and financial cost of malaria, including the economic impact of clinical disease and control strategies*
- *Give examples of current strategies for global malaria control, including individual precautions, population-based interventions, and new initiatives in vaccine development*

MALARIA IN HISTORY

Malaria, or a disease resembling malaria, has been known for approximately 4,000 years in literature and various other historical sources. The name, stemming from the Italian for "bad air," has surely influenced human populations for longer than recorded history and continues to cause illness and death to this day. Malaria symptoms were noted in ancient Chinese writings dating back to 2700 BC. There are many Greek references to the disease from the 4th century BC onward. Later, several Roman writers attributed malarial diseases to swampy areas. References to malaria, coming as the result of a bite of certain insects, were discussed in the *Susruta*, an ancient Sanskrit medical treatise.

The first recorded treatment is from a 2nd-century Chinese text, found in a tomb, known as the "52

Remedies." Treatment included the Qinghao plant, or *Artemisia annua* (sweet wormwood), that seemed to reduce fevers associated with the illness. In 1971, the active ingredient, Artemisin, was discovered and named by Chinese scientists. What we now call quinine was used by indigenous peoples in Peru and was brought to light by Spanish Jesuit missionaries during the treatment of the Countess of Chincon. Her fever was reduced and she survived. This treatment became known as cinchona or Peruvian bark. German scientist Hans Andersag discovered chloroquine in 1934, and in 1939 dichlorodiphenyltrichloroethane (DDT) was also discovered in Germany by Othmer Zeidler.

In 1880, Charles Luis Alfonse Laveran (a French Army surgeon) was the first to notice parasites in the blood of patients suffering from this febrile illness that would become known as malaria. The species name *Plasmodium* was given in 1886, and human parasites *falciparum, vivax, malariae,* and *ovale* were named in 1890 and 1893. It was in 1897 that Ronald Ross, a British officer in the Indian medical service, demonstrated that malaria came from infected mosquitoes, subsequently identified as various species of female *Anopheles*. Italian scientist Battista Grassi is also known to have independently demonstrated this vector at nearly the same time.[1]

IMPORTANCE AND DISTRIBUTION

Nearly 3.3 billion people, or approximately half of the world's population, are at risk for malarial infection each year. In the last 10 years there has been significant growth in the fight against malaria. The World Health Organization (WHO) Malaria Report 2011 suggested that it has observed decreasing total incidence, from between 230 and 400 million/year in 2000, down to 216 million cases/year of malaria in 2010. There was a corresponding decrease in the overall deaths from close to 1 million, down to an estimate of 655,000/year in 2010. Several trends in these data are troublesome though. Most deaths occur in sub-Saharan Africa, and approximately 90% of all-case deaths from malaria are in children under 5 years living in sub-Saharan Africa. This translates to one child dying every minute.[2]

Human immunodeficiency virus (HIV), tuberculosis, and malaria are the three greatest infectious disease killers at work in the world today. Both tuberculosis and HIV/AIDS caused more deaths (1.8 million people died of AIDS in 2010) than malaria in 2010, but there is a disproportionate effect on pregnant mothers and children under 5, with the highest rates of mortality in the world among these populations in sub-Saharan Africa, as already noted. Due to the investment in malaria control, there is an estimate of 1 million children's lives saved in sub-Saharan Africa in the past decade.[3]

There is a general consensus in the international community to try to meet the challenge of overcoming malaria as demonstrated by current global efforts. Part of this desire stems from a previous international campaign that was not successful in eradicating malaria or even limiting it in many parts of the world. This previous campaign ended in the late 1970s. It was not a complete failure, but in many critical areas of the world, especially in sub-Saharan Africa, there was minimal impact in limiting malarial illness and death.[4]

Over the past 10 years, overall incidence of malaria has steadied and then dropped slightly. We seem to be seeing some results of global eradication and control programs with falling total incidence and significant decreases in death rates as well (as much as 50% in some regions). The burden of disease, as demonstrated by Figure 9-1, is still quite concentrated in sub-Saharan Africa, both by total numbers and percentage of cases. During the past decade in Africa, there has been a one-third decrease in the incidence of malaria. At the same time, outside of Africa, 35 of 53 countries affected by malaria have reduced their incidence by 50%. Child mortality from malaria has decreased by 20% over these last 10 years. The Global Malaria Mapper, created by the Medicine for Malaria Venture and the WHO Global Malaria Programme, allows you to access comprehensive worldwide data from the WHO Malaria Report 2012, http://www.worldmalariareport.org/.

ORGANISM, LIFE CYCLE, AND TRANSMISSION

To be successful, malaria parasites must successively infect humans and then female *Anopheles* mosquitoes. Parasites that began in humans grow and multiply first in liver cells, then into red blood cells, and then into the bloodstream after destroying the red cells in which they live. These daughter parasites, or merozoites, are the particles that go on to invade other red cells and continue the cycle. A female *Anopheles* mosquito picks up some blood stage parasites, or gametocytes, during a blood meal. Following ingestion, parasites mate and

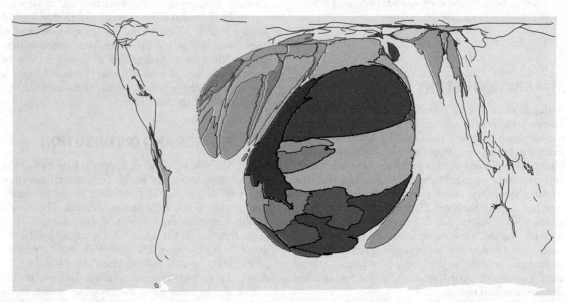

Figure 9-1. World map with incidence of malaria cases by country with countries sized by overall portion of global burden of disease World Mapper Malaria cases. http://www.worldmapper.org/display.php?selected=229.© Copyright SASI Group (University of Sheffield) and Mark Newman (University of Michigan).

migrate to the salivary glands where a new growth cycle begins. After 10 to 18 days of growth, sporozoites are injected into a new host during a subsequent blood meal, and the human infection begins again by parasitizing liver cells of the human host. Mosquitoes do not suffer from the presence of these parasites but instead act as the vector spreading the disease from human to human (Figure 9-2).

Several conditions must be present for malaria to be transmissible. First there must be climatic and temperature conditions allowing the *Anopheles* mosquito species to survive and multiply. Second, the proper conditions must exist to allow for immature parasites to complete their growth cycle in the mosquitoes themselves. For example, if the temperature drops below 68°F, this growth cycle cannot occur. (*P. vivax* can survive at lower temperatures.) Other factors also

influence transmission. Transmission will not readily occur at high altitudes, during cooler seasons, in deserts, or in areas where interrupted transmission has occurred through eradication of *Plasmodium* species. Transmission is much more intense in areas that are warmer and closer to the equator where *P. falciparum* dominates and where there are year-round conditions for malaria to replicate. There are areas in Europe and North America where *Anopheles* mosquito species live, but because of eradication via public health measures along with economic development, there are no *Plasmodium* species to transmit.

Clearly, transmission depends on multiple climatic factors that affect the concentration and survival of mosquito populations. There is seasonal variation; thus transmission is most intense in areas where *Anopheles* species can survive the longest. The 20 or so *Anopheles*

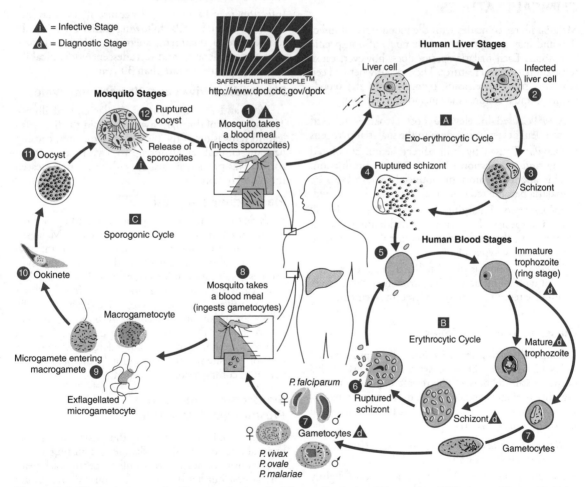

Figure 9-2. The malaria parasite life cycle. Centers for Disease Control and Prevention. DPDx Image Library. Malaria. http://www.dpd.cdc.gov/dpdx/HTML/ImageLibrary/Malaria_il.htm.

species also have particular transmission abilities and needs. The important vector species bite at night. All mosquitoes breed in water, but each prefers differing depths of water. Transmission is also more prevalent where the mosquitoes prefer humans rather than other animals. *Anopheles gambiae* is the dominant vector in Africa and the most efficient vector of all mosquitoes for human disease.

Another critical factor in transmission is human immunity. Moderate host immunity develops in areas of moderate to intense transmission, but it never provides complete protection. Severe disease is less likely with some level of immunity. Thus children are most at risk in high transmission zones; all age groups are at risk in areas with less transmission and lower immunity. Epidemics can occur quickly when some of these factors change suddenly, such as a flood in a normally dry region or an influx of malaria-naive refugees into a malaria-endemic region.

CLINICAL FEATURES

Malarial illness coincides with the blood stage of infection and may present with a wide range of nonspecific symptoms. Each malaria species does, however, cause some similar clinical features. These occur when red cell schizonts rupture, releasing pyrogens into the bloodstream. Similar features may include the following:

- *Fever:* Caused by elevated host cytokines released from leukocytes in response to the malarial pyrogens
- *Anemia:* Caused by both direct hemolysis of red cells and suppression of bone marrow production. This anemia is most pronounced in *P. falciparum* malaria because red cells of all ages may be infected
- *Splenomegaly:* Enlarging early in infections by all malaria species. If a patient has had many recurrent infections, the spleen may remain enlarged, leading to secondary hypersplenism
- *Jaundice:* Hemolysis of red cells may lead to jaundice in all types of malaria. *P. falciparum* may cause severe jaundice resulting from direct liver involvement.

Classical Stages of Fever

During well-established infections, the rupture of red cell schizonts may become synchronized. Why this occurs is still unknown. The release of pyrogens during this periodic schizogony leads to regular paroxysms of fever. This observation led to the traditional names of human malaria[5]:

- *Tertian malaria:* fever every third day (first day is number 1): *P. vivax* and *P. ovale*
- *Subtertian (malignant tertian) malaria:* fever slightly more frequent than every third day: *P. falciparum*
- *Quartan malaria:* fever every fourth day: *P. malariae*

Clinically, this periodicity often fails to develop and should not be used as a sign of clinical diagnosis. The important implication, however, is that patients with symptomatic or even severe malarial infection may be a febrile at any specific time, and the presence or absence of fever does not necessarily correlate with the severity of disease.

Natural History of Malaria Infection

Plasmodium falciparum

Death from a single acute infection is not an uncommon event. Those who survive develop some level of immunity and have a residual anemia. Recurrent symptomatic events may occur periodically over the course of a year before dying out. This recurrence, called *recrudescence,* is caused by the persistence of blood forms in small numbers between events.

Plasmodium malariae

Infection may be prolonged because illness may not occur for several weeks following initial infection. In the absence of treatment, anemia and hypersplenism may be considerable, and recrudescence of clinical illness may occur for more than 30 years.

Plasmodium vivax and Plasmodium ovale

P. vivax and *P. ovale* cause a similar clinical illness. The presence of dormant hypnozoites in the liver may lead to reinvasion of the blood by merozoites, causing periodic clinical *relapse* for up to 5 years, even if the patient was previously treated with drugs that cleared the blood of parasites.

Plasmodium knowlesi

P. knowlesi is an emerging human pathogen only documented in Southeast Asia, particularly Malaysia, where it may be the most common cause of malarial illness in children. Reports have described severe syndromes resulting from infections with *P. knowlesi,* but most cases present with a nonspecific febrile illness and a universal thrombocytopenia. They generally follow an uncomplicated course responding to first-line therapies. The most common complication that occurs is respiratory distress and relates directly to the level of parasitemia at presentation.[6] Anemia is also a common complication in children.

Syndromes Caused by *Plasmodium falciparum*

P. falciparum is set apart from other plasmodia species by its ability to cause severe disease, accounting for the vast majority of more than a million deaths each year. The largest burden of disease falls on children under 5 living in endemic areas because they are exposed recurrently but are still developing immunity. Severe disease may also occur in adults from areas where transmission is unstable in whom very little immunity develops or in travelers to any area who lack or have lost any preexisting immunity. In those with severe disease, the syndromes described next predominate and may occur in isolation or in any combination.

Change in Level of Consciousness

Changes in the level of consciousness, including coma, may occur alone or as a component of other syndromes, including hypoglycemia, acidosis, severe anemia, or as a result of a seizure or a postictal state. If the patient remains unconscious despite attempts to address these complications, he or she may have cerebral malaria. Even in a patient with a parasitemia, another diagnosis may be responsible for the presenting clinical syndrome. Bacterial meningitis, encephalitis, severe pneumonia, or a head injury may also present with changes in level of consciousness.

Cerebral Malaria

Cerebral malaria is a diffuse disturbance in cerebral function characterized by a decreased level of consciousness and commonly seizures. The onset may be either gradual or sudden, occasionally preceding other signs of disease, including fever. Limb flaccidity, hypertonicity, posturing, or opisthotonos may accompany coma. Seizure activity may be either generalized or represented by the smallest of repetitive muscle movements. A strict definition includes a patient's inability to localize painful stimuli and the persistence of coma despite the correction of other potential causes.

A distinctive retinopathy has been recently described. Bedside direct ophthalmoscopy with a short-acting mydriatic may observe areas of whitening of the macula, the extramacular optic fundus, and patchy whitening of small vessels. In an autopsy study, the presence of this retinopathy was the best available clinical predictor of malaria as the cause of death.[7] Other less distinctive retinal changes may include white-centered hemorrhages or papilledema.

A detailed pathogenesis of cerebral malaria is not yet clear, but it is likely to include multiple factors. The large burden of sequestered mature parasites in the brain may cause a detrimental metabolic environment to adjacent tissues in which oxygen, glucose, and other nutrients are consumed by parasites that in turn release toxic products, including lactate. This new metabolic environment stimulates the release of host cytokines that further contribute to the development of coma and other complications. Histopathologic changes include a large burden of erythrocytes containing parasites in capillaries and venules of many organs, including the brain. Because more than 90% of patients who recover do not sustain any permanent neurologic sequelae, it is thought that in general

this sequestering of erythrocytes is not completely occlusive. However, 5% to 10% of patients are left with some form of neurologic impairment, including hemiparesis, cerebellar ataxia, amnesia, diffuse spasticity, or epilepsy, suggesting that, at least in some cases, the microcirculation may be completed occluded. If antimalarial drugs and supportive care are provided promptly, about 80% of patients with cerebral malaria recover. However, a coma may persist for a few days after the initiation of treatment, especially in adults.

Severe Anemia

Severe anemia is a common complication, especially in young children living in areas where transmission is high. It may be found incidentally while presenting for unrelated complaints, or it may be the cause of presenting syndromes, including breathlessness, weakness, or a decreased level of consciousness. The clinical presentation may be more affected by the rate of hemoglobin decline than the absolute hemoglobin concentration. Multiple mechanisms for anemia coexist. Large-scale destruction of erythrocytes occurs when schizonts rupture as well as further hemolysis of both parasitized and nonparasitized cells via autoimmune mechanisms. The release of host cytokines leads to a direct suppression of bone marrow production reflected by the absence of a significant reticulocytosis that would be otherwise expected in a hemolytic anemia. Additionally, phagocytosis occurs in the bone marrow and peripheral circulation of both parasitized and apparently uninfected erythrocytes.

Acidosis

A number of factors may contribute to the development of tissue anoxia. The sequestration of parasitized erythrocytes may impair tissue perfusion; combined with anemia, hypovolemia and hypotension leads to localized anaerobic metabolism and the production of lactic acid. Deep breathing initially compensates for the resulting metabolic acidosis but may be insufficient to prevent a falling pH. Dyspnea is therefore the leading presentation of acidosis in children, and if associated with severe anemia or impaired consciousness, mortality may be around 20% to 30%. Mortality may be reduced through rapid fluid volume replacement, using whole blood if necessary.

Hypoglycemia

Hypoglycemia is a common complication of all *P. falciparum* infections, but children and pregnant women are particularly susceptible. The pathogenesis of hypoglycemia in malaria is also multifactorial but includes the direct suppression of hepatic gluconeogenesis by host cytokines and the consumption of glucose by parasites. Treatment of malaria with quinine or quinidine may cause hypoglycemia because these drugs stimulate the pancreas to release insulin. For this reason, parenteral infusions of these medications should be administered using fluids containing dextrose.

Other Syndromes

In severe infections with *P. falciparum,* significant intravascular hemolysis may be associated with hemoglobinuria and acute renal failure. This syndrome was historically known as Blackwater fever. Hemoglobinuria may be precipitated by a drug or dietary factor in patients with glucose-6-phosphate dehydrogenase (G6PD) deficiency. This type of hemolysis predominantly affects older erythrocytes. Some degree of disseminated intravascular coagulation is also common in *P. falciparum* infection and may be severe enough to cause bleeding.

MALARIA IN PREGNANCY

Approximately 50 million women live in malaria-endemic areas, and over half of these women live in sub-Saharan Africa. Women in this region have a much higher incidence of severe malaria leading to approximately 10,000 maternal deaths and 200,000 perinatal deaths of children each year.[8]

Because of poorly understood mechanisms, pregnant women have reduced immune response in pregnancy and thus more difficulty clearing malarial infection. Malaria parasites also sequester and replicate in the placenta and can be passed to the newborn (congenital malaria). Pregnant women have a risk of severe malaria that is three times greater than nonpregnant women and have a higher risk of dying from complications of severe malaria.[9]

Malarial infection in pregnancy can lead to miscarriage, low-birth-weight (LBW) infants, congenital infections, premature deliveries, perinatal death, and preventable LBW babies.[9]

LBW associated with malaria in pregnancy accounts for a third of all LBW children delivered annually. Mechanisms of fetal injury associated with severe malaria in pregnancy include placental insufficiency,

---

BOX 9-1. A VOICE FROM AFRICA

Edna looked tired. She had made the 5-hour walk to our district mission hospital several times as her pregnant belly grew. Edna's home was far down the escarpment of the Rift Valley in western Kenya, at least 2,000 feet below our hilltop hospital. I remembered the last agonizing time I had made that hike, with insufficient water and exuberant medical students from America. The moment of realization that home was back at the top of the hill is still a daunting memory.

As I strain to hear the baby's faint heartbeat through my fetoscope, a well-used metal trumpet pressed against my ear, I can feel Edna's rapid breathing, much faster than I'd expect in a veteran hill climber, even when pregnant. The skin of her ankles admits my soft push, leaving small finger-size dimples. I look at Edna's face and see small beads of sweat forming on her forehead, her normally pink conjunctiva pale white against her deeply dark skin.

Turning to Edna's chart I notice that although completing 34 weeks of pregnancy so far, she hasn't been seen in 2 months. This is important because she has missed the second dose of sulfadoxine-pyrimethamine normally given to patients entering their third trimester. Her first dose, given at her first obstetric appointment, is well documented. This widespread WHO initiative, the Intermittent Presumptive Therapy in Pregnancy (IPTp), has had dramatic effects on the incidence of malarial disease in Africa and especially on the complications during pregnancy and health of the newborn.

As I wait for confirmation of my clinical suspicion of malaria from the lab, I remember that although Edna survived many bouts of malaria as a young child, developing a partial immunity to the severe effects, her current pregnancy has left her especially vulnerable. Her body, in an immunologic effort not to reject her growing baby, has inadvertently reduced her protection against malaria. She will develop some immunity to the current parasites in her blood, but not in time to prevent the hemolysis that I expect to find reflected in her hemoglobin.

Inpatient parenteral therapy will be financially burdensome on this poor farmer. With the assistance of the WHO, the Kenyan Ministry of Health has provided both clear guidelines for treating Edna and access to low cost artemisinin-based combination therapies (ACTs). Artemether-lumefantrine, our first-line oral ACT, is well tolerated and will reduce her parasite load faster than intravenous quinine. Some iron tablets and her daily diet of sukumawiki, a green leafy plant with a name that translates as "pushing the weak," will gradually raise her hemoglobin in time for her delivery. With relatives close to town, Edna will stay a few days and visit before starting the long walk down to her valley home.

Source: Paul Larson, MD

severe maternal anemia, maternal hypoglycemia, and high output cardiac failure due to severe anemia.[10]

IMMUNITY IN MALARIA

Acquired immunity to malaria infections is not a sterilizing immunity but a partial immunity that seems to limit the incidence of severe malarial disease. Incidence of severe malaria and symptoms seem to definitely decrease as a person's age and number of infections increase, but there still seems to be a similar number of malaria parasites noted in the bloodstream. Certainly, part of the problem leading to only partial immunity is lack of cross-immunity when presented with antigenic variations even within the same *P. falciparum* family.[1]

NONIMMUNE PROTECTIVE FACTORS IN MALARIA

Aggressive malaria transmission may have helped shape the human genome. For example, the hemoglobin S trait is present in up to 25% of people in certain areas of sub-Saharan Africa. This sickle cell trait seems to decrease the risk of severe malaria significantly, although malaria infection is still possible. In contrast, hemoglobin SS disease, or sickle cell disease (SCD), and malaria can be a deadly combination, for children in particular. Although rates and severity of infection seem to be similar, SCD children have a much higher mortality with infection.[11] The presence of hemoglobin E and C is also noted to be protective. The mechanism is unclear but seems to involve the shape and adherence of the erythrocytes to endothelial cells and monocytes, truncating reactions creating conditions that lead to severe malaria.

Heterozygous thalassemias also lead to natural protection against malaria because *P. falciparum* has a hard time growing and replicating within the conditions of the cells. Fetal hemoglobin, or hemoglobin F, also seems to be protective. There is a decrease of this hemoglobin after the first few months of life and increased susceptibility to malaria. G6PD deficiency also leads to between a 45% and 58% decrease in severe malaria. This is the most common enzymopathy in humans, and the mechanism of protection is not well understood. There seems to be similar parasite densities in G6PD-deficient males and females but slightly more protection from severe malaria in males than females. There is also some evidence of blood group O being protective from severe malaria and some similar proof that Duffy antigen negativity also gives protection, specifically against *P. vivax* but not against the other three types of malaria-causing plasmodium species.[1] Duffy antigens are largely absent in West Africa.

Some new and fascinating information indicates that skin plays a more significant role in infection than understood previously. There is a suggestion that skin-infecting sporozoites initiate rapid suppression of immunity, making the following stages more tolerable to local defenses. This could explain susceptibility to reinfection by mosquito bites and has direct consequences for vaccine development and treatment in general.[12]

DIAGNOSIS

The confirmation of malaria disease, as distinct from asymptomatic malaria infection or other malaria-like illnesses, provides significant diagnostic challenges. Individual clinical features cannot accurately predict malaria illness in febrile patients from endemic areas, although the presence of splenomegaly makes malaria more likely. In nonimmune patients returning from endemic areas, the presence of fever, splenomegaly, hyperbilirubinemia, or thrombocytopenia makes malaria more likely.[13]

Misdiagnosis of malaria is common in both uncomplicated and severe disease. If the parasite burden is low, sensitivity of many available tests may be insufficient to be clinically useful. In this case test results may be falsely negative, leading to underdiagnosis of disease. Underdiagnosis may also occur in endemic areas where many patients may not reach a health facility. In nonendemic areas, health professionals may simply fail to consider the possibility of malaria.

Likewise, the presence of parasites in the blood does not necessarily provide definitive proof of causality for the presenting clinical syndrome. Patients living in areas of high transmission may tolerate levels of parasitemia, without any associated malaria illness, thus making the parasites passengers and not the agents of disease.[7] The possibility of overdiagnosis may also arise from the use of an algorithm-based presumptive diagnosis, especially where laboratory confirmation is not available. This is compounded by the fact that many presenting symptoms are nonspecific, and other comorbid illnesses, especially invasive bacterial infection, HIV, or malnutrition, may contribute significantly to both morbidity and mortality. Many components of malarial illness are mediated by host mechanisms, which are common in these and other diverse infections.[14] The primary consequence of overdiagnosis may be failure to treat these other causes of life-threatening disease.

Direct Diagnosis

The gold standard for clinical diagnosis of malaria is by direct examination of blood by a dried Giemsa- or Fields-stained blood smear. In experienced hands, the thick film is the most sensitive test for determining the presence of parasites and therefore answering the question, "Does the patient have malaria?" The thick film is prepared so that the erythrocyte layer is 10 to 20 cells deep and lysed, allowing many more cells to be examined simultaneously. Parasites, however, appear distorted and may make the identification of specific features more challenging. The thin blood film is fixed and cells are intact. It examines a single layer of cells and allows parasite morphology and therefore parasite species to be more easily determined.

Serodiagnosis

Antibodies to malarial antigens may be present in the host blood for years following an acute infection. Most methods for the detection of these antibodies are unable to distinguish between antigens of different parasites species. Therefore, serodiagnosis is of limited value in the diagnosis of acute infections. It may be of value in excluding malaria as a cause of recurrent fever or in determining the burden of infection in population surveys. One technique in current use is the indirect fluorescent antibody test.

New Methods of Diagnosis

The diagnosis of malaria is an area of very active research, and many new approaches are being developed. Parasitized erythrocytes have a different specific gravity than uninfected cells and therefore may be separated via centrifuge with subsequent examination of specific layers after staining with a fluorescent dye. This technique is called the quantitative buffy coat. Polymerase chain reaction may also detect the presence of parasite DNA but is mostly used in research studies. The presence of specific parasite antigens (HRP-2 or pLDH) may be detected using rapid immunochromatographic techniques. These techniques are currently used in a number of commercially available rapid diagnostic tests (RDTs). Advantages with the use of RDTs are that no additional special equipment is necessary, minimal training is needed, the tests are stable at room temperature, and no electricity is required. These tests have a higher per test cost and cannot quantify the density of infection. A recent Cochrane review concluded that RDTs have sufficient sensitivity and specificity to replace direct microscopy or extend the access to diagnostic services for *P. falciparum* malaria in endemic countries.[15]

TREATMENT

Prompt supportive treatment is essential in the treatment of acute malaria.

- *Rehydration:* Replacement of fluid volume is especially important in the presence of vomiting, diarrhea, or deep breathing suggestive of acidosis.

- *Monitor blood glucose and correct hypoglycemia:* An infusion of 10 to 40 ml of 50% dextrose diluted in three times the volume of normal saline is one acceptable approach.

- *Correcting severe anemia:* Strong clinical indications for blood transfusion include a hemoglobin less than 4 g/dL or anemia accompanied by coma, acidosis, or high parasite burden. In general, hemoglobin concentration will rise rapidly following specific antimalarial chemotherapy.

- *Correcting acidosis:* Fluid volume replacement, blood transfusion, and specific antimalarial chemotherapy are usually sufficient, and the use of bicarbonate is discouraged unless very close monitoring in severe disease is available. If available, arterial blood gas assessment may aid in fluid replacement, and the severity of acidosis correlates with prognosis.

- *Fever:* The temperature of a febrile patient may be reduced with oral or rectal acetaminophen. Fanning or sponging with cool water may also be helpful.

- *Monitor urine production:* Decreased urine production is an indication of intravascular volume depletion or acute kidney injury. Mild elevations of serum creatinine are common with dehydration. Greater elevations should be carefully monitored as part of fluid balance correction.

- *Seizures:* Prolonged seizures may be aborted with parenteral or rectal diazepam, lorazepam, or intramuscular paraldehyde or phenobarbital.

Treat Comorbid Illness

If an alternative or an additional diagnosis is possible, the administration of additional therapies or tests, including antibiotics, blood culturing, or lumbar puncture may be justified. Bacterial meningitis, pneumonia, bacteremia, HIV, and malnutrition are important considerations and often coexist with malaria. Dual treatment may be a common and justified approach. Studies in sub-Saharan Africa report a consistent rate of comorbid invasive bacterial infection of 4.4% to 5% with associated case fatality rates of 32%. If there is uncertainty that malaria parasitemia is the sole cause of illness, routine treatment with parenteral antibiotics may be warranted.[14]

Specific Chemotherapy (Table 9-1)

Multiple factors must be considered in the selection of specific antimalarial chemotherapy with the goal of eliminating the parasitemia as rapidly as possible. Many countries have clear national policies for first- and second-line treatment. This may influence drug availability and often reflects the specific drug resistance patterns in specific locations. If such a national

Table 9-1. Drugs for the treatment of malaria[a]

Drug	Adult dose	Pediatric dose	Use in pregnancy	Side effects
Co-Artem (Artemether/ Lumefantrine)	Oral: 80/480 mg@ 0, 8, 24, 36, 48, 60 h	5–15 kg: (20/120) 15–25 kg: (40/240) 25–35 kg: (60/360) >35 kg: (80/480) Same schedule as the adult	US FDA Category C	Palpitations, abdominal pain, anorexia, nausea, asthenia, prolonged QT
Artesunate	IV: 2.4 mg/kg @ 0, 12, 24, 48 h	2.4 mg/kg IV @ 0, 12, 24, 48 h 10 mg/kg PR	Fetal risk cannot be ruled out: weigh risks vs benefits	Bradycardia, rash, pruritus, nausea, vomiting, headache, dizziness
Quinine	Oral: 600 mg q8h for 7–14 days IV: 20 mg/kg loading dose over 4-h infusion. Subsequent dose of 10 mg/kg q8h	IV: 20 mg/kg loading dose followed by 10 mg/kg q12h	US FDA Category C; may cause uterine contractions	Cinchonism, tinnitus, deafness, dizziness, nausea, vomiting, hypoglycemia, hypotension, thrombocytopenia, rash
Malarone (Atovaquone/ Proguanil)	Oral: 1000/400 mg daily for 3 d	5–8 kg: (125/50) 9–10 kg: (187.5/75) 11–20 kg: (250/100) 21–30 kg: (500/200) 31–40 kg: (750/300) >40 kg: (1000/400) Daily for 3 d	US FDA Category C	Well tolerated: abdominal pain, nausea, elevated liver function test, headache, cough
Chloroquine base and amodiaquine	Oral: 600 mg @ 0 h, then 300 mg @ 6, 24, 48 h	Oral: 10 mg/kg (max 600 mg) @ 0 h, then 5 mg/kg (max 300 mg) @ 6, 24, 36 h	US FDA Category C; compatible with breastfeeding; infant risk is minimal	Nausea, vomiting, headache, hypotension, itching
Mefloquine	Oral: 1250-mg single dose	Oral: 10–12.5 mg/kg at 0 h and 6–8 h	FDA Category B	Abdominal pain, vomiting, sleep disturbance
Fansidar (Sulfadoxine/ Pyrimethamine)	Oral: 3 × (500/25 mg tablet) single dose	Oral: 5–10 kg 0.5 tab 11–20 kg: 1 tab 21–30 kg: 1.5 tabs 31–45 kg: 2 tabs >45 kg 3 tabs	FDA Category C; widely used for IPT-Pregnancy	Sulfonamide-associated rashes, photosensitivity

FDA, Food and Drug Administration; IV, intravenous.
[a]Dosages expressed as total number milligrams per dose.

policy exists, it should be followed. In general, uncomplicated malaria may be treated with oral preparations. Complicated *P. falciparum* malaria requires parenteral therapy until there is clinical improvement and the patient can take oral medications.

Artemisinin Combinations

Artemisinin and the more potent dihydroartemisinin are derived from the plant *Artemisia annua*, a Chinese herbal remedy used for millennia to treat fevers. They form three active antimalarial components: Artesunate, Artemether, and Artemotil, which are all converted *in vivo* back to dihydroartemisinin. These drugs may be used for chloroquine-resistant or multidrug-resistant *P. falciparum* and both severe and uncomplicated disease. Artemisinin-based medications result in the fastest clearance of parasites from the blood and are as effective, less toxic, and more convenient than quinine in severe disease. No human toxicity has been reported in the clinical use of artemisinin-based medications.

Due to the widespread development of various drug-resistant species of malaria and a high rate of recrudescence when used alone, artemisinins should be used in combination with other drugs. These combinations are known as artemisinin-based combination treatments (ACTs). This is a similar approach to the now standard treatments in tuberculosis, leprosy, HIV, and many cancers, and it is intended to delay the development of resistance to this new class of antimalarials. Development of new ACTs is a very active area of clinical research, and artemisinin derivatives have now been combined with most of the alternative antimalarials. Many additional options may be available at the time of publication. Various combinations are being tested by every route of administration, for resource-limited locations, and for special populations, including pregnant women and children. ACTs are now considered first-line therapy for uncomplicated malaria in most countries where malaria is endemic. Although high cost continues to limit access in some areas, the Global Fund Affordable Medicines Facility–malaria (AMF-m) program promises to both reduce the cost of ACTs and reduce the use of artemisinin monotherapies, delaying the development of resistance.

Artemether-lumefantrine (Coartem/Riamet) was the first widely available Artemisinin combination therapy now in widespread use in Africa. The standard adult dose is 4 tablets twice daily for 3 days, taken with food to enhance absorption. See Table 9-1 for the schedule. Often available in patient-friendly blister packs, the dose may be adjusted for children.

Parenteral and rectal artesunate has been well demonstrated to be superior to quinine for the treatment of severe falciparum malaria with a significant reduction in the risk of death. It is now the treatment of choice in low-transmission areas and in the second and third trimesters of pregnancy. Ongoing clinical trials are evaluating its use in African children. Parenteral artesunate is available in the United States in cases where there is known intolerance of or contraindication to the use of quinidine and where it may be rapidly obtained from the Centers for Disease Control and Prevention.[16] Following the acute stage a full course of standard oral therapy should be given.

Quinine

Quinine and its isomer quinidine are equally effective natural alkaloids derived from cinchona bark. Only partially soluble in water, these compounds form salts that may be used to make preparations for either oral administration or injection. In most of the world, quinine remains the first-line treatment for severe *P. falciparum* malaria, especially in areas of chloroquine resistance or where parenteral artesunate is not available.

A common syndrome, called cinchonism, occurs with normal therapeutic dosing. This may include tinnitus, deafness, dizziness, nausea, and vomiting. Administration does not need to be stopped, unless symptoms are severe, because the syndrome will resolve spontaneously. Quinine is cardiotoxic and should not be given as a bolus. Other side effects of treatment may include hypoglycemia, hypotension, thrombocytopenia, or an erythematous rash. Quinine may also stimulate uterine contraction, which may lead to miscarriage in pregnant women. The benefits of treating malaria in pregnancy, however, far outweigh the risks of causing uterine contractions with therapeutic dosing. Once the patient is able to eat and drink, therapy should be changed to oral formulations or alternative first-line drugs.

Atovaquone-Proguanil (Malarone)

Malarone is effective for both prophylaxis and treatment of uncomplicated *P. falciparum* malaria but remains prohibitively expensive as a first-line therapy in developing countries.

Chloroquine

Chloroquine is a synthetic bitter white powder that forms salts with acids. Some available preparations include diphosphates (Aralen, Resochin, Avloclor) and sulphates (Nivaquine). It is an effective schizonticide with some anti inflammatory properties that help reduce some nonspecific symptoms like malaise, headache, and myalgia. Side effects include nausea, vomiting, hypotension, and generalized itching in black-skinned people. It is rarely used now in most areas due to widespread resistance.

Amodiaquine

Amodiaquine has some similarities to both chloroquine and quinine. Side effects, toxicities, and dosing is the same as chloroquine with the addition that agranulocytosis has been associated with its use for prophylaxis. Resistance patterns tend to be similar but not identical to chloroquine.

Mefloquine

Mefloquine is only available as an oral preparation. It is chemically related to quinine but has a long half-life of 21 days. Side effects that occur at rates comparable with other chemoprophylactic drugs include headache, dizziness, and sleep disturbance, including vivid dreams. Vomiting is common. Rare severe toxic neuropsychiatric effects with an incidence between 1/6,500 and 1/10,600 may include seizures or psychosis and are more likely to occur in women.[17] Persons with a history of seizure disorders or mental health illnesses are advised to avoid its use. The US Food and Drug Administration considers mefloquine Pregnancy Category B. It does not appear to impair performance while driving, flying, or diving.

Sulfadoxine-Pyrimethamine (Fansidar)

Fansidar remains a widely used therapy for uncomplicated *P. falciparum* malaria, despite the development of widespread resistance in Southeast Asia and Africa. This is due to the primary benefits of very low-cost and single-dose treatment. As with all antimalaria therapies described here, local resistance patterns and government treatment protocols should be known and adhered to.

The Problem of Relapse

As described earlier, clinical relapse may be caused by the persistence of hypnozoites of the *P. vivax* or *P. ovale* species. Current first-line chemoprophylactic drugs do not prevent this relapse, even if taken correctly. The relapse may be prevented, however, with the use of primaquine, a synthetic white powder and a weak schizonticide with action against both hypnozoites and gametocytes. Side effects include abdominal cramping and hemolysis in those with G6PD deficiency. This indication is referred to as presumptive antirelapse therapy.

Standby Emergency Therapy

Some guidelines, especially those from Europe, do not recommend routine chemoprophylaxis for short-term travelers with a low to moderate risk of malaria.[17]

Rather, it is recommended that these people bring a course of antimalarial treatment for self-administration in the event of an acute febrile illness where immediate medical care is not available. Due to the risk for inaccurate diagnosis and administration of unnecessary medications, plus the potential for severe complications of disease, this approach has not been widely adopted.

Chemoprophylaxis (Table 9-2)

Chemoprophylaxis is routinely recommended for non-immune travelers visiting endemic areas. In addition, pregnant women and patients with sickle cell disease residing within endemic areas should also consider prophylaxis. These medications are taken to prevent the development of clinical symptoms and work by either preventing the development of pre-erythrocytic schizonts in the liver or by directly destroying parasites entering red blood cells. The use of medications for prophylaxis is only part of a comprehensive personal approach to malaria prevention that includes risk assessment, bite avoidance, prompt diagnosis, and treatment. Several medications are available, and recommendations may vary by cost, home country, destination, age, pregnancy, and other risk factors. No agent is 100% effective in the prevention of clinical symptoms, and travelers should maintain access to alternative medications for treatment. Malaria should be considered in travelers that

Table 9-2. Chemoprophylaxis of malaria.

Drug	Adult dose	Pediatric dose (see adult schedule)
Doxycycline	100 mg/d, begin 1–2 d prior to, during, and 4 wk following last exposure	>8 y old: 2 mg/kg/d (max 100 mg)
Mefloquine	250 mg/wk, begin 1–3 wk prior to, during, and 4 wk following last exposure	<45 kg (>6 mo) 5 mg/kg >45kg (>6 mo) 250 mg
Malarone (Atovaquone-Proguanil)	250/100 mg daily 1–2 d prior to, during, and 7 d following last exposure	11–20 kg: (62.5/25) 21–30 kg: (125/50) 31–40 kg: (187.5/75) >40 kg: (250/100)
Chloroquine base	300 mg once weekly, 2 wk prior to, during, and 4 wk following last exposure	5 mg/kg (max 300 mg)
Proguanil	200 mg daily, 1 d prior to, during, and 4 wk following last exposure	<1 y: 25 mg/d 1–4 y: 50 mg/d 5–8 y: 100 mg/d 9–14 y: 150 mg/d >14 yrs: 200 mg/day
Primaquine base (presumptive antirelapse therapy)	30 mg (base)/d for 14 d *G6PD* deficiency: 45 mg base/wk for 6 wk	0.5 mg (base)/kg/d (max 30 mg) for 14 d
Tafenoquine	Not available	Not available

G6PD, glucose-6-phosphate dehydrogenase.

develop a fever after returning home, even if they took prophylaxis. A malaria slide should always be obtained in these patients, even if symptoms suggest another cause.

Doxycycline

Doxycycline is effective against all malaria species and especially useful in areas of chloroquine and mefloquine resistance. Its use is contraindicated in women who are pregnant or breastfeeding as well as in young children. Common side effects that must be considered include photosensitization and yeast infections among women.

Mefloquine

Mefloquine remains the prophylactic drug of choice in many areas chiefly due to the widespread development of chloroquine resistance and relative expense of alternatives. There is considerable experience in the tropics regarding the safety of mefloquine for long-term prophylaxis. Toxic effects and contraindications described earlier should also be considered. Travelers should initiate prophylaxis at least 2 weeks prior to arrival to establish a therapeutic drug level and continue for 4 weeks after leaving a malaria-endemic area. Consideration for initiating prophylaxis 3 weeks prior to departure allows for assessment of tolerability because adverse events occur early in dosing. This also allows sufficient time to select an alternative drug prior to departure.

Atovaquone-Proguanil

The drug combination of atovaquone and proguanil is effective against chloroquine-resistant *P. falciparum*. Also effective against the development of pre-erythrocytic schizonts in the liver, atovaquone-proguanil need only to be taken for 1 week after leaving a malaria-endemic area. Atovaquone-proguanil is the best tolerated drug overall, but cost may restrict its use for some travelers. There are insufficient data (although no theoretical risk) to make recommendations in pregnancy or breastfeeding.

Chloroquine

Due to the widespread development of resistance, the use of chloroquine as a single or combination agent is now limited, and travelers must be aware of resistance patterns at their destination. See the CDC website for the latest recommendations and resistance patterns (wwwnc.cdc.gov/travel/). Due to the potential development of retinal damage with long-term use, prophylaxis should be less than 6 years of continuous use.

Proguanil

Proguanil is used only in prophylaxis against malaria. It is generally, but not always, used in combination with chloroquine. Due to the development of resistance to both chloroquine and proguanil, its use is now limited. Proguanil is considered the safest of all antimalarials, including in pregnancy and young children. Side effects may include heartburn, epigastric pain, and mouth ulcers.

Primaquine

Primaquine is also considered by some country guidelines as a second-line primary prophylactic option. Persons considering the use of primaquine for this indication should be tested for G6PD deficiency due to the risk of severe hemolysis. As with all antimalarial drugs, knowledge of local resistance patterns is imperative to any decision making.

Tafenoquine

Tafenoquine is similar to primaquine and has been shown effective in randomized controlled trials. It may be administered either weekly or monthly and is well tolerated by those with G6PD deficiency. It is not yet available for commercial use.

Intermittent Presumptive Therapy

It has been demonstrated that pregnant women living in endemic areas who are given antimalarial drugs in the second half of pregnancy irrespective of the presence of symptoms or parasites have a decreased incidence of placental malaria and LBW infants. Although no longer recommended as therapy or chemoprophylaxis, the drug combination sulfadoxine-pyrimethamine (Fansidar) may still be used for this purpose. It is generally given as a single oral dose, two or three times in the second and third trimesters. Specific protocols may vary by country and comprise one part of control measures that also include case management and the use of insecticide-treated nets. Studies have also shown intermittent presumptive therapy (IPT) to be an effective control strategy in infants when administered at the time of routine immunizations with resulting reductions in the incidence of clinical malaria, anemia, and hospital admissions.[18]

Seasonal Intermittent Preventive Treatment

A newer approach to the prevention of complications of malaria infection is similar to IPT and involves the completion of a full course of antimalarial medication during seasons of high transmission in endemic countries, regardless of whether or not individuals have a confirmed infection. This approach has been found to be effective in preventing anemia in children and is an accepted alternative to IPT in pregnancy.[19] This approach is most likely to be successful in areas where high-intensity transmission occurs over a short time interval. Considerable study is required to establish this approach as complementary to existing control methods as well as confirm medication options and delivery mechanisms.

Drug Resistance

As we have previously discussed, the development of widespread resistance to specific antimalarial drugs has significantly affected their use in acute treatment, chemoprophylaxis, and targeted control programs. Knowledge of local resistance patterns is vital to both physicians making individual treatment decisions as well as policymakers establishing guidelines for large populations. Drug resistance has been confirmed in only two of the five human malaria parasite species: *P. falciparum* and *P. vivax*. Chloroquine-resistant *P. falciparum* first developed in the late 1950s and early 1960s but was limited to three or four locations in Southeast Asia, Oceania, and South America. It has subsequently spread to all areas of the world where falciparum is transmitted. Although less widespread, *P. falciparum* has also developed resistance to almost all other antimalarial drugs, including sulfadoxine/pyrimethamine, mefloquine, halofantrine, and quinine.

There have been recent reports that *P. falciparum* parasites from French Guyana were highly resistant to artemether, and some have demonstrated diminished *in vitro* sensitivity. In addition, the efficacy of ACTs has apparently decreased along the Thailand-Cambodia border, the epicenter of drug resistance in Southeast Asia.[20] These reports highlight the importance of developing robust strategies for monitoring and deterring the development of resistance to ACTs. Once such project is the Artemisinin-Resistance Containment Project, a joint effort of the WHO and the health ministries of Cambodia and Thailand.

Chloroquine-resistant *P. vivax* malaria was first described in 1989 among Australians living in Papua New Guinea. It is now well established in Southeast Asia, India, and South America. In Oceania, vivax malaria is also less susceptible to primaquine.

Some specific strategies to curtail the development and spread of resistance to current and new antimalarials include an array of electronic surveillance and survey tools. Monitoring resistance patterns in areas of intense transmission includes tests of therapeutic efficacy, *in vitro* testing, and drug-specific molecular markers for *P. falciparum* resistance. Preventing the development of resistance is also an important component of national treatment guidelines and drug manufacturing quality control initiatives. An outline of many of these programs is available from the WHO at www.who.int/drugresistance/malaria.

ECONOMIC AND SOCIOLOGICAL IMPACT

Malaria takes a high toll on households and health care systems, and it impedes economic development in endemic countries. It is estimated that malaria reduces gross domestic product (GDP) growth by approximately 1.3% per year in some African countries.[21] The WHO also estimates that malaria can decrease the GDP of some high-burden countries by over 1%. This disease disproportionately affects poor and marginalized people who cannot afford treatment or have limited access to health care.[22] Malaria also discourages foreign investment, increases people's out-of-pocket spending on health care, and impairs children's ability to learn, particularly those who survive severe illness.[21] The startling statistic of one child death every minute (in sub-Saharan Africa) clearly has broad-reaching daily economic, social, and psychological impact in these areas.

GLOBAL MALARIA ERADICATION

As a historical example, in the United States, elimination programs began in 1947. Prior to that, the US Public Health Service and Tennessee Valley Authority worked at malaria control programs in endemic regions. The 1947 campaign successfully ended in 1951 when malaria transmission was eliminated within the boundaries of the United States. Eradication efforts in the world varied throughout 1955 to 1978 with several successes but many failures, mostly in sub-Saharan Africa, and gave rise to the growth of drug-resistant malaria. Goals for these programs transitioned from eradication to reduction of the number of malaria-related cases and deaths, and reduction of malaria transmission. In the past 15 years, there have been increases and a renewed commitment to again pursue the possibility of malaria elimination and perhaps eradication in many areas. In 2010, 91 of the 106 malaria-endemic countries still had transmission. In 2010, Armenia was the most recent state to be declared malaria free.

The Rollback Malaria Program (RBM), initiated in 1998, via the strategic partnership of the WHO, UN Children's Fund, UN Development Program, and the World Bank, is currently the leader in initiating the global framework for malaria control and eradication. The secretary-general and executive director of RBM are housed in Geneva at the WHO headquarters. RBM is in the center of multiple necessary partners in order to coordinate all efforts at combating malaria and maximize the impact of the limited finances committed to Malaria (Figure 9-3).

The Global Fund, the largest single source of funding for malaria control, was founded in 2002 to combat the three most dangerous infectious diseases identified in our modern world: malaria, HIV/AIDS, and tuberculosis. Just over 50% of all financing for malaria control has come from The Global Fund since 2009. Total investment in malaria control is estimated

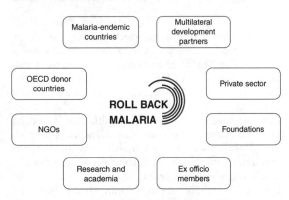

Figure 9-3. World Health Organization Roll Back Malaria constituents. NGO, nongovernmental organization; OECD, Organization for Economic Co-operation and Development. http://www.rollbackmalaria.org/mechanisms/constituencies.html.

to be peaking in the year 2011 at US$2 billion per year. There is some indication by trends that this total amount will begin to recede slightly in the next several years for various economic reasons. The remaining 49% of global funding for malaria control in 2010 primarily came from the Department for International Development in the United Kingdom, the President's Malaria Initiative in the United States, and the World Bank along with other assorted donors. The President's Malaria Initiative (PMI: started in 2005 by President Bush) contributions rose from $385 million in 2009 to $585 million in 2010. The World Bank Malaria Report notes there has been over US$1 trillion spent from the World Bank on malaria in the years 2000 to 2011.

The international development community has agreed to the global malaria action plan (GMAP). The 2015 targets of the GMAP include:

1. Reducing global preventable malaria deaths to near zero
2. Reducing global malaria deaths from 2000 levels by 75%
3. Reducing global malaria cases from 2000 levels by 75%
4. Meeting the Millennium Development Goal 6: To halt and begin to reverse the incidence of malaria and other major diseases
5. Eliminate malaria in 8 to 10 countries, either in pre-elimination phase or not.

The operational aspects of these targets include individual protection against mosquito bites and a reduction in intensity of local transmission of malaria.

The two interventions that are most powerful and have been most broadly applied are long-lasting insecticidal nets, or LLINs, and indoor residual spraying, or IRS. Insecticide-treated nets, or ITNs, include both LLINs and conventional netting later treated with insecticides. These nets (LLINs are preferred) have been recommended by the WHO since 2007 and seem to provide the greatest coverage for the least cost. IRS is the application of residual insecticides to the inside surfaces of dwellings or other household areas where mosquitoes tend to rest after a blood meal. Both of these methods work by decreasing the mosquito population and decreasing contact of the mosquitoes with humans. Larval control is another method used in certain areas where insecticides are added to standing water to kill larval stage mosquitoes. IRS and larval control must be carefully monitored because there is always the possibility of insecticide resistance. For example, some pyrethroid resistance has been seen in several areas of Africa. Each insecticide campaign should include efforts to monitor effectiveness of the chemical being used, vary these chemicals over time, and ensure that resistance in not emerging. Low-cost or free ITNs have been a significant part of the malaria control efforts over the past 5 years and are estimated to be available to 80% of the malaria-vulnerable populations.[23]

Appropriate diagnosis and treatment of malaria is also a critical portion of the plan to eradicate malaria. The first step should always be a prompt parasitologic confirmation of disease either by microscope or RDT. The most accurate treatment can then be applied in an attempt to avoid overuse of antimalarial medicines or improper use of medicine versus resistant or nonresistant types of malaria. The more recent notion of IPT has the promise to reduce malaria burden in certain target populations. This method has especially been used in pregnancy (known as IPTp) and has also been suggested for infants (IPTi). The intermittent preventive treatment protocols vary slightly but usually contain a complete therapeutic course for active malarial infection. They are taken in prevention, prior to any signs or symptoms of active infection.

All of these methods coordinated together and applied properly will limit resistance to medicine or insecticide use. Together, they have the possibility of greatly reducing malaria and potentially meeting the 2015 goals. One must always keep the economics of the strategies in mind because the total cost for these interventions as noted on the RBM GMAP (global malaria action plan) will average US$5.9 billion per year from 2011 through 2020. If the GMAP is successful, the cost after 2020 may decrease and is estimated to be somewhere in the neighborhood of US$3.3 billion[24] (Figure 9-4).

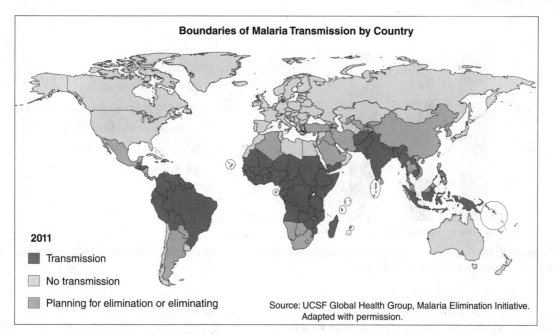

Figure 9-4. Boundaries of malaria transmission by country; 2011. Bardi JS. University of California. Malaria Elimination Maps Highlight Progress, Prospects.

Individual Precautions

Each year more than 125 million international travelers visit the 100 or more malaria-risk countries and regions. Thousands of visitors become ill after returning home. All nonimmune travelers when exposed to mosquito bites especially between dawn and dusk have a significant risk of developing malaria. The most at-risk travelers are children, pregnant women, and those who have lost any previous immunity by living away from endemic areas for more than 6 months. The WHO has an ABCD mnemonic to help travelers and advisers remember the basics of malaria protection.[25]

Awareness of risk, primary symptoms of malaria, the incubation period, and the possibility of delayed onset, is essential.

Bite avoidance of any insect but especially mosquitoes between dawn and dusk is critical.

Chemoprophylaxis with appropriate antimalarial drugs to prevent infection from developing into clinical disease.

Diagnosis and appropriate treatment for a fever that develops 1 week or more after entering an at-risk area and for 3 months after departure from that area are all-important.

In all cases, travelers should try to avoid mosquito bites by wearing appropriate clothing, using insecticide-treated bed nets, personal insect repellent,

and minimizing nighttime exposure. Depending on the length of exposure and the remoteness of destination, some individuals may consider bringing a course of standby emergency treatment. Pregnant women, children, and immune-suppressed travelers should consider carefully any travel into a region at risk for malaria transmission. They should consider carefully the necessity of the travel compared with the risks involved.

Vaccine Development Initiatives

Vaccine development has been difficult given the biology of malaria and the various lifecycle members each having genetically distinct strains. There are multiple scientific challenges to try to produce long-term immunity at a high level. The Malaria Vaccine Initiative, founded by the Gates Foundation to organize and push forward the development of malaria vaccines, identifies around 63 groups of scientists working on various aspects of vaccine development. Currently 41 of these efforts are in preclinical or clinical trials (Figure 9-5). The consensus goals in international development are to have a vaccine that is 50% effective by 2015 and eventually to have an 80% effective vaccine with longer term immunity by 2025.[26]

The RTS, S/AS01 vaccine is the only current vaccine in phase 3 clinical trials. Results have been promising, especially in the 5- to 17-month age category of

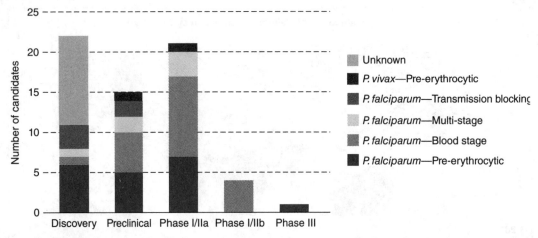

Figure 9-5. The progress of vaccine development. PATH Malaria Vaccine Initiative. http://www.malariavaccine.org/ images/globalmalariavaccineportfolio.jpg.

children, who seem to have a 50% reduction in the incidence of malaria in the first 12 months. Several initial concerns were a lack of reduction in death rate from malaria and a relatively significant rate of generalized seizures in the first week after administration of the vaccine.[27] There will be quite a bit more information and learning in this area in the years to come (Figure 9-5).

STUDY QUESTIONS

1. Why are local transmission patterns important in the development of partial immunity?

2. What factors affect the development of drug and insecticide resistance?

3. What are the primary obstacles to global malaria eradication as a major public health concern?

4. What global control strategies currently show promise for reducing morbidity and mortality in children younger than 5 years?

5. Describe the recent history of malaria worldwide with emphasis on the development of resistance and emerging human disease by species of *Plasmodia*.

REFERENCES

1. Mandell GL, Bennett JE, Dolin R. *Principles and Practice of Infectious Diseases.* 7th ed. Philadelphia: Elsevier, 2009: 3437–44.

2. World Health Organization. Q&A on Malaria, Mortality Estimates 2012. http://www.who.int/malaria/world_malaria_report_2011/WHOGMP_burden_estimates_qa.pdf.

3. The World Bank. Millennium Development Goals. Combat HIV/AIDS, Malaria and Other Diseases by 2015. http://www.worldbank.org/mdgs/diseases.html.

4. World Health Organization. World Malaria Report 2011, Fact Sheet. http://www.who.int/malaria/world_malaria_report_2011/WMR2011_factsheet.pdf.

5. Lalloo D, Molyneux M. Malaria. In: Gill G, Beeching N, eds. *Lecture Notes on Tropical Medicine.* 5th ed. Malden, MA: Blackwell Science, 2004:57.

6. Daneshvar C, Davis TM, Cox-Singh J. Clinical and laboratory features of human *Plasmodium knowlesi* infection. *Clin Infect Dis* 2009;49(6):852–860.

7. Koram KA, Molyneux ME. When is "malaria" malaria? The different burdens of malaria infection, malaria disease, and malaria-like illnesses. *Am J Trop Med Hyg* 2007;77(6):1–5.

8. World Health Organization. Malaria in pregnancy. http://www.who.int/malaria/high_risk_groups/pregnancy/en/index.html.

9. World Health Organization. Fact files: Pregnant women are particularly at risk of malaria. http://www.who.int/features/factfiles/malaria/malaria_facts/en/index8.html.

10. Warren, Kenneth S, Mahmoud, Adel AF. *Tropical and Geographical Medicine.* New York: McGraw-Hill, 1984:256.

11. McAuley CF, Webb C, Makani J, et al. High mortality from *Plasmodium falciparum* malaria in children living with sickle cell anemia on the coast of Kenya. *Blood* 2010;116(10):1663.

12. Guilbride DL, Guilbride PD, Gawlinski P. Malaria's deadly secret: a skin stage. *Trends Parasitol* 2012;28(4):142–150.

13. Taylor SM, Molyneux ME, Simel DL. Does this patient have malaria? *JAMA* 2010;304(18):2048–2056.

14. Gwer S, Newton C, Berkley JA. Over-diagnosis and co-morbidity of severe malaria in African children: a guide for clinicians. *Am J Trop Med Hyg* 2007;77(6):6–13.

15. Abba K, Deeks JJ, Olliaro P, et al. Rapid diagnostic tests for diagnosing uncomplicated *P. falciparum* malaria in endemic countries. *Cochrane Database Syst Rev* 2011:CD008122.

16. Rosenthal PJ. Artesunate for the treatment of severe falciparum malaria. *N Engl J Med* 2008;358:1829–1836.

17. Freedman DO. Malaria prevention in short-term travelers. *N Engl J Med* 2008;359:603–612.

18. Ponte JJ, Schellenberg D, Egan A. Efficacy and safety of intermittent preventive treatment with sulfadoxine-pyri-

methamine for malaria in African infants. *Lancet* 2009;374: 1533–1542.

19. Greenwood B: Review. Intermittent preventive treatment—a new approach to the prevention of malaria in children in areas with seasonal malaria transmission. *Trop Med Int Health* 2006;11(7):983–991.

20. Nosten F, White NJ. Artemisinin-based combination treatment of falciparum malaria. *Am J Trop Med Hyg* 2007;77(6):181–192.

21. The World Bank. Malaria Overview 2012. http://web.worldbank.org/WBSITE/EXTERNAL/TOPICS/EXTHEALTHNUTRITIONANDPOPULATION/EXTPH/0,,contentMDK:22792430~pagePK:148956~piPK:216618~theSitePK:376663,00.html.

22. World Health Organization. Fact Files: Malaria causes significant economic losses in high-burden countries. http://www.who.int/features/factfiles/malaria/malaria_facts/en/index9.html.

23. World Health Organization. World Malaria Report 2011. http://www.who.int/malaria/world_malaria_report_2011/en/.

24. Roll Back Malaria, Part II. The Global Strategy. http://www.rbm.who.int/gmap/2-5.html.

25. World Health Organization. International Travel and Health. Geneva: WHO Press, 2012:148.

26. Path-Malaria Vaccine Initiative. Accelerating Malaria Vaccine Development. http://www.malariavaccine.org/malvac-state-of-vaccine-dev.php.

27. RTS,S Clinical Trials Partnership. First results of phase 3 trial of RTS, S/AS01 malaria vaccine in African children. *N Engl J Med* 2011; 365:1863–1875. http://www.nejm.org/doi/full/10.1056/NEJMoa1102287.

FURTHER READING

Gill G, Beeching N, eds. *Lecture Notes on Tropical Medicine.* 5th ed. Malden, MA: Blackwell Science, 2004.

US Centers for Disease Control and Prevention. Malaria 2012. http://www.cdc.gov/malaria/index.html.

World Health Organization. Guidelines for Treatment of Malaria. 2nd ed., 2010. http://www.who.int/malaria/publications/atoz/9789241547925/en/index.html.

World Health Organization. Malaria 2012. http://www.who.int/malaria/en/.

Tuberculosis and HIV/AIDS

10

Lisa V. Adams and Godfrey B. Woelk

LEARNING OBJECTIVES

- *Describe the global epidemiology of tuberculosis and HIV/AIDS*
- *Understand how tuberculosis is transmitted, diagnosed, and treated*
- *List the components of the DOTS strategy, the Stop TB Strategy, and the Global Plan to Stop TB*
- *Discuss the current challenges to controlling tuberculosis in resource-limited settings and the recent advances in diagnosis, treatment, and prevention of tuberculosis*
- *Describe the history, pathogenesis, diagnosis, and transmission of HIV/AIDS*
- *Describe the treatment of HIV/AIDS including the prevention and management of opportunistic infections*
- *Outline the policy and operational issues on treatment rollout, with particular reference to low- and middle-income countries*
- *Discuss HIV/AIDS prevention strategies and their potential effectiveness and limitations at different stages of the epidemic*
- *Know where to find additional resources for both tuberculosis and HIV/AIDS*

INTRODUCTION

Tuberculosis (TB) and human immunodeficiency virus/acquired immunodeficiency syndrome (HIV/AIDS)—one a scourge nearly as old as humankind itself and the other a disease that emerged only 3 decades ago—are responsible for a significant burden of today's global morbidity and mortality. When occurring separately, each is a challenge to cure or treat, but when occurring together they constitute a deadly pair. In many parts of the world, especially in many resource-limited settings, they are inextricably linked and have required a joint health sector programmatic response. Because of the large overlap that exists between both epidemics in the poorest parts of the globe, these diseases have been grouped in a single chapter. TB and HIV/AIDS are considered first separately and then together in this chapter.

Global Epidemiology of Tuberculosis

TB is ubiquitous. Approximately a third of the world's population—more than 2 billion people—is infected with *Mycobacterium tuberculosis* (MTB). Under ordinary circumstances, about 10% of people infected with MTB develop active TB disease during their lifetime. The World Health Organization (WHO) estimates there were 8.8 million new cases of TB in 2010, with roughly 65% of these cases reported to public health programs and the WHO.[1] In the same year there were an estimated 1.5 million deaths due to TB (roughly a quarter of which were HIV-associated), making it the leading cause of death from a curable infectious disease.[1,2]

The vast majority of TB patients—over 80%—live in just 22 countries in the world. The list of 22 high-TB burden countries is dominated by the resource-limited countries of sub-Saharan Africa and Asia (Table 10-1) with India and China accounting for 40% of the notified cases in 2010. Strengthened TB control efforts and international investments have paid off. The absolute number of TB cases and TB incidence rates have been falling for at least the last 5 years (Figure 10-1).[1] In the 2 decades between 1990 and 2010, significant decreases in global prevalence and mortality rates were observed. With approximately 75% of TB cases in resource-limited countries occurring among those in their most economically productive years (between the ages of 15 and 54), the

Table 10-1. Countries with a high burden
of tuberculosis.

1. India
2. China
3. Indonesia
4. Pakistan
5. Bangladesh
6. Philippines
7. South Africa
8. Democratic Republic of Congo
9. Ethiopia
10. Nigeria
11. Vietnam
12. Myanmar
13. Russian Federation
14. Thailand
15. Afghanistan
16. Kenya
17. Mozambique
18. Cambodia
19. Brazil
20. United Republic of Tanzania
21. Uganda
22. Zimbabwe

Data from World Health Organization. Global Tuberculosis
Control 2011. Geneva: WHO, 2011. WHO/HTM/TB/2011.16.
(*Reproduced with permission.*)

human and economic toll on these countries has been
devastating.

The persistence of TB through the years is multifactorial, with key factors being a history of neglect
by governments and poorly managed TB control programs, poverty, population growth, and migration.
In the last 3 decades, the HIV epidemic has contributed to the rising number of TB cases in sub-Saharan
Africa. HIV is a significant risk factor that increases
the likelihood of progression from TB infection to
disease from 10% over a lifetime to 10% each year.
TB is the leading cause of death among HIV-infected
individuals, accounting for about a quarter of AIDS
deaths worldwide. In some of the worst affected
countries in sub-Saharan Africa, over 70% of patients
with acid-fast bacilli (AFB) smear-positive pulmonary
TB are also infected with HIV.[1]

The emergence of significant levels of multidrug-
resistant TB in some parts of the world has also hampered global efforts to control TB. Strains of TB that
are resistant to standard (first-line) anti-TB medications have been documented in every country; however,
certain hot spots in Asia and Eastern Europe harbor
the greatest burden of drug-resistant TB. Confirming
our worst fears, the emergence of TB strains resistant to nearly all anti-TB drugs, termed extensively

drug-resistant TB (XDR-TB), has been reported in
83% of the countries that have tested for it.[3,4]

Global Epidemiology of HIV/AIDS

The global epidemiology of HIV infection is not so
different from that of TB. Recurring themes include
the heavy case burden borne by sub-Saharan Africa
and the relationships between HIV infection and
poverty, prior lack of access to effective prevention
strategies and treatments, and the fact that HIV is
also killing those in their most productive years, in
many cases wiping out generations in the hardest hit
countries.

About 34 million (31.4 to 35.9 million) people were
living with HIV in 2011, more than ever before due
to the effects of antiretroviral therapy, which prolongs
life. AIDS resulted in the deaths of about 1.7 million
(1.5 to 1.9 million) in 2011, and an additional 2.5
(2.2 to 2.8 million) people were newly infected in
the same year.[5] Sub-Saharan Africa remains the worst
affected area, with approximately 23.5 million HIV-
infected inhabitants, roughly two-thirds of the total
global burden.[5] However, the numbers of people
infected with HIV in Eastern Europe and Central and
East Asia have also grown in the past few years. The
proportion of HIV-infected adults who are women
continues to increase, reaching 50% globally and
58% in sub-Saharan Africa.[5]

Heterosexual sex is the primary means of HIV transmission worldwide, although in some regions injection
drug use (often combined with an exchange of sex for
drugs) is still a major route of transmission. Efforts to
control HIV/AIDS were originally focused on preventing new infections, but in the past decade they have
included the scale-up of care and treatment programs
to provide life-prolonging antiretroviral therapy.

TUBERCULOSIS

Pathogenesis of Tuberculosis

TB is caused by the bacterium *Mycobacterium tuberculosis. M. bovis, M. caprae, M. africanum, M. microti,
M. pinnipedii,* and *M. canettii* are very similar genetically to MTB, and together they comprise the MTB
complex.[6] Although any of the MTB complex organisms may cause TB, MTB is the most common,
especially in the tropics. MTB is an obligate aerobic,
non-spore-forming, nonmotile bacillus with large
lipid content in its cell wall. MTB grows slowly, with
a generation time of approximately 15 to 20 hours as
compared with less than 1 hour for most common
bacteria. MTB bacilli are referred to as AFB because
of the ability of their lipid-rich cell walls to retain
red carbolfuchsin stain even after decolorization with

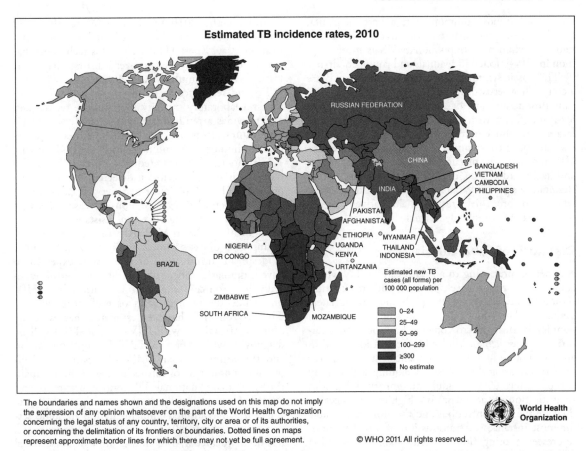

Figure 10-1. Distribution of tuberculosis in the world in 2010. *Source:* Data from World Health Organization. Global Tuberculosis Control 2011. Geneva: WHO, 2011. WHO/HTM/TB/2011.16.

acid and alcohol during the Ziehl-Neelsen staining procedure.

MTB is transmitted when a person with active TB coughs, sneezes, or talks and expels MTB bacilli into the air. These respiratory secretions contain droplet nuclei that become aerosolized and can linger in a contained airspace for up to 8 hours. Droplet nuclei are tiny, generally only 5 μm to 10 μm in diameter, which allows them to be transported to the terminal air spaces when inhaled. Once deposited in the terminal air sacs, the MTB bacilli are taken up by alveolar macrophages. Through hematogenous or lymphatic spread or by direct extension, MTB bacteria may spread to virtually any organ in the body. In most cases, the bacteria are "walled off" by macrophages and other cells that contain the infection through granuloma formation. In some cases, particularly in children, initial infection with MTB can result in primary disease that has the hallmarks of hilar or mediastinal lymphadenopathy with or without a visible

opacity, the "primary lesion," in the lung. If successfully contained, the MTB will continue to grow very slowly over the person's lifetime. This scenario is latent TB infection. Left untreated, MTB will stay dormant and never cause active disease in 90% of people who are otherwise healthy. If a person is HIV infected, this risk of developing active TB increases from a 10% lifetime risk to a 10% annual risk.

If the person's immune system is not able to contain the MTB infection, the bacteria begin to multiply more rapidly, and the person will develop active TB. In addition to HIV infection, poor nutrition, diabetes mellitus, chronic renal failure, and certain medications (e.g., steroids) can result in varying degrees of immune suppression that will increase the likelihood of progression from latent TB infection to active TB disease. Pulmonary TB is the most common form of the disease, accounting for over 80% of cases (in populations without large numbers of HIV-infected individuals). Extrapulmonary TB can affect any organ other than the lungs, but most commonly affected are the pleura, lymph nodes, spine, genitourinary tract, nervous system, or abdomen. Extrapulmonary TB is more common in HIV-infected individuals and young children.

The classic symptoms of active pulmonary TB are a cough that persists for more than 2 weeks with sputum production and occasional hemoptysis, weight loss, and fevers with night sweats. Chest pain and fatigue are also commonly seen. Fever and weight loss are more common in TB patients who are also HIV-infected. On physical examination, weight loss and tachycardia (due to the fever) may be noted. Respiratory signs are variable and may include crackles, wheezes, or bronchial breathing; alternatively, breath sounds may be completely normal.

Diagnosis of Tuberculosis

Any person presenting to a health care facility with a cough for 2 or more weeks in a TB-endemic country should be suspected of having TB and appropriately evaluated. The patient should submit three sputum samples for smear microscopy (and mycobacterial culture where available). Under ideal conditions (and in areas without a high HIV prevalence), sputum smear microscopy using Ziehl-Neelsen staining will identify approximately 65% of adult pulmonary TB cases.[7] Identification of these cases is a high priority because they are the most infectious and therefore responsible for most instances of transmission of TB. Immunofluorescence using fluorochrome stain is becoming widely available and is the preferred smear microscopy method. MTB can be identified more quickly using this method because smears can be scanned under a lower magnification. Results of smear microscopy, regardless of the stain used, are recorded based on the number of TB bacilli observed on the slide, which reflects the severity of the disease and the infectiousness of the patient.

Laboratory culture of MTB, considered the gold standard or definitive test for MTB disease, can require up to 8 to 12 weeks using standard culture technique (e.g., solid media with Lowenstein-Jensen media) for MTB growth to be detected. Liquid media using automated equipment such as the BACTEC system (Beckton Dickinson, Sparks, MD) can detect MTB growth as early as 2 to 3 weeks after inoculation, but its expense has limited its availability in resource-limited settings. Because of the lag time to obtain results, mycobacterial culture is not helpful in making rapid individual diagnoses but can be useful in detecting paucibacillary disease in HIV-infected individuals. Although access to mycobacterial culture is increasing in TB-endemic countries, it is rarely available at laboratories outside of academic centers or the country's national reference center(s).

In December 2010, the WHO endorsed the use of a new automated cartridge-based nucleic acid amplification assay, Xpert MTB/RIF.[8] This technology has several distinct advantages over existing diagnostic tests. The assay simultaneously detects the presence of MTB and resistance to rifampin, requires less training and laboratory capacity than culture techniques, and provides a result much more quickly—in about 90 minutes versus weeks to months with current culture technology. A multi-country study involving 1,730 patients demonstrated that Xpert MTB/RIF is both sensitive and specific; it detected 98% of smear-positive and 73% of smear-negative TB cases, and it correctly identified 99% of non-TB cases.[9] Its performance in detecting rifampin resistance is equally strong, with the Xpert MTB/RIF assay correctly identifying 98% of cases with rifampin-resistant bacteria.[9] Widespread introduction of this test is expected to have a dramatic impact on TB disease control, especially in resource-limited settings with a high HIV prevalence and/or high rates of multidrug resistant TB (MDR-TB). It has been estimated that twice the number of patients with HIV-associated TB will be diagnosed with Xpert MTB/RIF implementation, and three-times as many MDR-TB patients.[8] Rollout and monitoring of this technology is now a main thrust of many national TB control programs and WHO. Cost (especially of the cartridges which are single use) has limited implementation in some settings but as of mid-2012, more than 700 instruments had been procured in 67 countries through concessional pricing.[10]

Chest radiography is often used to aid in the diagnosis of pulmonary TB when none or only one of the sputum smears examined is positive for AFB or to evaluate concomitant lung pathology in a patient with extrapulmonary TB. Chest x-rays are more helpful in diagnosing TB in children, who, due to their paucibacillary disease and insufficient tussive force for producing sputum, usually have AFB-negative sputum smears. In adults, a chest x-ray may show one or more infiltrates, particularly in the upper lung lobes, with or without cavitation, fibrosis, or retraction. However, no radiographic findings are absolutely diagnostic of pulmonary TB, and even a normal chest x-ray cannot rule out the diagnosis. This is especially true in HIV-infected individuals, where the chest x-ray appearance is often atypical (e.g., normal) in those with severe immunocompromise.

The tuberculin skin test (TST, also referred to as the PPD test because it is composed of purified protein derivative) is rarely used to diagnose TB in adults in resource-limited settings. The TST has both poor sensitivity and specificity for active TB disease (the TST has been shown to be negative in up to 25% of patients with culture-confirmed TB), and its interpretation is complicated in areas where HIV infection is prevalent (increasing the potential for false negative results) and where Bacille Calmette-Guérin (BCG) vaccine is used (increasing the potential for false positive results).

Published data on two commercial ex vivo interferon-gamma release assays (IGRAs)—the T.SPOT. *TB* (Oxford Immunotec) and QuantiFERON-TB Gold In-Tube (Cellestis/Qiagen)—suggest that these rapid tests have a higher specificity than TST for detecting TB.[11,12] These tests detect T-cell responses to two MTB-specific antigens (ESAT-6 and CFP-10) and therefore, unlike the TST, they are not subject to false-positive results in BCG-vaccinated persons. Both tests require only a single blood draw for specimen collection. Evaluation of these tests has focused on their use in detecting latent infection rather than TB disease. The current US recommendation is that IGRAs can be used in place of TST in all situations but that IGRAs are preferred in persons who have been BCG vaccinated or who are in groups that historically have low rates of return for TST reading (e.g., homeless persons). The tuberculin skin test is preferred in young children because of the lack of consistent IGRA use data in this population. For all other groups, there is no preference. Their use is currently limited in the field setting by the need for relatively rapid specimen transport to a laboratory with the appropriate equipment and a trained technician. In addition, their current market-value costs are prohibitive for resource-limited countries.

In the absence of typical laboratory and radiographic findings, a small portion of patients will be diagnosed on the basis of the treating physician's clinical judgment.

Extrapulmonary TB, representing approximately 20% of all TB cases, presents a greater diagnostic challenge. Without the benefit of the standard sputum smear test for AFB and because of the limited availability of mycobacterial culture, the initial diagnosis is often presumptive, based on clinical findings, and confirmed retrospectively by a positive response to anti-TB treatment. Where available, diagnosis may also rely on the results of specialized diagnostic tools such as ultrasound, biopsy, or aspiration. If extrapulmonary TB is suspected or confirmed, the patient should also be evaluated for pulmonary TB. Children younger than 2 years are at risk for developing serious disseminated forms of TB, specifically miliary or disseminated TB or TB meningitis.

Treatment of Tuberculosis

Treatment of TB requires a multidrug regimen for at least 6 months. When taken without interruption, the standard regimen using first-line drugs will cure over 90% of patients with drug-susceptible TB. TB treatment is divided into two phases: the 2-month initial phase, when rapid bacterial killing occurs, and the 4-month continuation phase, when further sterilizing activity occurs. The two most effective drugs against TB in our arsenal are isoniazid and rifampin. Both bactericidal agents, they are used throughout TB treatment. Pyrazinamide, also bactericidal, is only active in an acid environment and therefore only effective during the 2-month initial phase of therapy. A fourth agent, ethambutol, is added to the regimen to prevent the emergence of drug resistance should the primary strain have underlying resistance to any of the other three drugs used.

Treatment regimens based on patient characteristics have been standardized by the WHO (Table 10-2). Different regimens are used for patients suspected of having drug-resistant TB (see "The Problem of Drug Resistance," later in this chapter). In general, adults and children, regardless of their HIV status, are treated similarly. Whenever possible, fixed-dose combination tablets should be administered because their use will facilitate correct prescribing and patient adherence and simplify drug ordering and stock control. Anti-TB drugs can be obtained by countries at low or no cost from the Global Drug Facility, a program administered by the Stop TB Partnership in Geneva. A 6-month course of anti-TB therapy costs as little as US $30.

Monitoring patients on therapy to ensure a therapeutic response is achieved is crucial. Patients with positive AFB-sputum smears or mycobacterial cultures should have follow-up sputum smears and cultures examined after the initial phase of therapy and again toward and at the end of therapy. New monitoring recommendations for patients who have a positive Xpert MTB/RIF test are being developed but will likely include similar follow-up.

The Role of Bacille Calmette-Guérin Vaccine

The BCG vaccine, a live bacterial vaccine first used in 1921, is currently given to about 100 million children each year.[13] Determination of its efficacy in preventing various forms of TB has yielded variable and inconsistent results. In a meta-analysis of efficacy studies, BCG vaccine was found to have an overall 51% protective effect against all forms of TB, a 64% protective effect against TB meningitis, and a 78% protective effect against disseminated TB.[14] However, this analysis did not exclude studies with "mycobacteria-experienced" patients (i.e., patients who have or may have had prior mycobacterial infection). In mycobacteria-naïve patients (i.e., those without prior mycobacterial infection, such as newborns), BCG efficacy is much higher, at 80%.[15]

Table 10-2. Tuberculosis treatment regimens.

Standard Regimens for New TB Patients	Intensive Phase Treatment	Continuation Phase
New patients with presumed, or known, to have drug-susceptible TB	2 months of HRZE[a]	4 months of HR
New patients in settings where the level of isoniazid resistance among new TB cases is high and isoniazid susceptibility testing is not done (or results are not available) before the continuation phase begins	2 months of HRZE[a]	4 months of HRE

[a]WHO no longer recommends omission of ethambutol during the intensive phase of treatment for patients with non-cavitary, smear-negative pulmonary or extrapulmonary TB who are known to be HIV-negative. In tuberculous meningitis, ethambutol should be replaced by streptomycin.

H = isoniazid, R = rifampicin, Z = pyrazinamide, E = ethambutol, S = streptomycin.

Daily dosing during both the intensive and continuation phases is considered optimal but three times weekly during the continuation phase is an acceptable alternative for any new TB patient receiving directly observed therapy. Three times per week therapy during both the intensive and continuation phases is an acceptable alternative if the patient is receiving directly observed therapy and is not living with HIV or living in an HIV-prevalent setting.

Standard Regimens for Previously Treated Patients (depending on the availability of routine drug susceptibility testing (DST) to guide the therapy of individual retreatment patients)

DST	Likelihood of MDR (patient registration group[a])	
Routinely available for previously treated patients	High (failure[b])	Medium or low (relapse, default)
Rapid molecular-based method	DST results available in 1–2 days confirm or exclude MDR to guide the choice of regimen	
Conventional method	While awaiting DST results[c]: Empirical MDR regimen *Regimen should be modified once DST results are available.*	2HRZES/HRZE/5HRE *Regimen should be modified once DST results are available.*
None (interim)	Empirical MDR regimen *Regimen should be modified once DST results or DRS data[d] are available.*	2HRZES/HRZE/5HRE for full course of treatment. *Regimen should be modified once DST results or DRS data are available.*

[a]The assumption that failure patients have a high likelihood of multidrug resistance (MDR) (and relapse or defaulting patients a medium likelihood) may need to be modified according to the level of MDR in these patient registration groups.
[b]And other patients in groups with high levels of MDR. One example is patients who develop active TB after known contact with a patient with documented MDR-TB. Patients who are relapsing or returning after defaulting from their second or subsequent course of treatment probably also have a high likelihood of MDR.
[c]Regimen may be modified once DST results are available (up to 2–3 months after the start of treatment).
[d]Drug resistance surveillance data.
Notes:

1. A country's standard MDR regimen is based on country-specific DST data from similar groups of patients.
2. In the country's standard regimens, the 8-month retreatment regimen should not be "augmented" by a fluoroquinolone or an injectable second-line drug; this practice jeopardizes second-line drugs that are critical treatment options for MDR patients. Second-line drugs should be used only for MDR regimens and only if quality-assured drugs can be provided by DOT for the whole course of therapy. In addition, there must be laboratory capacity for cultures to monitor treatment response, as well as a system for detecting and treating adverse reactions before embarking on MDR-TB treatment.

Adapted from Treatment of Tuberculosis Guidelines, 4th ed., WHO, 2010.

Currently, the WHO recommends administering a single dose of BCG vaccine at birth to all infants living in areas where TB is highly endemic as well as to infants and children at particular risk of exposure to TB in countries with low endemicity.[13] Furthermore, BCG vaccination should to be given at birth to all infants regardless of HIV exposure, especially considering the high endemicity of TB in populations with high HIV prevalence. Only those known to be HIV-infected or with severe immunosuppression from another cause should not receive BCG vaccine due to the risk of developing severe or fatal disseminated BCG disease.[16] There are no data to support BCG revaccination or booster inoculations.[13] BCG's effectiveness in protecting infants and young children from life-threatening forms of TB suggests that it may be playing a role in preventing even higher rates of TB globally, but it is clearly an insufficient measure to eradicate TB globally.[7]

Controlling Tuberculosis

The goals of TB control are to reduce morbidity and mortality from the disease until TB no longer poses a threat to the public's health. To achieve this, it is necessary to ensure the accurate and timely diagnosis and successful treatment of each patient with active TB disease, particularly those capable of transmitting the disease. This will prevent both further transmission to uninfected individuals and the emergence of drug-resistant TB strains.

The DOTS Strategy to Control Tuberculosis

Historically, attempts to treat TB were highly ineffective and could take several years. Some improvements in lessening the TB burden in industrialized countries were achieved through better nutrition, less crowded living conditions (which decreased the likelihood of close contact to and shared airspace with others with infectious TB), and the sanatoria movement (which removed infectious TB patients from the community); however, TB was still associated with a 50% mortality rate. In the 1950s, tuberculosis treatment was revolutionized by the development of new drugs that, given in combination, cured tuberculosis and eliminated the need for lengthy hospitalizations. However, despite the availability of effective treatment, tuberculosis remained a public health problem.

Years after the development of anti-TB drugs, it became apparent how difficult it is for patients to complete their full course of therapy. The practice of directly observed therapy (DOT), in which a trained individual watches patients take each dose of their medicines, was developed to address this problem. By ensuring regularity and completion of treatment,

patients whose treatment is observed have been shown in some settings to have decreased mortality from tuberculosis compared with those whose treatment is not observed.[17] In addition, the discovery of the highly effective drug rifampin made it possible to cure the majority of TB cases in 6 to 9 months. The new rifampin-containing regimen became known as short-course therapy. These two dramatic breakthroughs in TB treatment formed the basis of the DOTS approach: directly observed therapy, short course.

However, short-course therapy administered under direct observation was still not enough to control tuberculosis; an even more comprehensive approach was needed. Developed by Dr. Karel Styblo of the International Union Against Tuberculosis and Lung Diseases (IUATLD) based on his work in Africa in the 1980s, the DOTS strategy was launched in 1994 and quickly became the internationally accepted approach to tuberculosis control. Endorsed by the WHO, the DOTS strategy is a five-pronged comprehensive approach that builds on the administration of therapy under direct observation (Table 10-3).

The DOTS strategy helped to turn the tide in TB control in the last two decades. However, as the TB epidemic evolved, the DOTS strategy no longer addressed the most pressing issues affecting tuberculosis control: namely, tuberculosis control in HIV-endemic settings and treatment of multidrug-resistant (MDR) TB. In addition, the DOTS strategy has been criticized for placing too much emphasis on treating smear-positive patients, leaving a sizable proportion of patients (i.e., AFB-smear-negative patients, children, and patients with extrapulmonary disease) as a low priority, and therefore there was little support for the detection of smear-negative cases.[18] Similarly, sole reliance on the 100-year-old technique of smear microscopy provided little impetus for investment in

Table 10-3. The DOTS strategy.

The five components of the DOTS strategy are as follows:
1. Sustained political commitment
2. Case detection by quality-assured sputum smear microscopy
3. Treatment of TB cases with standard short-course chemotherapy regimens under proper case-management conditions, including direct observation of treatment
4. Uninterrupted supply of quality-assured anti-TB drugs
5. Recording and reporting system enabling outcome assessment and management of program effectiveness

Note: The DOTS strategy is an all-or-none approach; all elements must be implemented.

newer and more sensitive and specific diagnostic measures. Lastly, DOT, once a cornerstone of TB treatment, has also been challenged. Some studies have shown that similar cure rates can be achieved when treatment is self-administered, countering the dogma that DOT is essential to TB control.[19,20] Programs rolling out antiretrovirals in resource-limited settings are demonstrating that patients can take long courses of therapy (lifelong in the case of antiretrovirals) with appropriate support and education but without the need for direct observation. Whereas DOT in some settings is arranged to support patients, it has been criticized as punitive and burdensome in other settings. It is becoming clear that no one-size-fits-all approach can be accepted in every situation.

Based on the growing understanding of TB control needs, additional policy framework and clinical guideline documents were developed to provide guidance to TB control programs that build on the DOTS strategy.

The Stop TB Strategy and the Global Plan to Stop TB 2006–2015

Launched on World TB Day in 2006, the Global Plan to Stop TB 2006–2015 provides a road map for accelerated progress toward controlling TB with the goal of significantly reducing the global burden by 2015 (Table 10-4).[21] The cost of implementing this plan—US$56 billion—is the largest sum requested

Table 10-4. The Global Plan to Stop TB 2006–2015.

Vision: A TB-free world
Goal: To dramatically reduce the global burden of TB by 2015 in line with the Millennium Development Goals (MDGs) and the Stop TB Partnership targets

Objectives
- Achieve universal access to high-quality care for all people with TB
- Reduce the human suffering and socioeconomic burden associated with TB
- Protect vulnerable populations from TB, TB/HIV, and multidrug-resistant TB
- Support development of new tools and enable their timely and effective use
- Protect and promote human rights in TB prevention, care, and control

Targets
- MDG 6, Target 8: Halt and begin to reverse the incidence of TB by 2015
- Targets linked to the MDGs and endorsed by the Stop TB Partnership:
  - By 2015: reduce prevalence and deaths due to TB by 50% compared with a baseline of 1990
  - By 2050: eliminate TB as a public health problem

for TB control to date. The 2006 Global Plan was updated in 2010.[22] The foundation of the plan is the Stop TB Strategy (Table 10-5).[23] This new six-point strategy builds on the successes of DOTS while also explicitly addressing the key challenges facing TB such as TB/HIV co-disease, drug-resistant TB, and TB in

Table 10-5. The Stop TB Strategy.

1. Pursue high-quality DOTS expansion and enhancement
   - Secure political commitment, with adequate and sustained financing
   - Ensure early case detection and diagnosis through quality-assured bacteriology
   - Provide standardized treatment with supervision and patient support
   - Ensure effective drug supply and management
   - Monitor and evaluate performance and impact
2. Address TB-HIV, MDR-TB, and the needs of poor and vulnerable populations
   - Scale-up collaborative TB/HIV activities
   - Scale-up prevention and management of multidrug-resistant TB (MDR-TB)
   - Address the needs of TB contacts and of poor and vulnerable populations
3. Contribute to health system strengthening based on primary health care
   - Help improve health policies, human resource development, financing, supplies, service delivery, and information
   - Strengthen infection control in health services, other congregate settings, and households
   - Upgrade laboratory networks, and implement the Practical Approach to Lung Health (PAL)
   - Adapt successful approaches from other fields and sectors, and foster action on the social determinants of health
4. Engage all care providers
   - Involve all public, voluntary, corporate, and private providers through Public-Private Mix (PPM) approaches
   - Promote use of the International Standards for Tuberculosis Care (ISTC)
5. Empower people with TB and communities through partnership
   - Pursue advocacy, communication, and social mobilization
   - Foster community participation in TB care, prevention, and health promotion
   - Promote use of the Patients' Charter for Tuberculosis Care
6. Enable and promote research
   - Conduct programme-based operational research
   - Advocate for and participate in research to develop new diagnostics, drugs, and vaccines

vulnerable populations. The Stop TB strategy also recognizes the need and includes a call for universal access to high-quality TB care, further TB advocacy to support the development of new tools to prevent, detect, and treat TB, and empowerment of TB patients.

Evaluating Tuberculosis Control Activities: Global Targets

Setting and evaluating success toward agreed on goals has been an essential component of modern TB control. At the heart of the DOTS strategy is the evaluation of patient outcomes to assess the effectiveness of TB control activities. This process—referred to as cohort analysis—allows the determination of, among other outcomes, the treatment success rate of a cohort of patients who started treatment in the same quarter or year. In 1991, the World Health Assembly set the goals of 70% case detection and 85% treatment success as country-level targets to be achieved by 2000, then postponed until 2005.

More recently, the Millennium Development Goals set targets in 2000 for TB control: to reverse the rise in TB incidence globally by 2015 and to halve the 1990 prevalence and death rates in most regions by 2015. Both sets of targets are the benchmarks by which National Tuberculosis Programs (NTPs) now measure their overall success. Furthermore, the Global Plan to Stop TB, as mentioned previously, has set ambitious goals beginning with a vision of a TB-free world (Table 10-4).

The Problem of Drug Resistance

Drug-resistant TB is wholly a human-made phenomenon. With TB, the public health consequences of inadequate or incomplete treatment are worse than with no treatment. Drug-resistant strains emerge through spontaneous mutation of the bacilli and will be selected as the dominant strain whenever inappropriate therapy (e.g., therapy with a single agent) is used. Single-drug exposure can occur due to improper prescribing, irregular drug supply, incorrect administration, or poor drug quality. Today, we are paying the price for poor TB control efforts in the past. The rapidly rising rates of drug-resistant TB in many countries are due in large part to previous poor treatment adherence—specifically, a failure of patients to take drugs consistently and/or to complete the prescribed course of treatment. Treatment of drug-resistant TB is more complicated than treatment of drug-susceptible TB; specifically, it is longer, less effective, and vastly more expensive. Consequently, the very ability of public health systems to control TB is threatened by the rising rates of drug-resistant cases.

MDR-TB is defined as MTB resistant to at least isoniazid and rifampin—our two most powerful anti-TB drugs. Treatment of MDR-TB requires treatment with second-line drugs, which are generally from the following classes: aminoglycosides, polypeptides, fluoroquinolones, and carbothioamides; the category also includes cycloserine and para-aminosalicylic acid. Regimens to treat MDR-TB strains should contain at least four drugs to which the organism is known (or highly likely) to be susceptible. A typical initial phase for MDR-TB treatment may contain five or more drugs including an injectable agent that is given for a minimum of 6 months. Under ideal program conditions, MDR-TB cure rates can approach 70%. In general, second-line drugs are less effective and more toxic than first-line drugs. When rifampin can no longer be used because of resistance, treatment must be extended to 18 to 24 months to achieve cure. In addition, treatment of MDR-TB can be 100 times more costly than treatment of drug-susceptible TB.

The WHO estimates there were 290,000 new cases of MDR-TB among the notified TB patients in 2010.[1] Only 16% of these, or 46,000, were identified and started on treatment.[1] The most recent report of the WHO/IUATLD Global Project on Anti-Tuberculosis Drug Resistance Surveillance evaluated drug-resistant TB data collected from 93 settings between 2002 and 2007.[24] As was shown in the three previous surveys, MDR-TB was found in all regions of the world. Based on information compiled throughout the global project (using data from 114 countries and two Special Administrative Regions of China), it is estimated that MDR-TB represents 5% of all TB cases. In addition, patients who had received some treatment for TB in the past were more likely to have drug-resistant TB (an estimated 15% of retreatment cases are MDR-TB), and they have resistance to more drugs than previously untreated patients.[24] With a few exceptions, the MDR-TB burden in most countries is stable or declining.

In response to the growing problem of drug-resistant TB, the DOTS-Plus strategy was created in 1998.[25] Because the first priority in controlling MDR-TB is preventing its further emergence, a solid DOTS-based program must be in place before instituting DOTS-Plus. However, in MDR-TB hot spots such as Estonia, Latvia, and certain areas of Russia and China, where rates of MDR-TB have already reached high levels, additional measures, including the treatment and cure of resistant cases using second-line drugs, are needed to control MDR-TB. DOTS-Plus includes the designation of specialized treatment centers for MDR-TB, special clinical guidelines for management of MDR-TB patients with second-line drugs, and actions to make second-line drugs available for such treatment. Similar to the Global Drug Facility provision of first-line drugs, the Green Light Committee was established to provide quality-assured second-line drugs at reduced costs to carefully monitored programs.

DOTS-Plus has been shown to be cost effective in a variety of settings, and reasonably high cure rates (approximately 70%) have been achieved.[26] By September 2005, just 6 years after its launch, over 10,000 patients with MDR-TB had received treatment through 35 programs in roughly 29 countries. In recognition of the success of DOTS-Plus projects worldwide, the WHO published updated guidelines in 2006 on the management of MDR-TB.[26] Compiled by a team of international experts; these guidelines build on the extensive data collected over the years and represent the best available knowledge on the management of MDR-TB. In compliance with the new Global Plan to Stop Tuberculosis to treat all patients with TB, this document represents a significant shift in policy toward MDR-TB management: rather than a luxury reserved for programs with appropriate resources or for those experiencing the highest levels of drug resistance, management of MDR-TB is now an integral activity of an NTP.

In 2006, the emergence of a highly resistant strain of MTB associated with a high mortality rate was described in a report of 53 mostly HIV-infected patients from KwaZulu-Natal, South Africa.[27] This new strain—termed XDR-TB—is defined as MTB resistant to isoniazid, rifampin, and to two additional drug classes (fluoroquinolones and either aminoglycosides or capreomycin). Results from a survey of supranational reference laboratories conducted from 2000 to 2004 revealed that 20% of isolates were MDR-TB and 2% were XDR-TB. Population data from industrialized nations, Eastern Europe and Russia, and the Republic of Korea showed that 7%, 14%, and 15% of their reported MDR-TB cases, respectively, were XDR-TB.[28] XDR-TB poses a significant obstacle to global TB control; if allowed to propagate, it could result in an epidemic of potentially untreatable TB.

In 2009, clinicians in Iran described their experience with 15 patients with TB that was resistant to all anti-TB medications tested.[29] In 2011, a report of four patients in India was also published and garnered significant media attention.[30] In both reports, the respective authors referred to these cases as "totally drug resistant TB," or TDR-TB. Subsequently, the WHO issued a statement that it does not recognize the term *totally drug resistant TB* because it has not been clearly defined and limitations of current in vitro drug susceptibility testing (DST) for second-line drugs do not allow us to confirm MTB strains as totally drug resistant.[31] In contrast, MDR-TB has been well studied, DST methods and interpretation of results outlined, and a consensus reached on its definition. At this time it is unknown how *in vitro* DST results for the remaining second-line drugs will correlate with clinical response in a patient. Consequently, the WHO advises against using these results to guide individual patient care.

Current Challenges to Tuberculosis Control in Resource-Limited Countries

TB control activities must be considered in the context of the country's health system. If ignored, these factors may thwart efforts to control the disease; however, if leveraged appropriately, they can contribute to the goals of the NTP.

Role of the Private Sector In many countries, particularly in Asia, a substantial private health care sector exists and is the source of care for a sizable proportion of TB patients. If the role played by the private sector is not recognized by the NTP and the opportunity for collaborating with private practitioners is not seized, many patients will be treated outside of the auspices of the NTP without any assurances of quality or adherence to international guidelines for diagnosing and treating TB. As a result, diagnosis may be delayed, which can have an adverse outcome for the patient and will allow continued transmission of TB in the community.

Increasingly, NTP leadership is acknowledging the potential for private sector involvement and building collaborative relationships with private practitioners to support their involvement in NTP activities. A few countries, notably the Philippines and India, have established sophisticated public-private partnership schemes that outline different levels of engagement and collaboration—from simple referral mechanisms to full participation in the diagnostic and treatment activities supervised by the NTP. In most of sub-Saharan Africa, public-private collaborations are newer ventures. This area of involvement is constantly evolving as both the public and private sectors explore potential collaborations based on their specific country and health system context.

Issues of Access and Community-Based Care Health care access is an issue not only in rural areas, where health outposts may be understaffed or nonexistent, but also in urban areas, where overcrowded health facilities are unable to handle the large patient volume. In response, programs that train and use community health workers to extend the health care system's reach have been created. Beginning with the WHO-coordinated Community TB Care in Africa project in 1996, the experience and results of numerous models of community-based care have been shared among policymakers, NTPs, community-based organizations, and nongovernmental organizations (NGOs). In rural villages as well as urban slums, together these agencies have contributed to the development of innovative methods of providing patient-centered care and patient- and community-level education as well as contributing to the identification of TB patients—all of which allow the NTP to expand the availability of services that are reflective of the community's needs. It is essential that all community-based efforts be designed and executed in close collaboration with the NTP.

Health Care Worker Shortage Most resource-limited countries are experiencing some degree of health care worker shortage. The shortage is most severe in the countries of sub-Saharan Africa, where limited resources significantly contribute to the shortage. Because of poor working conditions, unlivable wages, and concerns about health worker safety, many local physicians and nurses emigrate and seek employment in Europe and the United States, resulting in the well-described brain drain phenomenon. Fueling this problem is active recruitment by these high-income countries to fill some of their own gaps in health care personnel. With only one physician or less per 100,000 population in high-TB burden countries such as Ethiopia, Tanzania, and Uganda, these countries fall short of the WHO-recommended minimum of 20 physicians per 100,000 population.[32] In addition, many health care workers who remain in-country are tempted away from clinical care delivery to work for one of the numerous international NGOs in their country (often for a higher salary) to serve in nonclinical management or public health roles. This internal brain drain further compromises the country's health care delivery capacity. A response to the shortage of health care workers is outside the scope of NTP activities and requires a systematic and sustained directive led by the Ministry of Health involving all health care partners, to which the NTP can contribute through appropriate capacity building and the provision of incentives for retaining TB control clinical staff.

A Dangerous Duo: Poverty and Stigma Both poverty and stigma challenge the success of TB control. TB is both caused by and a cause of poverty. On average, a person with TB loses a third of his or her annual income. Additionally, the poor are overrepresented among TB patients. The stigma associated with TB can be powerful and is only worsened in countries where TB is closely linked to HIV/AIDS. Patients with TB have been ostracized from their families and communities, and being witness to this behavior can lead people with a protracted cough to delay seeking care.

Efforts to address both the stigma of TB and its relationship to poverty have been undertaken by governments, NTPs, the WHO, and NGOs. Addressing poverty in TB control requires a multifaceted approach across several sectors to address economic impoverishment and the accompanying vulnerabilities and marginalization. The health system must be willing to undertake a pro-poor and equity-based approach to address the special needs of the most disadvantaged groups.[33] This approach, coupled with public education activities to address stigma (such as media campaigns

and the use of celebrity TB survivors, which have been successful in some countries), is needed to address these significant challenges to TB control efforts.

Tuberculosis and Diabetes Like HIV, diabetes increases one's risk for progressing from latent TB infection to TB disease. Another similarity is the negative feedback one disease has on the other, with TB worsening glycemic control and diabetes worsening the clinical course of TB. The prevalence of diabetes in some TB-endemic communities, especially in some Asian countries, is making diabetes the most common risk factor for developing TB disease. As has occurred with HIV-associated TB, a coordinated response supporting collaboration between TB and diabetes services and providers is essential. Mechanisms for collaboration and policy development for patients with TB and diabetes are being developed based on the models for integrated TB and HIV care, and bidirectional screening for both diseases is recommended. The WHO and the Union Against Tuberculosis and Lung Disease have published guidance for a collaborative framework for the management and control of TB and diabetes to begin to address this emerging issue.[34]

On the Horizon

Potential New Diagnostic Tests

Both sputum smear microscopy and the TST, the two 100-year-old TB diagnostic tests most commonly used in resource-limited settings, lack the sensitivity and specificity desirable in a diagnostic test. Mycobacterial culture, albeit a more sensitive test, is still an imperfect tool because of the delay in the availability of results. And although the introduction of Xpert MTB/RIF holds promise to increase TB case detection and retention dramatically (due to the short turnaround time to results), cost is likely to limit its use; currently, it is reserved for high-risk patients, namely HIV-infected and those suspected of having drug-resistant TB in specialized urban centers. The ideal TB diagnostic test would be a simple and accurate point-of-care (POC) technology that could be used at remote health centers without the need for sophisticated laboratory expertise or equipment.

Recent efforts on advancing TB diagnostics offer hope. Scientific research in this area has been renewed by the contributions from disciplines such as molecular biology, nanotechnology, immunology, and genomics. This work is shifting diagnostic development from the biologic to the molecular level.[35] Use of specimens other than sputum that are easier to collect (e.g., urine or stool) are being explored. Accessibility, affordability, and sensitivity are the three key characteristics that will determine the impact of future diagnostics for TB.[35]

New Drugs and Treatment Regimens

A faster and simpler therapy for TB is essential to achieve successful TB control globally. Sequencing of the MTB genome in 1998 led to advanced efforts to find novel ways to combat this pathogen. Recent public-private collaborations, led by the Global Alliance for TB Drug Development, have ensured swift movement of potential compounds through the development pipeline. New compounds, such as the diarylquinoline, bedaquiline,[36] recently approved by the Food and Drug Administration, and delamanid OPC-67683 hold promise for effective, shorter TB treatment with no evidence of cross-resistance.[37,38] Specifically, the addition of delamanid to standard therapy was shown in a randomized controlled trial to improve sputum culture conversion at 2 months in patients with MDR-TB.[38] In addition, results from a 2012 phase 2 clinical trial conducted in South Africa demonstrated excellent early bactericidal activity of a new combination therapy using the new TB drug candidate PA-824 plus moxifloxacin and pyrazinamide.[39] This combination may lead to a shortened course of therapy and be compatible with antiretroviral medications. This trial was unusual because typically, due to regulatory requirements and competition between companies, new drugs are developed consecutively. However, the Global TB Alliance supported this new approach to test drugs produced by competing pharmaceutical companies in combination in a single clinical trial. Follow-up studies using this new regimen are underway in several different countries.

New Vaccine Candidates

Given the lack of adult protection afforded by the current bacillus Calmette-Guérin (BCG) vaccine, a new vaccine against TB is greatly needed. Research is being conducted on potential live mycobacterial vaccines (using highly attenuated strains of MTB), inactivated vaccines (using nontuberculous mycobacteria), and subunit vaccines (using individual components of MTB). As with TB diagnostics, scientific contributions from multiple fields such as immunology and biotechnology have furthered progress toward a safe and effective vaccine against TB. Currently, 12 vaccine candidates are being studied in clinical trials. Seven of these are being evaluated as boosters to primary BCG vaccination; three are recombinant BCG variants that could possibly replace the current BCG vaccine.[40]

A breakthrough in TB vaccine research was made in 2010. Results from a phase 3 clinical trial showed that administration of an inactivated *M. vaccae* vaccine given in multiple doses to HIV-infected, BCG-vaccinated adults in Tanzania was associated with a significant decrease in the development of definite TB disease.[41] This vaccine could have a significant impact in reducing HIV-associated TB. At present, further study of this vaccine is underway including a modified production method for scale-up. Additional vaccine candidates are expected to enter clinical trials in the near future.

BOX 10-1. TUBERCULOSIS IN CHILDREN: ENDING THE NEGLECT

It is difficult to estimate accurately the global burden of TB in children due to the lack of a standard pediatric case definition and the challenges in confirming the diagnosis in young children (due to their inability to produce sputum). Best estimates suggest that children with TB represent 11% of the total burden of disease.[42] However, among the 4.5 million cases reported in 2010 from the 22 highest TB-burden countries, cases among those under age 15 comprised only 4% of the total.[42] These data help quantify the extent to which TB in children is under-diagnosed. With the prior emphasis on sputum smear–positive TB patients under the DOTS strategy, childhood TB cases were less of a public health priority. Children, especially infants, are prone to developing disseminated forms of TB such as miliary TB or TB meningitis, which are associated with higher mortality rates. Once diagnosed, children tend to tolerate anti-TB therapy well and can have good outcomes. Despite the evidence-based international recommendations for the use of isoniazid preventive therapy in children who are HIV-infected or contacts to adult TB cases, uptake of this practice has been slow. TB also has an impact on children by robbing them of one or more of their parents; in 2009, an estimated 9.7 million children were orphans due to parental deaths from TB.[1]

Fortunately, childhood TB is now receiving increased attention by policymakers, clinicians, and TB researchers. Recent advocacy by both child health and TB experts is helping to end the neglect of childhood TB. At an international meeting of concerned clinicians, researchers, and activists, a call to action for childhood TB was issued to outline the necessary steps to "ensure that all children exposed to TB or suffering from TB are correctly managed and receive the appropriate treatment."[43]

HIV/AIDS

AIDS first came to the attention of the public health community in the United States in 1981.[44–46] The clustering of cases of rare skin (Kaposi sarcoma) and lung (*Pneumocystis carinii* pneumonia) diseases in young, apparently healthy, homosexual men sounded warning bells of an unusual condition. Prior to that, Kaposi sarcoma, a skin cancer, had largely been confined to older men and women from the Mediterranean and African regions. *Pneumocystis carinii* pneumonia had usually been observed among those whose immune systems had been severely suppressed due to treatment or illness, such as cancer patients or destitute and sickly elderly men. Because AIDS appeared first among homosexual men, the initial epidemiologic investigations focused on lifestyle practices.

Soon after, AIDS cases were reported in entirely different populations in the United States and Europe, such as injection drug users (IDUs),[47] hemophiliacs,[48–50] recipients of blood transfusions,[51,52] newborn infants,[53,54] and a few travelers from central Africa who went to Europe for medical treatment.[55] Initially, drugs were implicated as a potential cause because homosexuals often used sexual performance–enhancing drugs such as amyl or butyl nitrate ("poppers"). At the same time, it was hypothesized that AIDS might be caused by immune reactions resulting from frequent immunostimulation by foreign proteins and tissue antigens from sperm and blood products. Similar to healthy homosexuals, hemophiliacs and IDUs were often found to have inverted ratios of infection-fighting cells. This was thought to result from frequent immunostimulation.

However, the observation of AIDS in the other disparate populations and the emerging epidemiology of the disease suggested an infectious cause.[56] The search for an infectious cause of AIDS eventually focused on viruses, particularly those that were known to cause immunosuppression. It was eventually postulated that a variant human T-cell lymphotrophic retrovirus (HTLV) might be the causative agent of AIDS.[57–61] The reasoning was that the recently discovered (in 1980) HTLV-1 was the only known virus at the time that infected T helper lymphocyte cells.[57] Moreover, HTLV was known to be transmitted through the same routes as the causative agent of AIDS: sexual contact, blood, and from mother to baby.[60] Eventually a variant of HTLV, termed HIV-1 (human immunodeficiency virus type 1), was isolated in 1983.[60,61]

Pathogenesis, Diagnosis, and Transmission

HIV infection causes AIDS through the depletion and eventual exhaustion of immune responses, leading to clinical illness and eventually death in most people. The virus binds on a receptor, penetrates the cell, organizes the infected cell to be able to make the viral genetic material, synthesizes proteins for virus particles, assembles the virus particles, and releases them from the cell. HIV is a retrovirus; this class of virus integrates with the genetic material of the host cell, which is unlike the actions of most other types of viruses. In this way, HIV establishes a permanent infection within the body. The virus attacks lymphocytes, white blood cells that are part of the body's immune defense system. In particular, the T4 helper or inducer lymphocytes that activate B cells to produce antibodies and regulate other cells to fight infections in different ways are invaded. This type of cell contains a significant amount of CD4 surface protein, the cell receptor to which HIV binds. In addition, macrophages, cells that engulf and destroy viruses, and dendritic cells also contain CD4 proteins, making them targets for invasion by HIV.

Thus HIV seems to damage the immune system by the weakening of the CD4 lymphocyte response in the following ways:

- Through invasion of the dendritic cells that stimulate the CD4 lymphocytes to respond to foreign organisms
- Through invasion of the CD4 lymphocytes and the suborning of the cell reproductive processes to produce more virus, with the subsequent destruction of the CD4 lymphocytes
- By facilitating uninfected CD4 lymphocytes to clump around infected CD4 cells, thus immobilizing them. The infected macrophages are not killed: most continue to produce HIV virus particles, and some establish a latent state of HIV infection. Although the body mounts a vigorous immune response to the virus through the production of antibodies, the sheer rapid replication of the virus, its latency, and virus variation eventually leads to the exhaustion and ultimate collapse of the immune system. The variability of the virus is particularly problematic because it has led to immunologically distinct subtypes that vary by region, making vaccine development difficult.

Two main types of HIV exist: HIV-1 and HIV-2. HIV-1 is more predominant and can be classified into three groups: group M, the "major" group; group N, the "new" group; and group O, the "outlier" group. Group O seems to be restricted to west-central Africa, and group N, which was discovered in 1998 in Cameroon, is extremely rare. Over 90% of HIV-1 infections are in group M, and there are at least nine genetically distinct subtypes (or clades): A, B, C, D, F, G, H, J, and K. In addition, two viruses of different subtypes in the same person can sometimes create a new hybrid virus, circulating recombinant forms (CRFs). For example, the CRF A/E is a mixture of subtypes A and E. Many people refer to the CRF A/E as "subtype E." Subtypes B and C are the most widespread viruses, with subtype C predominant in southern and eastern Africa, India, and Nepal, and subtype B most common in the Americas, Australia, Europe, Japan, and Thailand. Subtype C has caused the world's worst epidemic and accounts for about half of all infections. New subtypes will emerge as virus recombination and mutation continues to occur, and the current subtypes and CRFs will continue to spread to new areas with the global pandemic.

The geographic distribution of some of the current subtypes appears to be associated with specific modes of transmission, particularly subtype B, which is possibly more readily transmitted by anal intercourse and intravenous drug injecting (via blood, essentially). Subtypes C and CRF A/E, in contrast, appear to be more efficiently transmitted through vaginal intercourse (a mucosal route). The different subtypes appear to affect disease progression as well. Studies in Senegal and Uganda found that patients infected with subtype C, D, or G developed AIDS earlier and died sooner compared with patients infected with subtype A.[62,63]

HIV infection is diagnosed through the detection of antibodies. The most common HIV antibody test is an enzyme-linked immunosorbent assay (EIA or ELISA test). The current ELISA tests are more than 99.9% accurate. ELISA tests are also available for saliva (e.g., OraQuick, OraSure Technologies, Bethlehem, PA), and there are now antibody tests that can give results in less than 30 minutes (the rapid tests). Examples of these are Uni-Gold Recombigen HIV (Trinity Biotech, Dublin, Ireland) and Determine HIV 1/2 (Abbott Diagnostic Division, Hoofddorp, The Netherlands). The tests can detect HIV-1 and HIV-2, and the major subtypes of group M.

Although the antibody test is very accurate, there are times when it can produce false-positive or false-negative results. A false-positive result obviously can be very distressing to the individual concerned. Aside from a transcription or a laboratory error, the most likely reason for this is that the prevalence of HIV in the population concerned may be very low. Despite the accuracy of a test, screening in populations with low prevalence will result in a high proportion of false positives. This is an argument why, aside from the cost, general screening for HIV in, for example, the United States, where the prevalence is less than 1%, has not been advisable. Recently, however, the Centers for Disease Control and Prevention has recommended that HIV screening be widely offered to adults.

A more troublesome concern has been the occurrence of false negatives. Aside again from transcription or testing protocol errors, false negatives for HIV can occur for two reasons. The most common is when the individual has been infected but the body has not yet begun the manufacture of antibodies. After initial infection, production of antibodies can take as long as 6 months (although in most cases it is 2 to 6 weeks), so that during that time, the individual will test negative on the ELISA tests, which test for antibodies, yet will actually be HIV positive. This period, known as the window phase, is a dangerous time as with initial infection there is a large amount of circulating virus, making the individual particularly infectious. The immune system has not yet begun to effectively suppress viral replication because it is still in the process of identifying the invader and producing the appropriate antibodies. Newer HIV tests now screen for both antibody *and* antigen, which should make earlier diagnosis possible and more accurate with fewer false negatives. The window phase should be less a concern in the future.

The course of HIV infection and ultimately AIDS goes from a largely asymptomatic phase to that of severe disease and death over a period of 10 to 15 years or more. There is, however, significant individual variability in the disease progression. Table 10-6 shows the progression of HIV infection to AIDS.[64] In full-blown AIDS, where the immune system has been severely weakened, another reason for a false-negative finding with an ELISA test is that so few antibodies are being produced that the test can no longer detect them. False negatives can also occur in the rare instances of individuals who never mount an immune response.

Because HIV increasingly damages the immune system, signs and symptoms of various infections become visible. In babies this occurs faster than in adults; although the signs and symptoms vary, one of the first signs of HIV disease in babies may be a general failure to thrive and grow. In general, the clinical manifestations of AIDS can be grouped into opportunistic infections (OIs), that is, infections by microorganisms that would not normally cause disease in healthy individuals (e.g., *Pneumocystis jiroveci* pneumonia,* funguses, and to some extent tuberculosis); cancers (e.g., Kaposi sarcoma, a skin cancer that can also involve mucous membranes and be disseminated to the viscera), weight loss, and mental impairment.

The WHO Staging System

The WHO has developed a four-phase clinical staging system to describe HIV progression in adults and

---

*This is the current name for this organism, but the acronym PCP, for *Pneumocystis carinii* pneumonia, remains in use.

Table 10-6. The progression of HIV infection to AIDS.

Stage	Description
HIV infection	Initial infection with HIV (i.e., through sex or blood contact).
Window period (2–6 weeks; occasionally several months)	No signs or symptoms of disease; no detectable antibodies to HIV.
Seroconversion (brief period that occurs after 2 to 6 weeks, up to a few months)	The development of antibodies. This may be associated with flu-like illness, glandular fever-like illness, or occasionally encephalitis. Illness at seroconversion is sometimes called acute HIV syndrome. About 50% of people experience this illness.
Asymptomatic HIV (duration from less than 1 year to 10 to 15 years or more)	ELISA tests are positive, but there are no apparent signs or symptoms of illness. The incubation period may be associated with persistent generalized lymphadenopathy (PGL), persistent swollen glands.
HIV/AIDS-related illnesses (duration months or years)	Increasing signs and symptoms of disease because HIV is damaging the immune system. Initially not life threatening, but becomes progressively so with the course of the disease.
AIDS (usually less than 1 to 2 years in the absence of treatment)	The terminal stage of HIV infection. The immune system is severely weakened, allowing life-threatening opportunistic infections, including cancers.

From Jackson H. *AIDS Africa: Continent in Crisis.* Harare, Zimbabwe: Southern Africa HIV/AIDS Information Dissemination Service, SAfAIDS, 2002: 43. Adapted with permission.

adolescents (Table 10-7).[65] The WHO staging system is useful in resource-limited countries because it reduces the need for CD4 testing. CD4 testing is potentially expensive, requiring equipment (a capital cost) and reagents (a recurrent expense); for many resource-limited countries, it is unaffordable on a national scale presently. In recent years however, costs have declined, and with the advent of relatively inexpensive and easy to use POC testing machines, which facilitate same-day results, and reduce the need for logistics of transporting time-sensitive samples, CD4 testing has become more widely available and utilized in resource-limited countries. The increasing availability of CD4 testing has made the WHO staging system less useful because the emphasis now is on "treatment as prevention," starting HIV-infected persons on treatment as early as possible. This emphasis is for two reasons. First is that enrolling HIV-infected individuals on antiretroviral therapy (ART) as early as possible reduces the potential transmission of HIV because effective treatment significantly reduces the amount of circulating virus. On a large scale, this has the potential effect to reduce HIV infection at the community level, hence the term *treatment-as-prevention*. The second reason for treating HIV-infected individuals as soon as possible after infection is that treatment will reduce damage to the immune system and thus prolong and improve the quality of life. Also notable is that different regions appear to have different prevalences of OIs. In developing countries, the most prevalent HIV-related infection is TB.

HIV Transmission

HIV transmission occurs when the HIV-contaminated fluid of an infected person comes into contact with the bloodstream or mucosal lining of an uninfected person. The three modes of transmission are birth, blood, and sex. Perinatal transmission can occur during pregnancy, delivery, or through breastfeeding.

Transmission during pregnancy can occur when the mother has high levels of circulating virus (viremia) due to seroconversion or to her precipitating into AIDS, and particularly during the third trimester, when small tears sometimes occur in the placenta, facilitating the entry of cells from the mother's bloodstream into the baby's. HIV transmission during delivery is also enhanced by viremia; by the occurrence of sexually transmitted diseases at the time, particularly syphilis and herpes simplex (HSV2); the prolonged rupture of membranes; and trauma (cuts and tears) during the process. Delivery is a particularly risky time for HIV transmission to the infant because of the infected maternal secretions.

Breastfeeding mothers can also transmit HIV to their infants. Again, this is facilitated by the mother's viremia and by cuts and sores on the mother's nipples and in the child's mouth. In the absence of treatment, about a third of babies born to and breastfed by HIV-positive mothers will become HIV positive, with about a third becoming infected during pregnancy, a third during delivery, and another third through breastfeeding.

Table 10-7. WHO clinical staging system for HIV infection and disease.

Clinical stage 1: Asymptomatic
1. Asymptomatic/acute HIV infection
2. Persistent generalized lymphadenopathy (PGL)
3. History of acute HIV infection
And/or performance scale 1: asymptomatic, normal activity

Clinical stage 2: Early (mild) disease
1. Weight loss, <10% of body weight
2. Minor mucocutaneous (skin) problems (e.g., seborrheic dermatitis, prurigo, fungal nail infections, recurrent oral ulcerations, angular cheilitis)
3. Herpes zoster within the past 5 years
4. Recurrent respiratory tract infections (e.g., bacterial sinusitis)
And/or performance scale 2: symptomatic, normal activity

Clinical stage 3: Intermediate (moderate) disease
1. Weight loss, >10% of body weight
2. Unexplained chronic diarrhea, >1 month
3. Unexplained prolonged fever (intermittent or chronic), >1 month
4. Oral candidiasis (thrush)
5. Oral hairy leukoplakia
6. Pulmonary tuberculosis within the past year
7. Severe bacterial infections, (e.g., pneumonia, pyomyositis)
And/or performance scale 3: bedridden <50% of the daytime during the last month

Clinical stage 4: Late (severe) disease, AIDS
1. HIV wasting syndrome (weight loss >10% body weight, with diarrhea >1 month or chronic weakness and prolonged fever >1 month)
2. *Pneumocystis jiroveci* pneumonia
3. Toxoplasmosis of the brain
4. Cryptosporidiosis with diarrhea, >1 month
5. Isosporiasis with diarrhea, >1 month
6. Cryptococcosis, extrapulmonary
7. Cytomegalovirus (CMV) disease of an organ other than the liver, spleen, or lymph nodes
8. Herpes simplex virus (HSV) infection; mucocutaneous, >1 month, or visceral
9. Progressive multifocal leukoencephalopathy (PML)
10. Mycoses (e.g., histoplasmosis, coccidioidomycosis)
11. Candidiasis of the esophagus, trachea, bronchi, or lungs
12. Atypical mycobacteriosis, disseminated
13. Nontyphoidal *Salmonella* septicemia
14. Extrapulmonary tuberculosis
15. Lymphoma
16. Kaposi sarcoma (KS)
17. HIV encephalopathy (progressive disabling cognitive and/or motor dysfunction, interfering with activities of daily living)
And/or performance scale 4: bedridden >50% of the daytime during the last month

---

The prevention of maternal-to-child transmission (PMTCT)* of HIV was one of the first antiretroviral prevention interventions implemented in low-resource countries. This was made possible particularly with the efficacy of single-dose nevirapine (NVP), the low cost of the drug, and the practicalities of implementation. NVP given in a single dose to the mother in labor and a single dose to the baby at 2 to 3 days old reduces transmission by about 47%.[64,66] The mother can also be given a tablet to take home when labor begins (many mothers in resource-limited countries have their babies at home), and the baby can be dosed 3 days after the birth, perhaps when having a BCG vaccination. However, certain controversies have remained regarding the PMTCT program.

One of the controversies has been that, until recently, antiretroviral therapy was not offered to the parents when the mother tested positive in the antenatal care clinic, yet she was given NVP to prevent transmission to her baby. Consequently, in many programs, the uptake of the PMTCT program was low because the number of mothers agreeing to counseling and testing was low. With the introduction of opt-out testing, in which mothers first have a group talk on PMTCT and then are tested unless they specifically decline, the number of mothers being tested has increased significantly.[†]

Another controversy with the PMTCT program in many countries is the use of NVP. Even single-dose NVP has the potential to cause resistance, and some countries have abandoned its use altogether.

Some have moved to longer course regimens, whereas others have added another antiretroviral drug. These adjustments add to the cost of the program and to the logistics of implementation.

Another controversy is breastfeeding. The use of NVP does not prevent the transmission of HIV through breastfeeding. Ideally, HIV-positive mothers should not breastfeed. However, in many less resourced countries, this is not feasible because the cost of formula feeding is beyond the reach of most mothers, and clean water may not be accessible or available. Mothers are also stigmatized if they do not breastfeed because breastfeeding is very important in many cultures. Exclusive breastfeeding, however, is less risky than mixed feeding (breast and formula or even water and porridge). In the absence of formula feeding, current infant feeding guidelines recommend exclusive breastfeeding for the first 6 months, with

---

*This is also known as the prevention of parent-to-child transmission (PPTCT) to emphasize that both parents are responsible for the potential transmission of HIV to the baby.
†In a town adjacent to Harare, the capital of Zimbabwe, 98% of mothers attending antenatal care in the period from July 2005 to June 2006 were tested. Prior to opt-out testing, only 26% of mothers were tested in 1999 to 2002.

complementary feeding then introduced, and breast-feeding for 12 months.

Most countries now no longer use single-dose NVP for PMTCT because more efficacious prophylactic regimes are available that address the breastfeeding period also. Based on the WHO 2010 recommendations, these are provision of triple therapy (ART) for HIV-positive pregnant women with a CD4 count 350 cells/mm^2 or less or in WHO clinical stage 3 or 4.[67] One regimen (option A) for healthier HIV-positive pregnant women is zidovudine (AZT) prophylaxis from at least 14 weeks of pregnancy for at least 4 weeks until delivery. Breastfeeding infants would get NVP from birth until a week after breastfeeding is stopped. Another regimen (option B) for these women is the provision of triple therapy (three ART drugs) for the duration of pregnancy (from 14 weeks) until the cessation of breastfeeding. Infants would be given NVP or AZT for 4 to 6 weeks of age. Increasingly there is a trend toward a third option; enrolling all HIV-positive pregnant women (irrespective of CD4 count or WHO stage) on triple therapy for life.[68]

Transmission of HIV through blood can be through blood transfusion, through contaminated needles, or through other medical procedures and delivery. The highest risk of HIV transmission is through transfusion of HIV-infected blood (90%), and although blood for transfusion is screened for HIV in almost all countries now, there is still a risk because of the window period and because the screening tests are not perfect.

Transmission through contaminated needles can be through the sharing of needles during injection drug use or through accidental needle sticks between HIV-infected persons and health workers. Injection drug use is a very efficient mode of HIV transmission. According to the UNAIDS 2006 report, injection drug use accounts for 80% of HIV cases in Eastern Europe and Central Asia.[69] The reason for this efficiency is that during the process of injecting the drug, blood is drawn into the syringe to check that the needle has reached a vein, and then the contents of the syringe are injected repeatedly into the vein to ensure that all the drug goes in. If someone else then uses the same needle and syringe, traces of blood (and virus) are readily passed directly into the next person's bloodstream.

Transmission through needle-stick injuries and other medical procedures (e.g., surgery, deliveries, blood splashes) is low. Various studies show a range of HIV infection from 0.13 to 0.39 cases per 100 exposures by cut or needle-stick injury among health staff.[70]

Sexual transmission of HIV is the most common mode globally. About 70% of HIV infections worldwide are contracted through vaginal sexual intercourse.[64]

Anal intercourse (male-to-male sex or male-to-female sex) is the most risky form of intercourse because it often involves a slight tearing of the anus, thus involving the exchange of both semen and blood. In countries such as the United States, Australia, Western Europe, and parts of South America, men who have sex with men, most of whom practice anal intercourse,[71] constituted the initial risk profile for HIV.

Medical Care and Treatment of HIV/AIDS

Medications and Opportunistic Infections

ART is the most effective means of preventing OIs, and many programs link the prevention and treatment of OIs with ART. With the goal of universal access, rapid progress has been made to make ART more widely available (8 million received ART in 2011, a 20-fold increase since 2003), with 68% of women and 47% of men in low- and middle-income countries on treatment. Globally, however, only 28% of children have treatment coverage, compared with 54% of adults.[72] The prevalence of OIs varies by region; for example, TB is the most common OI globally and particularly in sub-Saharan Africa and Asia, whereas PCP is the most common OI in North America and Europe. Table 10-8 presents OIs that have primary and secondary prophylactic medications. ART is taken for life, and generally drugs for OI prophylaxis are taken for life, although they could be stopped if CD4 counts can be measured regularly and the immune system recovers. These activities need to be integrated into daily living.

The prevention and treatment of OIs should be complementary via a holistic approach. The efficacy of many medications is enhanced when the individual is well nourished, has good hygiene, is not stressed or tired, has a positive approach to life, and has access to an acceptable standard of living. Addressing food security and poverty, as well as access to medical care, is an important principle underlying effective medical care and treatment of HIV/AIDS. The prevention and treatment of OIs should include prevention of reinfection (abstinence and/or condom promotion), psychosocial support (counseling and support groups), and nutrition care and support.

Many people in resource-limited countries suffer from underlying nutrition deficiencies, particularly micronutrients, which are exacerbated with the acquisition of HIV. This situation then increases vulnerability to OIs and facilitates the progression to AIDS. In addition, the individual needs good nutrition to be able to better tolerate many of the antiretroviral drugs.

Counseling and Antiretroviral Therapy

Counseling should also be part of the care and treatment of HIV/AIDS. The counseling should involve

Table 10-8. Major opportunistic infections for which primary or secondary prophylactic drugs are available.

Condition	Treatment drugs	Prophylaxis
Candidiasis (oral, esophageal, vaginal)	Fluconazole	Treatment of individual episodes rather than prophylaxis because resistance is common
Cytomegalovirus (CMV—ocular, gastrointestinal, disseminated)	Ganciclovir or foscarnet	Valganciclovir, Foscarnet
Cryptococcus (meningitis, pneumonia, disseminated disease)	Amphotericin B deoxycholate and/or flucytosine	Fluconazole
Histoplasmosis (pneumonia, disseminated disease)	Itraconazole or amphotericin B deoxycholate	Itraconazole
Herpes virus (skin, genital, oral, esophageal, ocular, disseminated)	Valacyclovir Acyclovir	Valacyclovir Famciclovir Acyclovir (but risk of resistance development)
Mycobacterium avium complex (MAC—pulmonary, disseminated)	Clarithromycin plus ethambutol	Azithryomycin or Clarithromycin
Mycobacterium tuberculosis (pulmonary, extrapulmonary, disseminated)	Isoniazid, rifampin; pyrazinamide, ethambutol	Isoniazid (9 months) where positive skin test (latent TB infection)
Pneumocystis carinii pneumonia (PCP)	Trimethoprim-sulfamethoxazole (TMP/SMX, co-trimoxazole)	TMP/SMX
Toxoplasmosis (central nervous system)	Pyrimethamine and sulfadiazine plus leucovorin	TMP/SMX
Penicilliosis[a]	Amphotericin B, then itraconazole	Itraconazole
Leishmaniasis[a]	Amphotericin B	Amphotericin B
Isospora belli[a]	TMP and SMX	TMP and SMX
Chagas disease[a]	Benznidazole	Benznidazole

[a]Geographic opportunistic infections of special consideration.
From Centers for Disease Control and Prevention. Guidelines for prevention and treatment of opportunistic infections in HIV-infected adults and adolescents: recommendations from CDC, the National Institutes of Health and the HIV Medicine Association of the Infectious Diseases Society of America. *MMWR* 2009;58(RR-4):1–207. http://www.cdc.gov/mmwr/pdf/rr/rr5804.pdf. (*Adapted with permission.*)

consideration of what a positive result might mean in the patient's life, whom the result will affect (e.g., a spouse or regular sexual partner), to whom and how the patient will tell his or her results, and what long-term support services are available. There should also be ongoing counseling; this might include knowledge of HIV and AIDS, adherence to drug regimens, coping with stigma, repeated illness episodes, and death and bereavement. Terminal and bereavement counseling should include finances and signing powers, and, for dependents, wills and funeral arrangements.

Counseling, nutrition, and the treatment and prevention of OIs form an important part of the care of people living with HIV/AIDS, the heart of which should be ART. As stated earlier, with the advent of ART the incidence and prevalence of OIs have been reduced. The first antiretroviral drug marketed was azidothymidine or zidovudine (AZT/ZDV). It belongs to a class of drugs called nucleoside reverse transcriptase inhibitors (NRTIs). These drugs block HIV reverse transcriptase and prevent the copying of the viral genetic code (RNA) into the genetic code

(DNA) of infected host cells by imitating the building blocks of the DNA chain. The resulting DNA is incomplete and cannot create new virus. Table 10-9 lists the currently approved HIV antiretroviral drugs. The nonnucleoside reverse transcriptase inhibitors (NNRTIs) block HIV reverse transcriptase and prevent the copying of infected host cells by binding to the enzyme and making the active site ineffective. A more recently marketed drug class is the protease inhibitors. These drugs block the enzyme protease and prevent the assembly and release of HIV particles from infected cells. The integrase inhibitor raltegravir has now become part of the alternative first-line regimens in the United States and will become important worldwide. To avoid the rapid development of resistance, drugs are given in combination. Drugs that are in current use for first-line therapy in low- and middle-income countries include AZT, lamivudine (3TC), nevirapine (NVP), and efavirenz (EFV). Recommendations change frequently, and it is always good to check the WHO Website for current recommendations.

Table 10-9. Currently approved HIV antiviral drugs.

Drug class	Chemical/generic name	Trade name
Multi-class combination products	Efavirenz, emtricitabine, and tenofovir disoproxil fumarate	Atripla
	Emtricitabine, rilpivirine, and tenofovir disoproxil fumarate	Complera
	Elvitegravir, cobicistat, emtricitabine, tenofovir disoproxil fumarate	Stribild
Nucleoside reverse transcriptase inhibitors	Azidothymidine/zidovudine (AZT, ZDV)	Retrovir
	Dideoxyinosine/didanosine (DDI)	Videx
	Dideoxycytidine/zalcitabine (DDC) (no longer marketed)	HIVID
	Lamivudine (3TC)	Epivir
	Stavudine (D4T)	Zerit
	Abacavir (ABC)	Ziagen
	Abacavir and lamivudine	Epzicom
	Abacavir, zidovudine, and lamivudine	Trizivir
	Emtricitabine (FTC)	Emtriva
	Lamivudine and zidovudine	Combivir
	Tenofovir disoproxil fumarate (TDF)	Viread
	Tenofovir disoproxil fumarate and emtricitabine	Truvada
Nonnucleoside reverse transcriptase inhibitors	Delavirdine (DLV)	Rescriptor
	Efavirenz (EFV)	Sustiva
	Etravirine	Intelence
	Nevirapine (NVP)	Viramune
	Rilpivirine	Edurant
Protease inhibitors	Amprenavir (APV)	Agenerase
	Atazanavir sulfate (ATV)	Reyataz
	Darunavir (DRV)	Prezista
	Fosamprenavir (FPV)	Lexiva
	Indinavir (IDV)	Crixivan
	Nelfinavir mesylate (NFV)	Viracept
	Lopinavir and ritonavir (LPV/RTV)	Kaletra
	Tripranavir (TPV)	Aptivus
	Ritonavir (RTV)	Norvir
	Saquinavir (no longer marketed)	Fortovase
	Saquinavir mesylate (SQV)	Invirase
Fusion inhibitors	Enfuvirtide (T20)	Fuzeon
Entry inhibitors –CCR5 co-receptor antagonist	Maraviroc (MVC)	Selzentry
HIV integrase strand transfer inhibitors	Raltegravir (RAL)	Isentress

In resource-limited countries, first-line ART uses the older classes of drugs (the NRTIs and NNRTIs) because of the cost of protease inhibitors. Cost is an important consideration in ART. Even though the cost of HIV drugs has decreased considerably, the cost of providing ART to all who need it in many African countries is huge and not easily affordable. The WHO estimates that in the least developed countries, where populations are living on less than $1 per day, ART still costs about $100 per person per year. In addition, many health systems in limited resourced countries are weak and need to be strengthened to be able to roll out ART nationally; this entails a cost even greater than that of the drugs. There are insufficient numbers of doctors, nurses, counselors, and laboratory personnel, and these cadres need to be trained, motivated, and retained. Patient monitoring and adherence to treatment are critical to the success of the ART program; consequently, national health systems need to be able to routinely carry out CD4 and viral load testing to be able to assess the immune system function and the amount of HIV virus that can be detected. Enormous capital and recurrent costs are associated with equipping national health systems to be able to provide these monitoring functions. Low-cost diagnostic tools are in development for at least CD4 measurement and viral load.*

The WHO has developed guidelines as to when to treat and to assist in monitoring. Patients with a positive HIV test, clinical stage 3 or 4, and/or a CD4 count less than 350 are eligible for treatment in most countries in sub-Saharan Africa. In the United States, patients are eligible for ART if they have a positive HIV test. However, patients with HIV and TB are eligible for ART irrespective of CD4 count with the new "treatment as prevention"policy.[73] Although treatment efficacy or failure is assessed on clinical grounds: essentially, whether the patient is getting better, gaining (or not losing) weight, and is not experiencing opportunistic illnesses; a more valid measure is viral load. By the time patients are symptomatic, their immune systems may already be severely compromised. The correlation between the CD4 count and the clinical signs and symptoms is not perfect, and there are reports of patients with very low CD4 counts still being able to function normally.

Despite these challenges, enormous progress has been made in enrolling eligible patients onto ART. In sub-Saharan Africa where the need is greatest, 56% of those eligible have access to the drugs, and over 6 million have enrolled in treatment.[74] This represents a 100-fold increase in treatment access in less than a decade with a significant decrease in the cost of the drugs ($1,200 to less than $100 per annum). This demonstrates the impact of increased resources through the U.S. President's Emergency Fund for AIDS Relief (PEPFAR), the Global Fund, and organizations that have negotiated sharp reductions in the price of the drugs, such as the Clinton Foundation.

Prevention of HIV/AIDS

HIV/AIDS prevention remains the key to the control of the epidemic. Various prevention strategies have been tried over the years; these strategies vary according to the stage of the epidemic. When the HIV prevalence is still low (less than 1%) and the epidemic is confined to high-risk groups, different preventive interventions are used compared with when the epidemic has become generalized in the population. In generalized epidemics, there should be a focus on population- or community-level change because simply concentrating on high-risk groups will no longer be effective. High-risk groups, from which epidemics can spread to become generalized, include commercial sex workers (CSWs), men who have sex with men

(MSMs), IDUs, and mobile men (migrant workers, military personnel, truck drivers, etc.).

In the early stages of the epidemic, targeting of high-risk groups can slow the epidemic and prevent it from becoming generalized. Some countries, by acting early and vigorously, have been able to do this. Examples include Senegal, Thailand, and Australia. Despite being a predominantly Muslim country, Senegal was able to reduce the incidence and prevalence of HIV by encouraging condom use among CSWs through the legalization of commercial sexual activities, education on and provision of condoms, and the regular examination for and treatment of sexually transmitted infections (STIs).[75] Similarly, Thailand has been successful by developing interventions for CSWs and the army. Thailand adopted a 100% condom use policy for CSWs, which was enabled by the commercialized nature of sex work (the existence of brothels), allowing for the enforcement of this policy.[76,77] The implementation of this policy was facilitated through peer education programs for the CSWs.[77] Peer education was also the means through which behavior change among young men in the Thai army was facilitated and HIV prevalence reduced.[78] In Australia, the epidemic among IDUs was reduced through a policy of needle exchange.[79] A program in Sydney, Australia, included bleach distribution, community outreach, and expanded drug treatment. The needle exchange policy, which remains controversial in some countries, is predicated on a harm reduction approach, whereby the prevention of illness and death through HIV, and the possibility of transmission to others, is considered more important than prosecution for illicit drug use. Table 10-10 summarizes the evidence regarding various HIV/AIDS prevention interventions.

Abstinence, Faithfulness, and Condom Use

The abstinence, faithfulness, and condom use (ABC) policy remains the cornerstone of many HIV/AIDS prevention programs. Abstinence is a controversial strategy because there is widespread consensus that youth should abstain but less consensus about providing the knowledge and skills (including information on condom use and where they can be obtained) necessary to protect themselves should they not abstain. Moreover, although the message of abstinence until marriage has increased the age of sexual debut,[80] there is a tendency for "catch-up"—the rapid acquisition of HIV soon after becoming sexually active. Young women may not benefit from the strategy of abstinence because, despite being abstinent until marriage, a number of them become infected by their husbands soon after marriage.

Faithfulness is a key prevention strategy, especially in the context of multiple concurrent relationships in a generalized epidemic. The high risk of HIV transmission during the acute stage of infection makes this form

---

*See UNITAID 2012 HIV/AIDS Diagnostic Technology Landscape. 2nd ed., June 2012 (http://www.unitaid.eu/resources-2/news/9-uncategorised/345-technical-reports)

Table 10-10. Summary of the evidence base of interventions for HIV prevention.

Intervention/ Program area	Impact at population level	Impact at individual level	Comments
Abstinence	Temporary impact on young people through delayed debut, but tendency to have more rapid HIV acquisition in their 20s: "catch up" observed; less relevance for adults	While observed, 100% effective	"ABC" formulation has considerable baggage and has had less relevance for women. However, all three prongs are relevant and need reformulating for greater complementarity; avoid either/or formulation.
Be faithful	Appears to have been key to reduced incidence and prevalence in Uganda, Kenya, and Zimbabwe	100% effective *if* fully maintained by two HIV-negative people (or in a polygamous union)	Concurrent relationships appear to be a key epidemic driver because of very high infectivity in acute/incident infection.
Condoms, male	Appear not to have had strong impact in generalized epidemics (though central to concentrated, sexually driven epidemics elsewhere)	At least 80% to 90% protective if consistently and correctly used: the most protective device currently available for individual protection	Challenge is to achieve correct and consistent use (over 80%). Easiest in commercial sex, and then casual sex; least in more stable partnerships, concurrent or not.
Condoms, female	Contribute to number of protected sex acts where available	Highly protective against HIV, STIs and pregnancy	Advantage of female use.
STI treatment	Limited impact on HIV prevention because only targets bacterial STIs and misses 50% of those needing treatment (asymptomatic)	Untreated STIs greatly increase HIV transmission risk; more so if ulcerous	Only reaches small proportion of infected individuals; increasingly in southern Africa, viral STIs predominate, not bacterial, and treatment misses these.
STI control and prevention	More impact in concentrated than generalized epidemics, but crucial for young people in generalized epidemics	As above	Greater potential to reach large numbers, especially important for young people.
HSV2	Recent infection with HSV2 doubles the risk of HIV transmission, with recent infection with HSV2 more risky than chronic infection	HSV2 treatment reduces HIV shedding and thus reduces infectivity	Research is under way into HSV2 suppression.
Male circumcision	Strong observational data of protective impact at population level; includes correlation with lower incidence and prevalence of HIV in African and other populations; three randomized controlled trials completed; all demonstrated strong protection	50% to 75% protective for men, possibly some direct protection for women; many other health benefits for males (e.g., for penile cancer, some STIs, phimosis) and for females (especially reduced risk of cervical cancer)	Countries vary in their readiness to consider male circumcision where it is not traditionally practiced. UNAIDS and WHO have developed tools, guides, and manuals for safe male circumcision practice and programming. Progress has been slow, and there are challenges with implementation. New procedures being tested that need less highly trained health workers.

(Continued)

Table 10-10. Summary of the evidence base of interventions for HIV prevention. *(Continued)*

Intervention/ Program area	Impact at population level	Impact at individual level	Comments
Counseling and testing	Little population-level impact shown, although essential as an entry point to care and treatment, and for PMTCT	Some behavior change shown in discordant couples and in HIV-positive clients	Concern that "know your status" campaigns must link with effective and available posttest services for HIV-positive and HIV-negative clients, or they may not be effective.
Behavior change interventions for young people	Talloires' consultation in 2004: strongest evidence for behavioral impacts of radio with other media and TV/radio with other media; certain designs of curriculum-based sex and HIV education shown to be effective for young people in school when adult led, with no evidence of increased sexual activity	Increased individual access to youth- (and gender-) friendly health services also shown to be important for general SRH in various studies. Young men and women recognized as essential to reach with effective multipronged strategies	Data indicate behavior changes through different strategies that are likely to have an impact on HIV incidence in young people. Community interventions with young people: weak evaluation designs and incomplete information, so not possible yet to assess impact clearly of different approaches. Look out for Talloires' final report.
Microbicides	South African RCT using a 1% tenofovir (antiretroviral drug) gel demonstrated a protective effect of 39%	Not clear what level of protection; hoped at least 50%	Trial needs to be repeated in other settings. Other microbicide candidates under development.
Treatment as prevention	RCT HPTN 052 demonstrated a 96% protective effect among discordant couples	Approach not only treats individual with HIV disease but is able to virtually prevent transmission	Considerable enthusiasm for this approach because antiretroviral drug prices have become significantly cheaper. However, most transmission occurs soon after infection, before knowledge of status. Also, health system implementation challenges.

STI, sexually transmitted infection; HSV2, herpes simplex virus 2; PMTCT, prevention of maternal-to-child transmission; RCT, randomized controlled trial; SRH, sexual and reproductive health.
Updated from the Southern African Development Community (SADC) Expert Think Tank Meeting on HIV Prevention in High Prevalence Countries in Southern Africa; May 10–12, 2006; Maseru, Lesotho. *(Adapted with permission.)*

of sexual networking extremely dangerous, and concurrency is an important driver of the HIV/AIDS epidemic in southern Africa.[81,82] Because concurrency typically involves stable relationships with one or more partners outside the primary relationship, there is a diminished likelihood of condom use with these partners.

Condoms have been proven to be effective against HIV transmission,[83] but condom use is usually low in marriage and other long-term stable partnerships. Access to condoms is still low, and UNAIDS estimates there is only 19% condom coverage in sub-Saharan Africa.[69] Female condoms, which have the potential for providing a female-controlled prevention method, have been insufficiently programmed and scaled up for population impact.

Condoms, of course, also protect against other STIs. Control and treatment of STIs is an important strategy to prevent HIV; however, treatment is likely to be more effective when the epidemic has not yet become generalized. In a generalized epidemic, STIs are less important as facilitators of HIV. In many countries where genital herpes (HSV2) is the dominant STI, it is not yet clear what treatment will reduce the risk of HIV from this infection. HSV2 has emerged as a major risk factor for HIV transmission and acquisition.

Voluntary Medical Male Circumcision

Three trials in South Africa, Kenya, and Uganda were stopped early because they demonstrated a protective effect for men ranging from 50% to 75%. There is a further trial in Uganda examining the effect of voluntary medical male circumcision (VMMC) on HIV/ infected men, and there is also some evidence of the protective effect of circumcision on male-to-female transmission.[84–86]

Voluntary Counseling and Testing and HIV Testing and Counseling

Voluntary counseling and testing (VCT) has been the mainstay prevention strategy in much of sub-Saharan Africa, even in the absence of ART. However, aside from being effective for couples, and possibly for HIV-positive persons, its efficacy on a population-wide basis is not clear. With more widely available treatment programs, VCT has become important as an entry point for such programs and for the prevention of maternal-to-child transmission of HIV.

In health facilities, the standard has become "opt-out" testing, HIV testing and counseling (HTC). As part of care, patients are routinely tested for HIV. For example, in antenatal care, sexually transmitted disease, and TB clinic settings, clients are tested unless they specifically request not to be. HTC has been enormously important in increasing the number of people diagnosed with HIV and getting them into care.

Treatment as Prevention

A landmark trial, HPTN 052, demonstrated the efficacy of antiretroviral (ARV) drug therapy as a prevention strategy. Participants who were enrolled on ARV as soon as they were diagnosed showed a 96% reduction in transmission of HIV to their sexual partner.[87] Subsequently, treatment guidelines are being revised, with recommendations, for example, that all pregnant HIV-positive women be placed on ARV for life irrespective of CD4 count, and calls for all HIV-positive people to be placed on ARV. However, with only 54% of the people who need it currently on ART and with the weak health care systems and funding gaps, it is unclear that this is the most effective strategy. Moreover, the health benefits of enrolling people with CD4 counts higher than 500 on ART are unknown, as 052 demonstrated a clear benefit only for participants with CD4 counts of 200 to 500. The START trial findings are likely to be available in 2015 and should provide information to answer this question.[88]

Behavior Change Interventions

Mass media approaches and certain curriculum-based HIV and sex education designs for in-school youth are effective in producing behavior change among young people.[89] Behavior change approaches should be theory driven. The theories range from those that are individually focused (i.e., the health belief model and the theory of reasoned action/planned behavior)[90]

to those that focus on groups and communities (i.e., the ecological model and the theory of the diffusion of innovations).[91] The theory of reasoned action/ planned behavior emphasizes beliefs, attitudes, intentions, and subjective norms as important in behavior, whereas the diffusion of innovations theory, which seeks to explain how new ideas and practices spread in a community, gives attention to knowledge, persuasion, decision making, implementation, and confirmation. A number of theories are used in combination in developing behavior change approaches.

Microbicides

Microbicides have generated a lot of interest, particularly as a female-controlled prevention method that, unlike the female condom and to some extent the diaphragm, is invisible to the partner. Until 2000, there was excitement that microbicides would soon become an important HIV prevention tool because there was an effective candidate product: nonoxynol-9. However, studies showed that nonoxynol-9 irritated the vagina and hence had the potential to increase HIV transmission.[92] This product was subsequently abandoned. Work continued on other candidate microbicides, and in 2010 a South African trial (CAPRISA 004) announced that a microbicide containing 1% tenofovir gel reduced HIV acquisition by an overall 39% among women who received the gel compared with women who received a placebo gel.[93]

Combination Prevention

Recently, combination prevention has engendered significant support. Combination prevention was defined by UNAIDS as programs that are "rights-based, evidence-informed, and community-owned programmes that use a mix of biomedical, behavioral, and structural interventions, prioritized to meet the current HIV prevention needs of particular individuals and communities so as to have the greatest sustained impact on reducing new infections."[94] PEPFAR, the largest funder of HIV and AIDS services in the world, supports combination prevention interventions such as Treatment as Prevention, PMTCT, HTC, condoms, male circumcision (VMMC), and Prevention for Key Populations (Most at-Risk Populations) such as IDUs, MSMs, and CSWs.

Role of Advocacy

Advocacy—lobbying or campaigning for a particular decision or perspective—is extremely important in HIV/AIDS prevention. It involves information, education, and communication strategies; groups and individuals to partner with or lobby; and a position or decision to advocate. Individuals or groups who are highly visible, organized, networked, and influential can be powerful advocates. Uganda was able to reduce

---

BOX 10-2. ACCESSING HIV/AIDS CARE IN LOW- AND MIDDLE-INCOME COUNTRIES: SOME OF THE CHALLENGES

Tandi came to the clinic because she was experiencing a chronic cough she had had for some time. She had lost a lot of weight—her bones were beginning to stick out—and she had had a skin disease, the marks of which were still visible over her face and much of her upper body. She had a fever and felt sick. To be able to come to the clinic, she had borrowed money for the fee. After waiting 2 hours, she was finally seen by the sister-in-charge.

After examination, the sister-in-charge referred her to the hospital, where she would be seen by a doctor. The sister-in-charge wanted to call an ambulance for her because she was concerned that Tandi was too weak and ill to go on her own. Tandi refused, however, for she did not have money to pay the ambulance. Instead, she would take the cheaper public transport even though she would have to take two buses. When Tandi eventually got to the hospital, it was nearly evening. She had to queue again, and pay again. Tandi waited in the queue for 3 hours.

When a doctor examined her, he told her that he needed to order some tests for her to see how well her body's defense (immune) system was functioning and to find out what was causing her cough. He told her the likely costs of these tests. However, Tandi had already spent all the money she had borrowed. In fact, she had been hoping that she could save some of it to buy food for herself and her two children, ages 6 and 10. The doctor then gave her a prescription for some medicines, which included an antibiotic called Bactrim. At the hospital pharmacy, they only had the Bactrim. They told Tandi to go and buy the other medicines. Tandi then set off home, walking, because she had no more money.

Two days later, after the neighbors had found her collapsed in bed, she was taken back to the hospital. The neighbors and friends had made a collection for her, which helped to pay for the hospital stay. When Tandi came out she was better. She had gained some weight, and the cough had become a little better. Her relatives and friends felt that she should go to her aunt in a rural area because the rent was due for her room and she could not pay for it. They hoped in the rural area she could go to a mission hospital where the fees were not as expensive.

---

its HIV infection rate because of the visible commitment of its president, together with a multisectoral approach and widespread societal involvement.[95] Advocacy is often linked to policy development, articulation, and implementation. Policies are frameworks that guide decision making. For example, policies on HIV and IDUs may include strategies for needle exchange or the provision of bleach to clean the injection equipment. A policy may also exist whereby all newly diagnosed TB patients are screened for HIV.

HIV/AIDS Programs

In many countries, nongovernmental organizations (NGOs) were the first to begin to respond to the HIV epidemic. Although many governments have begun to roll out prevention and treatment programs, HIV/AIDS prevention, and to some extent treatment, still remains a major focus for NGOs. However, governments are ultimately responsible for the well-being of their people. HIV/AIDS programs should meet the following criteria:

1. **The program should work within the framework of the national AIDS control program.** The national AIDS prevention and control bodies vary from country to country. Some countries have a national AIDS control program within the

Ministry of Health (MoH), where the functions of AIDS control are largely focused on program logistics and technical aspects. Other countries have tried to promote a multisectoral approach and tried to engage a range of stakeholders, including civil society, which are formed into a board of a coordinating agency that is a separate entity. The board directs and oversees the work of the executive director and his staff. In this model, a major function of the coordinating body, in addition to coordination, is advocacy. The actual programs (e.g., condom promotion) remain in the relevant section of the MoH.

Since 2004, UNAIDS has been promoting the Three Ones principle:

- One agreed-upon HIV/AIDS action framework that forms the basis for the partners working together
- One national AIDS coordinating authority, which has a broad-based multisectoral mandate
- One agreed-upon country-level monitoring and evaluation system

2. **All programs should have monitoring (assessment of whether and how the program activities are being carried out) and evaluation (assessment**

of the extent to which the programs are likely to make an impact) components. This means that there should be a baseline assessment before the program is implemented. Sometimes this has not been the case, and subsequently there were attempts, usually not very satisfactory, to evaluate this retroactively. The monitoring and evaluation system should fit into the national monitoring and evaluating system.

3. **To optimize the impact of any prevention control and treatment program, there should be a number of interventions implemented at the same time.** These should include voluntary counseling and testing (especially as an entry point to ART); ongoing counseling facilities and support groups; and information, education, and communication (IEC). Depending on the target groups, the IEC should involve abstinence, being faithful to one mutually faithful partner, and/or correct and consistent condom use. There should also be a sexually transmitted disease treatment and control intervention. If the target population includes women of childbearing age, there will be a need for a PMTCT program. Stigma continues to blight HIV/AIDS activities, and in some instances TB control, and efforts should be made to reduce stigma through advocacy activities, the support of opinion leaders and decision makers, and efforts to encourage greater openness.

4. **Especially in high-prevalence areas, there is a need for strong links with the TB control program.** Screening for TB as a standard procedure among individuals who test positive for HIV is being actively considered, as is screening for HIV among people who are found to have TB. In both instances, treatment should be available.

5. **In areas where there are high levels of AIDS-related illness and death, prevention, control, and treatment programs should be linked to mitigation activities.** These activities include home-based care for persons living with HIV/AIDS (PLWH) including discharge planning and links to hospital care services, orphan care, nutrition support, income generation activities, and poverty alleviation.

HIV/AIDS AND TUBERCULOSIS: TWO DISEASES, ONE PATIENT

The links between TB and HIV are well established. HIV has been an important driver of the TB epidemic in much of the world, especially in sub-Saharan Africa, and increasingly in Asia and South America. TB is the leading cause of morbidity and mortality among those with HIV infection. The overlap has resulted in the phrase "two diseases, one patient" to

remind health care workers that although health services may be administered by separate disease control programs, they may be treating the same patient.

Tuberculosis and HIV appear to enjoy a dangerous biologic synergy. Untreated HIV results in progressive immunodeficiency that predominantly affects cell-mediated immunity, which increases the risk for developing OIs such as TB. As immune suppression from HIV progresses, so does the frequency and severity of OIs, which are associated with overall increased mortality rates. In recent years, it has also been shown that HIV-infected individuals with TB disease had higher adjusted mortality rates and incidence of non-TB OIs than HIV-infected individuals who did not have active TB.[96] It has been postulated that the immune activation induced by TB leads to a burst of HIV replication and, subsequently, irreversible, accelerated HIV disease progression. Thus TB and HIV participate in a negative feedback loop, each negatively affecting the other.

Recognizing this undeniable overlap and the need for a coordinated response to both epidemics, in 2002 the Strategic Framework to Decrease the Burden of TB/HIV was developed. In the document reporting this framework, it was acknowledged that "tackling tuberculosis should include tackling HIV as the most potent force driving the tuberculosis epidemic; [similarly,] tackling HIV should include tackling tuberculosis as a leading killer of PLWH."[97] This seminal manual has been followed by several others over the years to provide policy guidance and implementation guidelines for collaborative TB/HIV activities.

The key concepts of a coordinated TB/HIV strategy include the following: (1) establishing mechanisms for collaboration at the policy and planning levels and for integrated delivery of TB and HIV services, and conducting surveillance of patients with TB/HIV co-disease; (2) decreasing the TB burden among PLWH by intensified screening for TB, initiating early ART, and using isoniazid preventive therapy among PLWH; and (3) decreasing the burden of HIV among TB patients by provider-initiated HIV testing of those diagnosed with TB, counseling about HIV prevention, and ensuring HIV care and support.[98,99] Guidelines that describe what joint TB/HIV activities to implement, how to implement them, and by whom are available from WHO to support national TB control and HIV/AIDS control program managers in operationalizing this strategy.

Establishing Mechanisms for Collaboration on Controlling Tuberculosis and HIV

Collaboration between the national programs for TB control and HIV/AIDS control should occur at every level—from the central offices at the national level down to the district or facility level. At the national level, joint coordinating and planning bodies or committees should exist. Surveillance to capture the HIV prevalence among TB patients should be conducted. Evidence of joint activities at the facility level, where a student is most likely to encounter the product(s) of joint planning and coordination, may be through integrated and, ideally, seamless services for patients with TB and HIV provided at the same location and time. Care that is fragmented suggests a lack of adequate planning and coordination from control program managers.

Decreasing the Burden of Tuberculosis in People Living with HIV/AIDS

Intensifying case finding for TB in practical terms is usually done through routine screening of HIV-infected persons for active TB at the time of their HIV diagnosis. WHO recommends screening adults and adolescents living with HIV using a clinical algorithm that assesses for current cough, fever, weight loss or night sweats; patients that report one or more of these symptoms should be evaluated for TB and other diseases.[100] Similarly, children living with HIV should be screened for poor weight gain, fever or current cough, and for a history of contact with a TB case.[100] The value of routine collection of sputum samples for smears and cultures is also being studied. Screening for TB should be performed at every medical visit at either the HIV testing center or by referring the patient to a TB diagnostic site.

PLWH in whom active TB has been excluded are often tested for latent TB infection (LTBI) by TST. Currently, the WHO recommends that HIV-infected adults, adolescents, and children over 12 months of age who have an unknown or positive TST status and are unlikely to have active TB should receive at least 6 months of isoniazid preventive therapy (IPT) to decrease the risk of TB infection progressing to TB disease.[100] Provision of IPT is now considered a part of comprehensive HIV care. The duration of benefit from IPT is limited to approximately 2.5 years,[101] most likely due to recurrent reinfection in TB-endemic settings.

Infection control measures to reduce the risk of TB transmission in health care and congregate settings (e.g., prisons, military barracks) are recommended. Mechanisms to recognize suspected cases of TB and promptly diagnose and initiate treatment among those confirmed are essential to reducing TB transmission. Separation of people suspected of having TB from others (particularly HIV-infected persons) until a diagnosis can be confirmed is an effective, and generally feasible, option. Whenever possible, natural ventilation should be maximized. Every health care and congregate setting should develop and implement its own infection

control plan. The WHO provides guidelines for national and subnational TB infection control activities and for implementing practical infection control measures in health care facilities.

Decreasing the Burden of HIV Among Tuberculosis Patients

Many patients do not know their HIV status at the time they are diagnosed with TB. In settings where the HIV prevalence among TB patients is greater than 5%, patients diagnosed with active TB disease should receive provider-initiated HIV testing (i.e., it is provided as the standard of care, and patients must decline testing). Health care workers for TB control programs should include HIV prevention methods and education to reduce sexual, parenteral, and vertical transmission of HIV as part of their routine care or make appropriate referrals. Cotrimoxazole preventive therapy to prevent secondary bacterial and parasitic infections is also recommended by the WHO for HIV-infected adults and children. Specifically, cotrimoxazole preventive therapy has been shown to reduce mortality rates in HIV-infected TB patients.[102] HIV-infected TB patients should have access to general HIV/AIDS care and support, which includes clinical management (prophylaxis, diagnosis, treatment, and follow-up for OIs), nursing care (promoting hygiene and nutrition), palliative care, home care (including education for household members), counseling, and social support.

All HIV-infected TB patients should be started on ART soon after starting TB treatment. Co-treatment of TB disease and HIV is complicated by drug–drug interactions between certain anti-TB medications and ARVs (see later).

Treating Tuberculosis and HIV/AIDS Together

In PLWH who are diagnosed with TB and not yet on ART (as often occurs when TB and HIV are diagnosed simultaneously), the priority is to initiate treatment for TB. While the optimal time to start ART is unclear at present, recent clinical data suggest earlier initiation of ART (within 2 to 4 weeks after starting TB treatment) is associated with decreased HIV disease progression[103] and lower mortality.[104] If indicated, treatment for both HIV and TB can be started concomitantly, but careful management is needed.

Co-treatment of HIV-associated TB requires careful management due to drug–drug interactions between rifampin and some NNRTIs and protease inhibitors (PIs). Specifically, rifampin stimulates the cytochrome P450 liver enzyme system that metabolizes NNRTIs and PIs and therefore can lead to decreased blood levels of NNRTIs and PIs. Similarly, NNRTIs and PIs can activate or inhibit this enzyme system, leading to altered levels of rifampin. The results can be higher or lower blood levels of these medications, causing ineffective, suboptimal therapeutic levels or increased risk for drug toxicity. When anti-TB treatment and ART are used concomitantly, TB can be treated with a rifampin-containing regimen and ART should include efavirenz and two NRTIs.

When a patient with HIV-associated TB who has been started on ART and TB treatment simultaneously experiences a paradoxical worsening with exacerbation of symptoms, signs, or radiographic manifestations of TB, immune reconstitution inflammatory syndrome should be suspected. This paradoxical reaction occurs from a reconstitution of the immune system and may be accompanied by a high fever, lymphadenopathy, expanding central nervous system lesions, and worsening of chest x-ray findings.[105] Other possible causes (including TB treatment failure) must be excluded in the evaluation. Prednisone may be helpful in severe paradoxical reactions, although evidence to support its use is lacking.

STUDY QUESTIONS

1. What are the pros and cons of currently available diagnostic tests for TB?
2. Why is TB treatment difficult to complete?
3. What are the main challenges today to controlling TB globally?
4. Why is the prevention of HIV/AIDS of such significant public health importance in transitional and low- and middle-income countries?
5. What are the policy and operational issues in PMTCT and ART rollout in low- and middle-income countries?
6. What HIV/AIDS prevention strategies are likely to be effective in countries without a generalized epidemic?

RESOURCES

International Tuberculosis Organizations

- WHO, Stop TB Department: www.who.int/gtb/.
- Stop TB Partnership: www.stoptb.org/.
- International Union Against Tuberculosis and Lung Disease (The Union): www.theunion.org.
- KNCV Tuberculosis Foundation: www.kncvtbc.nl/Site/ Professional.aspx.
- The Global Fund to Fight AIDS, Tuberculosis and Malaria: www.theglobalfund.org.

Selected Tuberculosis Literature

- An Expanded DOTS Framework for Effective Tuberculosis Control (WHO/CDS/TB/2002.297) http://www.who.int/gtb/publications/dots/index.htm.
- Global Tuberculosis Control 2011 (WHO/HTM/TB/2011.16) http://www.who.int/tb/country/en/index.html.
- The Global Plan to Stop TB 2006–2015 and 2011–2015 http://www.stoptb.org/global/plan/.
- The Stop TB Strategy: Building on and enhancing DOTS to meet the TB-related Millennium Development Goals http://whqlibdoc.who.int/hq/2006/WHO_HTM_STB_2006.368_eng.pdf.
- Treatment of Tuberculosis Guidelines, 4th ed. (WHO/HTM/TB/2009.420). http://whqlibdoc.who.int/publications/2010/9789241547833_eng.pdf.
- Management of Tuberculosis: A Guide to the Essentials of Good Clinical Practice, Technical Consultants of The Union, 6th ed., 2010. http://www.theunion.org/index.php?id=158&cid=44&fid=57&task=download&option=com_flexicontent&Itemid=70&lang=en.
- WHO policy on collaborative TB/HIV activities: guidelines for national programmes and other stakeholders (WHO/HTM/TB/2012.1, WHO/HIV/2012.1). http://whqlibdoc.who.int/publications/2012/9789241503006_eng.pdf.
- Guidelines for intensified tuberculosis case-finding and isoniazid preventive therapy for people living with HIV in resource-constrained settings. http://www.who.int/tb/challenges/hiv/ICF_IPTguidelines/en/index.html.
- Implementing Collaborative TB-HIV Activities: A Programmatic Guide, P. I. Fujiwara, R. A. Dlodlo, O. Ferroussier, et al, 2012. http://www.theunion.org/index.php?id=758&cid=2091&fid=57&task=download&option=com_flexicontent&Itemid=70&lang=en.
- Multidrug and extensively drug-resistant TB (M/XDR-TB): 2010 global report on surveillance and response (WHO/HTM/TB/2010.3). http://whqlibdoc.who.int/publications/2010/9789241599191_eng.pdf.
- Anti-tuberculosis drug resistance in the world, Report no. 4 (WHO/HTM/TB/2008.394). http://whqlibdoc.who.int/hq/2008/WHO_HTM_TB_2008.394_eng.pdf.

Selected HIV/AIDS WebSites

- AIDS Action (USA): www.aidsaction.org. A network of 3,200 AIDS service organizations sharing information and experiences.

- AIDS and Africa: www.aidsafrica.com.
  Provides wide-ranging information on HIV/AIDS in Africa.
- AIDSETI (AIDS Empowerment and Treatment Initiative):
  http://www.usdfa.org/index.cfm?views=Proj_Aidseti.
  An international activist organization, with two-thirds of its membership living with HIV. It advocates and lobbies for increased treatment access.
- Centers for Disease Control and Prevention (US Department of Health and Human Services):www.cdc.gov.
  Focuses on health and treatment-related issues and surveillance.
- Education International: http://old.ei-ie.org/efaids/en/index.php.
  Dedicated to school health and HIV/AIDS prevention, documenting the widespread ideas and experiences of Education International and its partners.
- Family Health International: www.fhi.org.
  Works to improve reproductive and family health around the world.
  Global AIDS Alliance (GAA): www.globalaidsalliance.org.
  A transnational alliance of partner organizations.
- Global AIDS Interfaith Alliance: www.thegaia.org.
  Facilitates HIV prevention strategies in developing countries through religious and interfaith organizations.
- Global Fund to Fight HIV/AIDS, Tuberculosis and Malaria: www.globalfundatm.org.
  International funding mechanism to expand the response to these diseases.
- Global Health Council: www.globalhealth.org/.
  The world's largest membership alliance dedicated to improving health worldwide.
- Health Economics and HIV/AIDS Research Division, Natal University: www.heard.org.za/.
  Undertakes research, publication, policy analysis, planning, and information services on socioeconomic development and HIV/AIDS. In particular, produced AIDS Briefs and AIDS Toolkits on HIV/AIDS and sectoral impacts and responses that can be downloaded from the Web.
- Health link Worldwide (formerly AHRTAG): www.healthlink.org.uk.
  Works to improve the health of poor and vulnerable communities by strengthening the provision, use, and impact of information.
- International AIDS Economic Network (IAEN): www.iaen.org.
  Provides analysis on the economics of HIV/AIDS prevention and treatment in developing countries.
- International AIDS Vaccine Initiative: www.iavi.org.
  AIDS vaccine advocacy coalition.

- International Association of Physicians in AIDS Care: www.iapac.org.
  Provides information on clinical management and public health policy.
- International Centre for Research on Women: www.icrw.org.
  Works to improve the lives of women in poverty, advance women's equality and human rights, and contribute to economic and social well-being.
- International Labour Organisation: www.ilo.org.
  Labor organization of the United Nations (UN), with a focus on HIV/AIDS and the world of work.
- Programme for Appropriate Technology in Health: www.path.org.
  International nonprofit organization to improve health, especially the health of women and children.
- SAfAIDS (Southern Africa HIV and AIDS Information Dissemination Service): www.safaids.net.
  Information service on HIV/AIDS in southern Africa.
- Save the Children UK: www.savethechildren.org.uk.
  Supports children in need and is prioritizing HIV/AIDS. The Website introduces the organization's work. Among other publications, it has produced *Learning to Live: Monitoring and Evaluating HIV/AIDS Programmes for Your People,* a wide-ranging practical handbook for policymakers and practitioners.
- Teaching-aids at Low Cost: www.talcuk.org.
  Provides low-cost materials on HIV/AIDS regarding wide-ranging development issues, with a catalog of books, slides, videos, and participatory teaching aids.
- UNAIDS: www.unaids.org.
  UN coordination agency on HIV/AIDS to lead, strengthen, and support an expanded response to the epidemic; extensive links to UNAIDS, cosponsors, and many other Websites on wide-ranging areas of focus; UNAIDS publications include the Best Practice Collection series with Technical Updates, Case Studies, and Key Materials.
- UNDP (UN Development Programme): www.undp.org.
  Development agency of the UN, with an HIV/AIDS program concerning human rights, poverty, and development.
- UNODC (UN Office on Drugs and Crime): www.unodc.org.
  The drug control arm of the UN, including a focus on intravenous drug use and HIV/AIDS.
- UNESCO: www.unesco.org.
  UN focal agency for education, science, and culture, with wide-ranging publications and information on these areas, including a focus on HIV/AIDS.
- UNFPA (UN Population Fund): www.unfpa.org.
  Focus on sexual and reproductive health and population and development; publications include the

annual State of the World's Population and a series of HIV Prevention Briefs.

- UNICEF: www.unicef.org.
  UN's children's fund, with a strong focus on HIV/AIDS and children, including parent-to-child transmission; publications include the annual update State of the Children.

- UNIFEM: www.unwomen.org.
  Works to promote gender equity and equality and women's rights; focuses on gender issues and HIV/AIDS.

- World Health Organization: www.who.org.
  Health agency of the UN, with wide-ranging information related to health care, surveillance, transmission and prevention, voluntary counseling and testing, and other areas.

- World Bank: www.worldbank.org.
  Apart from a wide focus on economic development and HIV/AIDS, the World Bank has a multicountry HIV/AIDS Program for Africa (MAP). MAP aims to significantly increase access to HIV/AIDS prevention care and treatment programs.

- Youth Against AIDS: http://youthagainstaids.wordpress.com.
  Global network of support for young AIDS activists.

REFERENCES

1. World Health Organization. *Global Tuberculosis Control: WHO Report 2011.* Geneva: WHO, 2011. WHO/HTM/TB/2011.16.

2. World Health Organization. *Tuberculosis, Fact Sheet No. 104,* March 2012. http://www.who.int/mediacentre/factsheets/fs104/en/.

3. Centers for Disease Control and Prevention. Emergence of *Mycobacterium tuberculosis* with extensive resistance to second-line drugs—worldwide, 2000–2004. *MMWR* 2006;55(11):301–305.

4. World Health Organization. *Towards Universal Access to Diagnosis and Treatment of Multidrug-Resistant and Extensively Drug-Resistant Tuberculosis by 2015: WHO Progress Report 2011.* Geneva: WHO, 2011. WHO/HTM/TB/2011.3.

5. World Health Organization, UNAIDS, UN Children's Fund. *Progress Report 2011. Global HIV/AIDS Response. Epidemic Update and Health Sector progress towards Universal Access.* Geneva: WHO/UNAIDS/UNICEF, November 2011. http://www.unaids.org/en/media/unaids/contentassets/documents/unaidspublication/2011/20111130_ua_report_en.pdf.

6. Raviglione MC, O'Brien RJ. Tuberculosis. In: Long D, Fauci A, Kasper DL, et al., eds. *Harrison's Principles of Internal Medicine.* 18th ed. New York: McGraw-Hill, 2012: 1340.

7. World Health Organization. *Treatment of Tuberculosis Guidelines.* 4th ed. Geneva: WHO, 2010. WHO/HTM/TB/2009.420.

8. World Health Organization. WHO endorses new rapid tuberculosis test: A major milestone for global TB diagnosis and care [news release], December 8, 2010. http://www.who.int/mediacentre/news/releases/2010/tb_test_20101208/en/index.html.

9. Boehme CC, Nabeta P, Hillemann D, et al. Rapid molecular detection of tuberculosis and rifampin resistance. *N Engl J Med* 2010;363(11):1005–1015.

10. World Health Organization. WHO monitoring of Xpert MTB/RIF roll-out. http://www.who.int/tb/laboratory/mtbrifrollout/en/index.html.

11. Lalvani A, Pathan AA, McShane H, et al. Rapid detection of *Mycobacterium tuberculosis* infection by enumeration of antigen-specific T cells. *Am J Respir Crit Care Med* 2001;163(4):824–828.

12. Mazurek GH, LoBue PA, Daley CL, et al. Comparison of a whole-blood interferon gamma assay with tuberculin skin testing for detecting latent *Mycobacterium tuberculosis* infection. *JAMA* 2001;286(14):1740–1747.

13. World Health Organization. Safety of BCG vaccine in HIV-infected children. *Wkly Epidemiol Record* 2007;82(3):17–24.

14. Colditz GA, Brewer TF, Berkey CS. Efficacy of BCG vaccine in the prevention of tuberculosis: meta-analysis of the published literature. *JAMA* 1994;271(9):698–702.

15. Larkin JM, von Reyn CF. BCG and new vaccines against tuberculosis. In: Schlossberg D, ed. *Tuberculosis and Nontuberculosis Mycobacterial Infections.* 5th ed. New York: McGraw-Hill, 2006:117–122.

16. Hesseling AC, Rabie H, Marais BJ, et al. Bacille Calmette-Guerin vaccine induced disease in HIV infected and HIV uninfected children. *Clin Infect Dis* 2006;42(4):548–558.

17. Jasmer RM, Seaman CB, Gonzalez LC, et al. Tuberculosis treatment outcomes: directly observed therapy compared with self-administered therapy. *Am J Respir Crit Care Med* 2004;170(5):561–566.

18. Médecins Sans Frontières. *Running Out of Breath? TB Care in the 21st Century.* Geneva: Médecins Sans Frontières, March 2004.

19. Pope DS, Chaisson RE. TB treatment: as simple as DOT? *Int J Tuberc Lung Dis* 2003;7(7):611–615.

20. Zwarenstein M, Schoeman JH, Vundule C, et al. Randomised controlled trial of self-supervised and directly observed treatment of tuberculosis. *Lancet* 1998;352(9137):1340–1343.

21. STOP TB Partnership and World Health Organization. *The STOP TB Strategy: Building and Enhancing DOTS to Meet the TB-Related Millennium Development Goals.* Geneva: WHO, 2006. WHO/HTM/STB/2006.37.

22. World Health Organization. *The Global Plan to Stop TB 2011–2015: Transforming the Fight Towards Elimination of Tuberculosis.* Geneva: WHO, 2010.

23. Stop TB Partnership and World Health Organization. *Global Plan to Stop TB 2006–2015: Actions for Life Towards a World Free of Tuberculosis.* Geneva: WHO, 2006. WHO/HTM/STB/2006.35.

24. World Health Organization/International Union Against Tuberculosis and Lung Disease Global Project on Anti-Tuberculosis Drug Resistance Surveillance. *Anti-Tuberculosis Drug Resistance in the World: Fourth Global Report.* Geneva: WHO, 2008,WHO/HTM/TB/2008.394.

25. Iseman MD. MDR-TB and the developing world—a problem no longer to be ignored: the WHO announces 'DOTS Plus' strategy. *Int J Tuberc Lung Dis* 1998;2(11):867.

26. World Health Organization. *Guidelines for the Programmatic Management of Drug-Resistant Tuberculosis.* Geneva: WHO, 2006. WHO/HTM/TB/2006.361.

27. Gandhi NR, Moll A, Sturm AW, et al. Extensively drug-resistant tuberculosis as a cause of death in patients co-infected

with tuberculosis and HIV in a rural area of South Africa. *Lancet* 2006;368:1575–1580.

28. Shah NS, Wright A, Bai GH, et al. Worldwide emergence of extensively drug-resistant tuberculosis. *Emerg Infect Dis* 2007; 13(3):380–387.

29. Velayati AA, Masjedi MR, Farnia P, et al. Emergence of new forms of totally drug-resistant tuberculosis bacilli: super extensively drug-resistant tuberculosis of totally drug-resistant strain in Iran. *Chest* 2009;136:420–425.

30. Udwadia ZF, Amale RA, AjbaniKK, Rodrigues C. Totally drug-resistant tuberculosis in India. *Clin Infect Dis* 2012; 54(4):579–581.

31. World Health Organization. WHO Stop TB Department. Drug-resistant tuberculosis, Frequently Asked Questions, January 2012. http://www.who.int/tb/challenges/mdr/tdrfaqs/en/.

32. World Health Organization. *World Health Statistics 2012*. Geneva: WHO, 2012.

33. World Health Organization. *Addressing Poverty in TB Control—Options for National TB Control Programmes*. Geneva: WHO, 2005. WHO/HTM/TB/2005.352.

34. Stop TB Department and Department of Chronic Diseases and Health Promotion, World Health Organization, and the International Union Against Tuberculosis and Lung Disease. *Collaborative Framework for Care and Control of Tuberculosis and Diabetes*. Geneva: WHO, 2011. WHO/HTM/TB/2011.15.

35. World Health Organization. *Pathways to Better Diagnostics for Tuberculosis: A Blueprint for the Development of TB Diagnostics*. Geneva: WHO and New Diagnostics Working Group of the Stop TB Partnership, 2009.

36. US Food and Drug Administration. FDA News Release, December 2012. http://www.fda.gov/NewsEvents/Newsroom/PressAnnouncements/ucm333695.htm.

37. Andries K, Verhasselt P, Guillemont J, et al. A diarylquinoline drug active on the ATP synthase of *Mycobacterium tuberculosis*. *Science* 2005;307:223–227.

38. Gler MT, Skripconoka V, Sanchez-Garavito E, et al. Delamanid for multidrug-resistant pulmonary tuberculosis. *N Engl J Med* 2012;366:2151–2160.

39. Diacon AH, Dawson R, von Groote-Bidlingmaier F, et al. 14-day bactericidal activity of PA-824, bedaquiline, pyrazinamide, and moxifloxacin combination: a randomised trial. *Lancet* 2012;380(9846):986–993.

40. Kaufmann SH. Fact and fiction in tuberculosis vaccine research: 10 years later. *Lancet Infect Dis* 2011;11(8):633–640.

41. von Reyn CF, Mtei L, Arbeit RD, et al, for the DarDar Study Group. Prevention of tuberculosis in Bacille Calmette-Guérin-primed, HIV-infected adults boosted with an inactivated whole-cell mycobacterial vaccine. *AIDS* 2010; 24(5): 675–685.

42. Perez-Velez CM, Marais BJ. Tuberculosis in children. *N Engl J Med* 2012;367(4):348–361.

43. STOP TB Partnership. Call to Action for Childhood TB. http://www.stoptb.org/getinvolved/ctb_cta.asp.

44. Gottlieb MS, Schorff R, Schanker HM, et al. *Pneumocystis carinii* pneumonia and mucosal candidiasis in previously healthy homosexual men: evidence of a new acquired cellular immunodeficiency. *N Engl J Med* 1981;305:1425–1431.

45. Masur H, Michelis MA, Greene JB, et al. An outbreak of community-acquired *Pneumocystis carinii* pneumonia: initial manifestation of cellular immune dysfunction. *N Engl J Med* 1981;305:1431–1438.

46. Siegal FP, Lopez, C, Hammer GS, et al. Severe acquired immunodeficiency in male homosexuals, manifested by chronic perianal ulcerative herpes simplex lesions. *N Engl J Med* 1981; 305:1439–1444.

47. CDC Task Force on Kaposi's Sarcoma and Opportunistic Infections. Epidemiologic aspects of the current outbreak of Kaposi's sarcoma and opportunistic infections. *N Engl J Med* 1982;306:248–252.

48. Davis KC, Horsburgh CR Jr, Hasiba U, et al. Acquired immunodeficiency syndrome in a patient with hemophilia. *Ann Intern Med* 1983;98:284–286.

49. Poon MC, Landay A, Prasthofer EF, et al. Acquired immunodeficiency syndrome with *Pneumocystis carinii* pneumonia and *Mycobacterium avium-intracellulare* infection in a previously healthy patient with dings. *Ann Intern Med* 1983; 98:287–290.

50. Elliott JL, Hoppes WL, Platt MS, et al. The acquired immunodeficiency syndrome and *Mycobacterium avium-intracellulare* bacteremia in a patient with hemophilia. *Ann Intern Med* 1983;98:290–293.

51. Curran JW, Lawrence DN, Jaffe H, et al. Acquired immunodeficiency syndrome (AIDS) associated with transfusions. *N Engl J Med* 1984;310:69–75.

52. Jaffe HW, Francis DP, McLane MF, et al. Transfusion-associated AIDS: serological evidence of human T-cell leukemia virus infection of donors. *Science* 1984;223:1309–1312.

53. Oleske J, Minnefor A, Cooper R Jr, et al. Immune deficiency syndrome in children. *JAMA* 1983;249:2345–2349.

54. Rubinstein A, Sicklick M, Gupta A, et al. Acquired immunodeficiency with reversed T4/T8 ratios in infants born to promiscuous and drug-addicted mothers. *JAMA* 1983; 249:2350–2356.

55. Clumeck N, Mascart-Lemone F, de Maubeuge J, et al. Acquired immune deficiency syndrome in black Africans. *Lancet* 1983;1:642.

56. Francis DP, Curran JW, Essex M. Epidemic acquired immune deficiency syndrome: epidemiologic evidence for a transmissible agent. *J Natl Cancer Inst* 1983;71:1–4.

57. Essex M, McLane MF, Lee TH, et al. Antibodies to cell membrane antigens associated with human T-cell leukemia virus in patients with AIDS. *Science* 1983;220:859–862.

58. Gelmann EP, Popovic M, Blayney D, et al. Proviral DNA of a retrovirus, human T-cell leukemia virus, in two patients with AIDS. *Science* 1983;220:862–865.

59. Essex M, McLane MF, Lee TH, et al. Antibodies to human T-cell leukemia virus membrane antigens (HTLV-MA) in hemophiliacs. *Science* 1983;221:1061–1064.

60. Gallo RC, Sarin PS, Gelmann EP, et al. Isolation of human T-cell leukemia virus in acquired immune deficiency syndrome (AIDS). *Science* 1983;220:865–867.

61. Barre-Sinoussi F, Chermann JC, Rey F, et al. Isolation of a T-lymphotropic retrovirus from a patient at risk for acquired immune deficiency syndrome (AIDS). *Science* 1983;220:868–871.

62. Kanki PJ, Hamel DJ, Sankale JL, et al. Human immunodeficiency virus type 1 subtypes differ in disease progression. *J Infect Dis* 1999;179:68–73.

63. Laeyendecker O, Li X, Arroyo M, et al. The effect of HIV subtype on rapid disease progression in Rakai, Uganda.

Abstract 44 LB. Presented at: 13th Conference on Retroviruses and Opportunistic Infections, February 2006.

64. Jackson H. *AIDS Africa: Continent in Crisis*. Harare, Zimbabwe: Southern Africa HIV/AIDS Information, 2002.

65. World Health Organization. *Clinical Guidelines for HIV/AIDS*. Geneva: WHO, 2002.

66. Guay LA, Musoke P, Fleming T, et al. Intrapartum and neonatal nevirapine compared with zidovudine for prevention of maternal to child transmission of HIV-1 in Kampala, Uganda: HIVNET 012 randomised trial. *Lancet* 1999;354:795–802.

67. World Health Organization. *Antiretroviral Drugs for Treating Pregnant Women and Preventing HIV Infections in Infants: Recommendations for a Public Health Approach*, 2010 version. Geneva: WHO, 2010. http://www.who.int/hiv/pub/mtct/guidelines/en/.

68. World Health Organization. *Programmatic Update: Executive Summary of the Use of Antiretroviral Drugs for Treating Pregnant Women and Preventing HIV Infection in Infants*. Geneva: WHO, April 2012. http://www.who.int/hiv/pub/mtct/programmatic_update2012/en/.

69. Joint United Nations Programme on HIV/AIDS (UNAIDS). *2006 Report on the Global AIDS Epidemic*. Geneva: UNAIDS, 2006:114.

70. Ward DE. *The AMFAR AIDS Handbook: The Complete Guide to Understanding HIV and AIDS*. New York: W.W. Norton, 1999.

71. Joint United Nations Programme on HIV/AIDS (UNAIDS). *2002 Report on the Global AIDS Epidemic*. Geneva: UNAIDS, 2002.

72. Joint United Nations Programme on HIV/AIDS (UNAIDS). *Global Report: UNAIDS Report on the Global AIDS Epidemic 2012*. Geneva: UNAIDS, 2012.

73. WHO Programmatic Update Antiretroviral Treatment as Prevention (TASP) of HIV andTB, June 2012. http://whqlibdoc.who.int/hq/2012/WHO_HIV_2012.12_eng.pdf.

74. UNAIDS. HIV Treatment Now Reaching More Than 6 Million People in Sub-Saharan Africa. Geneva: UNAIDS Press Release, July 6, 2012. http://www.unaids.org/en/resources/presscentre/pressreleaseandstatementarchive/2012/#jul.

75. Meda N, Ndoye I, M'Boup S, et al. Low and stable HIV infection rates in Senegal: natural course of the epidemic or evidence for the success of prevention? *AIDS* 1999;13:1397–1405. Also see http://www.who.int/inf-new/aids3.htm and http://www.africarecovery.org.

76. Henenberg RS, Rojanapithayakorn W, Kunasol P, et al. Impact of Thailand's HIV control programme as indicated by the decline of sexually transmitted diseases. *Lancet* 1994;344:243–245.

77. World Health Organization. Thailand achieves sustained reduction in HIV infection rates. In: *Health: A Key to Prosperity. Success Stories in Developing Countries*. Geneva: WHO, 2000. http://www.who.int/int-new/aids1.htm.

78. Celentano DD, Nelson KE, Lyles CM, et al. Decreasing incidence of HIV and sexually transmitted diseases in young Thai men: evidence for success of the HIV/AIDS control and prevention program. *AIDS* 1998;12:F29–F36.

79. Des Jarlais DC, Friedman S, Choopanya K, et al. International epidemiology of HIV/AIDs among injecting drug users. *AIDS* 1992;6:1053–1068.

80. Asiimwe-Okiror G, Opio AA, Musinguzi J, et al. Change in sexual behaviour and decline in HIV infection among young pregnant women in rural Uganda. *AIDS* 1997;11:1757–1763.

81. Hankins C. Changes in patterns of risk. *AIDS Care* 1998;10:S147–S153.

82. Morris M, Kretzschmar M. Concurrent partnerships and the spread of HIV. *AIDS* 1997;11:641–648.

83. Weller S, Davis K. *Condom Effectiveness in Reducing Heterosexual HIV Transmission*. Chichester, UK: John Wiley and Sons, 2004.

84. Auvert B, Taljaard D, Lagarde E, et al. Randomized, controlled intervention trial of male circumcision for reduction of HIV infection risk: the ANRS 1265 trial. *PLoS Med* 2005;2(11):e298.

85. Gray R, Kigozi G, Scrwada D, Makumbi F, et al. Male circumcision for HIV prevention in men in Rakai, Uganda: a randomized trial. *Lancet* 2007;369:657–713.

86. Gray RH, Kiwanuka N, Quinn TC, Sewan Kambo NK, et al. Male circumcision and HIV acquisition and transmission: cohort studies in Rakai, Uganda, Rakai Project Team. AIDS 2000;14(15):2371–2381.

87. Cohen M, Chin YQ, McCauley M. et al. Prevention of HIV-1 infection with early antiretroviral therapy. *N Engl J Med* 2011;365(6):493–505.

88. Babiker AG, Emery S, Fätkenheuer G, et al. Considerations in the rationale, design and methods of the Strategic Timing of Antiretroviral Treatment (START) study. http://clinicaltrials.gov/ct2/show/NCT00867048.

89. Kaisernetwork.org HealthCast. *HIV Prevention Among Young People: Measuring the Impact* [Webcast]. Washington, DC: World Bank, September 8, 2004. http://www.kaisernetwork.org/health_cast/hcast_index.cfm?display=detail&hc=1263.

90. Ajzen I, Fishbein M. *Understanding Attitudes and Predicting Social Behavior*. Englewood Cliffs, NJ: Prentice-Hall, 1980.

91. Rogers E. *The Diffusion of Innovations*. 4th ed. New York: The Free Press, 1995.

92. US Government Accountability Office. *HHS: Efforts to Research and Inform the Public About Nonoxynol-9 and HIV*. Washington, DC: US Government Accountability Office, March 2005. GAO-05-399.

93. Abdool Karim Q, Abdool Karim S, Frohlich S, et al. Effectiveness and safety of tenofovir gel, an antiretroviral microbicide, for the prevention of HIV infection in women. *Science* 2010;329(5996):1168–1174.

94. Joint United Nations Programme on AIDS, UNAIDS. *Combination HIV Prevention. Tailoring and Coordinating, Biomedical, Behavioral and Structural Strategies to Reduce New HIV Infections. A UNAIDS Discussion Paper*. Geneva: UNAIDS, September 2010.

95. Kebaabetswe P, Norr KF. Behavior change: goals and means. In: Essex M, Mboup S, Kanki PJ, et al., eds. *AIDS in Africa*. 2nd ed. New York: Kluwer Academic/Plenum Publishers, 2002:514–526.

96. Badri M, Ehrlich R, Wood R. Association between tuberculosis and HIV disease progression in a high tuberculosis prevalence area. *Int J Tuberc Lung Dis* 2001;5(3):225–232.

97. World Health Organization. *Strategic Framework to Decrease the Burden of TB/HIV*. Geneva: WHO, 2002. WHO/CDS/TB/2002.2, WHO/HIV_AIDS/2002.2.

98. World Health Organization. *Interim Policy on Collaborative TB/HIV Activities*. Geneva: WHO, 2004. WHO/HTM/TB/2004.330, WHO/HTM/HIV/2004.1.

99. World Health Organization. *WHO Policy on Collaborative TB/HIV Activities: Guidelines for National Programmes and Other Stakeholders.* Geneva: WHO, 2012. WHO/HTM/TB/2012.1, WHO/HIV/2012.1.

100. World Health Organization. *Guidelines for Intensified Tuberculosis Case-Finding and Isoniazid Preventive Therapy for People Living with HIV in Resource-Constrained Settings.* Geneva: WHO, 2011.

101. Quigley MA, Mwinga A, Hosp M, et al. Long-term effect of preventive therapy for tuberculosis in a cohort of HIV-infected Zambian adults. *AIDS* 2001;15(2):215–222.

102. Zachariah R, Spielmann MP, Chinji C, et al. Voluntary counseling, HIV testing, and adjunctive co-trimoxazole reduces mortality in tuberculosis patients in Thyolo, Malawi. *AIDS* 2003;17:1053–1061.

103. Sinha S, Shekhar RC, Singh G, et al. Early versus delayed initiation of antiretroviral therapy for Indian HIV-infected individuals with tuberculosis on anti-tuberculosis treatment. *BMC Infect Dis* 2012;12(1):168.

104. Karim SA, et al. Initiating ART during TB treatment significantly increases survival: results of a randomized controlled clinical trial in TB/HIV-co-infected patients in South Africa. Paper presented at: Conference on Retroviruses and Opportunistic Infections (CROI), Montreal, 2009. http://www.retroconference.org/2009/Abstracts/34255.htm.

105. World Health Organization. *TB/HIV: A Clinical Manual.* 2nd ed. Geneva: WHO, 2004. WHO/HTM/TB/2004.329.

The Neglected Tropical Diseases

11

Gregory Juckett

LEARNING OBJECTIVES

- List the neglected tropical diseases (NTDs) of the developing world and the factors contributing to their being "neglected"
- Discuss the many links between NTDs and poverty and how the Millennium Development Goals might break these links
- Review the symptoms, diagnosis, treatment, and control measures for 13 chronic NTDs and one acute NTD (dengue)
- Discuss the application of various disease control strategies (vector control, mass drug administration, vaccination, reservoir elimination, etc.) to NTDs

INTRODUCTION

The neglected tropical diseases (NTDs) are chronic infections affecting the poorest people of the world, living in sub-Saharan Africa, Asia, and Latin America (Table 11-1). Because most health care workers in developed countries are unfamiliar with NTD diagnosis and treatment, these are summarized in Tables 11-2 and 11-3. The term *neglected tropical diseases* was first introduced in the 1980s as the "great neglected diseases of mankind" by the late Dr. Ken Warren. These chronic, disabling but rarely fatal diseases not only afflict the poor, but they also keep them in poverty. Many NTD victims are stigmatized by their illness and unable to find employment. These are the diseases with the horrific photos in the tropical medicine texts, and in many cultures the stigma is intensified by the condition being attributed to witchcraft or a curse. Although none are as deadly as

the three most important tropical diseases, malaria, tuberculosis (TB), and acquired immune deficiency syndrome (AIDS), if taken together the total disability of just 13 of these "lesser" diseases approaches that of HIV/AIDS and exceeds that of malaria and TB.[1] NTDs are "neglected" only because the suffering from these ancient scourges is largely confined to the so-called third world, effectively veiling their existence from wealthier nations. Many Americans are amazed to learn that they still exist. In the words of the World Health Organization (WHO), they are "not adequately addressed either nationally or internationally." There is also little financial incentive for pharmaceutical firms to develop or distribute new drugs or vaccines in the absence of a ready market for them, especially because most NTDs occur in the 2.7 billion people making less than $2 US per day.[2] Before philanthropic interests made them priorities, NTDs were literally "out of sight and out of mind."

Although only the 13 "classic" chronic NTDs proposed by Peter Hotez and one acute viral disease, dengue fever, are covered in this chapter, this by no means suggests that many other diseases are not equally neglected.[2] In addition to dengue, the WHO adds cysticercosis, echinococcosis, fascioliasis, rabies, and yaws to Hotez's list. The WHO considers the soil transmitted helminths as one NTD instead of three (Hotez) for a total of 17 conditions. There are also WHO "neglected conditions" such as snakebite and podoconiosis (nonfilarial elephantiasis).[3] Indeed it has been suggested that all tropical diseases other than the "big three" of HIV, malaria, and TB are neglected. Many diseases of the tropics have limited therapeutic options and remain in great need of further research.

The Link Between Poverty and Disease

The common factor with all the NTDs is poverty. How people live determines how they get sick and

Table 11-1. The 13 chronic neglected tropical diseases[1,2] and dengue.

Disease	Prevalence (in millions)	Areas of prevalence
Roundworm (Ascariasis)	807	Developing world (moist climates)
Whipworm (Trichuriasis)	604	Developing world (moist climates)
Hookworm (Necator, Ancylostoma)	576	Developing world (moist climates)
Schistosomiasis	207	Sub-Saharan Africa, Latin America
Lymphatic filariasis	120	India, Southeast Asia, Sub-Saharan Africa, East Asia-Pacific
Trachoma	84	North and Sub-Saharan Africa, Middle East, South Asia, East Asia-Pacific (dry climates)
Onchocerciasis	37	Sub-Saharan Africa, limited areas of Latin America
Leishmaniasis	12	India and South Asia (visceral), Latin America (cutaneous), Sub-Saharan Africa
Chagas disease	8–9	Latin America
Leprosy	0.4	India, Sub-Saharan Africa, Brazil
Human African trypanosomiasis	0.3	Sub-Saharan Africa
Buruli ulcer	0.05	Sub-Saharan (West) Africa
Dracunculiasis	0.01	Sub-Saharan Africa
Dengue	Acute illness and epidemics Incidence: 50–100 million cases annually	Southeast Asia, Caribbean, Latin America, Africa

Adapted from *Forgotten People, Forgotten Diseases* (Table 1.3) Peter Hotez[1]. Hotez PJ. Forgotten People, Forgotten Diseases: The Neglected Tropical Diseases and Their Impact on Global Health and Development. Washington, DC: ASM Press, 2008.

even how they die. These diseases thrive in crowded, dirty environments where there is little sanitation, a scarcity of potable water, and extensive exposure to the elements. Most people with NTDs depend on agriculture or herding to survive and spend much of their life outdoors. They live in crowded substandard housing (contributing to Chagas disease), are in contact with fecally contaminated soil (hookworm), bathe in snail-infested rivers (schistosomiasis), and are bitten by numerous insect vectors.

It makes sense that the elimination of poverty is therefore the best single approach to ending these diseases. Introducing privies or flush toilets is the surest way to eliminate soil-borne helminthic infections. Hygiene eradicates trachoma. Safe drinking water stops guinea worm. Bed nets and window screens dramatically reduce insect-borne diseases.

Affluence enables travelers from wealthy countries to "cocoon" themselves from most of these environmental threats. Travelers to these regions can be shielded by expensive insect repellents, air-conditioned hotels, bottled water, sturdy footwear, vaccinations, and antibiotics, but few if any of these resources are available to the impoverished local population. Although most of the diseases discussed in this chapter have specific control measures, a temporary lapse in implementation (due to regional conflict or loss of funding) has often resulted in their resurgence. The only permanent solution is the eradication of poverty.

The United Nations Millennium Declaration (2000) lists eight specific Millennium Development Goals (MDGs) to eliminate extreme poverty, hunger, and disease by 2015.[4] These include eliminating extreme poverty and hunger, achieving universal primary education, promoting gender equality and empowering women, reducing childhood mortality, improving maternal health, combating HIV/AIDS, malaria, and *other diseases*, ensuring a sustainable environment, and developing global partnerships for development. Lifting people out of poverty is the most effective way of ending the grip of NTDs on their lives. Although criticized as overly idealistic, these goals have spotlighted such issues, and many MDGs have received extensive funding from governmental (e.g., Presidents Emergency Plan for AIDS Relief, or PEPFAR) and philanthropic (e.g., Bill and Melinda Gates Foundation) organizations.

THE NEGLECTED TROPICAL DISEASES

Helminth Infections: Ascariasis (Roundworm), Trichuriasis (Whipworm), and Hookworm

The first three NTDs are soil-transmitted helminthic infections, affecting perhaps a billion people.[5] Many children are coinfected by all three of these worms (polyparasitism). Intestinal worms stunt the growth

Table 11-2. Neglected tropical disease diagnostic tests.

Disease	Diagnostic tests
Roundworm (Ascaris)	Stool O&P (eggs)
Whipworm (Trichuris)	Stool O&P (eggs)
Hookworm (Necator, Ancylostoma)	Stool O&P (characteristic eggs and sometimes larvae), CBC (iron deficiency anemia)
Schistosomiasis	Stool O&P (*S. mansoni*) or spun urine O&P (*S. haematobium*), Schistosoma antigen testing (available CDC), + eosinophilia; liver biopsy + exudative granulomata
Lymphatic filariasis	Blood parasite smear drawn at appropriate time, +LF antigen test, ultrasound (filarial dance)
Trachoma	Clinical appearance (WHO trachoma grading system)
Onchocerciasis	Six skin snips from iliac crests, biopsy of nodule, slit lamp examination of eye, CDC serologic testing (Onchocerca antigen tests)—serology unable to distinguish past from present infection,+ eosinophilia
Leishmaniasis	Microscopy of lesion biopsy or tissue smear, immunochromatographic test strip for leishmanial anti-K39 antibody, PCR, Montenegro (leishmanin) skin test (unable to distinguish current from past infection)
Chagas disease	Serologies for chronic infection: ELISA testing (e.g., Chagatest ELISA Recombinante) or Ortho *T. cruzi* ELISA Test System), then Chagas Radioimmune Precipitation Assay (Chagas RIPA) as confirmatory test
	Thin and thick blood smears (+ acute infection only); xenodiagnosis (development in triatomid bug) used historically
Leprosy	Confirmed by skin biopsy or microscopic exam of earlobe fluid (+ acid-fast bacteria typical only in multibacillary disease), still often a clinical diagnosis; + lepromin skin test only in tuberculoid leprosy (no culture possible)
Human African trypanosomiasis	Blood smear (East African form) or microscopy of lymph node aspirate (West African form); latter usually not seen in blood smear; serology used in research
Buruli ulcer	Clinical appearance, PCR standard for confirming diagnosis
Guinea worm (Dracunculiasis)	Clinical: ulcerated extremity with visible worm (rarely mimicked by onchocerciasis)
Dengue fever	RT-PCR for viremia (first 5 days of infection); DENV Detect IgM Capture ELISA for IgM antibodies after 5 days; four fold antibody increase in acute and convalescent serum samples; tourniquet test for dengue hemorrhagic fever

CBC, complete blood count; ELISA, enzyme-linked immunosorbent assay test; IgM, immunoglobulin M; O&P, ova and parasite examination; PCR, polymerase chain reaction; RT-PCR, reverse transcriptase polymerase chain reaction; WHO, World Health Organization.

of impoverished children in Africa, Asia, and Latin America. They are especially prevalent in the humid tropics where adequate rainfall and poor hygiene create ideal environments for these parasites. Together they are suspected of being a leading cause of child growth retardation.[6]

Ascaris

Ascaris, or roundworm, infections are especially common in areas of poor sanitation, where human feces contaminate the soil. These abundant roundworms are acquired by ingesting embryonated eggs, after which the larvae pass through the lungs to develop in the small intestine. Children are especially prone to heavy infections, which retard appetite, growth, and school performance, occasionally causing intestinal

obstruction. Migration of these worms into the bile ducts or pancreas may cause acute cholecystitis or pancreatitis.

Trichuris

Trichuris, or whipworm, infections commonly coinfect children with *Ascaris* and are acquired in a similar fashion, although these worms develop in the large intestine without passing through the lungs. They are associated with colitis and rectal prolapse.

Hookworm

The most important of the three helminth infections is hookworm. These parasites rob their victims of blood, producing profound iron deficiency anemia and fatigue. Both hookworm species, *Necator americanus* and the

Table 11-3. Treatment of neglected tropical diseases

Disease	Treatment
Roundworm (*Ascaris*)	Albendazole 400 mg or mebendazole 500-mg single dose
Whipworm (*Trichuris*)	Mebendazole 500 mg once or albendazole 400 mg qd × 3 d
Hookworm (*Ancylostoma, Necator*)	Albendazole 400 mg or mebendazole 500-mg single dose
Schistosoma haematobium/mansoni	Praziquantel 40 mg/kg/d in 2 divided doses × 1 d
Schistosoma japonicum	Praziquantel 60 mg/kg/d in 3 divided doses × 1 d
Lymphatic filariasis (LF)	Diethylcarbamazine 6 mg/kg/d in 3 doses × 12 d
Trachoma	Azithromycin 20 mg/kg single dose up to 1 g maximum
Onchocerciasis	Ivermectin 150 µg/kg once, repeated every 6–12 months until asymptomatic
	Doxycycline 100 mg qd × 6 wk may be added several days after the ivermectin dose[19]
Leishmaniasis	
Cutaneous	Sodium stibogluconate 20 mg Sb/kg/d IV or IM × 10–28 d or observation
	Liposomal amphotericin B superior to sodium stibogluconate
Mucocutaneous	Liposomal amphotericin B 3 mg/kg/d IV d1–5, 13, 21 or
Visceral	Sodium stibogluconate 20 mg Sb/kg/d IV or IM × 28 d or
	Miltefosine 2.5 mg/kg/d PO(max 150 mg/d) × 28 d (India)
Chagas disease	Nifurtimox 8–10 mg/kg/d in 3–4 doses × 90–120 d or
	Benznidazole 5–7 mg/g/d in 2 doses with food × 30–90 d
Leprosy paucibacillary or tuberculoid form, <5 skin lesions	Dapsone 100 mg qd and monthly rifampin 600 mg × 6 mo (finish 6 packs in 6–12 mo)
Multibacillary or lepromatous form, 6+ lesions, + smear	Dapsone 100 mg qd and clofazimine 50 mgqd, with monthly rifampin 600 mg and clofazimine 300 mg, × 12+ mo (finish 12 packs in 12–18 mo)
	Reference: *A New Atlas of Leprosy*[30]
Human African trypanosomiasis	
West African	Early West African: Pentamidine 4 mg/kg/d IM × 7 d or suramin 100–200 mg IV (test dose) then 1g IV on days 1,3,7,14,21
	Late West African: Eflornithine 400 mg/kg/d IV in 4 doses × 14 d or melarsoprol 2.2 mg/kg/d IV × 10 d
East African	Early East African: Suramin (doses as above)
	Late East African: Melarsoprol 2–3.6 mg/kg/d IV × 3 d, after 7 d: 3.6 mg/kg/d × 3 d; repeat again after 7 d
Buruli ulcer	Rifampin 10 mg/kg and streptomycin 15 mg/kg administered daily × 8 wk (some experimental regimens substitute clarithromycin for streptomycin)—a paradoxical reaction (temporary exacerbation) sometimes noted
	Reference: Converse et al[32]
Guinea worm (Dracunculiasis)	Manual extraction using stick; no medical treatment
Dengue fever	Hydration and supportive care (no pharmacologic treatment)

IM, intramuscular; IV, intravenous; PO, by mouth; qd, daily; Sb, antimony.
From reference 21.

less abundant *Ancylostoma duodenale*, are acquired from contact with fecally contaminated soil. Larvae penetrate the skin, often causing a pruritic "ground-itch" rash. They then migrate to the lungs, are coughed up and swallowed, and attain maturity in the small intestine where they survive for decades. Hookworm anemia results in a sallow complexion, and many cultures refer to it as "yellow disease."

Control

Transmission of all of these soil-transmitted helminthes is most effectively stopped by modern sanitation, which prevents fecal contamination of soil. Latrine use is a first step that is much more feasible than indoor plumbing for impoverished communities. Because any skin exposure to infected soil can result in hookworm infection, proper footwear is at best only a partial solution. Regular deworming of all schoolchildren with benzimidazoles (BZAs) is a practical interim solution, especially in high-incidence areas where infection rates exceed 50%.[7] In 2001, the WHO adopted resolution 54.19, urging regular deworming of at least 75% of at-risk schoolchildren by 2010.[8] Single-dose albendazole 400 mg or mebendazole 500 mg every 6 to 12 months is safe and effective, although these programs fail to reach preschoolers and children not attending school. BZA resistance is well known in veterinary use and emerging in human infection, necessitating an urgent need to develop new drugs. Unfortunately, there are few antiparasitic drugs in development. The newest alternative drug for human use is tribendimidine, which was approved in China in 2004.[9]

Vaccination against hookworm infection would be a major milestone on the road to eradication because it would prevent reinfection in areas of poor hygiene. The Human Hookworm Vaccine Initiative was established in 2000 with the goal of developing both effective hookworm and *Schistosoma* vaccines.

Schistosomiasis (Bilharzia)

Schistosomes are blood flukes that afflict over 200 million people, most (97%) of whom live in Africa.[10] Endemic areas of less importance include Brazil, Yemen, Southeast Asia, and the Philippines. Substantial eradication has already occurred in China and Egypt. Three principal species exist: *Schistosoma haematobium*, residing in bladder vessels and causing urinary schistosomiasis in Africa (63% of cases); *S. mansoni*, residing in the greater mesenteric vessels (intestinal schistosomiasis, 35%); and *S. japonicum*, residing in the lesser mesenteric vessels (Asian intestinal schistosomiasis, now less than 1%).[11] Other species, such as *S. mekongi* and *S. intercalatum*, are far less significant.

These flukes depend on freshwater snails, an intermediate host, to complete their life cycle, hence the alternative term *snail fever*. Another name, *bilharzia*, is derived from Theodor Bilharz, who first described urinary schistosomiasis in the 19th century. The infection is acquired from entering snail-infested water. Free-living cercariae (larval flukes) are released from snails and swim until they come in contact with and penetrate human skin. Some victims develop a pruritic rash or cercarial dermatitis ("swimmer's itch") at the sites of penetration, but this is variable. After entry, the cercariae lose their tails and migrate through the lungs and liver, eventually making their way to the bladder or mesenteric vessels, where they develop into blood-feeding permanently paired adults. An intense immune response to schistosome egg production may provoke an acute febrile illness termed *Katayama fever* in previously nonexposed travelers, but more commonly the infection is insidious. Although the flukes themselves remain largely invisible to the immune system (they mask their presence by shrouding themselves with their host's antigens), their spined eggs provoke significant inflammation as they penetrate through the bladder and intestinal walls. In the case of *S. haematobium*, this results in hematuria (sometimes termed *male menstruation*), bladder granulomas (which may cause hydronephrosis and renal failure), squamous cell cancer of the bladder, and female genital lesions (which increase the risk of HIV transmission). In the case of *S. mansoni* and *S. japonicum*, granulomas of the intestinal wall and liver develop leading to colitis, hepatosplenomegaly, and hepatic fibrosis. Hepatocellular carcinoma is a later, fatal complication.[12]

Eggs are excreted in the urine (*S. haematobium*) or stool (*S. mansoni*, *S. japonicum*), and the species can be easily identified by the spine's location on the egg (terminal in *haematobium*, lateral in *mansoni*, absent in *japonicum*). When human waste enters fresh water, the eggs hatch into miracidia that seek out snails to parasitize.

Vaccines against schistosomiasis would help prevent the continual threat of reinfection after treatment. Only one schistosomal prototype vaccine (*Bilhvax* for *S. haematobium*) has undergone successful human trials.[13] Although the vaccine was safe and effective, there are as yet no schistosome vaccines in clinical use.

The turning point in the war on schistosomiasis came with the discovery of praziquantel (Biltricide) by Bayer Pharmaceuticals in the mid-1970s. Praziquantel is effective for most flatworms (flukes and tapeworms), although resistance is starting to emerge.[14] Mass treatment programs with donated praziquantel 40 mg/kg/day, sometimes combining this therapy with albendazole for roundworm infection, have been effective and well tolerated.[14] The Schistosomiasis Control Initiative (SCI), funded by the Gates Foundation, has led these mass drug administration efforts. Single-dose praziquantel is often sufficient to eradicate infection. Molluscicides to kill snails in ponds, rivers, and streams have been used in conjunction with praziquantel in many areas. This integrated approach is termed *preventive chemotherapy and transmission control*, and similar strategies are used for controlling many NTDs.

Filarial Infections: Dracunculiasis, Lymphatic Filariasis, and Onchocerciasis

Dracunculiasis

Dracunculiasis, caused by the Guinea worm *Dracunculus medinensis*, is an ancient human scourge on the verge of eradication, with a 99% incidence reduction within the past 2 decades.[15] This unusual nematode is acquired from drinking water that contains parasitized water fleas (copepods). Once fleas are ingested, the larvae within them survive to migrate to the host's subcutaneous

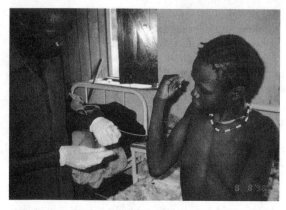

Figure 11-1. Guinea worm extraction in Sudan. (*Photo by Beth Grayson.*)

tissues where they may grow into yard-long worms (Figure 11-1). Guinea worm infection is incapacitating, producing a burning painful blister that induces victims to soak their limbs in cool water, often the very step-well from which their village receives its water supply. Immersion bursts the blister, releasing thousands of eggs that are ingested by water fleas. Unfortunately, there is no effective drug for this condition. The only cure is extraction of the worm by painstakingly winding it around a stick, a process that takes days.

Once widespread through the dry tropics in South Asia, Africa, and the Middle East, this parasite is now found primarily in Sudan. This is largely due to the efforts of the Carter Foundation's Dracunculiasis Eradication Program (DEP), which has exploited several "weak links" in its life cycle. Guinea worm parasitizes only humans, and its life cycle is easily interrupted by filtering drinking water through cloth or a nylon filter, keeping infected people out of the drinking water source, and using larvicides like Temephos (*Abate*), which kills water fleas. Armed conflict in Sudan has made it difficult to work in this region and cease-fires had to be arranged to continue the work. The eradication of Guinea worm in Africa appears to be imminent. This would make it the second disease to be truly eradicated after smallpox. It should be added that eradication is not the same as elimination. *Eradication* means that the global prevalence of the disease is now zero and that public health control measures no longer need to be continued (e.g., smallpox). *Elimination* refers to a reduction *in a given area* to zero or global reduction to a negligible amount (e.g., polio). Public health measures still need to be continued.[16]

Lymphatic filariasis

Lymphatic filariasis (LF, or "elephantiasis") is primarily caused by two filarial species: *Wuchereria bancrofti* (90%) and *Brugia malayi* (10%). This disease is now found mostly in South Asia and Africa, with a few remaining holdout areas in the Pacific and the Americas (Haiti, Northeast Brazil).[17] Mosquitoes transmit the infection, with larval worms dropping from the mosquitoes' proboscis onto the skin before entering the bite site. After reaching the lymphatics, the larvae mature into thin undulating long-lived adults (their motion visible on ultrasound as a "filarial dance" within the lymphatics). Inflammation and scarring of the lymphatics, with recurrent secondary bacterial infections, eventually result in unsightly lymphedema of the legs or scrotal hydrocele in some victims. However, it is now unusual for LF to progress to the point where patients require wheelbarrows for scrotal transport. LF is sometimes confused with podoconiosis (nonfilarial elephantiasis) in which lymphatic damage results from the absorption of volcanic minerals through bare feet.[18] Wearing shoes prevents this condition.

Adult filarial worms produce sheathed larvae (microfilaria) that circulate in the blood only when their insect vector is active (either nocturnal or diurnal "periodicity"), thus optimizing their chances of reaching new hosts. Periodicity also determines the best time for diagnostic blood draws: blood samples for *Wuchereria* and *Brugia* are only positive if drawn at night, unless stimulated by small doses of diethylcarbamazine, whereas African eye worm (*Loa loa*) *microfilaria*, which are spread by a diurnal deer fly, are active only during the day. *Microfilaria* seen on blood smears can be speciated by a careful microscopic examination, and serologic tests are now available for confirmation.

Control of LF is through mass dosing with diethylcarbamazine (DEC), which is much more effective in killing the microfilaria than the adult worms and thus does not result in a permanent cure. However, DEC-fortified salt or tablets proved very effective in eradicating LF by interrupting its spread to new victims. DEC is unavailable in the United States except through the Centers for Disease Control and Prevention (CDC).

In Africa, ivermectin is preferred to DEC because it is safer when there is coinfection with onchocerciasis. Currently, single annual doses of either DEC or ivermectin (combined with albendazole to reduce the likelihood of resistance) are favored, but this treatment must be repeated for 5 or more years.[17] The Global Alliance to Eliminate LF has set the goal of eliminating LF by the year 2020 through mass drug administration, establishing new control programs, and insect bite precautions.

Onchocerciasis

Onchocerciasis, or "river blindness," is the third filarial NTD success story. *Onchocerca volvulus* is mostly found in sub-Saharan Africa, although there is also a spotty distribution in Guatemala and northern South America. Its vector is the *Simulium* black fly, which breeds in flowing streams. Like *Wuchereria*, the larval worms drop from the fly's mouthparts, but after entering through the bite, the female worms develop within palpable skin nodules (onchocercomas), where they persist for 2 to 15 years, whereas the nomadic male worms migrate in the skin. [19] The numerous microfilaria or larval worms are found in the skin (and anterior chamber of the eye) rather than the bloodstream. Tenting the iliac skin with a needle and snipping off small fragments will usually demonstrate microfilaria on microscopic examination, especially after the skin snips are incubated overnight in saline. Antigen testing, available from the CDC, is becoming more popular for diagnosis. An accurate antigen detection dipstick assay has been developed that would greatly simplify diagnosis. [20]

Onchocerciasis has two major clinical presentations: a very stigmatizing onchocercal skin disease (OSD), also known as *craw-craw* or *sowda*, which is common in African forest areas and the Americas, and river blindness, which is usually limited to African savannahs. In OSD, abundant microfilaria in the skin cause a papular dermatitis with intense, unrelenting itching, depigmentation ("leopard patches"), and loss of skin elasticity ("hanging groin"). River blindness arises from small corneal opacities (resulting from dying microfilaria in the eye) that coalesce until eventual blindness results. Whole villages have been abandoned due to this devastating disease.

Onchocerciasis control measures began in 1974 with the development of the Onchocerciasis Control Program (OCP). Initially efforts were directed at black fly control with extensive aerial spraying and the use of larvicides in streams. The plan was to arrest transmission for 20 years, by which time most of the adult worms would have died out. Another breakthrough came with the development of ivermectin (*Mectizan*), which was found to be very effective at killing microfilaria, although not the adults. Ivermectin treatment consists of 150 µg/kg once with repeat dosing every 6 to 12 months. [21] Higher doses are not any more effective. Although not an outright cure, annual doses of ivermectin did interrupt transmission and augmented the spray program. Merck continues to donate ivermectin (*Mectizan*) to the OCP because it is still necessary to maintain treatment until all adult worms die. A new drug called moxidectin is able to kill the adult worms and is undergoing human trials. [22]

Distributing annual doses of ivermectin to patients in remote African villages proved a daunting task. A community drug distribution system had to be developed (now dubbed Community Directed Treatment with Ivermectin, or CDTI) because many patients were hard to locate during team visits. This same system has been adapted to distribute other much needed drugs and bed nets.

An additional option for onchocerciasis control is emerging with the discovery that this filarial parasite, and many other invertebrates (including many insects, such as bedbugs), depend on the endosymbiotic rickettsial bacteria *Wolbachia*. Treatment with doxycycline 100 mg daily for 6 weeks induces longterm sterility in the female worms. [23] Although OSD is related to the host response to microfilarial antigens, vision loss appears to be provoked by the immune response to *Wolbachia* bacteria, released from dying microfilaria in the eye. [19]

Trachoma

Trachoma is a recurrent bacterial eye infection from *Chlamydia trachomatis* that eventually results in blindness. Trachoma means "rough" in Greek, referring to the rough appearance of the upper tarsal conjunctiva. It is usually found in arid, impoverished areas of Africa and Asia, where flies and poor sanitation contribute to repeated eye infections in children (Figure 11-2). Eventually this results in eyelid scarring and inward-turning eyelashes (trichiasis) that damage the cornea. An estimated 15% of the world's blindness is due to this infection. [24] The environment that fosters trachoma has been described as having either "6 D's" (dryness, dust, dirt, dung, discharge, and density) or "5 F's" (flies, feces, faces, fingers, and fomites). [25] The International Trachoma Initiative (ITI) has developed a comprehensive strategy known as SAFE for trachoma control. [24] S stands for surgery to correct trichiasis. A small slit is incised in the eyelid and the skin is pulled back to evert the lashes. A is for antibiotic therapy, specifically single-dose azithromycin 20 mg/kg up to 1 g (donated by Pfizer), which has now replaced

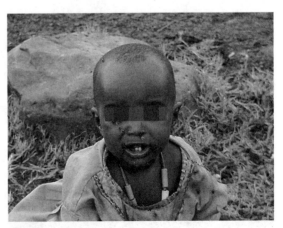

Figure 11-2. Child attacked by flies and at risk for trachoma.

tetracycline ointment as the most effective Chlamydia therapy.[26] F refers to facial hygiene or regular face washing. E is for environmental control such as access to clean water and latrine use to reduce fly populations. Trachoma diagnosis remains clinical, based on a WHO grading system. Countrywide campaigns with mobile surgical teams using the SAFE strategy have beaten back trachoma in many African countries. The disease was eliminated in Morocco in 2006.

Leishmaniasis

Leishmaniasis is caused by various intracellular protozoal parasites of the genus *Leishmania* that are spread by female sandfly bites. Leishmaniasis is prevalent in Latin America, the Indian subcontinent, the Middle East, the Mediterranean, and parts of Africa.[27] *Phlebotomus* sandflies act as *Leishmania* vectors in the Old World; *Lutzomyia* sandflies (Figure 11-3) play the same role in Central and South America. Some species of *Leishmania* are zoonotic infections of humans. The primary reservoirs of the disease are rodents (*L. major*), rock hyraxes (*L. aethiopica*), or dogs (*L. infantum*). This makes it difficult, if not impossible, to eradicate.

Leishmaniasis presents as three different clinical syndromes: cutaneous leishmaniasis (CL), mucocutaneous leishmaniasis (MCL), and visceral leishmaniasis (VL). Which type develops appears related to the temperature preference of the species involved. Some prefer the cooler environment of the skin ("dermotropic" CL species); others are more heat tolerant (VL species). MCL, usually caused by *Leishmania (Viannia) braziliensis* of the New World, appears to be intermediate between the two.[27]

When introduced to the body by an infected sandfly bite, flagellated *Leishmania* promastigotes are consumed by macrophages, and they lose their flagellae

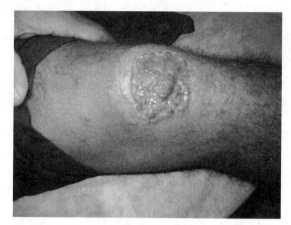

Figure 11-4. Cutaneous leishmaniasis in the Brazilian Amazon.

to become amastigotes. Instead of dying, however, they multiply in this hostile environment, infect even more macrophages, and either remain in the skin (CL) or invade the viscera (VL). Typical CL develops as an open persistent sore at the site of the bite, often after a lengthy incubation, with the base of the ulcer frequently described as having a "pizza-like" appearance. The slightly raised ulcer margins are often rolled and well demarcated (Figures 11-4 and 11-5). Eventually most of these ulcers heal, but only after many months, and with significant scarring. CL has many regional names that describe the sore: Baghdad boil, Ciclero ulcer (Brazil), bay sore (Caribbean), uta (Peru), or saldana (Iran). Many US servicemen have acquired "Baghdad boils" while serving in Iraq or Afghanistan.

The taxonomy of *Leishmania* is quite complicated, but there are several species complexes that produce

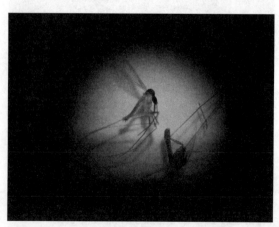

Figure 11-3. Sandfly, vector of leishmaniasis.

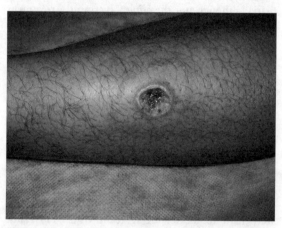

Figure 11-5. Cutaneous leishmaniasis in the Brazilian Amazon.

similar clinical syndromes. In the New World there is the *Mexicana* complex (*L. mexicana, amazonensis,* and *venezuelensis*) that causes self-limited CL. The New World *Braziliensis* complex belongs to the *Leishmania* subgenus *Viannia* consisting of L. (*V.*) *braziliensis, guyanensis, panamensis,* and *peruviana.* Cutaneous ulcers caused by the *Braziliensis* complex sometimes appear to heal, only to metastasize years later as the dreaded mucocutaneous form of the disease, which can destroy the nasal cartilage ("tapir nose") and produce severe facial deformities. MCL is usually known as *espundia,* Portuguese for "sponge."

Visceral leishmaniasis or *kala azar* (Hindi for "black disease") is most often caused by the mostly Old World *Donovani* complex (*L. donovani, infantum, chagasi*). *L. donovani* appears to be a human infection, not a zoonosis. VL is particularly common on the eastern Indian subcontinent and presents with fever, weight loss, splenomegaly, darkening of the skin, and anemia. It is often fatal without treatment, with a 75% to 95% case fatality rate.[27] *L. infantum* is found in southern Europe, with a reservoir in dogs, and it preferentially infects children or immunocompromised patients. It is easily spread by intravenous drug abuse and exacerbated by HIV infection. *L. chagasi* is now considered a South American variant of *L. infantum.*

The *Tropica* complex (*L. tropica, L. major, L. aethiopica*) is centered in North Africa, the Middle East, and western India. It is primarily cutaneous, although some cases may have visceral involvement. *L. tropica* causes dry facial lesions ("Baghdad boils") and is more common in urban areas. *L. major* and the similar *L. aethiopica* are common in rural areas and cause wet "oriental sores," being more likely to affect the extremities than the face. On biopsies of the ulcer edge, all Leishmania amastigotes are morphologically indistinguishable. They can only be speciated by isoenzyme analysis or monoclonal antibody testing. Polymerase chain reaction (PCR) testing is clinically superior where available.

Treatment of leishmaniasis is even more confusing than its classification. The mainstay of traditional therapy has been pentavalent antimony (sodium stibogluconate) that must be given parentally over 20 (CL) or 28 (VL) days, is unavailable in the United States (except from the CDC), and has toxic side effects.[21] Shorter 10-day courses of sodium stibogluconate have been used for *L. major, tropica,* and *mexicana.* Liposomal amphotericin B (*AmBisome*) for 5 days is a much less toxic therapy, but its great expense makes it unavailable to those who need it most. Recent donations of *AmBisome* are increasing access to this drug. Indian VL now can be effectively treated orally with miltefosine 100 mg daily for 28 days, a newer drug option originally developed for cancer treatment.[21] Miltefosine is a lifesaving innovation because at least half of Indian VL in Bihar State is now resistant to antimonial compounds.[27] It should be noted that cutaneous leishmaniasis does not always need treatment because more than 90% of the ulcers eventually heal after several (3 to 18) months.[27] New World CL ulcers caused by *L. (V.) braziliensis* are an exception because these could potentially progress to MCL even after healing. Many innovative CL therapies have been developed: intralesional pentavalent antimony, itraconazole, ketoconazole, paromomycin ointment (not available in the United States), cryotherapy, and heat treatments, but none are clearly superior. Unfortunately, the treatment of Leishmaniasis leaves much to be desired because it remains overly dependent on antiquated antimonial drugs. No mass treatment programs for leishmaniasis exist. Existing agents are far too toxic to use for disease prevention in at-risk populations. Sandfly (vector) control and the elimination of reservoir animals (stray dogs) have been the primary means of controlling Leishmaniasis. Insecticide-treated dog collars have been useful in the Mediterranean.[27]

Leishmania infection appears to confer lifelong immunity. An old practice called leishmanization involved intentional inoculation of the parasite on an inconspicuous area to prevent future facial ulcers and scarring.[28] Although no *Leishmania* vaccine is yet commercially available, several recombinant DNA antigen and protein CL vaccine prototypes exist due to the Leishmania Genome Project. Such a vaccine would offer the best hope for long-term disease control in endemic areas.[13]

Myobacterial Neglected Tropical Diseases: Leprosy and Buruli Ulcer

Leprosy

Leprosy, or Hansen disease (after G. Armauer Hansen, the Norwegian physician who discovered Hansen bacillus or *Mycobacterium leprae*), is the classic example of a dreaded stigmatizing disease. Victims have usually been ostracized since biblical times, although it is unclear if biblical leprosy is the same disease recognized as leprosy today. Once found worldwide, leprosy has declined precipitously in recent decades. By 2005 it had been eradicated in all but 10 countries, remaining a public health problem in Brazil, India, Nepal, and Central and Southern Africa (Angola, Central African Republic, Democratic Republic of the Congo, Madagascar, and Mozambique).[29] Most of the world's cases are now in India. Widespread use of bacillus Calmette-Guérin vaccine for TB appears to offer some cross-protection against leprosy, and this, along with effective multidrug therapy, has contributed to its decline. The US National Hansen's Disease Center in Carville, Louisiana, closed in 1997.

Mycobacterium leprae appears to be transmitted by nasal secretions, but unlike TB, which it closely resembles (acid fast positive rod, survival in macrophages), it requires more intense, prolonged contact, does not cause pulmonary disease, and cannot be cultured. Most of those infected never develop symptoms. For those who do, leprosy may manifest years later as a skin and peripheral nerve infection. The first manifestation of the disease is usually a hypopigmented or coppery anesthetic skin macule (Figure 11-6). The disease then develops along two major pathways (tuberculoid or lepromatous, with some additional "intermediate" cases), depending on the host's immune response. Most patients develop tuberculoid leprosy because they have a significant immune reaction to infection. The disease remains localized with relatively few bacteria (paucibacillary disease). Few skin plaques (one to five) with loss of sensation characterize this form. Patients who fail

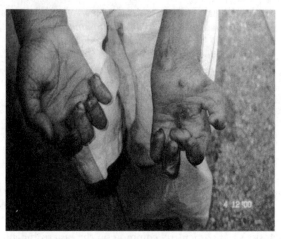

Figure 11-7. Advanced leprosy.

to develop a good immune response develop a widely disseminated multibacillary form of the disease known as lepromatous leprosy. Multibacillary leprosy results in multiple skin lesions (more than five), disfiguring leonine facies, and occasional blindness from corneal invasion. Loss of sensation in the digits results in repeated infections and auto-amputation of fingers and toes (Figure 11-7).

Leprosy is clinically diagnosed by noting hypertrophied peripheral nerves and counting the number of patches of anesthetic hypopigmented skin. Microscopic examination with acid-fast staining of a skin biopsy specimen or fluid expressed from earlobe slits (positive in multibacillary disease) can confirm the diagnosis. The lepromin skin test (similar to a tuberculin skin test for TB) has also been used, although lepromatous patients are likely to be anergic and thus fail to respond.[29]

Leprosy is now quite treatable with free multidrug treatment (MDT) blister packs containing daily doses of dapsone with monthly rifampin for 6 months for paucibacillary disease or daily dapsone and clofazimine with monthly rifampin/extra clofazimine for 12 months for multibacillary disease.[30] Late treatment arrests the disease but does not reverse the deformities already present. Therefore many cured patients continue to live in leprosy sanitariums because leprosy's stigma prevents them from returning home. Unlike TB treatment, however, it is still unclear how long leprosy MDT takes to eliminate transmissibility.

The Global Alliance for the Elimination of Leprosy was formed in 1999 with the hope of eliminating the world's remaining cases of human leprosy. Humans are the major host, but the nine-banded armadillo of the southern United States and Mexico can also carry this disease, making true eradication difficult. Armadillos

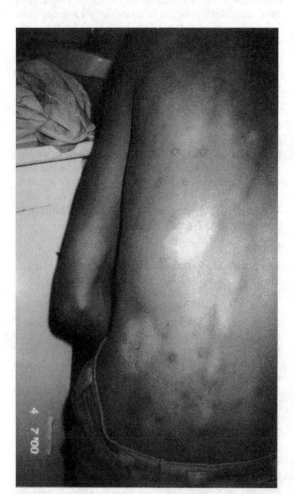

Figure 11-6. Hypopigmented anesthetic macules of leprosy in India.

have facilitated leprosy vaccine research because the organism cannot otherwise be maintained in the lab. Several prototype leprosy vaccines have been developed and are now in early clinical trials.

Buruli Ulcer

Buruli ulcer (BU) is a disfiguring ulcerative disease, primarily found in West Africa, caused by *Mycobacterium ulcerans,* an atypical mycobacterium in the *M. ulcerans* complex. However, scattered cases are found elsewhere in the tropics, including coastal Australia, Southeast Asia, China, and South America. It usually affects school-age children (ages 4 to 15), starting as a subcutaneous nodule that rapidly develops into a painless but nonhealing ulcer. About 80% of the lesions are on the extremities, with some cases complicated by contractures and osteomyelitis.[31] The ulceration results from a mycolactone cytotoxin produced by the bacteria, but locally the cause is all too often attributed to witchcraft, leading to further stigmatization. Swimming in ponds and rivers appears to be the major risk factor for acquiring the infection, and colonized aquatic insects are thought to carry the bacteria. The exact mechanism of transmission is still unknown. Minor skin trauma such as cuts or insect bites further increases susceptibility.[31] Although the diagnosis of Buruli ulcer is often clinical, PCR has now become the standard means of confirming the diagnosis.

Cure is difficult, with a high rate of relapse. Small lesions are usually surgically excised, with skin grafting when necessary. Since 2004, larger ulcers have been successfully treated with rifampin and streptomycin administered daily for 8 weeks.[32]

The WHO Buruli Ulcer Initiative began in 1998, but this mysterious disease has been difficult to research and eliminate. It is impractical to keep children away from the water. Buruli lesions have also been found in other mammals such as Australian possums. In one Australian case-control study, the odds of BU were halved by regular use of insect repellent, wearing long pants, and immediate washing of skin wounds. Risks were doubled for those with mosquito bites.[33] The best evidence to date suggests this infection is spread by environmental exposure, like anthrax. Vaccination has been considered as a possible solution, but no experimental vaccine is currently available.

Trypanosomal Diseases: Chagas Disease and Human African Trypanosomiasis

Chagas Disease

South American trypanosomiasis, or Chagas disease (named after Dr. Carlos Chagas, the Brazilian physician who discovered the causative agent *Trypanosoma cruzi*), afflicts impoverished people in Central and South America. The insect vectors are various species of triatomine bugs, sometimes called kissing or assassin bugs, which feed on blood at night and hide in roof thatch or cracked adobe walls during the day. Substandard housing is the most likely to be infested, and other resident mammals can also acquire the infection. Interestingly, Chagas disease is not transmitted directly but occurs when some of the insect's feces contaminate the bite site, usually through scratching the area. Infection can also be transmitted by eating raw meat from an infected animal, blood transfusion (US blood supply screening began in 2007) or even by drinking *acai* palm fruit juice, which may be contaminated by crushed triatomids hiding in the fruit.[34] Congenital cases also occur, including one recent birth in the United States.[35]

A self-limited local skin reaction termed a *chagoma* often occurs at the inoculation site. Swelling around the eye (Romañas sign) develops if inoculation occurs there. In the acute form of the disease, patients develop self-limited systemic symptoms such as fever, hepatosplenomegaly, myocarditis (with risk of fatal arrhythmias), and edema. A prolonged latent phase lasting years follows the acute illness. About a third of patients then progress to chronic Chagas disease, in which they develop cardiomyopathy, arrhythmias, megacolon, and megaesophagus.[36] The similarities to HIV have not gone unnoticed, and Peter Hotez has termed Chagas disease the "AIDS of the Americas." Death may occur from heart failure or arrhythmias.

Like Leishmania, *T. cruzi* sheds its flagellae after the acute stage and becomes an intracellular amastigote parasite. Diagnosis and treatment are difficult. Many cases present only after irreparable heart damage is done. Nifurtimox and benznidazole are two orphan drugs used as treatment options, but they are both toxic and require 1 to 3 months of daily dosing with no guarantee of a cure. New agents are urgently needed, but there is little financial incentive for research. Chagas disease control efforts have therefore relied on vector elimination by spraying pyrethrins inside homes and improving housing conditions. INCOSUR (*Initiativa de Salud del Cono Sud,* or Southern Cone Initiative) has led fairly successful eradication efforts in Argentina and Chile.

Chagas disease has recently become a concern in several southern states, including Texas, where many infected Latin American immigrants reside. Triatomid bugs exist in these states, although contact is less likely with better housing conditions. Blood transfusions from asymptomatic latently infected patients have rarely contaminated the US blood supply.

Human African Trypanosomiasis (Sleeping Sickness)

African sleeping sickness, or human African trypanosomiasis (HAT), is a devastating fatal protozoal infection spread by the bite of various tsetse fly (*Glossina*) species. There are three identical-appearing *Trypanosoma* species: *T. brucei gambiense* (causing West African or Gambian sleeping sickness), *T. brucei rhodesiense*, (East African or Rhodesian sleeping sickness), and *T. brucei brucei* (causing *nagana*, a wasting disease of cattle and other grazing animals).[37] Initially a skin chancre appears at the site of an infected tsetse fly bite. The trypanosomes migrate to the regional lymph nodes and then disseminate through the bloodstream as flagellated motile organisms.

The disease course depends on the species of parasite. West African disease is limited to humans and is fairly indolent with several years of fever, lethargy, and headache. Posterior cervical lymph nodes are enlarged (Winterbottom's sign), and lymph node aspirate is positive for parasites. Central nervous system involvement is initially manifested by psychiatric symptoms (paranoia, depression), followed by encephalitis, coma, and death.[38]

East African disease is a much more rapidly progressive zoonotic infection with death usually occurring within a year. Blood smears are positive with high parasitemia. The human diseases are separated geographically, although they overlap in Uganda. Nagana disease of cattle cannot affect humans because high-density lipoprotein in human blood is lethal to this subspecies.[39] However, livestock can also carry *T. brucei rhodesiense*, which may infect humans via tsetse fly bites.

Trypanosomes are able periodically to alter their surface antigens (antigenic variation) to stay one step ahead of the immune system. This "invisibility cloak" works for a while, and the patient sickens as the parasite multiplies asexually in the bloodstream. When the immune system catches up with the new antigens, the patient may temporarily improve, only to have the parasites switch their antigens again and repeat the cycle.

Therapy is toxic and difficult, with differing regimens for early and late disease, and for West and East African varieties. Melarsoprol is an arsenic-containing trypanosomal drug used for late stages that can cause a potentially fatal reactive encephalopathy. Other toxic drugs include suramin or pentamidine (for early disease) and eflornithine (late option for West African HAT).[21] These drugs are often difficult to obtain and poorly tolerated. Unfortunately, there is little financial incentive for new research into better treatments. Without treatment, both western and eastern forms of HAT are uniformly fatal, although the latter kills more quickly.

HAT has been eradicated from many areas due to spraying the tsetse fly vector. In West Africa, control is easier because there is no animal reservoir. Human treatment curtails the spread of disease. In the East African form, however, cattle and wildlife provide reservoirs for infection making this more of a challenge.

Dengue ("Break Bone") Fever

Dengue has become the most worrisome disease on the WHO's list of 17 NTDs, and it is now emerging in the United States with non-travel-related cases in Key West and Texas. Dengue may no longer be truly "neglected" because outbreaks are affecting tourism and raising public health alarms around the world. Unlike the mostly parasitic, rural, chronic NTDs discussed thus far, it is an acute arboviral (arthropod-borne virus) infection very common in urban areas. Dengue's day-feeding mosquito vectors, *Aedes aegypti* and *albopictus*, have a global distribution and can breed in the minute quantities of water found in tires and refuse, making vector control a constant challenge. Although most abundant in South and Southeast Asia, dengue is now at a 20-year high in the Caribbean and Central America.[40] Insect repellents are the only protection. There is as yet no vaccine or specific dengue remedy.

Dengue fever starts about 4 to 7 days after the infectious bite. Symptoms include high (often biphasic) fever for 5 to 7 days, headache, severe arthralgias, and a sunburn-like centripetal maculopapular rash in half of patients.[41] In light-skinned patients, the rash blanches with pressure and is often noted to have patches of pallor ("white islands in a sea of red"). The rash often follows the fever and resolves after several days.

Dengue is caused by four different flavivirus serotypes (DEN 1 to 4) with very little cross-protection between the different types. Most cases resolve uneventfully, but complications can occur. Dengue hemorrhagic fever (DHF) is a condition marked by fever, thrombocytopenia, leucopenia, increased vascular permeability, and hemorrhage. A positive tourniquet test after 5 minutes of blood pressure cuff constriction (more than 20 petechiae/square inch) confirms bleeding risk. Dengue shock syndrome (DSS), which occurs predominantly in children, is essentially DHF complicated by shock. A sudden drop in temperature accompanied by nausea and abdominal pain presages this condition. DSS mortality is high (12%) even with good hydration and care. Steroid use does not appear to reduce mortality.[42] Both DHF and DSS are thought related to a repeat dengue infection by a differing serotype.

Diagnosis is usually clinical, but dengue is easily confused with other infections such as chikungunya fever and leptospirosis. Early infection (viremia) in the first 5 days can be confirmed by reverse transcriptase-polymerase chain reaction (RT-PCR) testing. About a week after infection, immunoglobulin (Ig) M antibody (*DENV Detect IgM capture ELISA*) can be detected. As with other viral illnesses, a four-fold increase in antibody titers between acute and convalescent serum specimens is also diagnostic.[43] US dengue testing can be performed at the CDC Dengue Branch.

Vector control is the current mainstay of dengue control, but traditional spray and neighborhood cleanup programs have been supplemented by experimental programs (e.g., releasing genetically altered male mosquitoes that father wingless females). A new insecticide/larvicide, pyriproxyfen, sprayed where mosquitoes rest, first sterilizes the adult females and is then transported to breeding areas by the mosquitoes themselves. Ultimately, however, an effective dengue vaccine will be the best hope for long-term control. Several large-scale phase 3 clinical trials are currently in progress.

NEW STRATEGIES

Innovative new strategies will be necessary to control NTDs despite the relative success with vector control and mass treatment programs with specific drugs. Because many of these diseases share the same distribution and afflict the same populations, it would make sense to provide a single cocktail of drugs, hitting many NTDs at once, rather than setting up multiple duplicate distribution programs. A Rapid Impact Package (RIP) has been proposed that would contain a four-drug combination: albendazole (or mebendazole), praziquantel, ivermectin (or DEC), and azithromycin.[44] This would cover helminth infection, schistosomiasis, onchocerciasis, filariasis, and trachoma at almost half the expense of individual programs.[44] The cost for sub-Saharan Africa is estimated to be only $0.40 to $0.79 per person with a total 5-year program cost running between $1 and $2 billion.[2] Potential problems include suboptimal treatment and the eventual emergence of resistance.[45] Unfortunately, Chagas disease, African trypanosomiasis, and visceral leishmaniasis are not amenable to control by RIP and will continue to need careful surveillance, early treatment, and vector control.

The discovery of new drugs like ivermectin and praziquantel has saved countless lives. Although pharmaceutical companies have been very generous in donating these products to those needing them the most, research in developing newer drugs and vaccines for these remote exotic diseases has lagged behind. There is little financial incentive for companies to develop new interventions for diseases like leishmaniasis, Chagas disease, and African trypanosomiasis. Recent partnerships between the WHO, philanthropic foundations, and various governmental aid programs are starting to change this. There has been renewed interest in vaccine development for several diseases (e.g., hookworm, leishmaniasis, and dengue).[13] New drugs are needed to combat emerging resistance. Tribendimidine has in part been developed for its potential to treat helminth infections becoming resistant to benzimidazoles.[9] The discovery of *Wolbachia* bacteria in filarial worms effectively opened up new possibilities for sterilizing *Onchocerca* with the old standby drug doxycycline.[23] The old antimonial regimens for leishmaniasis are starting to be replaced by less toxic therapies like miltefosine, liposomal amphotericin B, paromomycin, and sitamaquine, although admittedly, leishmaniasis treatment is still fraught by controversy and confusion. Unfortunately, there are some NTD holdouts that resist easy solutions. Trypanosomal diseases are not only notoriously difficult to treat, but the few intermittently available medications are still antiquated and dangerous. BU treatment is equally difficult and uncertain. Diagnostic tests for many NTDs tend to be too challenging or expensive for the financially strapped clinics providing care for the poor, and new rapid diagnostic tests are urgently needed.

Ending the Neglect

In London, on January 30, 2012, a meeting was held entitled Uniting to Combat NTDs: Ending the Neglect and Reaching the 2020 Goals. The so-called London declaration endorsed at this meeting announced the massive support of the Gates Foundation and other donors to combat 17 NTDs around the world, and it reaffirmed the goals of WHO's Road Map on NTDs published earlier that month.[46] Essentially, the NTD field went from "rags to riches", greatly increasing the public heath community's confidence that NTDs could be controlled or eradicated. No longer would overseas aid for NTDs be limited to 0.6% of total health aid spending.[46] In addition to the ramped-up support from philanthropic and governmental sources, pharmaceutical industry donations amount to $2 to $3 billion of essential drugs each year.[46] Most NTD control programs depend on free access to donated ivermectin, praziquantel, albendazole, DEC, and azithromycin, all of which would be beyond the means of the marginalized populations that most need them. An open access global database for mapping and surveillance of NTDs is also being developed.[47] Accurate mapping of diseases such as schistosomiasis allows for better targeting of control interventions, thus saving limited resources.

The future for controlling, if not eradicating, many NTDs has never been brighter. In an optimistic 2012 editorial, David Molyneaux wrote that greater resources necessitate greater responsibility and offered four objectives.[46] The NTD public health community must effectively manage the increased donations, find new transparent ways of collaborating with each other, address the critical human deficits in NTD research and program management capacity, and avoid complacency as disease-specific goals and research targets keep changing. The next few decades offer unprecedented opportunities for lasting change, looking forward to a future when these long-dreaded diseases live on only in textbooks.

STUDY QUESTIONS

1. What factors have contributed to the neglected tropical diseases being overlooked for so many decades, and why has this started to change now?

2. Review the life cycles for various parasites and identify some "weak links" where this cycle could be interrupted by human intervention. An example of how these links can be broken is provided for guinea worm in the text.

3. What is the difference between disease elimination and disease eradication?

4. How do you pick the best stratagem (vector control, mass drug administration, vaccination) to use for a specific disease? If several strategies could be effective, how would you prioritize them?

5. Discuss the pros and cons of using a Rapid Impact Package of medications. Would you wish to add or subtract any drugs to or from this list?

REFERENCES

1. Hotez PJ. *Forgotten People, Forgotten Diseases: The Neglected Tropical Diseases and Their Impact on Global Health and Development*. Washington, DC: ASM Press, 2008.

2. Hotez P, Molyneux D, Fenwick A, et al. Control of neglected tropical diseases. *N Engl J Med* 2007;357:1018–1027.

3. WHO Neglected Tropical Disease List: http://www.who.int/neglected_diseases/diseases/en/.

4. United Nations Development Programme. "The Millennium Development Goals." http://www.undp.org/content/undp/en/home/mdgoverview/.

5. Bethony J, Brooker S, Albonico S, et al. Soil-transmitted helminth infections: ascariasis, trichuriasis and hookworm. *Lancet* 2006;367:1521–1532.

6. Crompton D, Nesheim M. Nutritional impact of helminthiasis during the human lifecycle. *Annu Rev Nutr* 2002;22:35–59.

7. Hall A, Horton S. Best practices—deworming: new advice from CC08. Copenhagen Consensus Center 2008:1–28. www.copenhagenconsensus.com.

8. Partners for Parasite Control. Resolution World Health Assembly 54.19. Geneva: WHO, 2001. Schistosomiasis and soil transmitted helminth infections. www.who.int/wormcontrol/about_us/en/.

9. Xiao S, Hui Ming W, Tanner M, et al. Tribendimidine: a promising, safe, and broad-spectrum antihelminthic agent from China. *Acta Trop* 2005;94(1):1–14.

10. Steinman P, Keiser R, Bos M, et al. Schistosomiasis and water resources development: systematic review, meta-analysis, and estimates of people at risk. *Lancet Infect Dis* 2006;6:411–425.

11. Hotez P, Bundy D, Beegle K, et al. Helminth infections: soil-transmitted helminth infections and schistosomiasis. In: Jamison D, Breman J, Measham A, et al, eds. *Disease Control Priorities in Developing Countries*. 2nd ed. Oxford: Oxford University Press, 2006: 467–482.

12. Ross A, Bartley P, Sleigh A, et al. Schistosomiasis. *N Engl J Med* 2002;346:1212–1220.

13. Bethony JM, Cole RN, Guo X, et al. Vaccines to combat the neglected tropical diseases. *Immunol Rev* 2011;239:237–270.

14. Fenwick A, Webster J. Schistosomiasis: challenges for control, treatment and drug resistance. *Curr Opin Infect Dis* 2006;19:577–582.

15. Hopkins D, Ruez-Tiben E, Downs P, et al. Dracunculiasis eradication: the final inch. *Am J Trop Med Hyg* 2005;73:669–675.

16. Dowdle W. The principles of disease elimination and eradication. *MMWR* 1999;48(SU01):23–27.

17. Ottesen E. Lymphatic filariasis: treatment, control and elimination. *Adv Parasitol* 2006;61:395–441.

18. World Health Organization. Podoconiosis. www.who.int/neglected_diseases/diseases/podoconiosis/en.

19. Udall D. Recent updates on onchocerciasis: diagnosis and treatment. *Clin Infect Dis* 2007;44:53–60.

20. Ayong L, Tume C, Wembe F, et al. Development and evaluation of an antigen detection dipstick assay for the detection of human onchocerciasis. *Trop Med Int Health* 2005;10:228–233.

21. The Medical Letter. Drugs for Parasitic Infections. *Treatment Guidelines from the Medical Letter* 2007 (last modified February 2008);5(Suppl):e1–e15.

22. Cotreau M, Warren S, Ryan J, et al. The antiparasitic moxidectin: safety, tolerability and pharmacokinetics in humans. *J Clin Pharm* 2003;43:1108–1115.

23. Hoerauf A, Mand S, Volkmann L, et al. Doxycycline in the treatment of human onchocerciasis: kinetics of Wolbachia endobacteria reduction and of inhibition of embryogenesis in female Onchocerca worms. *Microbes Infect* 2003;5(4):261–273.

24. Kasi P, Gilani A, Ahmad K, Janjua A. Blinding trachoma: a disease of poverty. *PLoS Med* 2004;1:e44.

25. Hotez P. The blinding neglected tropical diseases: onchocerciasis (river blindness) and trachoma. In: Hotez PJ. *Forgotten People, Forgotten Diseases: The Neglected Tropical Diseases and Their Impact on Global Health and Development*. Washington, DC: ASM Press, 2008: 55–68.

26. Solomon A, Holland M, Alexander N. Mass treatment with single dose azithromycin for trachoma. *N Engl J Med* 2004;351:1962–1971.

27. Piscopo T, Azzopardi C. Leishmaniasis. *Postgrad Med J* 2006;82:649–657.

28. Khamesipour A, Dowlati Y, Asilian A, et al. Leishmanization: use of an old method for evaluation of candidate vaccines against leishmaniasis. *Vaccines* 2005;23(28):3642–3648.

29. Rinaldi A. The global campaign to eliminate leprosy. *PLoS Med* 2005;2:e341.

30. McDougall A, Yuasa Y. *A New Atlas of Leprosy*. Tokyo: Sasakawa Memorial Health Foundation, 2001.

31. Merritt, R., Walker E, Small P, et al. Ecology and transmission of Buruli ulcer disease: a systematic review. *PLoS Negl Trop Dis* 2010;4(12):e911.

32. Converse P, Nuermberger E, Almeida D, Grosset J. Treating *Mycobacterium ulcerans* disease (Buruli ulcer): from surgery to antibiotics, is the pill mightier than the knife? *Future Microbiol* 2011;6(10):1185–1198.

33. Quck T, Athan E, Henry M, et al. Risk factors for *Mycobacterium ulcerans* infection, South-eastern Australia. *Emerg Infect Dis* 2007;13:1661–1666.

34. Nobrega A, Garcia M, Tatto E, et al. Oral transmission of Chagas disease by consumption of acai palm fruit, Brazil. *Emerg Infect Dis* 2009;15(4):653–655.

35. Centers for Disease Control and Prevention. Congenital transmission of Chagas disease—Virginia 2010. *MMWR* 2012; 61(26):477–479.

36. Teixeira A, Nitz M, Guimaro M, et al. Chagas' disease. *Postgrad Med J* 2006;82:788–798.

37. Hotez P. The kinetoplastic infections: human African trypanosomiasis (sleeping sickness), Chagas' disease, and the leishmaniases. In: Hotez PJ. *Forgotten People, Forgotten Diseases: The Neglected Tropical Diseases and Their Impact on Global Health and Development*. Washington, DC: ASM Press, 2008: 81–102.

38. Fevre E, Picozzi K, Jannin S, et al. Human African trypanosomiasis: epidemiology and control. *Adv Parasitol* 2006; 61: 168–221.

39. Pays E, Vanhollebeke B, Vanhamme L, et al. The trypanolytic factor in human serum. *Nat Rev Microbiol* 2006;4:477–486.

40. Jelinek T, Muhlberger N, Harms G, et al. Epidemiology and clinical features of imported dengue fever in Europe: sentinel surveillance data from TropNetEurop. *Clin Infect Dis* 2002; 35:1047–1052.

41. Wilder-Smith A, Schwartz E. Dengue in travelers. *N Engl J Med* 2005;353:924.

42. Tassniyom S, Vasanawathana S, Chirawatkul A et al. Failure of high dose methylprednisolone in established dengue shock syndrome; a placebo controlled double blind study. *Pediatrics* 1993;92:111.

43. Rigau-Perez J, Gubler G, Vorndam A, et al. Dengue surveillance—United States, 1986–92. *MMWR CDC Surveil Summ* 1994;43:7.

44. Molyneaux D, Hotez P, Fenwick A. Rapid Impact Interventions: how a policy for integrated control of Africa's neglected tropical diseases could benefit the poor. *PLoS Med* 2005; 2(11):e336.

45. Smits H. Prospects for the control of neglected tropical diseases by mass drug administration. *Expert Rev Anti Infect Ther* 2009;7(1):37–56.

46. Molyneaux D. Editorial: The 'Neglected Tropical Diseases': now a brand identity; responsibilities, context and promise. *Parasit Vectors* 2012;5:23.

47. Hurlimann E, Schur N, Boutsika K, et al. Toward an open-access global database for mapping, controls, and surveillance of neglected tropical diseases. *PLoS Negl Trop Dis* 2011;5(12):e1404.

Emerging Diseases and Antimicrobial Resistance

12

Arif R. Sarwari and Rashida A. Khakoo

 ## LEARNING OBJECTIVES

- *Recognize emerging and reemerging infectious diseases as threats to global health*
- *Raise awareness of the national and international response*
- *Learn about global issues of antimicrobial resistance of a variety of organisms and their spread*
- *Understand various concepts of antimicrobial resistance*
- *Learn about the impact of antimicrobial resistance among patients and communities*
- *Expand knowledge regarding prevention and control strategies directed against problems of antimicrobial resistance*

CASE STUDY OF AN EMERGING INFECTION

Severe Acute Respiratory Syndrome

Severe acute respiratory syndrome (SARS) is a prototypical emerging infectious disease that, largely because of global travel, instead of remaining an obscure respiratory infection in South China became a global public health crisis. By the time the outbreak ran its course, over 8,000 cases were identified from 29 countries with an overall 10% fatality rate.

Global attention toward the outbreak was first drawn in March 2003 with the recognition of cases of severe acute respiratory illness among patients in the Guangdong province of China, Hong Kong, Vietnam, Singapore, and Canada. The World Health Organization (WHO) issued a global alert and coined the term severe acute respiratory syndrome (SARS) for the disease. By April 2003, the WHO had to take the unprecedented step of issuing a travel advisory for the Guangdong Province and for Hong Kong, later broadened to other countries. Eventually, the etiologic agent was identified as a novel coronavirus (SARS CoV), likely a virus that jumped species from the civet (catlike delicacy in China) to humans. The initial zoonotic transmission was followed by subsequent nosocomial and human-to-human transmission perpetuating a widespread global epidemic. Most patients presented with fever, cough, shortness of breath, and reported either close contact with a person with SARS or a history of travel or residence in an area with recent local SARS transmission. The chest radiograph would reveal findings of pneumonia or acute respiratory distress syndrome, with some cases progressing on to require ventilatory support. Supportive treatment remained the mainstay of clinical care.

Initial cases of SARS were reported from Guangdong Province, China, in November 2002 with almost 800 cases noted by February 2003. A physician with SARS contributed to the subsequent widespread dissemination of the disease by traveling from Guangdong to a hotel in Hong Kong and infecting 10 other individuals who then traveled widely, perpetuating outbreaks in their countries of destination.[1] Most severe illness occurred in adults, with children, if infected at all, developing a milder illness. Patients older than 60 years had a higher mortality, with a case fatality rate up to 43%. Twenty-nine countries in Asia, Europe, and North America were affected with 83% of the reported cases hailing from China and Hong Kong. Table 12-1 depicts the timeline of the SARS outbreak.

Although most disease transmission occurred by droplet spread (requiring face-to-face contact), airborne transmission with droplet nuclei was strongly

Table 12-1. Timeline of the SARS outbreak.

Nov. 2002	First cases reported in Southern China
Feb. 2003	Up to 792 cases reported from Guangdong Province, China
March 2003	Index case of symptomatic physician traveling to Hong Kong
April 2003	Transmission to others living in same hotel as index case
May 2003	Widespread dissemination to Singapore, Vietnam, Canada, Thailand
June 2003	Global alert issued by WHO (March 12)
July 2003	1,622 cases reported from 13 countries, with 58 deaths
	WHO issues travel advisory to China, Hong Kong, Taiwan, and Toronto
	5,663 cases reported from 26 countries, with 372 deaths
	Travel advisories lifted for Toronto
	8,360 cases reported from 29 countries, with 764 deaths
	WHO lifts last remaining travel advisory for China
	100 days into the outbreak (June 19)
	8,447 cases reported from 29 countries, with 811 deaths
	Major epidemic in Asia ended
	WHO declares SARS outbreak contained worldwide

From www.who.int/csr/sars/en/.

suspected as the cause of cases in a large apartment complex in Hong Kong.[2] Transmission to health care workers was a common feature of the outbreak. This was likely precipitated by the high levels of viral shedding in nasopharyngeal aspirates early, and in stool later in the disease course, with possible environmental contamination. Infection control guidelines requiring that hospitalized patients be isolated in negative pressure rooms and that all health care workers wear masks, gowns, gloves, and protective eyewear helped finally control the epidemic.

DEFINITION AND BACKGROUND OF EMERGING DISEASES

The global spread of infectious disease can be traced back to the 16th century when Spanish explorers reportedly introduced smallpox, typhus, and measles to the susceptible population of the New World and returned with syphilis. This introduction of new diseases resulted in catastrophic depopulation with approximately 50 million deaths among the native South Americans. There have subsequently been a number of major epidemics, but by the mid-20th century, primarily with the rapid advances in sanitation and public health, infectious diseases were believed to be a problem of the past. In the United States, infectious disease mortality rates, per 100,000 population, fell from 500 in 1900 to 50 in 1960.[3] This success was reflected in statements such as "one can think of the middle of the twentieth century as the end of one of the most important social revolutions in history, the virtual elimination of infectious disease as a significant factor in social life."[4]

This optimism, unfortunately, was short lived as infectious diseases staged a dramatic comeback with more than 30 new diseases, including the HIV/AIDS pandemic, emerging in just the past 4 decades.[5] In addition, old foes like malaria and tuberculosis threatened to return with a vengeance. Among these and other infections, our options for control started shrinking as drug resistance started spreading. In fact, in the United States, between 1980 and 1992, the death rate from infectious diseases increased 50%.[3] Attention toward these emerging and reemerging infections was first drawn by a landmark 1992 report by the Institute of Medicine.[6] This report drew attention to the fact that pathogenic microbes can be resilient and dangerous foes. Although it is impossible to predict their individual emergence in time and place, we can be confident that new microbial diseases will continue to emerge. Based on this report, these diseases were defined as "New, reemerging or drug-resistant infections whose incidence in humans has increased within the past two decades or whose incidence threatens to increase in the near future."

This concept of emerging infections is flexible, reflecting not only the temporal and geographic interactions between humans and microbes, but also the ability of the medical community to identify them. The relationship between humans and microbe is seldom stable. New threats are ever present, confronting public health authorities as well as physicians.

The Institute of Medicine report identified some key factors explaining why infectious diseases emerge or reemerge. These include the following:

1. Global travel
2. Globalization of the food supplies and centralized processing of food
3. Population growth and increased urbanization and crowding
4. Population movements due to civil wars, famines, and other human-made or natural disasters
5. Irrigation, deforestation, and reforestation projects that alter the habitats of disease-carrying insects and animals
6. Human behaviors, such as intravenous drug use and risky sexual behavior

Table 12-2. Major agents of infectious disease identified over the past 4 decades.

Year	Infectious agent identified
1975–1979	Parvovirus B19, *Cryptosporidium parvum*, Ebola, *Legionella pneumophila*, *Campylobacter* spp.
1980–1984	*Borrelia burgdorferi*, HIV, *Escherichia coli* 0157:H7, *Helicobacter pylori*
1985–1989	*Ehrlichia* spp., hepatitis C and E virus
1990–1994	*Vibrio cholera* 0139, *Bartonella henselae*, Sin nombre virus, human herpes virus 8/Kaposi sarcoma, herpes virus
1995–1999	Prions, influenza A H5N1, enterovirus 71, West Nile virus
2000–2004	SARS-coronavirus, human metapneumovirus
2005–2009	Pandemic influenza A H1N1

7. Increased use of antimicrobial agents and pesticides, hastening the development of resistance
8. Increased human contact with tropical rain forests and other wilderness habitats that are reservoirs for insects and animals that harbor unknown infectious agents

Table 12-2 lists some of the major agents of infectious disease identified over the past 4 decades.

Examples of Emerging and Reemerging Infectious Diseases

Although there are many examples of new, emerging, and reemerging illnesses, only those of particular importance worldwide are discussed here. Agents of bioterrorism have assumed great recent importance and are also included.

Dengue

Dengue virus infection is an example of an emerging infection with a wide distribution, now found in all continents except Europe and Antarctica (Figures 12-1 and 12-2). With over 100 million annual infections worldwide among the 2.5 billion individuals at risk, the dengue viruses are arguably the most important arthropod-borne viruses from a medical and public health perspective.[7] A flavivirus, there are four antigenically related but distinct dengue virus serotypes carried by the principal mosquito vector *Aedes aegypti* that is well adapted to the urban environment.

Both epidemic and endemic transmission is maintained through a human-mosquito-human cycle, and no evidence for a significant animal reservoir exists, unlike yellow fever or West Nile virus. Susceptible individuals become infected after a bite from the infected female *Aedes* mosquito and become viremic toward the end of a 4- to 6-day incubation period.

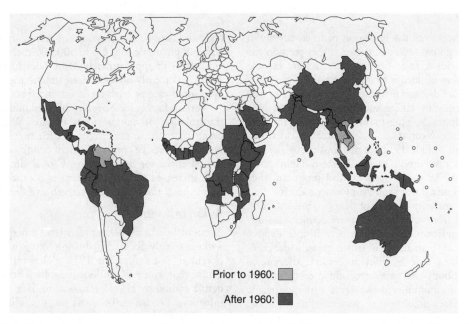

Prior to 1960:
After 1960:

Figure 12-1. Global distribution of cases of Dengue, before and after 1960. http://www.who.int/csr/disease/dengue/impact/en/index.html. (*Reproduced, with permission, from WHO. Global Alert and Response. Impact of Dengue.*)

Average annual number of DF/DHF cases reported to WHO & average annual number of countries reporting dengue

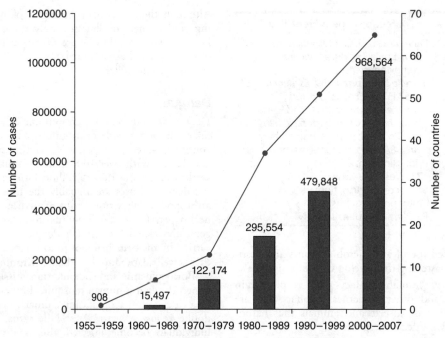

Figure 12-2. Average annual number of dengue fever/dengue hemorrhagic fever cases reported to the World Health Organization and average annual number of countries reporting dengue. http://www.who.int/csr/disease/dengue/impact/en/index.html. (*From WHO. Global Alert and Response. Impact of Dengue.*)

Viremia persists until the resolution of fever, usually in 7 days. Mosquitoes become infected if they feed on the viremic individual, and after 8 to 12 days are capable of transmission of disease for the duration of their life-span. They are daytime urban feeders and prefer to bite humans, frequently taking multiple blood meals in a single breeding cycle. Thus transmission among multiple family members is common. *Aedes aegypti* are widely distributed from latitude 45° N to 35° S. Although greatly restricted in distribution in the Western Hemisphere during the 1970s yellow fever control programs, they now have reinfested nearly all their former habitats.

The vast majority of cases of dengue virus infection globally are from areas with hyperendemic transmission: the continuous circulation of multiple dengue virus serotypes, particularly in urban areas. Most clinical cases occur among children because the prevalence of antibody rises with age, and most adults are immune. This immunity, however, is serotype specific and may, in fact, predispose to more fulminant disease. Instead of a self-limiting, nonspecific, febrile viral illness, individuals with antibodies to one dengue virus serotype but infected with another serotype are more likely to manifest the complications of hemorrhagic

fever and dengue shock syndrome secondary to a capillary leak phenomenon. Up to 500,000 such cases occur annually with approximately 25,000 deaths worldwide. There is currently no specific treatment available; however, some vaccine trials are in advanced stages.

Various factors have been implicated in the increased transmission of dengue virus of late. Warmer temperatures increase the length of time that a mosquito remains infective, and crowded conditions increase the potential for transmission. Global climate change with increased global temperatures is expected to further expand the range of *A. aegypti* and dengue virus.

Avian Influenza

Avian influenza H5N1 represents an emerging disease with currently focal distribution but with explosive potential, not unlike the 1918 global influenza pandemic that killed 20 million people. The 1918 pandemic caused by H1N1 remains, to date, the greatest infectious disease outbreak in history. This virus was an avian strain that adapted to infect and transmit among humans. Of the three influenza pandemics in the 20th century, two were caused by human-avian reassortment viruses (H2N2 in 1957 and H3N2 in 1968). Genetic reassortment between avian and human viruses leading to a new virus capable of pandemic spread may occur in coinfected persons or intermediate hosts like pigs that have receptors for both avian and human influenza viruses.

After its initial identification in May 1997 in a young boy who died of influenza in Hong Kong, sporadic transmission of avian influenza H5N1 to about 200 humans in Asia had raised concerns about an imminent pandemic.[8] The virus is now endemic among bird and poultry populations in Eurasia and likely spread by migratory birds. There are concerns that the virus will adapt to a strain capable of sustained human-to-human transmission, unlike the current strain where almost all cases are secondary to direct contact with poultry.

Like most new influenza strains, the current H5N1 strain also emerged in Southeast Asia and rapidly spread westward, reaching Turkey by 2006. This spread has continued despite the culling of domestic and agriculture poultry flocks. Over 600 human infections have been confirmed in 15 countries including Thailand, Vietnam, Indonesia, Cambodia, China, Turkey, Azerbaijan, Egypt, and Iraq with a 50% case-fatality rate. Human cases from 2006 compared with 1997 show that the virus has undergone some antigenic changes (i.e., antigenic drift).

Clinical presentation may include symptoms related to both the respiratory and gastrointestinal systems. Most patients present with fever, upper respiratory symptoms, diarrhea, and pneumonia as documented by chest radiographs. Laboratory abnormalities may include elevated aminotransferases and pancytopenia with complications and death resulting from respiratory failure and multiorgan dysfunction.

The H5N1 avian influenza virus is resistant to amantadine and rimantadine but susceptible to the neuraminidase inhibitors oseltamivir and zanamivir. The latter are most effective early in the course of illness. Unfortunately, strains with a high level of oseltamivir resistance have already been identified from a few Vietnamese patients. In addition to treating the patient, household contacts are recommended to receive postexposure prophylaxis with oseltamivir 75 mg daily for 7 to 10 days.

The WHO and governments across the world have actively prepared for a pandemic by investing in vaccine development, stockpiling medication, and developing grassroots plans to cater to large numbers of patients. As of September 2012, the WHO had retained the avian influenza pandemic alert at phase 3. The following is a description of the six phases of pandemic alert:

Phase 1: Interpandemic phase; low risk of human cases
Phase 2: New virus in animals but no human cases; high risk of human cases
Phase 3: Pandemic alert; no or very limited human-to-human transmission
Phase 4: Clusters of human cases suggesting increased adaptability of the virus; evidence of increased human-to-human transmission
Phase 5: Larger clusters of human cases over longer periods; evidence of significant human-to-human transmission
Phase 6: Pandemic; efficient and sustained human-to-human transmission

West Nile

The West Nile virus, another flavivirus, suddenly emerged in North America in August 1999. It was first identified as an outbreak of viral encephalitis in New York with 62 cases and 7 deaths.[9] The virus has since progressively spread westward, and 2005 saw activity detected in 48 states and the District of Columbia. An arbovirus extensively distributed throughout Africa, the Middle East, Europe, South Asia and Australia, the North American strain is believed to have been imported from the Middle East, likely through air travel. In the United States, the peak of the outbreak was in 2003 when all but three states in the continental United States reported a total of 9,862 cases, 2,866 with neuroinvasive disease. Like other arboviral encephalitides, peak incidence was seen in late summer or early fall. In summer 2012, there was another surge in infections with the state of Texas hit particularly hard. Viral transmission has also spread to Canada, Mexico, the Caribbean, and Central America.

Mosquitoes of the *Culex* genus are the primary vectors with birds as the primary amplifying hosts, maintaining a bird-mosquito-bird cycle. Humans are incidental hosts and, unlike dengue, not important for transmission. Most are asymptomatic or present with a nonspecific febrile illness with only 1 in 150 infections resulting in meningitis or encephalitis, especially among the elderly. No specific treatment exists.

West Nile virus transmission in the United States has subsequently also been described with blood transfusions and organ transplantation, the latter often with catastrophic results.

Agents of Bioterrorism

In addition to the natural emergence and reemergence of disease, some biologic agents have the potential to be used deliberately to inflict mass casualties. Among weapons of mass destruction, biologic weapons are more destructive and cheaper to produce than chemical weapons, and they may be as lethal as nuclear weapons. It is estimated that the aerosolized release of 100 kg of anthrax spores upwind of Washington, D.C., would result in between 130,000 and 3 million deaths, similar to a hydrogen bomb.[10] In 2001, the United States experienced a bioterrorism attack using anthrax powder distributed via the postal system.[11] Three cases of anthrax were confirmed in South Florida in October 2001 with 19 additional confirmed or suspected cases from New York City, New Jersey, Maryland, Pennsylvania, Virginia, Connecticut, and Washington, D.C. Eleven of these were cases of inhalational anthrax, most occurring in postal employees. The FBI investigation, code named Amerithrax, was formally concluded in February 2010 after the prime suspect took his own life before charges could be filed. This attack remains the worst biologic attack in US history.

Although the list of potential biologic agents is large, the Centers for Disease Control and Prevention (CDC) has identified a number of high-priority organisms as category A agents based on their potential for easy dissemination, person-to-person transmission, and ability to cause panic, social disruption, and high mortality. Category B agents are moderately easy to disseminate and cause moderate morbidity and low mortality; category C agents include emerging pathogens that could be engineered for mass dissemination in the future because of availability (Table 12-3). Preparedness and planning for a bioterrorism-related event involves strengthening existing systems for detection and response to naturally occurring epidemics, particularly the emerging and reemerging infections. Through strong epidemiologic training, development of a communications infrastructure, a network of diagnostic laboratories, and a respect for the threat of biologic terrorism, preparedness can be improved and the impact of epidemics, regardless of the origin, can be reduced.

GLOBAL RESPONSE TO THE PROBLEM

In response to the Institute of Medicine report, the CDC developed a strategic plan in 1994 that was subsequently updated in 1998.[12] Four interdependent goals were identified:

1. Surveillance and response
2. Applied research
3. Infrastructure and training
4. Prevention and control

Surveillance systems monitor emerging infectious pathogens and outbreaks of disease. A response is mounted when surveillance data or other information indicates a change in the incidence or distribution of an infectious disease, or when a new or variant strain of a pathogen has become a health threat. Through applied research, scientists answer questions about the etiology, transmission, diagnosis, prevention, and control of emerging infectious diseases. Research, surveillance, and response all depend on the public health infrastructure that supports, trains, and equips public health workers, and links them in national and global networks. Training the next generation of public health scientists is a crucial component of the public heath infrastructure. All of the CDC's efforts are ultimately directed at implementing the fourth goal: prevention and control. In many instances, the CDC acts as

Table 12-3. Potential bioterrorism agents by category.

Category A	Category B	Category C
Variola major (smallpox)	*Coxiella burnetii* (Q fever)	Nipah virus
Bacillus anthracis (anthrax)	*Brucella* spp. (brucellosis)	Hantavirus
Yersinia pestis (plague)	*Burkholderia mallei* (glanders)	Congo-Crimean hemorrhagic fever
Clostridium botulinum (botulism)	*Burkholderia pseudomallei* (meliodiosis)	(CCHF) virus
Francisella tularensis (tularemia)	*Chlamydia psittaci* (psittacosis)	Tick-borne encephalitis viruses
Filoviruses (ebola, marburg)	*Rickettsia prowazeki* (typhus)	Yellow fever
Arenaviruses (lassa, junin)	Alphaviruses (encephalitis viruses)	Multidrug-resistant tuberculosis
	Ricin toxin	(MDR-TB)
	Clostridium perfringens toxin	
	Staphylococcus enterotoxin B	
	Salmonella spp. (salmonellosis)	
	Shigella dysenteriae (shigellosis)	
	E. coli O157:H7 (enterohemmorrhagic *E. coli*)	
	Vibrio cholerae (cholera)	
	Cryptosporidium parvum (cryptosporidiosis)	

a catalyst, developing and evaluating prevention and control strategies that can be implemented by others.

The Global Emerging Infection Sentinel Network of the International Society of Travel Medicine, or GeoSentinel (www.istm.org/geosentinel/main.html) systematically surveys travelers as sentinels to herald the emergence of new pathogens early enough to develop appropriate public health responses to limit the dissemination of novel microbial threats. Compared with the conventional surveillance based on public health laboratories and local health departments, this is a provider-based consortium of 54 travel medicine clinics located in various countries.

Crucial to the global response has been the incorporation of information technology resources for the rapid dissemination of information. ProMED-mail (www.promedmail.org), a free e-mail list run by voluntary moderators, was established in 1994 and reports on disease outbreaks in plants, animals, and humans. In February 2003, ProMED-mail reported on the 300 cases of pneumonia in South China identified from November 2002, ultimately recognized as SARS and leading to the WHO-issued global alert by March 2003.

In January 1995, a peer-reviewed, public domain, indexed journal *Emerging Infectious Diseases* (wwwnc.cdc.gov/eid/) was launched with the objective of enhancing the knowledge of professionals in infectious diseases and related sciences. The quarterly journal tracks disease trends, analyzes new and reemerging infectious diseases, and disseminates information around the world.

The WHO, in 1995, created a new division, Emerging and Other Communicable Diseases Surveillance and Control, and it uses at least two instruments to disseminate information: the *Disease Outbreak News* (www.who.int/disease.outbreak-news) immediately alerts to outbreaks detected and verified by the WHO, and the *Weekly Epidemiological Record* (www.who.int/wer) is the WHO's principal instrument for alerting the world to changes in both the behavior of infectious diseases and recommended measures for control. How all these instruments came together was well exemplified by the SARS outbreak and its rapid containment.

IMPORTANT CONCEPTS ON ANTIMICROBIAL RESISTANCE

Antimicrobial resistance is widely recognized as a global public health problem. This problem continues to worsen with selective pressure exerted by inappropriate use of antimicrobials and the spread of resistant organisms in health care institutions and the community.

In health care settings, the incidence and prevalence of many resistant strains has been increasing, including but not limited to methicillin-resistant *Staphylococcus aureus* (MRSA), vancomycin-resistant enterococci (VRE), and extended-spectrum β-lactamase producing strains of aerobic gram-negative rods. There are increasing reports of multidrug-resistant strains of *Pseudomonas aeruginosa, Klebsiella pneumoniae, Acinetobacter baumannii,* and additional concern about *Staphylococcus* with intermediate sensitivity to glycopeptides and rare strains showing resistance to vancomycin.

Worldwide there is an increasing population of critically ill and immunosuppressed patients who often require and receive various courses of antimicrobials, further increasing problems of resistance. The issue of resistance to antimicrobials is not restricted to hospitals and other health care institutions. Organisms causing community-acquired infections have also demonstrated resistance as noted in the case study later in this chapter. Worldwide there is a problem of antimicrobial resistance of respiratory bacterial pathogens, including *Streptococcus pneumoniae, Haemophilus influenzae* and *Moraxella catarrhalis.* Organisms that cause sexually transmitted infections, such as *Neisseria gonorrhoeae,* and pathogens causing gastrointestinal infections, such as *Shigella* and *Salmonella,* have also demonstrated widespread resistance. Multidrug-resistant tuberculosis (MDR-TB) is defined as those infections caused by isolates that are resistant to both rifampin and INH. Data from the WHO in 2008 showed an estimated 390,000 to 510,000 cases of MDR-TB emerging globally. Among all reported tuberculosis cases globally, 3.6% are estimated to have MDR-TB; almost 50% are estimated to occur in India and China. Extensively drug-resistant tuberculosis (XDR-TB) is defined as tuberculosis caused by isolates resistant to second-line injectable drugs and fluoroquinolones in addition to INH and rifampin. Data from the WHO on testing for XDR-TB demonstrated that 9% of MDR-TB cases were found to have XDR-TB; a total of 77 countries have confirmed at least one case of XDR-TB (www.who.int/tb/challenges/xdr/faqs/en/). In the United States, data from the US National Surveillance System 1993–2008 showed the baseline prevalence of MDR-TB and XDR-TB was 12.6% and 0.38%, respectively. Worldwide MDR-TB has emerged as a threat to public health. (See Chapter 10 for more information on tuberculosis.)

Resistance is not restricted to bacteria but is also present in viruses, fungi, and protozoa. With the ongoing HIV pandemic and the expanding use of antiretroviral therapy, both primary and secondary resistance is being increasingly reported. Difficulty with adherence to antiretroviral therapy poses many challenging issues and frequently results in the development of acquired multidrug resistance. Primary drug resistance is also occurring, dictating the need for resistance testing in more patients, where available. In developing countries this issue can pose challenges. Acyclovir resistance of *Herpes simplex* has been reported in HIV-infected patients.[13] Recently resistance to foscarnet, an alternative drug, was also reported.[14] Fungal pathogens have also been reported to be resistant, particularly some of the nonalbicans species of *Candida* whose resistance to fluconazole has been well described. In the SENTRY Antimicrobial Surveillance Program, resistance of bloodstream isolates of *Candida* to fluconazole, echinocandins, and voriconazole was reported.[15] Occurrence of multi-drug-resistant *Plasmodium falciparum* continues to be a significant and serious problem worldwide.

The global spread of antimicrobial resistance can occur with increased travel. Infectious diseases have been known to travel faster and further than ever before. During the 1990s, resistant *S. pneumoniae* was identified in Spain and then rapidly found in Argentina, Brazil, Chile, China, Columbia, Malaysia, Mexico, Philippines, Cambodia, South Africa, Thailand, and the United States. The inappropriate use of antimicrobials also extends to their use in veterinary medicine and agricultural fields. Antimicrobials have been used in food animals in North America and Europe for half a century. There is continued debate about this issue and the impact of this type of antimicrobial use on human health. Commonly used agents include penicillins, tetracyclines, cephalosporins, fluoroquinolones, avoparcin (a glycopeptide related to vancomycin), and virginiamycin (a streptogramin related to quinupristin-dalfopristin). Antimicrobials are given to these animals for growth promotion and for therapy. The percentage of antimicrobials used for animals versus humans is not exactly known. It is estimated that 50% of all antimicrobials produced in the United States are administered to animals mostly for subtherapeutic uses.[16] The use of antimicrobials in food animals has been postulated to be associated with antimicrobial resistance among *Salmonella* and *Campylobacter* isolates from humans.[17] Widespread resistance to Streptogramin antimicrobials among *Enterococcus faecium* strains throughout the poultry production region on the US eastern seaboard has been reported.[18] White et al found that 20% of samples of ground beef obtained from supermarkets in the United States were contaminated with Salmonella.[19] Overall, 84% of these isolates were resistant to at least one antimicrobial. Another study found that at least 17% of chickens obtained in supermarkets in four states had strains of *Enterococcus faecium* that were resistant to quinupristin-dalfopristin.[20] Resistance to many antimicrobials has emerged among bacterial strains colonizing pet animals and also those causing infections. Increasing numbers of antimicrobials are used in pet animals.[21] Bacteria possess a large number of mechanisms for the development of resistance. They can undergo *mutations* in chromosomes and express a latent resistance gene or acquire new genetic material by different mechanisms including direct exchange of DNA via *conjugation* or by bacterial *transduction* and extra chromosomal plasmid DNA via *transformation*. The information encoded in the genetic material makes it possible for the organisms to develop resistance by production of antimicrobial inactivating enzymes, alteration of antimicrobial target sites, or preventing antimicrobial access to a target site. Transposons and plasmids (extrachromosomal DNA) provide the transfer of genes easily. In addition to exchanging genetic material, transposons and plasmids also may encode genes for the active efflux of antimicrobials. An organism may possess more than one mechanism of resistance. A few examples of organisms commonly causing infections and their mechanisms of resistance are detailed to enhance understanding of mechanisms.

Health care associated MRSA are generally multidrug resistant. The presence of the mec gene is a requirement for methicillin resistance. In susceptible *S. aureus*, β-lactams bind to penicillin-binding protein (PBP) 1 to 3. Mec A encodes for PBP 2a, which has a low affinity for β-lactam antimicrobials. Phenotypic expression of methicillin resistance in the laboratory varies, and it is important to follow guidelines for determining the presence of MRSA in the laboratory. The exact mechanism of intermediate-resistant strains of *S. aureus* to vancomycin (MIC 8 μg/ml to 16 μg/ml) is not known. Thickening of cell walls has been visualized by electron microscopy. It is postulated that vancomycin is trapped in the cell wall because of decreased cross-linking of peptidoglycan strands. Vancomycin resistance of *S. aureus* (MIC 32 μg/ml or higher) is thought to be due to synthesis of an alternative terminal peptide, D-ala-D-lac, instead of D-ala-D-ala. Vancomycin is unable to bind to this changed peptide.

Inactivation of β-lactam antimicrobials occurs with the production of β-lactamases. Initially described β-lactamases inactivated penicillin and narrow-spectrum cephalosporins. Extended-spectrum β-lactamases (ESBLs) were initially described in the 1980s. The family of ESBLs is heterogeneous.[22] Their activity against different oxyimino-β-lactams (cefotaxime, ceftazidime, and ceftriaxone) varies, but they do not inactivate cephamycins (cefoxitin, cefotetan, and cefmetazole) and carbapenems. ESBLs have been found in aerobic gram-negative organisms, predominantly *Escherichia coli* and *Klebsiella*. However, they also occur in other aerobic gram-negative rods. Identification of organisms producing ESBLs in the laboratory is important because they are heterogeneous and can be missed.

Resistance to antimicrobial agents is increasing with newer mechanisms of resistance. Carbapenem-resistant strains of Enterobacteriaceae have continued to emerge worldwide resulting in few or no options for treatment.[23] NDM-1 is a metallo-β-lactamase first identified in carbapenem-resistant *K. pneumoniae* in a patient from Sweden transferred from New Delhi in 2008.[24] In a short period, NDM-1 producing enterobacteriaceae have been reported from many parts of the world, and many were linked to the Indian subcontinent. Recently, there have been reports of isolations of bla (NDM-2) positive *A. baumannii* in the Middle East. This raises concern about emergence of a unique clone. Carbapenemase-producing strains are usually associated with many non-β-lactamase resistant determinants resulting in multidrug resistance.

Enterococci are intrinsically resistant to several antimicrobials. They have become resistant to additional antimicrobials. High-level resistance to ampicillin has been demonstrated in *E. faecium*. Intrinsic resistance of *E. faecium* to ampicillin is thought to be due to the presence of a cell wall with low affinity for PBPs. High-level resistance to ampicillin is postulated to be due to alterations of PBP_5 protein and increased expression of PBP_5. Enterococci show intrinsic resistance to low and moderate levels of aminoglycoside. Unfortunately, strains showing high-level aminoglycoside resistance have also been reported to cause infection. Streptomycin resistance can be caused by mutation or by the presence of a streptomycin-modifying enzyme. High-level resistance to gentamicin is due to the production of bifunctional enzymes. High-level resistance to gentamicin and streptomycin results in a lack of synergy with cell wall active antimicrobials.

High-level resistance of enterococci to vancomycin was first reported in Europe. Subsequently, VRE have been reported from many parts of the world. Vancomycin inhibits enterococci by binding to the D-alanyl-D-alanine terminus of cell wall protein. In the peptidoglycan, D-ala-D-ala is replaced with D-alanyl-D-lactate. Binding of vancomycin to this changed terminus is with significantly lower affinity. Different clusters of genes, Van A, B, and D, encode for high-level resistance to vancomycin. Van A is the most common type of vancomycin resistance. It also mediates cross-resistance to teicoplanin. The second most common type of vancomycin resistance is Van B. These organisms are usually sensitive to teicoplanin.

Linezolid and quinupristin-dalfopristin resistant isolates of *E. faecium* have also been reported. Mutations in the V domain of 23S rRNA appear to be related to resistance.[25] Linezolid-resistant strains have even been identified prior to exposure to linezolid. Resistance to quinupristin-dalfopristin occurs via a variety of mechanisms: antimicrobial-modifying enzymes, efflux pump, and modification of the target site.[26]

Decreased susceptibility of some organisms to antimicrobials might be difficult to detect during routine laboratory testing. Examples include decreased susceptibility of *S. aureus* to vancomycin, detection of resistance of *S. pneumoniae* to penicillin, and organisms with newer mechanisms of resistance, for example ESBLs. There are difficulties in the detection of carbapenemase in laboratories. Phenotypic tests such as the modified Hodge test are used in microbiology laboratories for the detection of carbapenemases. These show low sensitivity and specificity for detecting NDM. There was a recent report of the Carba NP test based on a technique designed to identify hydrolysis of the β-lactam ring of carbapenem.[27] This test was highly sensitive and specific.

Case Study of an Issue with Antimicrobial Resistance

Health-care-associated MRSA infections were initially reported in the 1960s. They have become prevalent pathogens causing health-care-associated infections. There were sporadic reports of community-acquired methicillin resistant *Staphylococcus aureus* (CA-MRSA) infections beginning in 1980. The current epidemic in the United States has been reported since 1999.[28] Initial reports in the United States occurred with infections among young children. Subsequently, infections were reported in prisoners, men who have sex with men, intravenous drug users, and those competing in contact sports. Currently, many people are seen with CA-MRSA skin infections with no underlying risk factors or specific epidemiologic circumstances. Skin infections can range from minor to severe, including necrotizing fasciitis. Skin infections caused by these organisms often have necrotic centers and have sometimes been misdiagnosed as "spider bites."[29] CA-MRSA has also been associated with severe pneumonia and sepsis including deaths in healthy persons. Over the last decade, there have been increased numbers of reports of invasive CA-MRSA infections reported in many parts of the world.

The Mec gene is required for *S. aureus* to express resistance. The Mec gene is part of a mobile chromosomal element called staphylococcal cassette chromosome (SCCmec). Five SCCmec types have been described. Most CA-MRSA have type IV SCCmec. Most CA-MRSA isolates in the United States have been reported as containing genes encoding Panton-Valentine leukocidin (PVL), a cytotoxin that causes leukocyte destruction and has been postulated to cause tissue necrosis. No difference in 30-day mortality was noted in patients when invasive infections were caused by PVL-positive and -negative CA-MRSA strains. In a recent study, it was reported that severity of invasive disease caused by CA-MRSA is likely related to the entire genotype rather than just PVL.[30] Some of the virulence characters are as described earlier. The pathogenesis of infections caused by CA-MRSA is also not clear, and in addition, we do not have data on host factors that are important for occurrence and transmission of infection. Patients with CA-MRSA pose challenges for clinicians. These patients are usually seen in the outpatient setting with skin and soft tissue infections, and spread of these organisms to health care facilities has occurred. Awareness and recognition of this problem is important. Traditionally used cephalosporins and antistaphylococcal penicillins are ineffective. Many isolates in the United States have been reported to be sensitive to trimethoprim-sulfamethoxazole, doxycycline, and clindamycin in addition to the usual drugs used for health-care-associated MRSA. There are no clinical trials to demonstrate whether clindamycin or trimethoprim-sulfamethoxazole is actually effective for these infections. Clindamycin presents an additional challenge. Strains that may be sensitive to clindamycin but resistant to erythromycin *in vitro* can contain genes encoding inducible resistance to clindamycin and have the potential to develop resistance while the patient is receiving treatment. If the strain demonstrates resistance to erythromycin and sensitivity *in vitro* to clindamycin, it is very important to check for inducible resistance before clindamycin is used. For serious infections, vancomycin is usually recommended. Alternative agents include daptomycin and linezolid. However, daptomycin cannot be used if there is an infection involving the lungs. The importance of drainage of infected foci and appropriate debridement cannot be overemphasized.

IMPACT OF ANTIMICROBIAL RESISTANCE

The issue and problem of antimicrobial resistance has received attention from a wide sector throughout the world, including health care professionals, governments, nongovernmental organizations, and the general public. An article by Cosgrove and Carmeli outlines some of these issues of impact.[31] Increasing antimicrobial resistance presents a major threat to public health.

The impact on the patient can be quite serious. Resistance can certainly result in the delay of administration of appropriate antimicrobials to the patient. Multidrug resistance of organisms can limit the choices available for the patient. Alternative agents may be more toxic or unavailable. Occasionally with multidrug-resistant strains, there might not be any options or some of the alternative agents may not be as effective. The patient is often placed in contact isolation on admission and upon subsequent admissions. The potential barrier to care from contact isolation

has been reported,[32] and the impact on health care workers has also been reported.[33] With increasing resistance of various organisms, empirical regimens change, and patients who may not have infection with resistant organisms on admission are administered empirical therapy to cover the possibility of resistant organisms.

Many methodological issues are outlined in the literature regarding the measurement of the impact of resistance. Often there are no controls for length of stay before the onset of infection with resistant organisms. The selection of an appropriate control group is essential. It is important to adjust for the severity of illness. The patients with infections caused by resistant organisms often have more severe underlying illnesses that may result in adverse outcomes. The assessment of severity of illness more than 48 hours before the first signs of infection is considered important. One must distinguish between all-cause mortality versus attributable mortality, and morbidity has to be determined carefully. MDR-TB, for example, is associated with increased morbidity and mortality. One reason for this is that an appropriate anti-TB regimen is not used early in the course of infection. In developing countries, where second-line treatments are not as easily available and where most cases occur, resistant organisms are likely to have a significant impact on death rates.

Understanding of the economic impact of antimicrobial resistance on society as a whole is limited. In addition to morbidity, mortality, and increased length of stay, antimicrobial resistance in *S. aureus,* Enterococcus, and gram-negative bacilli has also been associated with the increased cost of health care. A recent study demonstrated that antimicrobial resistance was associated with higher expense, greater length of stay, and higher mortality.[34]

One of the areas discussed is how to measure cost appropriately. There is an interesting paper by McGowan[35] on the economic impact of antimicrobial resistance. He discusses differing viewpoints of the various stakeholders, including physicians, health care businesses, the pharmaceutical industry, and the general public, as far as the economic impact is concerned. His paper provides an excellent perspective on assessing the economic impact of resistance. He comments on the follow-up work that is necessary to further define the optimal methods of measurement of this impact, including noting the specific perspective from which the assessment is being made.

CONTROL STRATEGIES TO COUNTER ANTIMICROBIAL RESISTANCE

Strategies to prevent, control, and improve antimicrobial resistance are critical. A single country cannot adequately address the problem. Collaboration and cooperation among various countries dealing with this issue is very important. In 2001, the WHO issued the Global Strategy for Containment of Antimicrobial Resistance. It was difficult to translate this strategy into public health action. In 2004, the WHO published another paper on the antimicrobial resistance containment and surveillance approach, a public health tool that outlines important areas of action.[36]

Surveillance

Surveillance systems can be helpful for monitoring the current situation but also for assessment of the impact of any intervention that is made. Surveillance programs together with decision support systems are useful for improving recommendations regarding empirical antimicrobial therapy in a variety of settings, including the development of appropriate guidelines. Data can be used for giving feedback to users of antimicrobials, helping direct more focused and appropriate infection control efforts, monitoring changes in resistance patterns, providing various comparisons, and carrying out interventions that help prevent the spread of resistant strains.

It is important to track the spread of resistant organisms globally through a variety of surveillance programs. There are numerous types of surveillance programs: local, national, and international. Masterson[37] lists the aims of surveillance programs as specific, measurable, accessible, realistic, and targeted.

Many countries have established national and regional surveillance collaborations; others have not. Many regional programs have been set up in the various WHO regions. Core components for global collaborations have been discussed. Systematic collection, consolidation, and evaluation of antimicrobial resistance data are important to define global problems. To support surveillance at various levels, the WHO Collaborating Center for Surveillance of Antibiotic Resistance developed and supports WHONET software for the management and sharing of microbiology results. In most countries, WHONET software is used as a core component of national surveillance programs. In developing countries, surveillance for antimicrobial resistance remains suboptimal.

Most laboratories worldwide are capable of performing antimicrobial susceptibility testing. However, help is still needed for many laboratories in terms of future training on quality control, dissemination of information, interpretive criteria, and harmonizing methodology worldwide.

WHO has initiated a global program for gathering information on resistant bacteria. WHONET[38] involves a network of microbiologists collecting antimicrobial resistance results in a common database. Quality control and proficiency testing are also included in the program. There are surveillance programs targeting specific organisms and specific antimicrobial agents. There are programs for health-care-associated infections such as the National Healthcare Safety Network in the United States. Some surveillance programs evaluate trends in the antimicrobial susceptibility of pathogens that cause lower respiratory infections. Data have been systematically collected for *S. pneumoniae*, *Haemophilus influenzae*, and *Moraxella catarrhalis*. The SENTRY program is a multinational antimicrobial surveillance program. It monitors the predominant organisms and antimicrobial resistance patterns of health-care-associated and community-acquired infections by using a network of sentinel hospitals. Surveillance programs by themselves are not adequate for preventing the occurrence and spread of antimicrobial-resistant organism infections. Sharing of this information with all the stakeholders and feedback of this information to the users of antimicrobials is critical in making a change. Molecular techniques have recently been included in the SENTRY program that should provide further information.[39] The data on the detection of increasing resistance have led to some changes in clinical prescribing practice. A decrease in the incidence of penicillin-resistant pneumococci was observed in Iceland. Resistance of *S. pneumoniae* has been controlled by prescription restriction of antimicrobials in Japan, Hungary, Finland, and Iceland. In European countries, antimicrobial resistance has been monitored in selected bacteria from humans since 1998 through the European Antimicrobial Resistance Surveillance System (EARSS), now called European Surveillance of Antimicrobial Consumption (ESAC). One of the indicator organisms in EARSS is *S. pneumoniae*. Previous results from EARSS in 11 European countries demonstrated a linear relationship between the use of β-lactamase antimicrobials and macrolides and the proportion of penicillin-resistant *Streptococcus pneumoniae* among all invasive *S. pneumoniae* isolates. Data demonstrated that resistance for *S. pneumoniae* followed a north-to-south gradient. Southern European countries had higher proportions of these organisms than countries of northern Europe. There was a correlation with antimicrobial use data and antimicrobial resistance.[40] A recent paper on surveillance data from ESAC from 35 countries still demonstrated a north-to-south gradient. Use of ESAC quality indicators resulted in improved antimicrobial use in several European countries; however, an increase in the use of broad-spectrum antimicrobials was noted.[41]

It is important to include quality improvement programs in the surveillance systems. Surveillance depends on enhancing epidemiologic and laboratory capabilities. Surveillance of the use of antimicrobials in veterinary practice, agriculture, and food animals is also important.

Improving the coordination of the various surveillance programs and distributing the best information for feedback and intervention is critical. It is also very important to use standardized laboratory methods and data elements so that sensitivity results and surveillance data can be compared across widely dispersed geographic areas. Linking of microbiologic, clinical, and pharmaceutical data are also important for the prevention and control of resistance. Just reporting the strains as susceptible, intermediate, or resistant can mask any emerging antimicrobial resistance problem. For example, an organism with a decrease in susceptibility may likely still be classified as susceptible. Clinical laboratories that provide data for antimicrobial resistance surveillance purposes should routinely participate in pertinent educational and proficiency testing programs and indicate methods that are used for surveillance.

APPROPRIATE ANTIMICROBIAL USAGE

Health Care Facility

The CDC in the Action Plan[42] defined appropriate antimicrobial use as "use that maximizes therapy by minimizing toxicity and development of resistance." The Antimicrobial Stewardship Programs (ASPs) have been in existence for a number of years. Recently a policy statement regarding this was published by the Society of Health Care Epidemiology of America, the Infectious Diseases Society of America, and the Pediatric Infectious Diseases Society of America.[43] This document outlines minimum requirements that include components of a multidisciplinary team, formulary restrictions, guidelines for management of common infections, interventions to improve use of antimicrobials, antimicrobial use surveillance and intervention, monitoring for drug-resistant pathogens, *Clostridium difficile* infections, and appropriate benchmarking and reporting. McGowan has outlined the outcomes of ASP, including improved patient outcomes, improved patient safety, reduced resistance, and cost. He also outlined the challenges of measuring impact.[44]

Computerized decision support systems developed by Pestotnik[45] at LDS Hospital in Salt Lake City have been used to support physicians in the choice of antimicrobial agents. These programs have been successful. The same group of investigators has demonstrated that computerized support was able to stabilize antimicrobial resistance background in their institution over several years. The approaches used also include streamlining, discontinuing antimicrobials on day 2 or 3 if the infection is not documented, or deescalating once susceptibility testing data are available and an appropriate change can be made. A number of approaches have been undertaken in the United States and other parts of the world in terms of the various components of the antimicrobial stewardship programs. These programs have demonstrated several times to have an impact on outbreaks caused by multidrug-resistant pathogens. One example is a decrease in ESBL-producing *Klebsiella* infections, VRE, and *C. difficile* infections. The data are more limited on the effect of antimicrobial restriction on the endemic resistance of organisms. However, it is still important to continue the programs and monitor these strains worldwide on a more long-term basis. In some parts of the world, particularly in developing areas, some but not all components of the antimicrobial stewardship program may be possible.

Programs to Promote Appropriate Outpatient Antimicrobial Drug Use

Antimicrobials are also used extensively in the ambulatory setting. Data on this use are not as extensive as that in inpatient use. As noted earlier, antimicrobial use has been monitored in Europe and many countries. In the United States, data show varied use in different states. For example, West Virginia ranked very high with 1.2 prescriptions for antimicrobial per capita, compared with a national average of 0.86. A recent study in Portland, Oregon, showed that many "low-risk" veterans received antimicrobials for acute respiratory tract infections; 87.8% were thought not to be indicated.[46] In developing countries, the problem of inappropriate use of antimicrobials in outpatients is also widespread. Problems are compounded by human resource issues, inadequate laboratory facilities for drug sensitivity testing, and counterfeit drugs. About 15% of all drugs are thought to be counterfeit, and this may be as high as 50% in some parts of Africa.

The recent guidelines for an ASP also included a section on Antimicrobial Stewardship in Ambulatory Health Care Settings and noted the importance of such programs and suggested funds for pilot programs.

Antimicrobial Use in Food Animals

The Interagency Task Force on Antimicrobial Resistance, with co-chairs from the CDC, the US Food and Drug Administration (FDA), the National Institutes of Health, and a number of other health care agencies, has recommended the following:

- Improvement and understanding of the risks and benefits of antimicrobial use and ways to prevent emergence and spread of resistance
- Development and implementation of principles for appropriate antimicrobial drug use in the production of food animals and plants

- Improved animal husbandry and food production practices to reduce the spread of infection
- A regulatory framework to address the need for antimicrobial drug use in agriculture and veterinary medicine while ensuring that such use does not pose a risk for human health

Many European countries stopped using penicillin, streptomycin, and tetracycline for growth promotion in the mid-1970s. The policy was expanded to other medically important antimicrobials in the 1990s and to all antimicrobials for growth promotion across the European Union in 2006.

In the United States, there have been ongoing discussions regarding the issue of antimicrobial use in food animals for growth promotion. In June 2012, the FDA established guidelines with a 3-year time frame for producers to eliminate use of antimicrobials in livestock for growth promotion. The plan also includes veterinary oversight for antimicrobial use.

Infection Control

Infection control principles and practices in the prevention of transmission of resistant organisms in the health care setting are critical. The importance of hand hygiene cannot be overemphasized. Alcohol-based gel is now available widely. However, adherence to hand hygiene continues to be a problem worldwide, and it has varied among health care professionals and institutions. Reasons perceived as contributing to poor hand hygiene adherence include:

- Time required to perform hand hygiene
- The effect of hand hygiene products on the skin
- Inadequate knowledge of the guidelines
- Workload

The influence of role model and group behavior on the reported levels of adherence is important. A campaign sponsored by the WHO since 2005 is promoting the use of alcohol-based hand rubs throughout the world. This campaign has been called, "Clean Care Is Safe Care" by the WHO. As of May 2012, 15,000 health care facilities from 156 countries have made a commitment for improving hand hygiene. This represents 10 million health care workers.

To decrease transmission, there is also an emphasis on the importance of the detection of patients who are colonized with resistant organisms, so appropriate isolation precautions can be in place before an infection develops.

In the United States, rates of central line associated bloodstream infections (CLABSI) and ventilator-associated pneumonia have decreased following the institution of specific control measures. In a report of 103 intensive care units (ICUs) in Michigan, there was a 66% reduction in CLABSI rates.

The increasing availability of molecular techniques for rapid diagnosis and testing for resistance would help to decrease empirical antimicrobial therapy. Rapid testing for MDR-TB is very valuable for early detection and appropriate therapy and decreasing transmission. Xpert MTB/Rif assay is a rapid molecular assay that can be used close to the point of care. This test was endorsed by the WHO in 2010. On August 7, 2012, the WHO announced a novel financing arrangement between the manufacturers of Xpert MTB/Rif, Cepheid, the Bill and Melinda Gates Foundation, and other agencies, including USAID, President's Emergency Plan for AIDS Relief (PEPFAR), and UNITAID. This arrangement will result in the reduced cost of the test cartridge and will take immediate effect in 145 high-burden low- and middle-income countries. This assay will provide improved rapid detection of TB, including rifampin resistance and will enable timely and appropriate care and hopefully decrease transmission of resistant organisms.

Infection control in the health care setting will also be enhanced by the development and use of other tests to improve rapid diagnosis, understanding of factors that promote the transmission of organisms, and future modifications of medical devices that will help reduce the risk of infection.

Vaccines

Vaccines have the potential to prevent infections and avoid dissemination within a population. Pneumococcal conjugate and influenza vaccine in children have resulted in reduction of antimicrobial use and could result in decreased resistance.[47] However we should also have constant surveillance for the emergence of nonvaccine serotypes causing infection. There is potential for different vaccines in the future, including those against *Staphylococci* and some of the enteric pathogens.

Education

In addition to the education of health care professionals, it is very important to educate the public regarding antimicrobial resistance and inappropriate antibiotic use. Education should include the importance of adherence to prescribed antimicrobials, including the use of directly observed therapy (DOT). DOT for tuberculosis has resulted in higher cure rates when there is a low level of multidrug resistance.

Health Care Regulations

Antimicrobial use can be affected by reimbursement policies, financial incentives, and health care regulations. In developing countries, there are issues of ease of availability of antimicrobials over the counter. Self-medication and poor adherence also occur. Since 1999 the Chilean Ministry of Health has enforced existing laws regarding the purchase of antimicrobials without a medical prescription. This regulatory agency has had a very positive impact on antimicrobial use in the outpatient setting. Separation of dispensing and prescribing of antimicrobials is important. An article in *Emerging Infectious Disease*[48] stated the example of the Korean government policy that prohibited physicians from dispensing drugs and pharmacies from prescribing drugs. This new policy decreased the prescribing of antimicrobial agents and selectively reduced inappropriate prescribing of these antimicrobials for patients with viral infections. The regulatory environment should also extend to prescription of antimicrobials for food animals and for veterinary practice.

SUMMARY

Despite earlier predictions of a world free of infectious diseases, the struggle for survival between humans and microorganisms will continue indefinitely, and new etiologic agents and infectious diseases will continue to emerge. The challenge lies in our recognition and response to their emergence. Examples such as SARS suggest an air of optimism in our global response strategies. However, antimicrobial resistance remains a global problem and a public health threat.

The problem of antimicrobial resistance is not restricted to only health care settings but has also spread in the community. The example of CA-MRSA is of concern, and recent data demonstrate its spread back into health care institutions. There are a variety of mechanisms of resistance, and new mechanisms continue to be described. Global strategies for combating antimicrobial resistance issues are available. The implementation of these strategies requires system and behavior changes. Extensive data are available on health-care-associated outbreaks and the institution of appropriate antimicrobial restriction and infection control measures to terminate the outbreak. More data on decreasing endemic resistance rates in health care institutions and communities are needed. Global hand hygiene initiatives are empowering. Global surveillance for resistant pathogens of epidemiologic importance is important. Despite many remaining issues regarding the various types of surveillance for antimicrobial resistance, a lot of progress has been made. Sharing of data and feedback on an ongoing basis to appropriate stakeholders and instituting necessary interventions is important. Global travel poses threats for the transmission and rapid spread of emerging infections and resistant organisms, and interventions require ongoing collaboration and cooperation between agencies and countries, including sharing of data. Some of the processes necessary for combating antimicrobial resistance are more difficult in resource-constrained environments, but they are necessary. Molecular techniques for rapid diagnosis of resistant pathogens will be critical.[49] A recent creative partnership for availability for use of a rapid diagnostic test for determining rifampin resistance in *Mycobacterium tuberculosis* in resource-constrained environments is exemplary. The use of antimicrobials in food animals remains a concern, and a global approach to this issue is critical. With increasing antimicrobial resistance and fewer antimicrobials in the development pipeline, we must strive to avoid the development of a post-antimicrobial era.

STUDY QUESTIONS

1. Change in land use such as deforestation and reforestation projects have been implicated in the emergence of infectious diseases. What specific examples can be cited for each?

2. With mass travel assuming such an important role in the global spread of infectious diseases, are there specific technological advances or interventions at airports or other ports of entry that can implemented to identify the ill traveler?

3. Resistance to antimicrobials is a global problem. What approaches have been most useful in studying this problem? Outline prevention strategies.

4. Resistance to antimicrobials in food animals is also a global issue. Give examples of antimicrobials that are used in food animals and associated with resistance and issues with human health.

REFERENCES

1. Tsang KW, Ho DL, Ooi GC, et al. A cluster of cases of severe acute respiratory syndrome in Hong Kong. *N Engl J Med* 2003; 348:1977.

2. Yu IT, Li Y, Wong TW, et al. Evidence of airborne transmission of the severe acute respiratory syndrome virus. *N Engl J Med* 2004;350:1731.

3. Armstrong GL, Conn LA, Pinner RW. Trends in infectious disease mortality in the United States during the 20th century. *JAMA* 1999;281:61.

4. Burnet FM, White DO. *Natural History of Infectious Diseases.* Cambridge: Cambridge University Press, 1962.

5. Fauci AS, Morens DM. The perpetual challenge of infectious diseases. *N Engl J Med* 2012;366:454.

6. Institute of Medicine. *Emerging Infections: Microbial Threats to Health in the United States.* Washington, DC: National Academy Press, 1994.

7. Scheld WM, Armstrong D, Hughes JM. *Emerging Infections.* Washington, DC: ASM Press, 1998.

8. Monto AS. The threat of an avian influenza pandemic. *N Engl J Med* 2005;352:323.

9. Nash D, Mostashari F, Fine A, et al. The outbreak of West Nile virus infection in the New York City area in 1999. *N Engl J Med* 2001;344:1807.

10. Office of Technology assessment, US Congress. *Proliferation of Weapons of Mass Destruction*. Washington, DC: US Government Printing Office, 1993: 53–55.

11. Centers for Disease Control and Prevention. Update: Investigation of bioterrorism—related anthrax and interim guidelines for exposure management and antimicrobial therapy, October 2001. *MMWR* 200;50:909.

12. Centers for Disease Control and Prevention. *Preventing Emerging Infectious Diseases: A Strategy for the 21st Century*. Atlanta: US Department of Health and Human Services, 1998.

13. Levin MJ, Bacon TH, Leary JJ. Resistance of *Herpes simplex* virus infections to nucleoside analogues in HIV-infected patients. *Clin Infect Dis* 2004;39:S248.

14. Lascaux AS, Caumes E, Deback C, et al. Successful treatment of acyclovir and foscarnet resistant herpes simplex virus lesions with topical imiquimod in patients infected with human immunodeficiency virus type 1. *J Med Virol* 2012;84:194.

15. Pfaller MA, Castanheira M, Lockhart SR, et al. Frequency of decreased susceptibility and resistance to enchinocandins among fluconazole-resistant bloodstream isolates of *Candida glabrata*. *J Clin Microbiol* 2012;50(4):1199.

16. Gorbach SL. Antimicrobial use in animal food—time to stop. Editorial. *N Engl J Med* 2001;345:1202.

17. Angulo FJ, Nargund VN, Chiller TC. Evidence of an association between use of anti-microbial agents in food animals and anti-microbial resistance among bacteria isolated from humans and the human health consequences of such resistance. *J Vet Med* 2004;51:374.

18. Hayes JR, Wagner DD, English LL, et al. Distribution of streptogramin resistance determinants among *Enterococcus faecium* from a poultry production environment of the USA. *J Antimicrob Chemother* 2005;55:123.

19. White DG, Zhao S, Sudler R, et al. The isolation of antibiotic-resistant salmonella from retail ground meats. *N Engl J Med* 2001;18:345.

20. McDonald LC, Rossiter S, Mackinson C, et al. Quinupristin-dalfopristin-resistant *Enterococcus faecium* on chicken and in human stool specimens. *N Engl J Med* 2001;18:1155.

21. Lloyd David H. Reservoirs of antimicrobial resistance in pet animals. *Clin Infect Dis* 2007;45:S148–S152.

22. Paterson DL, Bonomo RA. Extended-spectrum beta-lactamases: a clinical update. *Clin Microbiol Rev* 2005;18:657.

23. Gales AC, Castanheira M, Jones RN, Sader HS. Antimicrobial resistance among gram-negative bacilli isolated from Latin America: results from SENTRY Antimicrobial Surveillance Program (Latin America, 2008–2010). *Diagn Microbiol Infect Dis* 2012;73(4):354.

24. Yong D, Toleman MA, Giske CG, et al. Characterization of a new metallo-beta-lactamase gene, bla(NDM-1), and a novel erythromycin esterase gene carried on a unique genetic structure in *Klebsiella pneumoniae* sequence type 14 from India. *Antimicrob Agents Chemother* 2009;53(12):5046.

25. Raad II, Hanna HA, Hachem RY. Clinical-use-associated decrease in susceptibility of vancomycin-resistant *Enterococcus faecium* to linezolid: a comparison with quinupristin-dalfopristin. *Antimicrob Agents Chemother* 2004;48:3583.

26. Hershberger E, Donabedian S, Konstantinou K, et al. Quinupristin-dalfopristin resistance in gram-positive bacteria: mechanism of resistance and epidemiology. *Clin Inf Dis* 2004;38:92.

27. Nordmann P, Poirel L, Dortet L. Rapid detection of carbapenemase-producing *Enterobacteriaceae*. *Emerg Infect Dis* 2012;18:9.

28. Fridkin SK, Hageman JC, Morrison M, et al. Methicillin-resistant *Staphylococcus aureus* disease in three communities. *N Engl J Med* 2005;352:1436.

29. King MD, Humphrey BJ, Wang YF, et al. Emergence of community-acquired methicillin-resistant *Staphylococcus aureus* USA 300 clone as the predominant cause of skin and soft-tissue infections. *Ann Intern Med* 2006;144:309.

30. Wehrhahn MC, Robinson JC, Pascoe EM, et al. Illness severity in community-onset invasive *Staphylococcus aureus* infection and the presence of virulence genes. *J Inf Dis* 2012;205:1840.

31. Cosgrove SE, Carmeli Y. The impact of antimicrobial resistance on health and economic outcomes. *Clin Infect Dis* 2003;36:1433.

32. Evans HL, Shaffer MM, Hughes MG, et al. Contact isolation in surgical patients: a barrier to care? *Surgery* 2003;134:180.

33. Khan FA, Khakoo R, Hobbs GR, et al. Impact of contact isolation on health care workers at a tertiary care center. *Am J Infect Control* 2006;34:408.

34. Neidell MJ, Cohen B, Furuya Y, et al. Costs of healthcare- and community-associated infectious with antimicrobial-resistant versus antimicrobial-susceptible organisms. *Clin Infect Dis* 2012;55(6):807.

35. McGowan JE. Economic impact of antimicrobial resistance. *Emerg Infect Dis* 2001;7:286.

36. Gunner SS, Tapsall JW, Allegranzi B, et al. The antimicrobial resistance containment and surveillance approach—a public health tool. *Bull World Health Organ* 2004;82:928–934.

37. Masterson RG. Surveillance studies: how can they help the management of infection? *J Antimicrob Chemother* 2000;72:53.

38. Stelling JM, O'Brien TF. Surveillance of antimicrobial resistance: the WHONET program. *Clin Infect Dis* 1997;(Suppl 1):S157.

39. Pfaller MA, Acar J, Jones RN, et al. Integration of molecular characterization of microorganisms in a global antimicrobial resistance surveillance program. *Clin Infect Dis* 2001;32:S156.

40. Bronzwaer SL, Cars O, Buchholz U, et al. A European study on the relationship between antimicrobial use and antimicrobial resistance. *Emerg Infect Dis* 2002;8:278.

41. Adriaenssens N, Coenen S, Versporten A, et al. European surveillance of antimicrobial consumption (ESAC): quality appraisal of antibiotic use in Europe. *J Antimicrob Chemother* 2011;66(Suppl 6):vi71–vi77.

42. Centers for Disease Control and Prevention. A Public Health Action Plan to Combat Antimicrobial Resistance. Part 1: Domestic Issues. 2005 with revisions in 2011. http://www.cdc.gov/drugresistance/actionplan/aractionplan.pdf.

43. SHEA, IDSA, PIDS. Policy Statement on Antimicrobial Stewardship by the Society for Healthcare Epidemiology of America (SHEA), the Infectious Diseases Society of America (IDSA), and the Pediatric Infectious Diseases Society (PIDS). *Infect Control Hosp Epidemiol* 2012;33(4):322.

44. McGowan JE Jr. Antimicrobial stewardship—the state of the art in 2011: Focus on outcome and methods. *Infect Control Hosp Epidemiol* 2012;33(4):331.

45. Pestotnik SL. Expert clinical decision support systems to enhance antimicrobial stewardship programs: insights from the Society of Infectious Diseases Pharmacists. *Pharmacotherapy* 2005;25:1116.

46. Logan JL, Yang J, Forrest G. Outpatient antibiotic prescribing in a low-risk veteran population with acute respiratory symptoms. *Hosp Pract* 2012;40(1):75–80.

47. Wilby KJ, Werry D. A review of the effect of immunization programs on antimicrobial utilization. *Vaccine* 2012;30(46): 6509–6514.

48. Harbarth S, Samore MH. Antimicrobial resistance determinants and future control. *Emerg Infect Dis* 2005;11:794.

49. Tenover FC. Potential impact of rapid diagnostic tests on improving antimicrobial use. *Ann NY Acad Sci* 2012;1213:70.

Injury and Global Health

13

Jeffry P. McKinzie

LEARNING OBJECTIVES

- *Understand the global impact of injuries and their relative importance as a cause of morbidity and mortality worldwide*
- *Know the most common categories of intentional and nonintentional injuries, and their relative importance in the global burden of disease*
- *Identify recommended focus areas for future research in injury prevention*

INTRODUCTION

Injury is a leading cause of mortality worldwide, resulting in more than 5 million deaths annually.[1] Global mortality due to injury exceeds that of HIV/AIDS, tuberculosis, and malaria combined.[2] Deaths due to injury represent only the tip of the injury iceberg, however. For every person who dies from an injury, several thousand injured persons survive with permanent disability. Additional adverse consequences spill over to affect multiple individuals within the family and community of each injured person.

In 2004, injuries accounted for approximately 10% of the world's deaths and over 12% of the global burden of disease.[3] The relative importance of injuries within the global burden of disease is expected to rise even further, with injury becoming the third leading cause of death and disability by 2020.[4]

Accident versus Injury

In the past, the term *accident* was used to describe various categories of unintentional injuries, including those associated with road traffic collisions, falls, burns, and other causes. This traditional view implies that the events leading to injury are random, unavoidable, and unpredictable. Public health officials now recognize that injuries are preventable nonrandom events. After years of historical neglect, injury prevention has become a major area of emphasis within the public health arena. In 2000, the World Health Organization (WHO) established a Department for Injuries and Violence Prevention to promote global initiatives in injury prevention and control. The phenomenon of injury has now been taken out of the realm of chance "accident" and placed squarely within the framework of scientific study, where research is being conducted to design effective injury control interventions.

Classification of Injuries

Using the accepted conventions of the WHO,[5] injuries can be divided into two broad categories: intentional injuries and unintentional injuries. Intentional injuries are subdivided into self-inflicted injuries (i.e., suicide attempt or completion), interpersonal violence (i.e., homicide or intentional injury to others), and war-related violence. Unintentional injuries are further subdivided into road traffic injuries, poisoning, falls, fires, and drowning. Most public health experts and organizations, including the WHO, use this classification scheme in discussions of global injury surveillance and prevention.

Mortality versus Disability-Adjusted Life Years

Mortality due to injuries is a very important indicator of the magnitude of the problem. However, nonfatal outcomes with associated disability and other adverse sequelae must also be considered to fully appreciate the impact of injuries on global health. The disability-adjusted life year (DALY) is an epidemiologic indicator that has been developed to quantify the combined impact of disability and premature death due to illness or injury. One DALY is defined as 1 lost year of healthy life, either due to disability or premature death (see Chapter 2).

Injury Disparities

Although injuries are a leading cause of morbidity and mortality worldwide, the nature and scope of the problem varies considerably by region, age, sex, and socioeconomic status. For example:

- More than 90% of the world's deaths due to injuries occur in low-income and middle-income countries.[2]
- Injury mortality among men is almost twice that among women worldwide.[2]
- Males in Africa have the highest injury mortality rates, and women in the Americas have the lowest injury mortality rates worldwide.
- Young people between the ages of 15 and 44 years (the most economically productive segment of society) account for almost 50% of global injury mortality.[6]

The relative importance of different types of injuries also varies significantly based on geographic and demographic variables.

- Men have almost three times higher mortality rates from road traffic injuries and interpersonal violence than do women.[6]
- Children ages 0 to 14 years account for more than 50% of DALYs lost due to burn injuries and more than 50% of global mortality due to drowning.[6]
- Road traffic injuries are the leading cause of injury-related mortality in most regions except for Europe, where self-inflicted injuries predominate, and in the low- and middle-income countries of the Americas, where interpersonal violence is the most common cause of injury-related death.[5]

More research is needed to clarify the reasons for these disparities and develop strategies to reduce them.

Economic Burden

The global economic burden of injuries is enormous. For example, the annual cost of road traffic injuries alone is estimated at US$518 billion worldwide.[7] In low-income countries, the cost of caring for road traffic injuries is estimated to exceed the amount of development assistance these countries receive. At the individual and family level, medical costs associated with injuries can have a devastating effect on personal finances. This is especially true in low- and middle-income countries, where most injured persons are poor and scarce resources that are needed for other basic necessities must be diverted to pay for medical

care. In addition, because injuries disproportionately affect young healthy adults who are in their peak earning years, the loss of earning power due to injury-related death or disability further compounds the economic burden.

UNINTENTIONAL INJURIES

Approximately two-thirds of injuries worldwide are unintentional injuries, with road traffic injuries comprising the largest category.

Road Traffic Injuries

The coroner who attended the inquest of the first road traffic death in 1896 was reported to have said, "This must never happen again."[8] More than a century later, road traffic accidents have become the leading cause of injury-related death and disability worldwide. Approximately a quarter of all injury deaths are due to road traffic injuries. Over 90% of these deaths occur in low-and middle-income countries. Each year, road traffic crashes kill more than 1.2 million people and injure or disable up to 50 million people. Young people between the ages of 5 and 44 years and vulnerable road users (pedestrians, cyclists, and passengers on public transport) are at the highest risk.[9]

In recent decades, road traffic death rates have decreased significantly in high-income countries but have increased dramatically in low- and middle-income countries. There is considerable variation among different countries within the same region and economic classification, however. For example, from 1975 to 1998 in North America, the road traffic fatality rate decreased by 27% in the United States but by 63% in Canada. During the same period, road traffic fatality rates in Asia increased by 44% in Malaysia but by 243% in China. By 2020, road traffic fatalities are projected to increase by 83% in low- and middle-income countries, and to decrease by 27% in high-income countries. This will result in a predicted 67% overall increase in global road traffic deaths. Thus road traffic injuries are expected to become the sixth leading cause of death worldwide and the third largest contributor to the global burden of disease (DALYs lost) by 2020.[10]

Many factors contribute to the high number of road traffic injuries and deaths in the developing world, including:

- Large numbers of vulnerable road users, such as pedestrians and cyclists, who must share the road with larger vehicles
- Poorly equipped and maintained motor vehicles, which often lack basic safety features such as seatbelts
- Poorly designed and maintained roads with inadequate lighting

- Inadequate establishment and enforcement of traffic safety laws
- Lack of access to quality prehospital and hospital care for injured persons.

The WHO has identified the following five key areas for effective interventions that can reduce the burden of road traffic injuries worldwide: speed, alcohol, seatbelts, helmets, and visibility.[11]

Speed

Speed is a contributing factor in approximately 30% of road traffic fatalities. For every 1 km/hour increase in speed, there is a 3% increased risk of a crash resulting in injury and a 5% increased risk of a fatal crash. Effective interventions include setting and enforcing speed limits, improved road design, and utilization of traffic-calming measures such as speed bumps and traffic circles. For example, placement of speed bumps on an accident-prone stretch of highway in Ghana resulted in a 35% reduction in the number of crashes, a 76% reduction in serious injuries, and a 55% reduction in road traffic fatalities at that location.[11]

Alcohol

Blood alcohol concentrations greater than 0.04 g/dL significantly increase the risk of road traffic crashes. An alcohol-impaired driver has a 17-fold increased risk of being involved in a fatal crash than an unimpaired driver.[12] For any alcohol level, the risk of crash fatality increases with decreasing driver age and experience. Suggested interventions include setting and strictly enforcing blood alcohol concentration limits in drivers, mass media educational campaigns, and utilization of random breath testing. For example, since 1993 in Australia, widespread random breath testing has been credited with an estimated 40% reduction in alcohol-related deaths.[11]

Seatbelts

The use of seatbelts has saved more lives than any other road safety intervention. Seatbelts reduce the risk of fatal or serious injury in a crash by an estimated 40% to 65%. In addition, proper use of child restraints can reduce toddler deaths by 54% and infant deaths by 71%. Suggested interventions include establishment and enforcement of mandatory seatbelt and child restraint use, mass media educational programs, use of audible seatbelt reminders, and child restraint loan programs. For example, a well-publicized police enforcement campaign in the Republic of Korea resulted in an increase in seatbelt use from 23% in 2000 to 98% in 2001, accompanied by a 5.9% decrease in road traffic fatalities.[11]

Helmets

Head injuries are a major cause of death and disability among users of motorized two-wheel vehicles (mopeds and motorcycles). Nonhelmeted riders have a three-fold increased risk of head injury in a crash when compared with helmeted riders. The proper use of helmets has been shown to reduce the risk of serious or fatal head injury by up to 45%. Suggested interventions include establishment and enforcement of mandatory helmet laws, targeted educational campaigns, and development of safe inexpensive helmets that are comfortable in tropical climates. For example, enforcement of the helmet law in Thailand resulted in a five-fold increase in helmet use, accompanied by a 41% decrease in head injuries and a 20% decrease in deaths.[11]

Visibility

The abilities to see and be seen are fundamental requirements for the safety of all road users. Poor visibility of pedestrians and motor vehicles significantly increases the risk of road traffic injuries. In addition to being relatively unprotected in a crash, pedestrians and cyclists are harder to see than larger vehicles and are therefore more vulnerable to injury. Inadequate street lighting and insufficient use of reflective equipment and vehicle lights also contribute to poor visibility. Proposed interventions include improved street lighting, increased use of reflective clothing and equipment for pedestrians and cyclists, and requiring use of daytime running lights for motorized vehicles. Crash rates are 10% to 15% lower for vehicles using daytime running lights than for those that do not.[11]

Poisoning

The category of "poisoning" in the injury literature includes unintentional poisoning deaths and non-fatal outcomes. Intentional poisonings and adverse drug reactions are excluded.[13] In 2004, poisoning accounted for 6% of all injury deaths and 4% of DALYs lost due to injury. Overall, 91% of poisoning deaths occur in low- or middle-income countries.[3]

Europe is the only region where poisoning is a leading cause of death, with a third of all poisoning deaths worldwide occurring in this region.[4,6] Males in the low- and middle-income countries of Europe have a poisoning mortality rate approximately three times higher than the rate in either sex in any other region of the world, with alcohol poisoning accounting for a significant proportion of these cases. Adolescents and adults between 15 and 59 years of age account for over 60% of the global mortality due to poisoning.[6]

Preventive interventions aimed at reducing the global burden of poisoning injuries include:

- Educational campaigns to inform the public regarding the dangers of accidental poisoning and the importance of proper storage and use of medications and household chemicals

- Establishment and enforcement of laws that mandate the use of child-resistant packaging, adequate labeling, and safer formulations of medications and toxic substances
- Promotion of the use of carbon monoxide detectors in the home, and improving availability of these devices in low-income settings
- Establishment of poison control centers and promotion of their use by the public as a point of first contact following a potential toxic exposure.

In the United States, the introduction of child-resistant packaging, safer product formulation, and interventions by poison control centers and health professionals all contributed to a 45% decline in poisoning deaths among children from 1974 to 1992.[14,15] Further investigation is needed to identify ways to adapt these and other interventions for use in limited-resource settings.

Falls

An estimated 424,000 people die worldwide each year due to falls, excluding falls due to assault or intentional self-harm. Adults over the age of 60 years have the highest fall-related mortality rates in all regions of the world. Children account for significant fall-related morbidity, however, with almost 40% of total DALYs lost due to falls occurring in children.[16]

Interventions aimed at reducing the risk of injuries due to falls include:

- Public education about fall risk factors and how to modify them in the home
- Establishment and enforcement of laws that promote workplace safety, including fall prevention
- Promotion of exercise programs to improve strength and balance in the elderly
- Education of healthcare providers in how to reduce the risk of falls in the elderly through medication modifications, enhanced vision services, physical therapy, and other therapeutic interventions

Fires

Fire-related burn injuries are responsible for an estimated 195,000 deaths annually worldwide.[17] The vast majority of burn fatalities occur in low- and middle-income countries. Women in Southeast Asia have the highest rate of burn mortality worldwide.[17] Other groups with statistically higher rates of death due to burn injuries include women in the eastern Mediterranean region, males in low- and middle-income countries in Europe, and children under 15 years of age in Africa.[6] In addition, for every person who dies due to burn injury, there are many more who experience nonlethal burn injuries, often with permanent disabling sequelae and severe scarring. Most burn injuries occur at home or in the workplace. Women and children are most often injured at home, especially in communities where open fires are used for cooking, lighting, and heating. Men often sustain burn injuries in the workplace. Alcohol and smoking both contribute to the risk of burn injuries, especially when used in combination. One in four burn deaths in the United States are directly related to careless smoking, and almost half of all burn deaths involve combined alcohol abuse and smoking.[18] Low socioeconomic status is associated with a higher risk of burn injuries in both low-income and high-income countries. Contributing factors may include overcrowded living conditions, inadequate parental supervision of children, and lack of appropriate safety measures.

Scald burns due to contact with hot liquids are also a major source of burn injury. These burns typically occur in the home in association with cooking activities or due to excessively hot tap water. Water heated to 60°C (140°F) can cause a severe burn in 2 to 5 seconds in an adult and in less than 1 second in a child. However, it takes up to 5 minutes for a severe burn injury to occur in water heated to 49°C (120°F), allowing sufficient time for an exposed person to react and remove themselves from the exposure.

Despite advances in burn care in recent decades, primary prevention remains the best approach to reduce morbidity and mortality due to burn injuries. Suggested interventions include:

- Promotion of fire safety education in communities and schools
- Promotion of safer cooking stoves, less hazardous fuels, and enclosure of open fires
- Establishment and enforcement of fire safety standards in the workplace
- Promotion of safer design and construction for single-family and multifamily residential dwellings, incorporating the use of less flammable building materials, smoke detectors, sprinkler systems, and fire escape routes
- Lowering the temperature of hot water taps to 49°C (120°F).

Drowning

Drowning is the third leading cause of unintentional injury death worldwide. An estimated 380,000 people drown each year, with 96% of these deaths occurring in low- and middle-income countries. The incidence of drowning varies significantly by region. For example, the rate of drowning in Africa is more than eight times as high as in Australia or the United States.[19]

Major risk factors for drowning have been identified.[20] Males have a two-fold increased risk of drowning when compared with females. Factors contributing to the higher risk among males may include increased occupational and recreational exposure to water, and increased high-risk behavior (i.e., swimming alone, drinking alcohol before swimming). Young age is also a factor, with children under 5 years of age having the highest drowning mortality rates worldwide. Drowning deaths in children are often associated with inadequate adult supervision. Children who live in close proximity to unfenced bodies of water (swimming pools, ponds, irrigation ditches, wells) are at increased risk. Alcohol use increases drowning risk among adolescents and adults, and it also contributes to drowning risk in children due to alcohol-related impairment of adult supervision.

Interventions aimed at decreasing the incidence of drowning include:

- Promotion of "learn to swim" and water safety programs within communities
- Mandatory fencing of swimming pools and other water hazards
- Draining unnecessary accumulations of water
- Discouraging by legislation and/or education the use of alcohol while engaged in boating, swimming, or other water-related activities
- Establishing and enforcing boating safety regulations, including essential safety equipment and maximum passenger capacity

INTENTIONAL INJURIES (VIOLENCE)

The WHO defines *violence* as "the intentional use of physical force or power, threatened or actual, against oneself, another person, or against a group or community, which either results in or has a high likelihood of resulting in injury, death, psychological harm, maldevelopment, or deprivation."[21] This definition encompasses three broad categories of intentional injuries: self-inflicted injuries, interpersonal violence, and collective violence (war). Approximately a third of injuries worldwide are recognized as intentional; roughly half of these are self-inflicted injuries, and the other half are the result of interpersonal violence and war.[22] The incidence of all three categories of intentional injuries is expected to rise, with each category ranking within the 15 leading causes of death and disability worldwide by 2020.[4] More than 1.6 million people die annually due to violence, and many more are injured.[21] Survivors of violence often experience long-term sequelae, including physical, sexual, and mental health problems.

Self-Inflicted Injuries

An estimated 782,000 people committed suicide in 2008.[23] Suicide is sometimes misclassified and unrecognized in official death records due to the social stigma and taboos that are associated with suicide in many cultures. The rate of suicide in the global population varies significantly by age, sex, and geographic region.

- In general, males have a three-fold increased risk of suicide compared with females.
- Suicide rates increase with advancing age. The suicide rate for those age 75 years or older is three times higher than for people 15 to 29 years of age.
- The highest suicide rates worldwide are found among males in the low- and middle-income countries of Europe and among both sexes in the Western Pacific region.
- Women in China have a two-fold increased rate of suicide when compared with women in other parts of the world.[6]

In addition, cultural and religious values, socioeconomic status, and gender equality issues appear to play some role in the variability of suicide rates in different regions.

On average, the ratio of suicide attempts to suicide completions is 10:1. The likelihood that a suicide attempt will be fatal is directly related to the method chosen. The most lethal methods of suicide include gunshot, hanging, and jumping from a height. The attempt-to-completion ratio tends to be higher among people under 25 years of age who often choose a less lethal method, such as medication overdose.

Suicide attempts are often precipitated by stressful events or circumstances such as the loss of a loved one, divorce, unemployment, financial or legal problems, or problems in interpersonal relationships. These events are common life experiences, however, and most people who experience them do not commit or attempt suicide. Those who are driven to suicide often have preexisting risk factors that make them more vulnerable. Multiple risk factors have been identified that predispose an individual to suicide and self-injury, including:

- Mental illness, such as depression or schizophrenia
- Alcohol or substance abuse
- Physical illness, especially when painful or disabling
- History of physical or sexual abuse during childhood
- Access to the means to kill oneself (guns, medicines, poisons, etc.)
- History of a prior suicide attempt
- Social isolation[21]

Several approaches have been suggested to decrease the incidence of self-inflicted injuries and suicide, including:

- Early identification and treatment of mental illness and/or substance abuse disorders
- Community-based programs, including telephone hotlines, counseling centers, and support groups, especially targeting youth and elderly persons
- School-based interventions designed to identify at-risk youth and refer them to appropriate mental health services
- Media campaigns designed to raise public awareness of the problem and the availability of community resources for those at risk
- Legislative initiatives to restrict access to firearms

Interpersonal Violence

Interpersonal violence is a broad category of intentional injury that includes intimate partner violence, child abuse and neglect, abuse of the elderly, youth violence, sexual assault, and other forms of violence directed by one person or small group of persons toward another. The nature of interpersonal violence can be physical, sexual, psychological, or any combination of these. Deprivation and neglect are also considered forms of interpersonal violence.[21]

Homicide is the ultimate form of interpersonal violence. In 2010, an estimated 468,000 people died as a result of homicide worldwide.[24] For every person who is killed, however, many more survive their injuries, often with permanent physical, sexual, and psychological sequelae. Many survivors also go on to suffer repeated acts of physical and/or sexual violence.

As with other forms of injury, interpersonal violence does not affect all segments of global society equally. Most homicides occur in the low- to middle-income countries. Approximately two-thirds of homicide deaths in 2010 occurred in Africa and the Americas; only one-third occurred in Europe, Asia, and Oceania. When analyzed by population size, the homicide rate for Africa and the Americas is approximately twice the global average; that of Europe, Asia, and Oceania is roughly half the global average.[24] Three quarters of all homicide victims are males. The homicide rate among males tends to decline with advancing age, with the highest rate occurring in males ages 15 to 29 years.[21] Racial, cultural, and socioeconomic factors also play a role. For example, in the United States in 1999, the rate of homicide among African American youths age 15 to 24 years was twice that of their Hispanic counterparts, and over 12 times higher than their white non-Hispanic counterparts.[25]

Intimate partner violence occurs in all countries, all cultures, and in all levels of society. Some populations are at higher risk than others, however. Although women can be violent toward their male partners, the vast majority of partner violence is inflicted by men upon women. Surveys conducted among abused women reveal that many victims are subjected to multiple acts of violence over extended periods of time, and many suffer from a combination of physical, sexual, and psychological abuse. Women are at particularly high risk in societies where marked gender inequality exists and where sanctions against intimate partner violence are weak and poorly enforced. A significant number of homicides in women are due to partner violence. Studies from various countries reveal that 40% to 70% of female homicide victims were killed by their husband or boyfriend.[21]

Child maltreatment is any form of abuse or neglect that occurs in children under 18 years of age. Common forms of child maltreatment include physical, sexual, and emotional abuse. Although child maltreatment is recognized as a global problem, reliable estimates of its scope are lacking, especially in low- and middle-income countries. International studies suggest that roughly 20% of women and 5% to 10% of men have been sexually abused as children. Between 25% and 50% of children report having suffered physical abuse. Permanent impairment of physical and mental health often occurs in victims of child maltreatment.[26]

Elder maltreatment, as defined by the WHO, is "a single or repeated act, or lack of appropriate action, occurring within any relationship where there is an expectation of trust which causes harm or distress to an older person." This type of interpersonal violence may take many forms, including physical, sexual, and emotional abuse; financial abuse; abandonment and neglect; and loss of dignity and respect. It is estimated that 4% to 6% of elderly people have experienced some form of maltreatment at home. The number of cases of elder maltreatment is expected to rise as the aging of the population continues globally over the next several decades.[27]

Multiple common risk factors are associated with the various forms of interpersonal violence, including:

- Alcohol and substance abuse
- History of childhood exposure to violence in the home
- Family or personal history of divorce or separation
- Low self-esteem and poor behavioral control
- Poverty and income inequality[21]

Violence prevention requires a multifaceted approach. The finding that early childhood experiences play an important role in the subsequent risk of becoming a violence perpetrator suggests an important opportunity to intervene through programs that impact early childhood development and promote family stability. Suggested interventions designed to decrease the incidence of interpersonal violence include:

- Early identification and treatment of alcohol and substance abuse and mental disorders
- Improved surveillance for victims of violence within schools, healthcare facilities, workplaces, and communities, coupled with provision of services to ensure the care and future protection of these victims
- Providing community resources for family therapy and training in parenting skills
- Media campaigns designed to raise public awareness about violence prevention and stimulate community action
- Legislative initiatives to restrict access to firearms
- Establishment and enforcement of strict legal penalties for perpetrators of all forms of interpersonal violence[21]

Collective Violence (War)

Collective violence is defined by the WHO as "the instrumental use of violence by people who identify themselves as members of a group against another group or set of individuals, in order to achieve political, economic, or social objectives."[21] This category of violence includes armed conflicts between nations and groups, terrorism, gang warfare, genocide, and the use of rape and torture as weapons of war.

During the 20th century, an estimated 191 million people died as a direct or indirect result of armed conflict, making it one of the most violent periods in human history. More than half of these fatalities were among the civilian population. In 2008, armed conflict directly caused almost 200,000 deaths worldwide.[28] As with other forms of violent and nonviolent injury, the number of survivors far exceeds the number of deaths, with many survivors experiencing permanent physical and psychological sequelae. Torture and rape have been used as deliberate weapons of war in some conflicts to terrorize and demoralize communities. For example, during the conflict in Sierra Leone, many civilians suffered mutilation and severed limbs at the hands of armed forces. During the conflict in Bosnia and Herzegovina, the number of women raped by soldiers is estimated between 10,000 and 60,000 [21] (see Chapter 15).

In addition to the deaths and injuries that occur as a direct result of armed conflict, there are significant increases in morbidity and mortality indirectly related to conflict. Essential infrastructure, including health care, sanitation, shelter, transportation, and food supply are often disrupted during periods of conflict. This can result in famine and increased vulnerability to disease within the population. Increased mortality is often seen, especially among the most vulnerable populations, including infants and refugees. Prevention of collective violence and armed conflicts requires international effort and cooperation across multiple sectors. Goals of the global community should include:

- Reduction of poverty and inequality between groups in society
- Reduction in access to weapons, including biologic, chemical, and nuclear weapons
- Promotion and enforcement of international treaties and human rights initiatives[28]

FUTURE DIRECTIONS

Much progress has been made in recent decades in the field of injury prevention. However, there is much left to accomplish, and further progress is needed in three important areas:

- **Epidemiology:** Expanded research is needed to more accurately quantify the scope and magnitude of intentional and unintentional injuries, and to delineate risk factors and economic consequences of injury.
- **Prevention:** There is a need to design and evaluate injury prevention interventions, and to identify best practices for implementation among various target populations and geographic settings.
- **Advocacy:** Enhanced efforts are needed to promote education and awareness of injury prevention within the general public, and among policymakers and donor agencies.

SUMMARY

Injuries, both intentional and unintentional, are now recognized as leading causes of morbidity and mortality worldwide. The impact of injuries on the global burden of disease is expected to increase significantly in the coming decades. The causes of injuries are multifactorial, crossing all segments of society. Therefore, injury prevention initiatives must be multidisciplinary in nature, with involvement of public health officials, social scientists, educators, community leaders, politicians, mass media, and others. Significant progress in injury prevention and control has been made in the high-income countries of the developed world. As this progress continues, ways must be identified to adapt successful injury prevention strategies for use within the low- and middle-income countries where most injuries occur.

STUDY QUESTIONS

1. Using the accepted conventions of the WHO, outline the types of injuries discussed in this chapter.

2. List and discuss five key interventions to reduce road traffic injuries worldwide.

3. List and discuss five interventions to reduce morbidity and mortality from burns.

4. List and discuss five interventions to reduce the incidence of drowning.

5. What are some risk factors for suicide? Compare and contrast the importance of these factors in the developing world versus the industrialized world.

6. List and discuss five interventions to decrease the incidence of interpersonal violence.

REFERENCES

1. World Health Organization. *Violence, Injuries and Disability: Biennial Report 2010–2011.* Geneva: WHO, 2012.

2. World Health Organization. *Injuries and Violence: The Facts.* Geneva: WHO, 2010. http://whqlibdoc.who.int/publications/2010/9789241599375_eng.pdf.

3. World Health Organization. *The Global Burden of Disease: 2004 Update.* Geneva: WHO, 2008. http://www.who.int/healthinfo/global_burden_disease/2004_report_update/en/index.html.

4. Murray CJL, Lopez AD. *The Global Burden of Disease.* Cambridge, MA: Harvard University Press, 1996.

5. Peden M, McGee K, Krug E. *Injury: A Leading Cause of the Global Burden of Disease, 2000.* Geneva: World Health Organization, 2002.

6. Peden M, McGee K, Sharma G. *The Injury Chart Book: A Graphical Overview of the Global Burden of Injuries.* Geneva: World Health Organization, 2002.

7. Jacobs G, Aeron-Thomas A, Astrop A. *Estimating Global Road Fatalities.* Wokingham, Berks, UK: Crowthorne, Transport Research Laboratory, 2000 (TRL Report No. 445).

8. Shinar D. *Traffic Safety and Human Development.* Oxford, UK: Elsevier, 2007.

9. World Health Organization. *Global Status Report on Road Safety: Time for Action.* Geneva: WHO, 2009.

10. Peden MM. *The World Report on Road Traffic Injury Prevention.* Geneva: World Health Organization, 2004.

11. World Health Organization. *Safer Roads: Five Key Areas for Effective Interventions.* Geneva: WHO, 2004.www.who.int/features/2004/road_safety/en/.

12. World Health Organization. *Road Safety: Alcohol.* Geneva: WHO, 2004.www.who.int/violence_injury_prevention/publications/road_traffic/world_report/alcohol_en.pdf.

13. World Health Organization. *International Statistical Classification of Diseases and Related Health Problems, tenth revision. Vol. 1: Tabular List.* Geneva: WHO, 1992.

14. Liebelt EL, DeAngelis CD. Evolving trends and treatment advances in pediatric poisoning. *JAMA* 1999;282:1113–1115.

15. Rodgers GB. The safety effects of child-resistant packaging for oral prescription drugs: two decades of experience. *JAMA* 1996;275:1661–1665.

16. World Health Organization. *Falls: Fact Sheet No. 344.* Geneva: WHO, 2012. www.who.int/mediacentre/factsheets/fs344/en.

17. World Health Organization. *Burns: Fact Sheet No. 365.* Geneva: WHO, 2012. www.who.int/mediacentre/factsheets/fs365/en.

18. World Health Organization. *Facts About Injuries: Burns.* Geneva: WHO.www.who.int/violence_injury_prevention/publications/other_injury/en/burns_factsheet.pdf.

19. World Health Organization. *Drowning: Fact Sheet No. 347.* Geneva: WHO,2012. www.who.int/mediacentre/factsheets/fs347/en.

20. World Health Organization. *Facts About Injuries: Drowning.* Geneva: WHO.http://www.who.int/violence_injury_prevention/publications/other_injury/en/drowning_factsheet.pdf.

21. World Health Organization. *World Report on Violence and Health.* Geneva: WHO, 2002.

22. Murray S. Global injury and violence. *CMAJ* 2006;174(5):620–621.

23. World Health Organization. *Causes of Death 2008: Data Sources and Methods.* Geneva: WHO, 2011. www.who.int/gho/mortality_burden_disease/global_burden_disease_DTH6_2008.xls.

24. *2011 Global Study on Homicide: Trends, Context, Data.* Vienna: United Nations Office on Drugs and Crime, 2011. http://www.unodc.org/unodc/en/data-and-analysis/statistics/crime/global-study-on-homicide-2011.html.

25. Anderson RN. Deaths: leading causes for 1999. *Natl Vital Stat Rep* 2001;49(11):1–87.

26. World Health Organization. *Child maltreatment: Fact Sheet No. 150.* Geneva: WHO, 2010.www.who.int/mediacentre/factsheets/fs150/en.

27. World Health Organization. *Elder Maltreatment: Fact Sheet No. 357.* Geneva: WHO, 2011. www.who.int/mediacentre/factsheets/fs357/en.

28. World Health Organization. *Facts: Collective Violence.* Geneva: WHO, 2002. http://www.who.int/violence_injury_prevention/violence/world_report/factsheets/en/collectiveviolfacts.pdf.

OTHER USEFUL REFERENCES

Krug EG, Sharma GK, Lozano R. The global burden of injuries. *Am J Public Health* 2000;90:523–526.

National Center for Injury Prevention and Control (CDC) Website: http://www.cdc.gov/injury/index.html.

World Health Organization Violence and Injury Prevention Website: http://www.who.int/violence_injury_prevention.

World Health Organization. *Preventing Violence: A Guide to Implementing the Recommendations of the 'World Report on Violence and Health.'* Geneva: WHO, 2004.

Safe Kids USA Website: http://www.usa.safekids.org/.

World Health Organization. *World Report on Violence and Health: Summary.* Geneva: WHO, 2002.

Surgical Issues in Global Health 14

Eileen S. Natuzzi, Rooney Jagilly, Kathryn Chu, Doruk Ozgediz, Emmanuel Elobu, Kathleen Casey, Robin Petroze, Georges Ntakiyiruta, and Thomas E. Novotny

LEARNING OBJECTIVES

- *Define global surgery*
- *Describe the history of surgical care and issues in international health*
- *Describe the global burden of surgical disease including its impact on noncommunicable diseases and other disease control programs*
- *Discuss surgical capacity building as part of global health initiatives in resource-constrained environments*

INTRODUCTION

Today 84% of the world's population lives in developing countries where 93% of the world's disease burden exists but only 11% of global health research dollars are spent.[1] Although deaths in developing countries from communicable diseases such as tuberculosis (TB), malaria, and HIV/AIDS are slowly decreasing, the prevalence of noncommunicable diseases (NCDs) such as cancer, diabetes, cardiovascular disease, and chronic respiratory disease are steadily rising. With the urbanization of towns and cities in developing countries, traffic crashes and injuries have become more common place. A high baseline prevalence of communicable diseases, along with rising rates of NCDs and injuries, will create inordinate future health system demands and may impede overall progress on the Millennium Development Goals (MDGs). Many of these diseases require surgical treatment to save lives, decrease suffering, and prevent or end disability to restore health and livelihoods. At present, access to complete surgical care in most developing countries is not readily available.

The Alma-Ata Declaration of 1978 identified primary health care as the cornerstone to achieving "health for all." This historic document highlighted the gross inequities in health and access to care between people living in developed and developing countries. Although the Alma-Ata Declaration strongly supports primary care for all, it also "addresses the main health problems in the community, providing promotive, preventive, curative and rehabilitative services." Appropriate, cost-effective curative and rehabilitative surgical interventions are secondary and tertiary preventive services and a necessary response to diseases that elude primary prevention.[2]

The volume of major surgeries performed worldwide is estimated to be between 187.2 million and 281.2 million procedures per year. A total of 73.6% of these surgeries occur in high-income countries and 22.9% in countries in transition, and only 3.5% take place in developing countries where most of the world's population lives.[3,4] The imbalance in the numbers of operations performed per capita in developed countries versus developing countries is due largely to the lack of available surgical care in these resource-challenged nations.

This chapter has the following objectives regarding surgical care and global health:

- Define global surgery.*
- Present a historic overview of surgical issues in international health.
- Describe the global burden of surgical disease, including its impact on NCDs and other disease control programs.
- Discuss surgical capacity building as part of global health initiatives in resource-constrained environments.
- Discuss ways in which surgical providers can become integrated with global public health.

---

*In this chapter the term *international surgery* is used to describe broadly the delivery of surgical care. This care includes the delivery of anesthesia, obstetrics, and surgical nursing.

Definition of Surgery and International Surgical Care

The word *surgery* is an Anglicized derivation of the Latin word *chirurgia,* meaning "hand work." A *surgeon* is any health provider who treats surgical conditions through manipulation of tissues and provides invasive measures such as incisions and punctures with the intent to cure disease. Surgical care is not always invasive, and in some cases surgeons attend to a patient without performing an operation as in the treatment of splenic or liver injuries, fractures, and closed head injuries. Although an operation may not be performed in some of these cases, surgical expertise is needed. Surgery can be performed by a range of providers, including physicians with formal specialty training in surgical care and techniques, general practitioners with limited training in surgical care and techniques, and nonphysician health care providers who have had focused training in certain surgical techniques. In resource-constrained environments such as sub-Saharan Africa, many surgical and anesthetic services are limited to those provided by general practitioners or nonphysician health care providers. For the purposes of this discussion, *surgeon* refers to any physician with formal training in surgical care and techniques unless otherwise indicated.

International surgery, also referred to as global surgery,[†] is often represented as a humanitarian branch of medicine concerned with post disaster emergency care and with elective treatment of congenital anomalies such as cleft lip and palate, cardiac birth defects, and musculoskeletal deformities.[5] This work depends not only on the voluntary participation of trained specialists but also on the cooperation and understanding between donor and recipient nations. International surgery programs increasingly include education, research, capacity development, philanthropy, and advocacy. In addition, these programs include the delivery of anesthetic services, obstetric care, nursing care, and postoperative rehabilitative care. Global surgery fosters cooperation and understanding between nations. It includes north-to-south and south-to-north learning as well as south-to-south collaborations. It focuses on vulnerable populations even in high-income countries. One of the most notable deployments of international humanitarian surgical aid took

place in 2010 in response to the earthquake in Haiti. Medical teams from all over the world descended on Haiti to treat the injured. Shortly after the earthquake, Médecins Sans Frontières (MSF) dispatched the largest nonconflict surgical team in its history, treating over 550,000 Haitian patients and performing more than 4,000 surgical interventions in 10 weeks.[6] Although a high-profile disaster such as the Haiti earthquake is seen by many as humanitarian surgical care, it is the day-to-day surgical care needed in developing countries that is the true "disaster."

A Brief History of International Surgery

Surgical treatment dates back to as early as 10,000 to 5,000 BC. Early medical providers were known as healers, shamans, priests, barbers, and medicine men. Originally all medical providers were essentially surgeons as they treated wounds, drained infections, set broken bones, and stopped bleeding by applying hot metal or hot oil to wounds. Some of the oldest surgical procedures included the closure of lacerations using suture made of tendons threaded through needles made of sharpened bone. Trepanation, the act of drilling openings into the skull to release so-called evil spirits from the body dates back to the Mesolithic period (Figure 14-1).[7] Hieroglyphics in ancient Egypt and textbooks that were the foundation of Ayurvedic medicine (the Sushruta Samhita) describe many operations, including cesarean deliveries, rhinoplasty, craniotomy, and laparotomy performed while using wine and *Cannabis indica* as anesthetic agents.[8]

Wars and conquests throughout history have taken soldiers and their field surgeons to foreign lands, and care of battlefield injuries has provided surgery with some of its greatest technical advances as a result of working in very difficult field environments. These advances include improvements in anesthesia, in transportation and care of the injured, in achieving hemostasis and in treating sepsis. John Snow, the father of public health, also assisted in the development of surgical anesthesia as we know it today. Snow, well known for his epidemiologic work identifying the Broad Street pump handle as the source for London's 1854 cholera outbreak, was also an anesthetist and an advocate for the use of inhalation anesthesia during difficult childbirth.[9]

Colonial expansion brought surgical treatment to parts of the new world. As European colonialists, slave traders, and pirates moved throughout the Caribbean, Americas, and Pacific regions, they brought with them communicable diseases that would devastate native populations. In addition, they had new opportunities to understand tropical illnesses and apply medical and surgical treatments to a host of new maladies. Over time missionary physicians and surgeons

[†]The use of the term *global surgery* links the integration of surgical interventions, humanitarian aid, and the education and training of surgical workforces into global health strategies. Global health is a multidisciplinary strategy with the priority of improving health through training of health care workforces, incorporation of social justice, development fostering health care solutions as well as population-based prevention. International or global surgery is one of the disciplines that constitute global health.

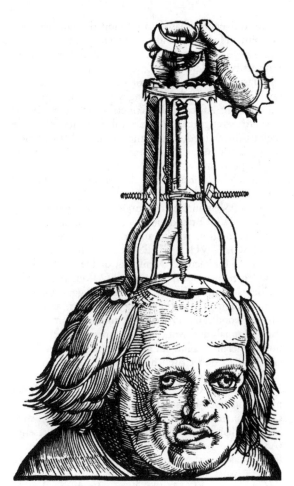

Figure 14-1. Trepanation (Courtesy of von Gersdorff H. *Feldbuch der Wundartzney*, 1517.)

were employed to keep the colonialists healthy and to assure the health of local human assets that were needed to sustain colonial economies.[10] They built, supported, and staffed hospitals in some of the most challenging locations. In addition to the Caribbean, Americas, and Pacific regions, colonialism in Africa fostered development of the Colonial Medical Service with training and research conducted at the London School of Tropical Medicine and Hygiene and other institutions. Medical and surgical teaching programs were established throughout the continent with early training programs flourishing in Sierra Leone, Nigeria, and Uganda.[11]

Early support for international medical and surgical education and public health training also came from the Rockefeller Foundation's International Health Board, the World Bank, the Pasteur Institute, and the World Health Organization (WHO). However, years of political and civil unrest in many of these sub-Saharan African countries left what were once grand academic medical institutions in disarray, and surgical services deteriorated as a result of deficient infrastructure and support. Médecins Sans Frontières (MSF), established in 1971 by a small group of French doctors in response to the Biafra crisis, filled a health care void created by war. MSF quickly added surgical services in 1983 after seeing the need for field operating theaters manned by expatriate surgeons who provided treatment for refugees from Chad and Liberia's wars. In a short period of time, MSF became one of the largest, most respected providers of international medical and surgical care in areas of civil unrest and natural disasters as well as in areas of nonconflict. Today MSF works in over 70 countries providing medical care, including general surgery, orthopedic surgery, obstetric emergency procedures, and surgical care for the injured.[12] The organization also advocates vigorously for human rights and health equity.

In the 1990s, investment in surgical service development in developing countries was minimized. In the World Bank's 1993 World Development Report, "Investment in Health," the Bank recommended governments in developing countries invest more heavily in "cost-effective programs that help the poor" through prevention rather than in direct medical care services.[13] The report emphasized the prevention and treatment of communicable diseases, including HIV/AIDs, malaria, and TB, all of which represented the most significant burdens of disease among developing countries. This report, authored along with the WHO, was very influential in defining the direction global health has taken today. Shortly after its release, a cascade of private health-directed philanthropy began. In 1999, Bill and Melinda Gates established the Gates Foundation, which stimulated an unprecedented effort to address specific diseases such as TB, HIV/AIDs, and malaria. In 2001, the MDGs were established and included mandates to reduce maternal and child mortality. The Global Fund to fight AIDs, Tuberculosis, and Malaria (GFATM) followed in 2002, and in 2003 the US Congress approved the establishment of the President's Emergency Plan for AIDs Relief (PEPFAR), which has committed over $63 billion to date, making it the largest health initiative addressing a single disease in US history. NCDs and injuries, neglected tropical diseases (NTDs), as well as health system strengthening, were not addressed in this global development agenda. The development of surgical services was not included as a goal of this unprecedented philanthropy because these services were perceived to be too expensive and therefore not cost effective. 20 years after the 1993 World Bank Report made the statement "Public money is spent on health interventions of low cost-effectiveness, such as surgeries for most cancers, at the same time that critical and highly cost-effective interventions such as treatment of TB or STDs remain underfunded,"[13] the mortality rates from cancers, injuries, and other NCDs in developing countries are increasing at alarming rates and the need for surgical interventions and horizontal health development programs has been recognized. Prevention strategies for these diseases include early detection and treatment as well as palliative care to relieve suffering. All of these can be accomplished through the addition of appropriate surgical services.

For years, teams made up of volunteer surgeons, operating room nurses, and technicians from developed countries have provided surgical care in many developing countries. Short duration surgical subspecialty groups like Operation Smile, Smile Train, Operation Hernia, Cure International, Orbis, and Children's Heartlink have filled the void of specialty surgical care for children living in developing countries who have cleft lip and palate, hernias, life-threatening congenital cardiac anomalies as well as other congenital musculoskeletal defects. Both military and civilian surgeons have been involved in international responses to natural disasters and wars such as Haiti, Banda Aceh, and conflicts in the Middle East and the Horn of Africa.[14] Even in conflict situations, more than 50% of the surgeries performed are for routine, nonviolent, usually obstetric or infectious problems, illustrating that even during war the need for general surgical care is great.[15,16]

The number of short surgical missions conducted in developing countries has grown over the past decade. These "outreach" or "mission visits" provide a valuable service, but many lack sustainability. The 2006 WHO Work Force Report recognized that these efforts were necessary until the local workforce improved. Nonetheless, concerns have been expressed over the quality, safety, appropriateness, and motives of these types of surgical missions.[17–20] Coordination of volunteer surgical outreaches with local providers, hospitals, and Ministries of Health is necessary to reduce duplication of efforts and burden on local staff. Follow-up care should also be planned in advance. The cost of conducting these short duration surgical missions is as difficult to estimate as is the total number of operations they provide. Maki et al conservatively estimated well over $250 million per year is spent on sending teams to provide care in developing countries.[21]

Programs such as the Pan-African Academy of Christian Surgeons (PAACS), established in 1997, and the Royal College of Surgeons of England have begun to address workforce shortage issues by committing to full time, in-country, primary surgical training programs in Gabon, Ethiopia, Cameroon, and Kenya.[22,23]

Many universities based in developed countries such as Johns Hopkins, Duke, University of California San Diego, University of California San Francisco, University of Michigan, University of Virginia, McMaster, and University of British Columbia have established academic exchanges with universities in sub-Saharan Africa, Latin America, and the Middle East to strengthen the surgical capacity of these regions through education and research.[24] Integration of academic surgical training along with outreach surgical care allows coordinated programs to create sustainable solutions while delivering much needed surgical services.

In 2005, as interest in surgical care strengthening grew, the WHO responded by establishing the Global Initiative on Emergency and Essential Surgical Care (GIEESC).[25] WHO GIEESC's mission is to create guidelines for member Ministries of Health to use in order to reduce death and disability from road traffic accidents, trauma, burns, injuries, pregnancy-related complications, domestic violence, disasters, and other surgical conditions in low-and middle-income countries. Manuals and workshops for training doctors and nonphysician surgeons in safe emergency surgical care and how to outfit rural hospitals with the minimum equipment needed to do so are available. Over the past 8 years, WHO GIEESC has grown and now includes input from over 400 surgeons working in more than 60 countries. Annual international surgery meetings such as the Alliance for Surgical and Anesthesia Presence (ASAP), the Bethune Round Table, and the Center for Global Surgery's Extreme Affordability Conference address issues pertinent to surgical capacity building and the surgical burden of disease. Professional organizations such as the American College of Surgeons' Operation Giving Back, the Royal Australasian College of Surgeons' International Program, Global Partners in Anesthesia and Surgery, and the Society of International Humanitarian Surgeons provide avenues for advocacy, information, research, volunteer opportunities, and education (Table 14-1).

In 2009, the US Global Health Initiative (GHI) expanded its portfolio of aid beyond disease specific acute care to include more sustainable aid by health system strengthening and the development of human resources for heath (HRH). Much of this work is funded through the National Institute of Health's (NIH) Medical Education Partnership Initiative (MEPI) grants. In addition to medical and public health education and training, MEPI grants support surgical education and research. Two MEPI grants were recently awarded to surgical capacity building programs in Mozambique and Rwanda.

Despite all of this initial work and a movement toward sustainable surgical capacity development, there are still significant challenges to the delivery of

Table 14-1. A list of international surgical organizations. These organizations encourage capacity building through the education of local surgeons.

World Health Organization Global Initiative for Emergency and Essential Surgical Care (WHO GIEESC)
Bellagio Essential Surgery Group
American College of Surgeons Operation Giving Back
Surgeons Over OverSeas
Alliance for Surgical and Anesthesia Presence
Global Partners in Anesthesia and Surgery
Pan-African Academy of Christian Surgeons (PAACS)
Canadian Network for International Surgeons
Royal Australian College of Surgeons International Program

Table 14-2. Global burden of disease. World Health Organization *International Classification of Diseases* (ICD) classification system based on mortality and disability.

Group 1: Infectious communicable diseases, perinatal, maternal, and nutritional disorders.
Group 2: Noncommunicable diseases: neoplasms, diabetes, cardiovascular disease, pulmonary, congenital anomalies, and psychiatric disorders.
Group 3: Intentional and unintentional injuries and violence.

surgical care in resource-constrained environments. Further efforts are needed in defining the enormous unmet surgical need in developing countries, its economic impact, as well as prospective studies that evaluate surgical capacity building programs.

BURDEN OF SURGICAL DISEASE

Describing the global burden of surgical need is important because a detailed analysis allows for measurement of frequency of disease (incidence and prevalence); its severity (mortality and disability); its consequence on populations (health, social, and economic impacts), and who is most affected (age, gender, socioeconomic position, region). This information assists with prioritization of strategies yielding the greatest benefit, identifying emerging trends, establishing spending priorities, and assisting in setting global health research agendas. In 1991, the World Bank commissioned the Global Burden of Disease Study (GBD) to quantify the burden of disease using mortality, disability, risk factors, and disease prevalence data projection by age, gender, and geographic region from 2000 to 2020. Diseases were classified into three broad groups based on the WHO ICD classification system (Table 14-2). Murray and Lopez published the first reports estimating the global burden of disease[26] with updates by the WHO in 2010. The Global Burden of Disease, Injury and Risk Factors 2010 Study, conducted by the Institute for Health Metrics and Evaluation, is the most comprehensive evaluation of disease burden to date. It includes analysis of more than 220 conditions and injuries, over 40 risk factors, and over 230 nonfatal health condition sequelae in 21 regions of the world. While death rates from infectious diseases such as malaria, AIDS, and TB are decreasing, there has

been a steady rise in chronic diseases such as diabetes, cancer, and cardiovascular disease as well as injuries. Hospital bed occupancies in developing countries are shifting from patients with predominantly infectious diseases to patients with diabetic complications, cardiovascular disease, cancers, and those debilitated by injuries such as femur fractures. This disease burden transition is due largely to population aging, reduced childhood mortality, and control of some communicable diseases. It is also the result of globalization and urbanization with behavior shifts toward poor diets, cigarette smoking, and decreased levels of activity. The prevalence of NCDs is expected to rise by more than 40% by 2030 and will account for an estimated 70% of deaths and 57% of disability-adjusted life years (DALYs) worldwide. Developing countries will be most dramatically impacted by increasing NCDs. Rates of injuries in developing countries are also increasing as these countries undergo urbanization, and traffic and factory production increase. Mortality, morbidity, and disability data collected by the GBD Study are the best estimates of the burden of disease, and they take into account the available sources of information in a country or region while correcting for bias. See Chapter 2 for more information on the burden of disease and Chapter 13 for information about injuries.

The prevalence of surgical conditions is not known. Many of the disease conditions described in the Global Burden of Disease Study analysis are amenable to surgical interventions if care is available, but many surgical conditions such as intestinal obstruction, gallbladder disease, appendicitis, and hernias are not included in the GBD data. Table 14-3 lists the medical conditions that would benefit from surgical intervention. The burden of surgical conditions (BoSC) is defined as disability, death, or illness that is wholly or partially curable by surgical intervention, and it includes all causes of surgical conditions. The BoSC, like the GBD, is expressed as DALYs. (See Chapter 2 for an explanation of the

Table 14-3. A sample list of prevalent diseases and disorders seen in low- to middle-income countries with surgical treatment options.

Disorder	Surgical treatment
NCDs	
Cancers: breast, cervical, colon, gastric, lung	Resection for cure, bypass for palliation
Chronic lung disease: asthma, COPD, emphysema	Lung volume reduction
Cardiovascular disease: acquired and congenital	Valve replacement, angioplasty
Diabetes: wound infections, limb loss, retinopathy	Debridement, amputation, laser retinal surgery, dialysis access
Thyroid masses due to iodine deficiency	Thyroidectomy
Communicable and NTDs	
Trachoma, Filariasis, Buruli ulcers	Excision, skin grafts, skin flaps, tarsal flap rotation
Ascariasis, induced bowel obstructions	Exploratory surgery, bowel resection, enterectomy
Tuberculosis: Pulmonary TB	Lung resection, decortication, plumage, thoracoplasty
Abdominal TB	Exploratory laparotomy, bowel resection or bypass
Potts disease (spine)	Debridement, fixation, rodding
Malaria: hypersplenism and spontaneous rupture	Splenectomy
Millennium Development Goals 4 and 5	
Ectopic pregnancy	Salpingectomy, salpingostomy
Dystocia, cephalopelvic disproportion, fetal distress	Emergency cesarean section
Obstetrical fistulas	Repairs
Congenital abnormalities:	
Cleft lip/palate	Repair
Club foot	Ponseti technique
Hernias	High ligation
Imperforate anus	Colostomy/definitive care
Branchial cleft, thyroglossal cyst	Excision
Random unpreventable diseases (many of these conditions are not included in the GBD data)	
Appendicitis	Appendectomy
Cholecystitis	Cholecystectomy
Necrotizing fasciitis	Debridement and reconstruction
Cellulitis and abscess	Incision and drainage
Incarcerated hernia	Repair and possible bowel resection
Foreign body: oral, nasal, ear	Removal possibly with exam under anesthesia
Miscellaneous mass	Excisional biopsy
Injury and violence	
Burns	Debridement, skin grafting, contracture release, escharotomies
Blunt trauma	Exploratory laparotomy, bowel, liver, spleen repair, flail chest fixation, fracture stabilization
Penetrating trauma	Exploratory laparotomy, bowel, liver, spleen removal. Repair of vascular, tendon, nerve injury

COPD, chronic obstructive pulmonary disease; GBD, Global Burden of Disease; NCD, noncommunicable disease; NTD, neglected tropical disease.

DALY.) The DALY measures mortality due to disease states as well as associated disability.

It is difficult to quantify surgically treatable conditions in developing countries because data collection and reliable reporting is limited. Most data come from hospital records and incomplete death registries. In 2006, Debas et al reported the first rough estimate of the global BoSC based on a survey of 18 surgeons working throughout all WHO regions. Surgically treatable conditions were estimated to be responsible for approximately 11% of all DALYs (Tables 14-4 and 14-5).[27] The authors recognized that their data underestimated the true burden of disease because they do not take into account the true total number of operations performed or the number of "surgical opportunities" missed due to lack of access to surgical care.[28] Weiser et al, estimated the annual volume of surgical interventions in developing countries to be 8 million, or just 3.5% of surgical care worldwide.[29] Bickler et al defined the burden of surgical disease based on the

Table 14-4. The breakdown of Debas' surgical burden of disease worldwide accounting for 11% of disability-adjusted life years.

Trauma (38%)
Cancer (19%)
Random unpreventable disease such as appendicitis or hernias (19%)
Congenital anomalies (9%)
Obstetric complications (6%)
Cataracts (5%)
Perinatal conditions (4%)

ability to address surgical need. They defined surgery as met surgical need (actual surgical care provided), unmet surgical need (potential surgical care), and unmeetable surgical need (unpreventable death or disability despite surgical care) (Table 14-6).[30] Current estimates of surgically treatable disease are based predominantly on met surgical need taking place in facilities such as hospitals, and they underestimate surgical conditions that go undiagnosed. With Bickler's classification, these "missed surgical care opportunities" are included in the data (Figure 14-2).[30]

To define accurately the true unmet burden of surgical disease, a global survey of surgically treatable conditions is needed. This would require complex, costly, and time-consuming data collecting from communities as well as health facilities. A recent population survey conducted in Sierra Leone by Surgeons Over Seas has done this. They reported one quarter of all people interviewed during a community cluster sampling study had a condition that would benefit from surgical assessment.[32] The authors have reported similar findings in Rwanda.[33]

Table 14-5. Surgical disability-related life years divided into Global Burden of Disease classification.[a]

Group	% DALYs in World[26]	% DALYs in Developing Countries[26]	% DALYs Surgical[27]
I	20.1	22.2	10
II	59.7	56.7	28
III	20.1	21.1	38

[a]Using estimated surgical disability-adjusted life years (DALYs) data from Table 67.2 in the second edition of DCPDC and Murray and Lopez's DALYs data for disorder groups in the world and developing regions, a need for surgical intervention across all areas of global health is demonstrated. The greatest potential surgical impact is in noncommunicable diseases and injuries.

Injuries are an increasing global public health problem and have resulted in over 5 million deaths and millions of people left with disabilities every year. The WHO estimates 90% of road traffic crashes and 90% of burns occur in developing countries. Trauma is the leading cause of death in children age 10 to 19, and 70% of burns occur in young children.[34] Timely trauma care can save lives at low cost. The addition of prehospital care in resource-constrained environments has reduced mortality from injury by more than 25%, and regular Advanced Trauma Life Support (ATLS) training can decrease mortality even further.[35,36] The improvement of trauma surgical care in developing countries could save between 1,730,000 and 1,965,000 lives a year in severely injured patients.[37]

The economic consequences of the increasing incidence of cancers in developing countries are projected to exceed $7 trillion by 2025 or $25 to $50 per person worldwide. Adding surgical interventions to prevention programs can reduce this economic impact. Table 14-7 lists GLOBOCANs 2008 data on incidences of the top six cancers in developing countries and estimates the percentage of these cancers that are surgically treatable if adequate surgical care is made available. Overall, 33% or 2,211,000 people living in developing countries diagnosed with cancer in 2008 would potentially benefit from surgical interventions, and without it they would die.

A number of papers have looked at the cost per DALY averted of providing essential surgical services. The cost per DALYs averted at four rural hospitals that included treatment of appendicitis, incarcerated hernia repair, and trauma care was estimated to be between $11 and $33 per DALY. The cost of providing hospital-based trauma and injury care was valued at roughly $78 per DALYs averted.[38-40] This cost analysis is on par with the cost of many primary public health interventions such as vitamin A distribution and immunization programs. An uncomplicated open appendectomy and hernia repair can be performed in a rural setting and cost less than $120, averting approximately 9.3 DALYs.[41] Treatment of peritonitis secondary to appendicitis can avert 27 DALYs.[42] This is nearly equivalent to the cost of providing combination antiretroviral medications to one person for a year.[43,44] The cost per DALY averted by cleft lip and palate repair surgery is estimated to be $73 per person.[45] Untreated cleft lip and palate defects in sub-Saharan Africa alone can translate into economic losses of between $252 and $441 million due to premature death, unrealized potential, and disability.[46] Although these economic data are helpful in determining where funding resources are spent, it does not take into account the social externality impacts, including productivity lost by family caretakers or out-of-pocket payments associated with transportation and treatments.

Table 14-6. Terminology describing and measuring the burden of surgical conditions and need for surgical care.[30]

Term	Definition	Unit of measure
Burden of surgical conditions	The disability and premature death that would exist in a population without any surgical care	DALYs
Met need for surgical care, averted	The disability and premature death in a population that has been prevented or corrected with surgical care	DALYs
Unmet need for surgical care, potentially avertable	The disability and premature death in a population that is preventable or correctable with surgical care	DALYs
Unmeetable need for surgical care, unavertable	The disability and premature death in a population that is unpreventable or uncorrectable with even the best surgical care	DALYs

DALY, disability-adjusted life year.

Economic impact is only one factor in determining resource allocation; human rights and dignity must also be included in policy making decisions. Minimizing suffering due to uncontrolled bleeding, loss of one's airway, or an open fracture must be acknowledged as a basic right. The socioeconomic consequences of untreated surgical conditions can compromise individuals, their families, and the community they live in. The loss of human capital through death or disability has an impact on family economics, especially if that person is the principal breadwinner. Health setbacks among poor families can result in adverse consequences such as pulling children out of school to provide care or reassigning their school fees to cover medical costs, shifting family farm work or other labors to children, and reducing family food consumption overall.[47–49] Untreated surgical conditions can diminish the size of the labor force, impacting local economies and development. Although the precise economic burden of specific surgical conditions has not been measured, it is estimated that the projected economic impact of major categories of diseases such as injuries or cancer, surgical conditions take an extraordinary economic toll on families.

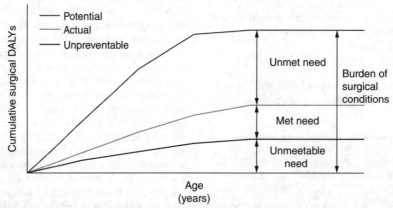

Figure 14-2. Diagram estimating the burden of surgical conditions and the unmet need for surgical care. Surgical disability and premature death in a population is a time-dependent function that relates to the incidence of surgical conditions and the quantity and quality of surgical care available. The potential, actual, and unpreventable curves represent the age-specific cumulative disability-adjusted life years (DALYs) with different levels of surgical care. Unmet surgical conditions are also referred to as "missed surgical care opportunities." See Table 14-6 for the definitions of surgical care and the burden of surgical conditions. (Adapted from Bickler S, Ozgediz D, Gosselin R, et al. Key concepts for estimating the burden of surgical conditions and the unmet need for surgical care. World J Surg 2010;34:374–380.)

Table 14-7. The 2008 incidence of the top six NCD cancers in LMICs using total number and age-standardized rates (ASR)per 100,000.[a]

NCDs	2008 incidence (ASR)	Treatable by surgery	Preventable
Cancers:			
Breast	691,521 (27.3)	81.6%[1]	+/−
Lung	884,359 (19.1)	45%[2]	+
Cervical	453,531 (17.8)	50%[3]	+
Stomach	713,907 (15.3)	85%[4]	+
Liver	626,548 (13.1)	25%[4]	+
Colorectal	506,558 (10.7)	80%[4]	+/−
All cancers	**7,107,273 (147.8)**	**33% (2,353,561)[b]**	

ASR, age-standardized rate; NCD, noncommunicable disease.

Age-standardized rate: A rate is the number of new cases or deaths per 100,000 persons per year. An age-standardized rate is the rate that a population would have if it had a standard age structure.

[a]Estimates of potential surgical interventions obtained from data in low-and middle-income countries and developed country reports. (*From GLOBOCAN 2008. http://globocan.iarc.fr/factsheets/populations/factsheet.asp?uno=902.*)

[b]The number of new cases (incidence) of cancer treated by surgical intervention.

[1]Groot MT, Baltussen R, et al. Cost and health effects of breast cancer interventions in epidemiologically different regions of Africa, North America and Asia. *Breast J.* 2006;12(Suppl 1):S81– S90.

[2] Hammerschmidt S, Wirtz H. Lung cancer: current diagnosis and treatment. *Dtsch Arztebl Int* 2009;106(49): 809–820.

[3]Duska LR, Toth TL, Goodman A. Fertility options for patients with stages Ia2 and Ib cervical cancer: presentation of two cases and discussion of technical and ethical issues. *Obstet Gynecol* 1998;92(4, Pt 2):656–658.

[4] Doherty G. *Current Diagnosis and Treatment: Surgery.* 13th ed. New York: McGraw-Hill, 2010.

By efficiently returning sick and injured people back to health after surgical emergencies, productivity is restored and financial demands on families decrease. Primary prevention of injuries and surgical conditions is arguably the most cost-effective way to avoid the negative consequences of premature death and disability, but the addition of cost-effective early diagnosis and restorative surgical treatments as secondary prevention will further decrease the disease burden in developing countries.

BOX 14-1. NONCOMMUNICABLE DISEASES: CANCER

NCDs have been described as a "slow-motion disaster" on its way to happening.[50] During the 2011 high-level United Nations and World Health Assembly meetings, the escalating problem of NCDs was discussed by member states and aid agencies.[51,52] The prevalence of diabetes in the Pacific Region is now over 40%. Global cancer deaths are predicted to increase from 7.1 million to 11.5 million, and global cardiovascular deaths will increase from 16.7 million to 23.3 million by 2030. A total of 53% of cancer cases and 60% of cancer deaths will occur in developing countries.[53]

• The most common cancers amenable to surgical interventions in developing countries include breast, cervical, gastric, liver, colon, and lung cancer.

• Cancers tend to present in advanced stages due to delays in accessing care and lack of screening programs. Many of these cancers are preventable.

• Early detection of cancers through low-cost screening programs will catch these diseases when they are potentially curable by excision.

• Screening programs in developing countries are a double-edged sword. Finding an increased number of early stage lesions that are curable by surgical intervention without strengthening the surgical capacity will frustrate both patients and providers.

BOX 14-2. MILLENNIUM DEVELOPMENT GOALS

Achieving MDG1 (Eradication of extreme poverty and hunger), 4 (Reduce child mortality), 5 (Improve maternal health), and 6 (Combat HIV/AIDS, malaria, and other diseases) can be augmented by the addition of surgical interventions to comprehensive health system programs.

- MDG 1: Eradication of extreme poverty and hunger is assisted by the inclusion of surgical care. Returning people back to a state of health and productivity has broad social, economic, and development impacts on not only a country but also on individuals and families. The World Economic Forum estimates the economic impact of untreated NCDs alone will exceed $47 trillion by 2030.

- MGD 4: Corrective surgery for congenital anomalies and perinatal conditions such as imperforate anus, cleft lip and palate, or clubfoot will decrease childhood disability and mortality.
- MGD 5: The ability to perform cesarean deliveries and repair obstetric fistulas will save lives and reduce morbidity. Less than 40% of hospitals in developing countries are able to perform lifesaving obstetric procedures due to the lack of training.
- MGD 6: Decrease the transmission of HIV/AIDs through male circumcision and by encouraging safe surgical techniques.

BOX 14-3. ROAD TRAFFIC ACCIDENTS, INJURY, AND VIOLENCE

Injuries account for over 5 million deaths worldwide with more than 90% of injury deaths occurring in developing countries. Millions more are left disabled, compounding economic losses. Injuries can occur due to war and violence; however, unintentional injuries, including road traffic crashes, drowning, burns, poisoning, and falls are the leading cause of death in young people, the most economically productive segment of a global population.

- Injuries kill more people than HIV, TB, and malaria combined.
- For adult men age 15 to 44, road traffic injuries rank second to HIV/AIDS as the leading cause of ill health and premature death worldwide.
- In high-income countries 1.7 deaths occur per 10,000 vehicles. Contrast that with over 50 per 10,000 vehicles in sub-Saharan Africa.
- Driver behavior (speeding, drinking, not using seatbelts), poorly maintained vehicles, and road infrastructure all contribute to higher death rates

per number of vehicles seen in developing countries.
- The proportion of prehospital deaths from injury is inversely related to a country's prehospital resuscitation and transportation capabilities.
- Developing countries lack organized prehospital trauma care and emergency services systems.
- Regular, affordable ATLS training is needed because less than 50% of staff members treating trauma patients in developing countries are current in their certification. The addition of regular ATLS in-services has been shown to decrease mortality by over 35%.
- WHO's Violence and Injury Prevention program (WHO VIP) has shown that emphasis on prevention paired with trauma services and protocols can reduce disability and fatalities.
- Surgical care in areas of conflict and disaster settings can save lives if mobilized early with adequate supplies and staff.

BOX 14-4. RANDOM UNPREVENTABLE DISEASES WITH SURGICAL TREATMENT

Some disease processes are random and not impacted significantly by prevention and education. Such conditions are referred to as random unpreventable diseases (RUDs) and generally are not accounted for in global burden of disease data. Many are treated by surgical interventions. The best examples of RUDs are appendicitis, congenital anomalies, and hernias.

- Appendicitis is the most common emergency surgical procedure performed, carrying a lifetime risk of 8% and responsibility for 10% of hospital admissions.
- In developing countries appendicitis most commonly presents with gangrene, abscess, perforation, and peritonitis due to delays in obtaining treatment.
- Hernias are 10 times more common in developing countries than in developed countries where more hernia surgeries are performed.

- Manual labor, farming, poor nutrition, and poverty contribute to the number of hernias, and delays in treatment result in large complicated inguinal-scrotal hernias.
- The number of inguinal hernia repairs and strangulated inguinal hernia repairs performed in Africa is low despite a high incidence of hernias. An estimated 18 to 56 per 100,000 surgeries have been performed in low- to middle-income countries; 130 to 260 per 100,000 hernia repairs occur in high-income countries.
- Up to 85% of children will require some surgical procedure by age 15, underscoring the need for safe pediatric surgery and anesthesia services and providers.[54]

SURGICAL CAPACITY BUILDING

There are significant but not insurmountable hurdles to overcome in order to establish and improve surgical care as an integral part of developing countries' health care systems. The capacity of a country to provide surgical care for its citizens has been described in reports from Pakistan, Afghanistan, the Solomon Islands, and many countries in sub-Saharan Africa.[55-63] The list continues to grow. Despite their geographic diversity, several common deficiencies have emerged from these reports:

1. A lack of infrastructure
2. Shortages of consumable supplies
3. Inadequate workforce numbers and development
4. Barriers or "patient factors"[‡] contributing to the inability to access surgical care
5. Cost of establishing surgical care
6. A perception that surgery is not compatible with public health goals

The next section of this chapter discusses each of these deficiencies in detail and includes solutions and programs that will correct these deficiencies.

Lack of Infrastructure and Inadequate Surgical Supplies

The lack of skills and equipment are the leading reasons patients are referred from district hospitals to tertiary care hospitals. Many district or provincial hospitals are located in isolated rural areas where there is unreliable electricity and running water. Operating theaters may not exist at these hospitals or may lack proper equipment such as lights, anesthesia machines, or autoclaves to sterilize equipment. In hospitals that have basic surgical instruments, a lack of proper maintenance severely shortens the effectiveness and lifespan of the equipment. Nearly all district hospitals in developing countries have problems with obtaining and maintaining adequate consumable surgical supplies such as gauze, suture, sterile gloves, antibiotics, pain medications, and anesthetic agents. The situation is further compounded by the remoteness of these hospitals and by poor hospital management skills. Supply shortages result in delays in treatment that impact lives and add financial burden to already poor families trying to procure supplies for their family member. The availability of surgical supplies, equipment, and human resources are also influenced by local political and economic factors in cases where operating budgets cross sector boundaries and require cooperation between the Ministries of Health and Finance. In addition, it is easier for donors, Ministries

---

[‡]"Patient factors" include fear, cultural and educational influences, and geographic obstacles as well as financial constraints.

BOX 14-5. DEVELOPING COUNTRY SURGICAL CAPACITY ASSESSMENT

Using the WHO Global Initiative on Emergency and Essential Surgical Care Situational Analysis Tool, the surgical capacity of developing countries listed here has been evaluated. Data are collected on the type of hospital, population served, infrastructure available, workforce, supplies, and procedures performed during on-site visits.

Afghanistan	Bangladesh	Botswana
Ethiopia	Gambia	Ghana
Liberia	Malawi	Mongolia
Mozambique	Niger	Nigeria
Pakistan	Rwanda	Nigeria
Solomon Islands	South Africa	Sierra Leone
Sri Lanka	Tanzania	South America
Vietnam	Zambia	Uganda

of Finance, and planners to embrace infrastructure projects as one-off investments; however, without the supply chain and repair structures built into these investments, they can quickly become dysfunctional and unable to sustain service delivery. Incentives for political leaders or bureaucrats to fix these deficiencies are limited because these leaders, at great expense to their country, often fly their own family members who have surgical problems to richer countries for treatment.

Because surgical care is hospital-centric, improving quality and delivery often requires improvements at both the individual hospital level as well as at the level of the health system. Tertiary care hospitals or national referral hospitals tend to be located in urban areas. These hospitals are usually the country's best equipped and staffed, thereby providing specialized and complex surgical services. But tertiary care hospitals can have inadequate services due to the lack of funding, equipment, or limited training. In rural areas, where most people live in developing countries, improving access to basic safe surgical care is important. Investments in infrastructure should include running water and a backup generator or solar power sources for hospitals. Not every district or provincial hospital needs a fully functioning surgical department. Key provincial hospitals should be identified for establishment of essential surgical care as determined by the Ministry of Health (MoH) and based on the population served, ease of access, connection to a tertiary care center, available funding, and political will for upgrades, supplies, and workforce expansion. The goal of these regional referral centers is to provide basic, safe, emergency surgical and obstetric care as outlined by WHO GIEESC. Protocols that guide staff on when and how to refer severely injured

or critically ill patients to tertiary care centers should be included. Technical assistance with management skills, financial oversight, medical supply chain procurement, as well as staff hiring and scheduling, should be included so that disruption of services is avoided.

International surgical programs are providing their surgical peers with the support and development they request, rather than what is believed to be necessary from the outside. A top-down approach toward strengthening surgical services is not necessarily the best approach because projects are sustained by personal and professional partnerships developed with the key persons who are responsible for day-to-day activities. These surgical development partnerships work toward keeping surgical interventions safe, environmentally responsible, culturally appropriate, cost effective, and with appropriate infrastructure. Not all technology used in developed countries belongs in resource-constrained environments, nor should old and discarded equipment be donated. Familiarity with the WHO Guidelines for Health Care Equipment Donations will prevent generosity from becoming waste.[64] New equipment or competently refurbished equipment should be procured with consideration given to cost, maintenance, and the assumption of local ownership by the health care system. Biomedical Engineering (BME) education and training on medical equipment care and development will help avoid the "implementation gap" that exists between health innovations and its deployment in developing countries. Partnerships between developed and developing countries BME training programs currently focus on local design constraints, maintenance deficiencies, and development solutions for the local environment.[65]

In an effort to create affordable surgical equipment, international surgery groups have begun applying so-called extreme affordability techniques to surgical supply development in order to reduce cost.[66,67] Surgeons working in resource-constrained environments, such as Dr. Awojobi Oluyombo from Nigeria, are forced by limited supplies and funds to build functional medical equipment from common items, such as a hematocrit centrifuge from the rear wheel of a bicycle.[68]

Public private partnerships (PPPs) formed between NGOs, governments, and corporations that manufacture surgical supplies have resulted in product development for resource-constrained environments that is less expensive and high quality. Disruptive innovations have been slowly reducing the cost of medical and diagnostic equipment worldwide and could be pushed further by utilizing south-to-south collaboration strategies whereby developing countries produce medical supplies for use in other developing countries.[69] An excellent example of the application of south-to-south collaborations is the Aravind Eye Care System. Cataracts are the leading cause of blindness worldwide, and in India more than 10 million people need cataract treatment, but the high cost of intraocular lenses (IOLs) needed for the surgery made the procedure too expensive. Aravind partnered with a local manufacturing company, Aurolab, to produce affordable IOLs and expand services to thousands of people living in developing countries.[70] This type of "local" manufacturing, along with the creation of an economy of scale, keeps the cost of procedures down, allowing treatment to be provided to patients who otherwise could not afford it. It fosters sustainability of supply as well as encouraging local production that bolsters industry and economy.

Inadequate Surgical Workforce

In developing countries there is a shortage of health care workforce at all levels and in every specialty area. This includes surgeons, anesthesiologists, operating room nurses, and technicians. In Africa there are 0.25 trained surgeons per 100,000 people as compared with 5.7 per 100,000 in the United States.[71,72] Shortages in the anesthesia workforce exist as well. In Uganda there are approximately 19 anesthesiologists for over 30 million people, and in Ethiopia there are 19 anesthesiologists caring for 82 million. To put this in perspective, there are more than 70,000 anesthesia providers in the United States alone. Inadequate numbers and training of surgeons, anesthesiologists, and nurses, as well as the lack of supplies, contribute to perioperative deaths, some estimated to be as high as 2.6%.[73] Severe shortages in biomedical technicians, pathology technicians, and medical technicians also impact quality of care.

Multiple factors contribute to the shortage of health workers, including so-called brain drain. Push factors contributing to emigration of health workers include poor remuneration and work conditions. Shortages in the health workforce in high-income countries and recruitment programs also pull health care professionals from developing countries. The cost of educating a surgeon in sub-Saharan Africa is approximately $5,000 US. Recruiting these new graduates has resulted in losses of over $2 billion in returns on investment of training these doctors.[74] The WHO Code of Practice on the International Recruitment of Health Personnel, established in 2010, addresses voluntary cooperative measures that decrease the impact emigration has had on health workforces.[75] Other factors contributing to shortages in the health workforce include a lack of training, inadequate numbers of health workers entering the workforce, career shifts, early retirement, and death. Medical universities in developing countries have not been able to train enough doctors, nurses, and technicians to meet their own demands, and along with the loss of health workers to high-income countries have resulted in such inadequate staffing that patient safety has been negatively impacted. The remaining health care workforce can easily become overworked, and staff can suffer from burnout, exhaustion, and demoralization. Surgical training is subject to further stressors because it is specialized and requires comprehensive specialized teaching. If surgical professors lack teaching and research skills, the clinic skills of new trainees suffer. Research in general is considered a luxury in the settings of limited resources and extensive unmet need. The omission of surgical research contributes to a dearth of context-specific treatment and prevention programs based on locally defined health issues.

Extension of surgical care to strategically identified district hospitals will require increases in resources, including expansion of the surgical workforce. This includes increasing the number of and support for the education of new and current surgeons, anesthesiologists, and nurses. Task shifting through the training of nonsurgeon physicians and nonphysician surgical and anesthesia technicians should be encouraged because it has been shown to be a cost-effective, safe, and expedient way to increase the workforce. Implementation of task shifting depends on the country's political will, endorsement by local medical and surgical associations, and appropriate regulations that define the training and scope of services these nonsurgeon cadres will provide.[76–78] Training of local biomedical engineers should also be included because medical equipment is an investment, and regular maintenance and repair is critical to delivering care.

Creating positive barriers to emigration, such as financial incentives for staff to obtain additional skills or sign-on bonuses to work in underserved rural hospitals, can help decrease the early loss of graduates from medical and nursing schools. In addition to reducing brain drain, education programs will improve the distribution and quality of care in rural settings. Achieving the goal of strengthening local medical education will require collaboration between the MoHs and Ministries of Finance, with input from medical universities and NGO partners. This collaboration will foster supportive work environments for the healthcare workforce. The Rwanda-Canada paradigm for surgical training, in keeping with the concept of "train the trainer," includes expatriate surgical faculty who serve as moderators and facilitators of education programs run by local surgeons. The curriculum is developed based on local needs. This type of partnership addresses the essential elements of medical education and surgical capacity building in developing countries: local ownership, leadership skill and career development, and accountability for program sustainability.[79] For doctors and health care specialists working in isolated and austere environments or in countries that do not have medical universities, a judicious combination of in-country as well as out-of-country training should be offered. In addition to focusing on surgical skills, local surgeons are encouraged to document their unique expertise in providing care in resource-constrained environments through publications and presentations, and to apply for research grants that allow them to address these issues. The new breed of "public health surgeons" is creating a workforce that prioritizes prevention, early detection, and treatment programs. Regional surgical associations can spearhead the expansion and promotion of these opportunities.

By nature surgeons are hospital based and therefore should contribute to hospital management by overseeing surgical services. Working along with hospital staff to keep track of supplies and place timely replacement orders will prevent disruptions in care. Local surgeons should teach not just new trainees but also the entire health care team, including their medical associates who will be a source of surgical referrals. Schedules, when workload allows, should allot adequate time for each of these duties along with clinical responsibilities.[80]

Barriers to Surgical Care

A number of patient factors contribute to delayed or failed access to obtaining timely surgical care. Grimes et al examined barriers to surgical care in developing countries.[81] Based on 52 reports on barriers to ophthalmology services, obstetrics and gynecology care, injury and burn care, and general surgical care, a number of barriers to seeking care have been defined. These factors, although unique in some respects to surgical

care, have many elements in common with HIV, TB, and other communicable disease treatment challenges.

Culture, Fear, and Educational Hurdles

People fear the unknown, and they fear pain. A person's prior experience or even observations or opinions may keep them and others they influence from seeking surgical treatment. The death of a family member while undergoing a surgical procedure can result in a perception that surgery is witchcraft, negatively influencing any future pursuit of surgical care. Or the community may lose confidence in the local health facility if outcomes are poor. Likewise, if a scheduled operation is cancelled or delayed, a patient may choose not to reschedule based on superstition or frustration. Cultural norms may also prevent people from seeking timely surgical care. In many cultures women are forbidden to travel alone, resulting in delays in seeking care as they wait for male family members to accompany them. If a sick family member is a child caretaker or gardener, the loss of their input in these areas can create problems at home and have economic consequences. Lack of education and trust in the health care system also contributes to barriers in seeking timely care.

Geographic Obstacles

The lack of surgical infrastructure, equipment, and expertise at district hospitals means that surgical services may not be available locally and require traveling a significant distance to the nearest facility that has adequate surgical services. A country made up of many islands that requires a long boat journey, a mountainous region made impassable by winter snows, or extensive flooding during the rainy season that washes out roads can make accessing facility-based care difficult. The lack of availability of passable roads, boats, planes, vehicles, and even work animals can contribute to the inability to travel, as can the cost. The clinical ability of primary care providers to recognize and act on surgical conditions is also problematic.

Financial Impact of Obtaining Care

Financial concern is one of the most significant barriers to obtaining surgical care. In one obstetric care study from Ghana, care offered at no charge resulted in women being 4.6 times more likely to seek professional health care. Financial barriers to care are the result of direct and indirect costs. Direct costs include surgical fees, drugs, supplies, diagnostic tests, transportation, food, and stay at the hospital. In India, as well as many other developing countries, family members must purchase surgical supplies and pharmaceuticals from the black market located just outside many hospitals and deliver them to physicians to initiate treatment for their loved one.

Tertiary care referrals are often delayed until funds can be obtained to cover costs. Indirect costs are those related to loss of work productivity and the need for a caretaker due to illness. This includes loss of income and time away for care and travel. A large percentage of people living in developing countries depend on subsistence living, such as farming and fishing, resulting in extremely modest incomes and limited resources. Any event that increases expenses can have a profound negative effect on individuals and their families. The financial burden associated with surgery can be tremendous, and these costs, combined with the loss of income and/or family care work, can render extended families destitute. In some countries 11% of the population suffers from poverty related to health care costs, and 5% are forced into extreme poverty. The use of National Health Accounts (NHAs) by developing countries allows them to identify their sources of health funding and to develop policies to address inequity of cost. Reducing out-of-pocket or direct payments to less than 15% to 20%, as recommended by the WHO, decreases financial catastrophe risk. Unfortunately, many of the poorest countries have out-of-pocket expenses that exceed 50% of total health expenditures.

Public education is needed about the availability and benefits of obtaining surgical care for obstetrics, injuries, burns, and congenital anomalies, in addition to education in preventing injuries, burns, and obstetric emergencies. Elimination of upfront cost for emergency care and subsidized elective surgical care is needed. In sub-Saharan Africa, abolition of user fees has had positive effects on utilization of health services, but planning and implementation of such programs is needed.[82] Conditional cash transfers for accessing treatment early and subsidized transportation funding have been shown to increase the use of facility services while deferring personal costs.[83] External aid funding tied to reducing or eliminating upfront costs can help. A clear delineation of which surgical interventions can be safely provided at district hospitals is accomplished through education of staff on criteria for referral to higher-level care by a trained medical transportation service. Expanding local providers' skill sets in essential emergency surgical care allows care to take place closer to home, reducing costs and encouraging access.

Cost of Establishing Surgical Care

There is a perception that providing surgical care in resource-constrained settings is too expensive and therefore should not be part of global health schemes. This perception likely stems from the cost of care in developed country health systems. Surgical services in the United States are very technology dependent and expensive. Over half of all money spent on medical devices worldwide is spent in the United States.[84] High-end technology-intensive procedures such as those using the DaVinci robot, ceramic hip replacements, gastric bypasses, and others have no role in resource-constrained countries that are in need of lifesaving and disability-preventing services provided by essential surgical interventions. Sadly, most health system strengthening programs in developing countries have omitted basic and appropriate surgical care because of this cost misconception. On the contrary, as mentioned earlier in this chapter, once established, surgical care in developing countries is just as cost effective as treating HIV/AIDs, TB, or vaccination programs.

International surgical organizations have worked on limited budgets consisting of mainly private donations, small grants, and in-kind donations from the very industries used within their own practices. These efforts have demonstrated that contrary to popular belief, surgical interventions can be provided at a reduced cost. Scale up of workforce, supplies, and infrastructure upgrades will initially be costly but once established should level off or decrease. The use of disruptive technologies, extreme affordability techniques, and south-to-south product manufacturing collaboration will assist in keeping costs low.

A Perception That Surgery Is Not Compatible with Public Health Goals

Surgical interventions may be seen as violating public health tenets: focusing on individuals rather than populations, and curative rather than traditionally preventive interventions. As mentioned earlier in this chapter, surgical treatment restores function for individuals and families improving community development, financial stability, and a sense of social justice using secondary or tertiary prevention approaches. Primary prevention of cancers, communicable diseases, maternal and child health problems, obstetric emergencies, and injuries are very cost effective, but they are not perfect. The surgical treatment of many diseases must also be considered as a component of comprehensive approaches to disease control and prevention. Primary prevention cannot be the sole means of addressing many of the diseases mentioned in this book, and to withhold surgical treatment where appropriate would be akin to withholding treatment for TB or HIV/AIDS.

Worldwide, surgeons have begun to incorporate public health principles into their daily work. Surgical training programs in the United States have integrated population health principles along with teaching the treatment of surgical diseases.[85] Including public health training for surgeons in developing countries will assist in creating advocacy for their fellow citizens by documenting the unmet surgical need and the resources needed to address it.[86,87] By leaving the operating theater to address prevention efforts by describing the diseases they see and feel, surgeons can contribute to changing unhealthy behaviors and disease impacts. They can also discuss health issues with their national leaders and guide them in ratifying, implementing, and supporting prevention measures like the Framework Convention on Tobacco Control (FCTC) and the WHO's Violence Prevention Plan.

CONCLUSION

This chapter discussed the importance of incorporating appropriate surgical care into global health programs in developing countries. In particular, it frames the role of surgery in the public health paradigm in the management of noncommunicable diseases, trauma and injury, MDGs 1, 4, 5, and 6, as well as other surgical conditions. The rationale to invest in surgical workforce and infrastructure improvements, and to address barriers in access to care is also provided. How surgeons should be involved in prevention and provide leadership in their hospitals and communities is described. Public health surgeons promoting prevention programs in developing countries can demonstrate how an integrated approach toward health saves lives and money.

Building or strengthening surgical programs in developing countries through partnerships is a slow, methodical process that must begin with establishing trust built on dialogue and mutual respect. Any development partnership must take into account the context-specific concerns of working in a resource-constrained environment as expressed by the local surgeons, the MoH, the Ministry of Education, and any other sectors impacting delivery of care. Surgical programs, like all aid programs, must align with the needs and goals of local health providers and the MoH in making education and surgical services congruent with the needs of the people and resources limitations. Local ownership of programs must be integral to the design. Open communication and, where feasible, coordination with other agencies providing development assistance for health (DAH) should take place via open and transparent sharing of records and reports as well as active participation in MoH and donor agency meetings.

To create stable surgical care programs in developing countries and allow sustainable work to flourish, long-term funding commitments are needed. Like HIV/AIDS programs, surgical capacity building programs initially go through an intense development phase as labor, task shifting, infrastructure, and skills are brought online. This initial phase will give way to the less costly and less intense maintenance or support phase as local surgical health care workers take responsibility for programs. Without consistent financial support, program gains can quickly be lost. A number of international surgical programs such as the Royal Australian College of Surgeons' (RACS) International Program and the Canadian Network for International Surgery (CNIS) receive consistent financial support from their government aid agencies, the Australian Agency for International Development (AusAID) and the Canadian International Development Agency (CIDA), respectively. The Clinton Health Access Initiative (CHAI), USAID, and the Rwandan MoH have established the Human Resources for Health Program, a program that will address the critical health care worker shortage in Rwanda, including that of surgeons.[88] The College of Surgeons of East, Central, and Southern Africa (COSECSA), a "college without walls," fosters postgraduate surgical education at regional, missionary, and district hospitals in nine countries in sub-Saharan Africa. It does this by standardizing training and assisting MoHs in implementing best practices.[89] PAACS and many other committed faith-based surgical training programs receive regular financial as well as spiritual support from their churches. Their hard work has begun to pay off. The PAACS program has graduated 18 surgeons since 1997, and most of these graduates are working in rural areas in Africa today.[23]

Slowly but surely the message that appropriate, essential surgical care should be included in global health programs is being heard. In 2008 and again in 2012, the Copenhagen Consensus Group, a think tank made up of economists and Nobel Prize laureates tasked with defining measures that impact some of the world's greatest problems, listed "strengthening surgical capacity" in developing countries as a top cost-effective measure that would significantly improve the well-being of the world's poor.[90] The addition of NIH MEPI grant funding and other sources of consistent funds will allow surgical programs in developing countries to grow and improve the delivery of care to the millions of people they are responsible for.

Untreated disease has a significant impact on daily life, productivity, and a developing economy. By definition, global health "places priority on improving health and achieving equity in health for all people worldwide. It emphasizes transnational health issues, determinants, and solutions; involves many disciplines within and beyond the health sciences and promotes inter-disciplinary collaboration; and it is a synthesis of population-based prevention with individual-level clinical care."[91]

Surgical providers can make a significant contribution to global health. The role of surgery in treating diseases in developing countries needs to be recognized for its effectiveness in eliminating suffering and pain from burns, injuries, and other surgical conditions. It is not a luxury; it is a human right that cannot be ignored. Surgical care that saves lives and restores health is essential and should be incorporated into current health system strengthening programs.

STUDY QUESTIONS

1. Name six deficiencies identified in the delivery of surgical care in developing countries and discuss how to improve them.

2. What roles have organizations such as Médecins San Frontières and the World Health Organization Global Initiative on Emergency and Essential Surgical Care played in surgical care and capacity building?

3. How does the addition of surgical care have the potential to impact death and disability rates due to injuries and road crashes, MDGs 1, 4, 5, and NCDs?

REFERENCES

1. Global Forum for Health Research, 10/90 research gap. 2011. http://www.globalforumhealth.org/about/1090-gap/

2. WHO, Declaration of Alma-Ata, 1978 http://tinyurl.com/7rpss7s.

3. Weiser T, Regenbogen S, Thompson K, et al. An estimate of the global volume of surgery: a modeling strategy based on available data. *Lancet* 2008;372(9633):139–144.

4. Tollefson T, Larrabee W. Global surgical initiative to reduce the surgical burden of disease. *JAMA* 2012;307(7):667–668.

5. Lett R. International surgery: definition, principals and Canadian practice. *Can J Surg* 2003;46(5):365–372.

6. Chu K, Stokes C, Trelles M, Ford N. Improving effective surgical delivery in humanitarian disasters: lessons from Haiti. *PLoS Med* 2011;8(4):e1001025.

7. Missios S. Hippocrates, Galen, and the uses of trepanation in the ancient classical world. *Neurosurg Focus* 2007;23(1):E1–E9.

8. Raveenthiran V. Knowledge of ancient Hindu surgeons on Hirschsprung's disease: evidence from Sushruta Samhita of circa 1200–600 BC. *J Pediatr Surg* 2011;46:2204–2208.

9. Paneth N. Assessing the contributions of John Snow to epidemiology. *Epidemiology* 2004;14(5):514–516.

10. Ajayi OO, Adebamowo CA. Surgery in Nigeria. *Arch Surg* 1999;134(2):206–211.

11. Burke-Gaffney H. The history of medicine in the African countries. *Med Hist* 1968;12(1):31–41.

12. Chu K, Rosseel P, Trelles M, Gielis P. Surgeon without borders: a brief history of surgery at Médecins Sans Frontières. *World J Surg* 2010;34:411–414.

13. World Bank. World Development Report 1993. http://tinyurl.com/3qdan9b.

14. Kushner AL, Groen RS, Kingham TP. Surgery and refugee populations. *Scand J Surg* 2009;98:18–24.

15. Chu K. Rethinking surgical care in conflict. *Lancet* 2010;375:262–263.

16. Chu KM, Trelles M, Ford NP. Quality of care in humanitarian surgery. *World J Surg* 2011;35(6):1169–1172.

17. Welling DR, Ryan JM, Burris DG, Rich NM. Seven sins of humanitarian medicine. *World J Surg* 2010;34:466–470.

18. Shein M. Commentary: Seven sins of humanitarian medicine. *World J Surg* 2010;34:471–472.

19. Abelson R, Rosenthal E. Charges of shoddy practices taint gifts of plastic surgery. *New York Times*. http://www.nytimes.com/1999/11/24/world/charges-of-shoddy-practices-taint-gifts-of-plastic-surgery.html?scp=5&sq=Charges+of+shoddy+practices+taint+gifts+of+plastic+surgery&st=nyt.

20. Wolfberg AJ. Volunteering overseas—lessons from surgical brigades. *N Engl J Med* 2006;354(5):443–445.

21. Maki J, Qualls M, White B, Kleefiels S, Crone R. Health impact assessment and short term medical missions: a methods study to evaluate quality of care. *BMC Health Svc Res* 2008; 8:121.

22. Lancet editorial. Global surgery—the final frontier? *Lancet* 2012;379:194.

23. Pollack JD, Love TP, Steffes BC, Thompson CD, Mellinger J, Haisch C. Is it possible to train surgeons for rural Africa? A report of a successful international program. *World J Surg* 2011;35:493–499.

24. Riviello R, Ozgediz D, Hsia RY, Azzie G, Newton M, Tarpley J. Role of collaborative academic partnerships in surgical training, education, and provision. *World J Surg* 2010;34: 459–465.

25. WHO Emergency and essential surgical care. http://www.who.int/surgery/mission/GIEESC2005_Report.pdf.

26. Murray CJ, Lopez AD. Alternative projections of mortality and disability by cause 1990–2020: Global Burden of Disease Study. *Lancet* 1997;349:1498–1504.

27. Debas HT, Gosselin R, McCord C, Thind A. Chapter 67. In: *Surgery, Disease Control Priorities in Different Countries.* 2nd ed. Washington, DC: World Bank, 2006: 1245–1258.

28. Gosselin R, Gyamfi Y, Contini S. Challenges of meeting surgical needs in the developing world. *J Surg* 2011;35:258–261.

29. Weisert T, Regenbogen S, Thompson K, et al. An estimate of the global volume of surgery: a modeling strategy based on available data. *Lancet* 2008;372(9633):139–144.

30. Bickler S, Ozgediz D, Gosselin R, et al. Key concepts for estimating the burden of surgical conditions and the unmet need for surgical care. *World J Surg* 2010;34:374–380.

31. Vos T. Improving the quantitative basis of the surgical burden in low-income countries. *PLoS Med* 2006;6(9):1–2.

32. Groen R, Samai M, Stewart K, et al. Untreated surgical conditions in Sierra Leone: a cluster randomized, cross-sectional, countrywide survey. *Lancet* 2012;380(9847):1082–1087.

33. Personal correspondence, Peter Kingham, Surgeons Over Seas.

34. Lavy C, Sauven K, Mkandawire N, et al. State of surgery in tropical Africa: a review. *World J Surg* 2011;35:262–271.

35. Husum H, Gilbert M, Wisborg T, Heng H, Urad M. Rural prehospital trauma systems improve trauma outcome in low-income countries: a prospective study from north Iraq and Cambodia. *J Trauma* 2003;54:1188–1196.

36. Ali J, Adam R, Butler AK, et al. Trauma outcome improves following the advanced trauma life support program in a developing country. *J Trauma* 1993;34:890–899.

37. Mock C, Joshipura M, Arreola-Risa C, Quannsah R. An estimate of the number of lives that could be saved through improvements in trauma care globally. *World J Surg* 2012; 36:959–963.

38. Gosselin R, Thind A, Bellardinelli BA. Cost/DALY averted in a small hospital in Sierra Leone: what is the relative contribution of different services? *World J Surg* 2006;30:505–511.

39. Gosselin R, Heitto M. Cost-effectiveness of a district trauma hospital in Battambang, Cambodia. *World J Surg* 2008;32: 2450–2453.

40. Gosselin R, Maldonado A, Elder G. Comparative cost-effectiveness analysis of two MSF surgical trauma centers. *World J Surg* 2010;34:415–419.

41. Shillcutt SD, Clarke MG, Kingsnorth AN. Cost-effectiveness of groin hernia surgery in the western region of Ghana. *Arch Surg* 2010;145(10):954–961.

42. Gosslein R, Thind A, Bellardinelli BA. Cost/DALY averted in a small hospital in Sierra Leone: what is the relative contribution of different services? *World J Surg* 2006;30:505–511.

43. Bendavid E, Leroux E, Bhattacharya J, Smith N, Miller G. The relation of price of antiretroviral drugs and foreign assistance with coverage of HIV treatment in Africa: retrospective study. *BMJ* 2010;341:c8218.

44. Hontelez JAC, de Vlas SJ, Tanser F, et al. The impact of the new WHO antiretroviral treatment guidelines on HIV epidemic dynamics and cost in South Africa. *PLoS* 2011;6(7):e21919.

45. Corlew D. Estimates of impact of surgical disease through economic modeling of cleft lip and palate care. *World J Surg* 2010;34:391–396.

46. Alkire B, Hughes C, Nash K, Vincent J, Meara J. Potential economic benefit of cleft lip and palate repair in sub-Saharan Africa. *World J Surg* 2011;35:1194–1201.

47. Zivin J, Thirumirthy H, Goldstein M. AIDS treatment and intrahousehold resource allocation: children's nutrition and schooling in Kenya. *J Public Econ* 2009;93(7–8):1008–1015.

48. Thirumirthy H, Zivin J, Goldstein M. The economic impact of AIDS treatment: labor supply in western Kenya. *J Hum Resour* 2008;43(3):511–552.

49. D'Adda G, Goldstein M, Zivin J, Nangami M, Thirumirthy H. ARV treatment and time allocation to household tasks: evidence from Kenya. *Afr Dev Rev* 2009; 21(1):180–208.

50. Rosenbaum L, Lamas D. Facing a "slow-motion disaster": the UN meeting on noncommunicable diseases. *N Engl J Med* 2011; 365(25):2345–2348.

51. NCD Alliance. UN high-level meeting puts NCDs on the map, falls short of setting goals or targets. http://www.ncdalliance.org/node/3517.

52. GTF CCC Report: Closing the cancer divide. http://gtfccc.harvard.edu/icb/icb.do?keyword=k69586&pageid=icb.page450139.

53. WCR 2008. http://www.iarc.fr/en/publications/pdfs-online/wcr/2008/index.php.

54. Bickler S, Telfer M, Sanno-Duanda B. Need for paediatric surgery care in an urban area of Gambia. *Trop Doct* 2003;33:91–94.

55. Kingham TP, Kamara TB, Cherian MN, et al. Quantifying surgical capacity in Sierra Leone: a guide for improving surgical care. *Arch Surg* 2009;144:122–127.

56. Blanchard RJ, Blanchard ME, Toussignant P, et al. The epidemiology and spectrum of surgical care in Pakistan. *Am J Public Health* 1987;77:1439–1445.

57. Contini S, Taqdeer A, Cherian M, et al. Emergency and essential surgical services in Afghanistan: still a missing challenge. *World J Surg* 2010; 34: 473–478.

58. Ozgediz D, Galukande M, Mabweijano J, et al. The neglect of the global workforce: experience and evidence from Uganda. *World J Surg* 2008; 32: 1208–1215.

59. Choo S, Perry H, Hesse AJ, et al. Assessment of capacity for surgery, obstetrics and anaesthesia in 17 Ghanaian hospitals using a WHO assessment tool. *Trop Med Int Health* 2010;15(9):1109–1115.

60. Iddriss A, Shivute N, Bickler S, et al. Emergency, anaesthetic and essential surgical capacity in the Gambia. *Bull World Health Organ* 2011;89(8):565–572.

61. Sani R, Nameoua B, Yahaya A, et al. The impact of launching surgery at the district level in Niger. *World J Surg* 2009; 33: 2063–2068.

62. Natuzzi ES, Kushner A, Jagilly R, et al. Surgical care in the Solomon Islands: A road map for universal surgical care delivery. *World J Surg* 2011; 35:1183–1193.

63. Kwon S, Kingham T, Kamara T, Sherman L, Natuzzi E, Mock C, Kushner A. Development of a surgical capacity index: opportunities for assessment and improvement. *World J Surg* 2012;36(2):232–239.

64. World Health Organization. WHO guidelines for health care equipment donations, 2000. http://www.who.int/medical_devices/publications/en/Donation_Guidelines.pdf.

65. Douglas T. Biomedical engineering education in developing countries: research synthesis *ConfProc IEEE Eng Med Biol Soc 2011*; 2011: 3628–3630.

66. Design That Matters. Extreme affordability. http://designthatmatters.org/.

67. DeVries CR, Price RR. *Global Surgery and Public Health.* Burlington, MA: Jones and Bartlett, 2011.

68. World Health Organization. Rising to the challenge of rural surgery. *Bull World Health Organ* 2010; 88:331–332.

69. Smith MD, Christensen CM. Disruptive innovation: can health care learn from other industries? *Health Affairs* 2007; 26(3):w288–w295.

70. Levine R. *Treating Cataracts in India. Case Studies in Global Health: Millions Saved.* Burlington, MA: Jones and Bartlett, 2007.

71. Lynge DC, Larson EH, Thompson MJ, Rosenblatt RA, Hart LG. A longitudinal analysis of the general surgery workforce in the United States, 1981-2005. *Arch Surg* 2008;143:345–350.

72. Chu K, Rosseel P, Giells P, Ford N. Surgical task shifting in Sub-Saharan Africa. *PLoS* 20096(5): e1000078.

73. Ouro-Bang'na Maman A, Kabore R, Zoumenou E, Gnassinge K, Chobli M. Anesthesia for children in sub-Saharan Africa—a description of settings, common presenting conditions, techniques and outcomes. *Pediatr Anest* 2009;19:5–11.

74. Mills E, Kanters S, Hagopian A, et al. The financial cost of doctors emigrating from sub-Saharan Africa: human capital analysis. *BMJ* 2011;343:d7031.

75. The WHO Global Code of Practice on International Recruitment of Healthcare Personnel. Sixty-Third World Health Assembly; WHA63.16, May 2010. http://www.who.int/hrh/migration/code/full_text/en/index.html.

76. Rosseel P, Trelles M, Guilavogui S, Ford N, Chu K. Ten years of experience training non-physician anesthesia providers in Haiti. *World J Surg* 2010; 34(3):453–458.

77. Chu K, Ford N, Trelles M. Providing surgical care in Somalia: a model of task shifting. *Conflict Health* 2011;5:12.

78. Mullan F, Frehywot S. Non-physician clinicians in 47 sub-Saharan African countries. *Lancet* 2007;370:2158–2163.

79. Deckelbaum D, Ntakiyiruta G, Liberman A, Razek T, Kyamanywa P. Augmenting surgical capacity in resource-limited settings. *Lancet* 2012;380(9843):713–714.

80. Luboga S, Galukande M, Ozgediz D. Recasting the role of the surgeon in Uganda: a proposal to maximize the impact of surgery on public health. *Trop Med Int Health* 2009;14(6): 604–608.

81. Grimes C, Bowman K, Dodgion C, Lavy C. Systematic review of barriers to surgical care in low-income and middle-income countries. *World J Surg* 2011;35:941–995.

82. Riddle V, Morestin F. A scoping review of the literature on abolition of user fees in health care services in Africa. *Health Policy Plann* 2011;26:1–11.

83. Lim S, Dandona L, Hoisington J, James S, Hogan M, Gakidou E. India's Janani Suraksha Yojana, a conditional cash transfer programme to increase births in health facilities: an impact evaluation. *Lancet* 2010; 375:2009–2023.

84. Suter LG, Paltiel AD, Rome BN, et al. Medical device innovation: Is "better" good enough? *N Engl J Med* 2011; 365(16): 1464–1466.

85. Crandall ML. Integrating population health into a general surgical residency curriculum. *Am J Prev Med* 2011; 41(4S3): S276–S282.

86. Loew J, Kingham TP, Casey KM, Kushner AL. Global surgery: thoughts on an emerging surgical subspecialty for students and residents. *J Surg Educ* 2010; 67(3):143–148.

87. Chu K. Open letter to young surgeons interested in humanitarian surgery. *Arch Surg* 2010; 145: 123–124.

88. Clinton Foundation up close. http://tinyurl.com/8zcdt36.

89. COSECSA. http://www.cosecsa.org.

90. Copenhagen Consensus Report 2012 and 2008. http://www.copenhagenconsensus.com/Default.aspx?ID=788.

91. Kaplan JP, Bond TC, Merson MH, et al. Towards a common definition of global health. *Lancet* 2009; 373: 1993–1995.

Humanitarian Assistance and Disaster Relief

15

Sheri Fink, Vera Sistenich, and Clydette Powell

LEARNING OBJECTIVES

- *Understand the history of international humanitarian assistance, including the key organizations involved and the principles and laws governing their work*
- *Know the most common causes of morbidity and mortality in populations affected by conflict, disaster and terrorism, and the key assessment strategies and public health interventions to consider*
- *Be familiar with prevention and preparedness approaches to disasters and acts of terrorism, and the roles and limitations of health interventions in conflict mitigation and humanitarian protection*
- *Be able to apply lessons learned to actual cases involving conflict, disaster, displacement, and terrorism*
- *Know where to go for updated information on the field of humanitarian assistance and its practice*

INTRODUCTION

A health professional who wishes to make a positive impact in a disastrous situation faces many challenges. To begin with, goals must be defined. Is the aim of humanitarian medical work to reduce death, sickness, and suffering during a period of acute vulnerability? Or does the work extend to promoting the sustainable development of health systems and advancing peace, justice, and the respect of human rights? What if the choice to engage in relief work is motivated by religious, political, or military objectives?

Whether or not the aims of the work are narrowly or broadly defined, practitioners need excellent technical skills in evidence-based medicine and public health to avoid doing more harm than good. They must become rapidly familiar with the particular health problems threatening the population in question and the available resources (structural, financial, human, and organizational) and strategies that exist to cope with them. The most effective aid workers elicit and prioritize the health concerns of those being served: respect, support, learn from, and, when appropriate, guide colleagues; coordinate efforts; maintain flexibility; and strive for equity and efficiency while ensuring that assistance also reaches the most vulnerable populations. These aid workers also dedicate themselves to serving others while taking care to maintain personal health and equanimity in the midst of unfamiliar and stressful situations.

Experienced aid workers realize that their work may put them in danger, and they contribute to individual and group security by respecting sound security protocols, maintaining positive interpersonal relationships (with officials, community members, and colleagues), and collecting and sharing relevant information. In sum, the consummate humanitarian health worker combines compassion, commitment, and integrity with technical proficiency in promoting the delivery of the most appropriate, evidence-based, and up-to-date preventive and curative health services—a tall order in what are often very challenging environments!

The potential dangers, stresses, frustrations, and, at times, monotony of humanitarian work should not be underestimated. Still, far from being a selfless exercise, the rewards of this work are many.

A HISTORY OF HUMANITARIAN WORK

The word *humanitarian* evokes a mysterious figure wearing a stained white coat and operating by candle light to the percussion of bombs and artillery rounds.

The epithet that graces the frontispiece of the NATO war surgery handbook only reinforces this romantic view of wartime medicine: "[H]ow large and various is the experience of the battlefield and how fertile the blood of warriors in the rearing of good surgeons."

In fact, the reality of most aid work differs radically from these images of adrenaline-charged, hands-on crisis medicine. More often effective relief work involves long-running efforts to prevent disease and facilitate access to care. Sometimes, far from being an ideal culture medium for medicine's greatest achievements, the stresses and strains of aid work try the good will and challenge the ethical compasses of those involved in it.

What Is a Humanitarian?

Many groups with different philosophies participate in relief work. Most believe that humanitarian assistance is about relieving suffering and saving lives in times of conflict and in other situations where the entities typically responsible for providing the basic services fundamental to life are not doing so.

The history of the Red Cross Movement is intertwined with the development of modern humanitarian work and law. Its founder, Henri Dunant, was a Swiss businessman who encountered thousands of soldiers of multiple nationalities lying wounded near Solferino, Italy, during the War of Italian Unification in 1859. Dunant assisted the wounded and wrote a book about the experience, highlighting the need for a cadre of pretrained volunteers ready to assist in emergencies and calling for the establishment of an international relief society.[1] His idea was that aid workers should be allowed to enter the battlefield unharmed as long as they agreed to remain neutral in a conflict.

The Red Cross Movement was born out of this idea, and *humanity, impartiality, neutrality, independence* and *volunteerism* are among the agency's central principles. The Geneva Conventions, discussed later in this chapter, provide the International Committee of the Red Cross (ICRC) with the mandate to protect and assist victims of both international and non-international armed conflict. Its activities include, among many others, aiding civilians and prisoners (e.g., visiting prisoners of war to assess their conditions, transporting messages between family members divided by conflict, and providing medical and surgical assistance), helping to reunite families and trace missing persons, and spreading knowledge about humanitarian law. The ICRC is based in Geneva, Switzerland, and its delegates are usually Swiss. In addition, nearly 200 countries maintain a Red Cross or Red Crescent society. These societies are members of the International Federation of Red Cross and Red Crescent Societies. All of these organizations together form the International Red Cross and Red Crescent Movement. To acknowledge Israel's national emergency society Magen David Adom, an additional distinctive emblem of equal status to the Red Cross and Red Crescent, a square-shaped red frame on its edge known as the Red Crystal, was introduced in 2005 to the Movement.[2]

When Red Cross delegates document violations of the laws of war, they typically make recommendations in confidence to the responsible authorities. This policy of confidentiality helps the organization maintain its unparalleled access, but does it have its limits? During World War II, ICRC delegates visited concentration camps and did not publicly reveal what they saw. Keeping silent about extreme, persistent human rights violations can break into complicity, and now the ICRC occasionally goes public with its findings when governments fail to heed its concerns. For example, the Red Cross repeatedly questioned the legality and humanitarian consequences of the U.S. practice of undisclosed detentions and alleged interrogation techniques it said amounted to torture at facilities in Guantanamo Bay, Cuba, and Bagram, Afghanistan, in the first decade of the 21st century. More recently, in 2010 the ICRC also condemned Israel's blockade of Gaza as a violation of the country's commitments under international law. Other relief organizations, such as the nongovernmental organization (NGO) Doctors Without Borders (in French, *Médecins sans Frontières*, or MSF) make "bearing witness" to human rights violations and advocating for populations at risk a central part of their humanitarian work. Often aid workers are the only independent outsiders to witness war crimes against civilians.

Who Else Provides Aid?

First and foremost, most assistance provided in conflict and disaster situations, particularly in the critical early days, is performed by local and national—rather than international—agencies and authorities. These include local health providers and health facilities, Red Cross and Red Crescent chapters, civil society organizations, militaries, police, and regular citizens. Too often their work is overlooked or sidelined by international actors coming in to "save the day."

United Nations (UN) agencies also play a major role in humanitarian assistance. Founded in 1948, the UN emerged from the Cold War in the early 1990s as a key organization for preventing and resolving international conflicts. The UN High Commissioner for Refugees (UNHCR) has a mandate to protect refugees under the 1951 Convention on the Status of Refugees and its 1967 Protocol. In recent years, the agency has also assisted the larger population of internally displaced persons (IDPs), who, unlike refugees, are displaced within their countries of origin. Table 15-1 describes the differences between refugees and IDPs. In 1997, the need for the UN to "act coherently" was recognized by then secretary-general Kofi Annan, who began reforming the agency to integrate humanitarian, peacekeeping, and political structures.[3,4] UN agencies and other groups involved in humanitarian work are listed in Table 15-2.

The hundreds of NGOs that exist have diverse histories and philosophies. Some of these nonprofit groups were born out of the Red Cross mold. Others offer assistance based on their members' religious convictions to serve the less fortunate. Government agencies, such as the US Agency for International Development (USAID) and the European Community Humanitarian Office, fund humanitarian assistance at least in part out of their cognition that promotes good will and good foreign relations in addition to its ability to improve lives.

Governments sometimes contract out assistance work to private for-profit companies as well as to nonprofits. Also, countries have offered the extensive logistical capacities of their militaries to assist in the aftermath of foreign disasters. Civil affairs units of armies involved in military actions in foreign countries may also provide aid to civilians, as Coalition forces did in Iraq.

From a national security perspective, promoting health can be a way to promote national or regional stability. The US Department of Defense has programs to support healthcare in overseas disasters and humanitarian emergencies in conjunction with USAID. However military goals and time frames often differ from development objectives, presenting collaboration challenges. Complexities in the civilian-military relationship are explored in Case Studies 1 and 2.

Local groups listed by the United States and other countries as terrorist organizations may also operate wings responsible for providing emergency assistance. For example, Kashmir-based militant groups ran many of the displaced person's camps following the 2005 Pakistan earthquake, and Hezbollah provided

Table 15-1. Definition of terms.

Refugee: Defined under international law as a person who "owing to a well-founded fear of being persecuted for reasons of race, religion, nationality, membership of a particular social group, or political opinion, is outside the country of his nationality, and is unable to or, owing to such fear, is unwilling to avail himself of the protection of that country; or who, not having a nationality and being outside the country of his former habitual residence as a result of such events, is unable or owing to such fear, is unwilling to return to it." Article 1, The 1951 Convention Relating to the Status of Refugees.
In 2011 there were an estimated 10.5 million refugees, according to the UNHCR's "The State of the World's Refugees 2012: In Search of Solidarity."

Internally Displaced Person (IDP): An IDP often flees his or her home for identical reasons as a refugee and faces similar difficulties. IDPs, however, are defined by not having crossed an internationally recognized border. IDPs do not enjoy the legal protections conferred by the 1951 Refugee Convention, but increasingly they are, in practice, being provided with similar assistance according to the UN's 1998 Guiding Principles on Internal Displacement. According to UNHCR, in 2011 there were as many as 27.5 million IDPs—there were many more IDPs than refugees because of an increase in non-international versus international armed conflicts.

Disaster: A situation or event involving the destruction of property, injuries, and deaths of multiple people, which typically overwhelms local capacity and necessitates outside assistance. Types of disasters include natural (e.g., hydro-meteorological, geological, biological), technological (e.g., mine explosion, chemical spill, other industrial accidents) and human-made (e.g., complex humanitarian emergency).

Complex Humanitarian Emergency (CHE): A disaster that comes about at least in part due to human design. CHE is usually used to describe a disaster that involves multiple components such as large-scale displacement of people in the context of conflict, war, persecution, economic crisis, terrorism, political instability, or social unrest.

Terrorism: There is no internationally agreed-upon definition of terrorism. A United Nations Global Counter-Terrorism Strategy adopted in September 2006 and reviewed in June 2012 describes terrorism as "activities aimed at the destruction of human rights, fundamental freedoms and democracy, threatening territorial integrity, security of States and destabilizing legitimately constituted Governments." Terrorism often refers to attacks on non-military targets, such as the deliberate bombing of civilians and the taking and killing of hostages. These kinds of attacks would, if conducted during wartime, violate the laws of war and thus constitute war crimes. Terrorism is sometimes defined as violent, threatening, or criminal acts perpetrated against human victims but aimed against larger targets, usually States, and intended to create fear or terror in the minds of a population.

Table 15-2. Entities typically involved in relief work.

The International Red Cross and Red Crescent Movement:
International Committee of the Red Cross (ICRC) (www.icrc.org), International Federation of the Red Cross and Red Crescent Societies (IFRC) (www.ifrc.org), national Red Cross societies
United Nations Agencies:
Many, including the World Health Organization (WHO) (www.who.int), United Nations Children's Fund (UNICEF) (www.unicef.org), Office for the Coordination of Humanitarian Affairs (OCHA) (ochaonline.un.org), United Nations High Commissioner for Refugees (UNHCR) (www.unhcr.org), World Food Programme (WFP) (www.wfp.org), United Nations Development Program (UNDP) (www.undp.org), United Nations Entity for Gender Equality and the Empowerment of Women (www.unwomen.org), United Nations Population Fund for Activities (UNFPA) (www.unfpa.org)
International non-governmental organizations (NGOs):
Many, including American Jewish World Service (AJWS) (www.ajws.org), American Refugee Committee (ARC) (www.arcrelief.org), CARE (www.care.org), Catholic Relief Services (CRS) (www.crs.org), Doctors of the World (also Médecins du Monde—MDM) (www.doctorsoftheworld.org), Doctors without Borders (also Médecins Sans Frontières—MSF) (www.doctorswithoutborders.org), International Medical Corps (IMC) (www.internationalmedicalcorps.org), International Rescue Committee (IRC) (www.rescue.org), Islamic Relief (IR) (www.islamic-relief.com), Mercy Corps International (MCI) (www.mercycorps.org), Oxfam International (www.oxfam.org), Save the Children (STC) (www.savethechildren.org), World Vision International (www.worldvision.org)
Local and national non-governmental and civil society organizations:
Many, different in each country
United States government entities:
US Agency for International Development (USAID) (http://www.usaid.gov)
Bureau of Population, Refugees and Migration (PRM) (www.state.gov/j/prm/)
Other governmental agencies:
Humanitarian Aid Department of the European Union (ECHO) (ec.europa.eu/echo/index_en.htm)
United Kingdom Department for International Development (DFID) (www.dfid.gov.uk/)
Japan International Cooperation Agency (JICA) (www.jica.go.jp/english/)
Intergovernmental organizations:
International Organization for Migration (IOM) (www.iom.int/)
Military operations:
Peacekeeping Forces
Monitoring Forces
Belligerent Forces (parties to a conflict)
Non-State Militant/Political Organizations
Civilian-Military Operations Center (CMOC)
Civil-Military Information Center (CMIC)
Local and national government organizations:
Ministries of Health
Ministries of the Interior

aid to victims of the 2006 war in Lebanon. Foreign aid workers should be prepared to encounter these groups in the field.

Coordinating Diverse Agencies

In complex emergencies, humanitarian needs exceed the capacity of a single agency. In recent years, more and more agencies have become involved in humanitarian work. However, in emergency after emergency, the greatest criticism of the international relief response has been its poor coordination. As part of its reform efforts, in 2005 the UN set out nine thematic "clusters" covering key areas of humanitarian assistance in crises,

including health, nutrition, and water/sanitation.* In the field, each cluster is led by a UN agency. The goal is to deliver humanitarian assistance in a cohesive and effective manner with a mandated and accountable lead agency. However evaluations of the cluster system suggest that although it has led to some improvements, it is costly and has many shortcomings.[5]

Although NGOs operate independently, most have agreed to adhere to a common code of conduct[6]

---

*The nine clusters are agriculture, camp coordination and management, early recovery, education, health, nutrition, protection, emergency shelter and water, and sanitation and hygiene. Two common clusters are emergency telecommunications and logistics.

and minimum standards.[7] On-the-ground humanitarian coordination is typically facilitated by the UN's Office for the Coordination of Humanitarian Affairs or by agencies set up by the governments of affected countries. Through the current coordination system, UN and non-UN actors engage in joint planning and prioritization of humanitarian response strategies and access shared funding pools. When arriving at an emergency, it is important to find out about interagency coordination meetings and look for Humanitarian Information Centers, which are often set up to provide a clearinghouse of information and maps and to keep tabs on "who's doing what where." With advances in satellite and communications technologies, there is an increasing role for technological experts to rapidly establish communications and information networks in emergencies.

The same agencies that respond to conflict-affected populations also tend to respond to major natural disasters. These often occur in parts of the world that are simultaneously affected by conflict, civil strife, and poverty.

Case Study/Dilemma 1: Iraq

In late 2002 and early 2003, humanitarian aid agencies prepared to provide assistance to Iraqis in the event of a US-led military offensive. NGOs disagreed about whether to accept US government funds to support their work. Some NGO leaders felt that taking the money would allow them to respond to a potential catastrophe, such as massive population displacement or a disease outbreak in a population that had already endured years of sanctions, isolation, and repression. Taking the funds might also give these NGOs a conduit to provide feedback to the United States about the needs of the civilian population. Other NGOs took sharply different positions. Their leaders argued that taking funding from a party to a conflict (a belligerent) would compromise the independence of the aid agencies and produce the appearance of taking sides in the conflict.

After the war began, the dilemma deepened. Aid workers disagreed among themselves about how they should relate to the US-led coalition and its civilian-military operations centers, which were involved in assisting Iraqi civilians. Aid workers cringed when the US-led coalition publicized their work as part of the coalition's effort to win Iraqi "hearts and minds." As insurgent attacks on aid workers grew, many worried about the blurring of the lines between the military, the political, and the humanitarian, not only in Iraq, but also in Afghanistan and other countries. Figure 15-1 depicts the medical services one American relief agency provided during the US-led

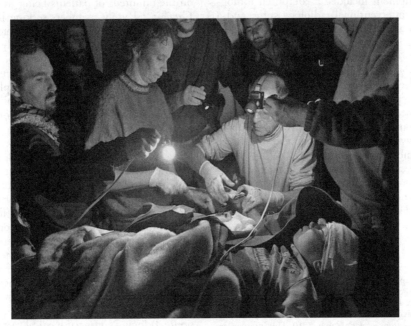

Figure 15-1. December 2001, Afghanistan: NGO personnel work under extremely austere conditions to stabilize a young Afghan boy. The boy was playing with an unexploded Russian heavy machine gun shell, which discharged, amputating his right hand. Apparently the boy's friend struck the firing pin of the shell with a rock causing the explosion. Reproduced, with permission, from Andrew Cutraro Creative LLC. www.cutraro.com.

bombing campaign in Afghanistan, ironically treating the wounds a small child sustained from the lingering munitions of a previous war.

Case Study/Dilemma 2: USNS *Comfort* After the Haiti Earthquake[†]

The 7.0 magnitude Haiti earthquake in January 2010 caused injuries estimated in the hundreds of thousands. Although Miami's hospitals were only a short flight away, at first only Haitians with US citizenship were allowed to enter the United States for care. The United States deployed a vast hospital ship, the USNS *Comfort,* to the harbor of Port-au-Prince and began treating the critically ill and injured 1 week after the earthquake. Its gleaming white topsides accented with red crosses were a conspicuous symbol of US generosity. The *Comfort* and its 1,000-plus physicians and staff provided a range of advanced medical and surgical services, many of which were unavailable elsewhere in the low-income country. A surge of approximately 254 patients arrived within the first 72 hours straining the ship's resources and personnel.[8] Over a period of 40 days, a total of 872 patients were processed, more than 800 of whom were admitted for longer than a day. More than half of them went to the operating room, with many patients undergoing surgery multiple times.[9] The ship's equipment included a computed tomography scanner, interventional radiology suite, and a large pharmacy and blood bank.

However, painful ethical dilemmas arose. First, there were many more patients who needed help than the *Comfort* and other hospitals and clinics could handle. How to decide which patients to treat? Should the *Comfort* accept a smaller number of patients who needed very specialized resource-intensive care that only the ship could provide? Or should some complex patients be allowed to die in an attempt to maximize the overall number of patients treated? Who should make these decisions? A multidisciplinary Health Care Ethics Committee convened even before arriving in Haiti and was frequently consulted during deployment.[10] Figure 15-2 depicts quandaries faced by American medical workers in Haiti.

Other dilemmas emerged. Representatives of the Haitian health ministry discouraged treating patients who would need advanced follow-up care of the type that could not be assured in Haiti after the *Comfort*'s departure. Should the ship's medical staff heed this advice? Or should they instead save these patients' lives and work to secure other resources for later care, taking advantage of the enormous outpouring of assistance and money available in the wake of the disaster? Some exceptions were made to the ministry's guidance. Ship staff also provided some training and supplies to onshore medical workers for follow-up treatment and hospice care.[11]

Although many of the medical needs and ethical quandaries in Haiti were anticipated, communications with family members and referring doctors were problematic. In the chaos of the disaster, helicopters often whisked the ill and injured from one medical site to another without documentation, leaving family members behind.[12] Family members were sometimes not permitted to travel to the *Comfort* with patients. Aboard the ship, only one in five patients had an accompanying escort. Healthcare workers had to make treatment and discharge decisions for children who arrived unaccompanied and could not give informed consent.

Initially there was no working phone number set up for relatives or referring doctors to call to check on the hundreds of patients being treated aboard the *Comfort*.[12] Family members seeking loved ones were anguished. In one case, a young man flown to the ship simply disappeared. His family was later told he was dead on arrival to the ship, but they never received his body, were not given documentation, and were not permitted to view photographs a ship official said were taken of him before he was allegedly transferred to an overwhelmed Haitian morgue, which had no records of having received him.

The *Comfort* entered arriving patients into an electronic medical records system, but it did not have a practice of funneling information on patient disposition back to referring clinics. One man was flown to the *Comfort* from a US government-run field hospital for treatment of a severely fractured femur. His family members were not allowed to accompany him and returned repeatedly to the site of the field hospital to ask what had happened to him. They despaired for weeks until the man, who was ultimately transferred from the ship for treatment at a hospital in Atlanta, Georgia, spoke with a US reporter, who phoned them.

Finally, how and when to end the expensive mission?[13] Bringing advanced medical care to a developing country that had little of it prior to a disaster presents inherent ethical questions: What level of care should be restored before it is acceptable to depart? What impact can such a level of care have on local healthcare

---

[†]Editors' note: Complex humanitarian emergencies are called complex for a reason. The Haitian situation was very difficult, and each aspect was complex and had many sides. In addition to the references cited here, this case study is based on reporting and interviews by author Sheri Fink from January-March, 2010. This information is very important and helps us understand how much we still have to learn. In this short space, however, we cannot begin to give a complete picture of the whole operation, nor can we give any official view from the US Navy. For more reading on this subject, several references are listed at the end of this case study.

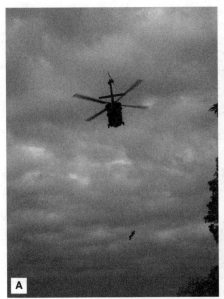
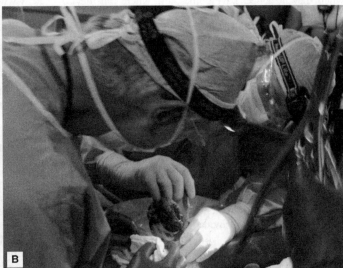
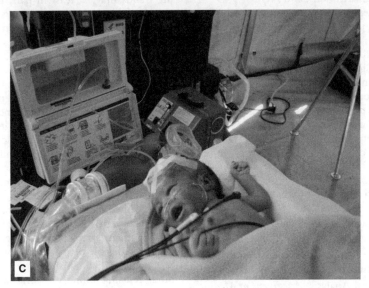

Figure 15-2. Collage of three pictures. (A) A soldier is lifted back into a navy helicopter after transporting a baby to a US government-run field hospital in Port-au-Prince, January 25, 2010. The baby arrived without family members and had untreated hydrocephalus, a condition unrelated to the earthquake requiring neurosurgery, a scarce specialty in Haiti prior to the earthquake. After a visit to the field hospital by CNN reporter and Atlanta neurosurgeon Dr. Sanjay Gupta, the baby was transferred to the USNS *Comfort* for a possible operation. (*Photo by Dr. Sheri Fink.*) (B) Dr. Chris Born, orthopedic surgeon from Rhode Island (left), and Dr. Carl Schulman, trauma surgeon from Miami (right), amputate the toes of a patient with gangrene at a US government-run field hospital in Port-au-Prince. Medical professionals faced dilemmas and tried to minimize amputations after being advised that Haitian amputees could be discriminated against and face challenges surviving in Haitian society after their operations. (*Photo by Dr. Sheri Fink.*) (C) A newborn baby with suspected neonatal tetanus is treated in the intensive care tent of a US government-run field hospital in Port-au-Prince, January 24, 2010. The field hospital ran short of oxygen, pediatric ventilators, and fuel for its generators, among other critical resources, leading to a scramble to procure more as medical professionals made life-and-death triage decisions. (*Photo by Dr. Sheri Fink.*)

practitioners? Where should patients be discharged when they no longer have homes, and where can they be transferred for needed ongoing treatment when local hospitals are overwhelmed? Moreover, should only acute "earthquake-related" health priorities be considered when timing a withdrawal, or should other needs be taken into account, such as those of patients with chronic medical problems that predated the earthquake and were inadequately treated in a low-income country, or the specter of ongoing injuries caused by earthquake debris, or the emergence of infectious epidemics like cholera?

The *Comfort* left Haiti 2 months after the earthquake, after senior leaders judged its humanitarian relief mission to be completed. At around the same time, all land-based field hospitals and clinics operated by the US Department of Health and Human Services, which had provided surgery, wound care, and childbirth services, also closed. Acute surgical needs were giving way to needs for rehabilitation and primary care best handled by the Haitian government, local medical institutions, and NGOs.

However, the departures were controversial. The Haitian government publicly supported these decisions. Government officials faced pressure from fee-for-service Haitian doctors who believed they had, paradoxically, lost needed business to foreigners providing free healthcare. In contrast, some aid workers and other Haitian doctors vehemently opposed the departures, pointing to the continuing need for skin grafts, complicated wound treatment, and the correction of surgeries performed hastily under less than optimal conditions.

Here are some other useful resources for more information:

1. Farmer P. Haiti after the Earthquake. Washington, DC: Public Affairs, 2011.

2. Katz JM. The Big Truck That Went By. New York: Palgrave, MacMillian, 2013.

3. *Time* magazine editors. Haiti tragedy and hope. New York: Time Home Entertainment, 2010.

4. Center for Naval Analysis. *Assessment of Medical Support for Haitian Relief Operations.* Alexandria, VA: CAN, April 2011. CRM D0024702.A4/1Rev.

5. US Navy Bureau of Medicine and Surgery. *Operation Unified Response-Haiti: Navy Medicine After Action Review.* Washington, DC: BUMED, May 2010.

6. Department of Health and Human Services. Haiti—USNS Comfort Medical and Surgical Support, 2010. www.hhs.gov/haiti/usns_comfort.html.

7. Pan-American Health Organization. *Health Response to the Earthquake in Haiti: January 2010: Lessons to Be Learned for the Next Massive Sudden-Onset Disaster.* Washington DC: PAHO, 2011. http://www2.paho.org/disasters/dmdocuments/HealthResponseHaitiEarthq.pdf.

8. Sternberg S. Haiti's 'Floating Hospital': Tough Questions on the USNS Comfort. *USA Today,* 2010. http://usatoday30.usatoday.com/news/health/2010-01-27-1Acomfort27_CV_N.htm.

9. US Naval War College. Humanitarian Assistance/Disaster Relief Conference. Rhode Island, May 2011. http://www.usnwc.edu/ha.

Humanitarians in an Age of Terrorism

Terrorism is a major concern for international aid workers, not only because it leads to morbidity and mortality among civilians, but also because aid workers themselves are increasingly the targets of terrorists. More than 100 aid workers per year have died in recent years, constituting a tripling over a decade, according to a UN study,[14] and the number of kidnappings has also markedly increased. These disturbing trends may, at least in part, be explained by the perceived blurring by belligerents of the humanitarian, political, and peacekeeping mandates of the UN that has come with the processes of UN integration and humanitarian coordination. In Baghdad, Iraq, in 2003, both the UN compound, which housed the UN's political and humanitarian wings, as well as the ICRC headquarters, were targeted by suicide bombers. Since 2005, violence against aid workers has grown more sophisticated and lethal and has been concentrated in a small number of volatile countries, including Afghanistan, Sudan, and Somalia.

For their protection in conflict zones, humanitarians have traditionally relied primarily on an invisible shield forged from tradition and from the "laws of war," which state that noncombatants, and particularly relief workers, are never legitimate military targets. Humanitarians typically prefer to avoid security measures that involve armed protection. Aid workers take pains to distinguish themselves from the military, often refusing military escorts, and trusting instead that their widely recognized neutral and impartial status will protect them.

Because belligerents have played on the vulnerability of relief workers—the fact that they are often soft targets without much in the way of armed protection—the magnitude and frequency of the attacks has forced a belief among some workers that the promise of protection given by the Geneva Conventions is inadequate. Some aid workers have felt compelled to use armed guards for protection and other pragmatic options to avoid having to withdraw and leave the embattled civilians they have traveled across the world to assist. Sadly, many aid agencies have withdrawn from countries where violence has surged in recent years such as Afghanistan, Pakistan, and Somalia because of security concerns and a sense that the "humanitarian space" needed to do their jobs according to their principles has been lost.

Legal Conventions Governing Humanitarian Practice

The major bodies of law that apply to humanitarian work, particularly in times of war and conflict, include international humanitarian law, refugee law, and human rights law.[15]

DILEMMA: IDENTIFYING EMBLEMS

IHL requires aid workers to identify themselves with certain emblems for their protection. However, in recent years, aid workers have been specifically targeted by militaries, other armed groups, and terrorists. Some agencies have removed all identifying marks from their clothing and their workplaces. What do you think?

To foster trust in beneficiaries, humanitarian workers long eschewed guns and guards, relying instead on the respect of international law and strong relationships with the community for protection. However attacks on aid workers have occurred frequently in recent years. Humanitarians must consider whether and when hiring private security forces or accepting military escorts will make them more secure and effective in their work, or conversely risk compromising their independence and their access to the most vulnerable populations. How would you decide the best way to ensure your team's security—both for international and national staff?

International humanitarian law (IHL) includes, most importantly, the Geneva Conventions of 1949 and Additional Protocols I and II (1977). In 2006, the Geneva Conventions achieved universal acceptance. In 2012, the world's youngest state, South Sudan, joined all others informally agreeing to abide by them. IHL requires that belligerents respect the four principles of *discrimination* between military and non military objects, *proportionality* (the degree of force used should be proportional to anticipated military advantage and should be weighed against the risk of "collateral" damage to civilians), *precaution* to minimize non-combatant risk, and *protection of noncombatants*.

Noncombatants include not only civilians having nothing to do with the fighting, but also injured and captured fighters, refugees, and humanitarian, medical, religious, and journalistic personnel carrying out their duties in the conflict area. IHL gives Red Cross workers and other humanitarians the right to assist war-affected populations without interference or harm, and also certain responsibilities: mainly to practice in accordance with medical ethics and not get involved with fighting (apart from self-defense or protection of patients).

Refugee Law (Convention on the Status of Refugees, 1951, and the Protocol Relating to the Status of Refugees, 1967) gives nations the duty to grant asylum, thus protecting refugees when their home countries have failed to do so.

Human Rights Law [based on the Universal Declaration of Human Rights, 1948; and many other instruments, including those related to genocide (1948), racial discrimination (1965), civil and political rights (1966), economic, social, and cultural rights (1966), women's rights (1979), children's rights (1989), torture (1984), and internal displacement (1998)], protects certain "non-derogable" rights that are not to be limited under any circumstances, including during time of war or national emergency. These include the rights to life; juridical personality and legal due process; and freedoms of religion, thought, and conscience. Human rights law also prohibits torture, slavery, and degrading or inhuman treatment or punishment in wartime as well as peace time.

The protection to be afforded noncombatants during war time is, at base, protection against suffering and death, whether from physical violence, wartime deprivations, or the violation of inalienable human rights. The responsibility for providing this protection rests primarily on states and members of armed forces. They in turn must allow humanitarian organizations to operate whenever noncombatant needs outstrip the ability of states or militaries to provide for them.

Medical aid workers operating in conflict-affected environments should observe *medical neutrality*. The concept derives from international human rights, humanitarian law, and medical ethics. It refers to the idea that medical professionals must uphold medical ethics (e.g., beneficence, autonomy, nonmalfeasance, and justice) and treat patients according to need, without discriminating based on nationality, religion, ethnicity, political views, or even their status as members of a particular military force. Healthcare professionals must not cause harm to their patients or participate in torture. Healthcare clinics or hospitals that are used by the military to store weapons or conduct attacks can lose their protected status.

Current Trends

In recent years, the number of refugees falling under the mandate of UNHCR has varied—from nearly

18 million in 1992 to just over 9 million in 2004 to 10.5 million in 2011. However, the number of IDPs worldwide has increased dramatically—from little over a million in 1982 to an estimated 27.5 million in 2011. Various factors may have contributed to this trend, for example more international recognition of IDPs as a group; the tendency of potential asylum countries to close their borders to refugees; and an increase in internal conflicts and civil wars where civilians are specifically targeted. It is important to note that situations of displacement have often stretched on for many years or even decades, highlighting the need for international healthcare assistance and—more importantly—efforts to attain just and durable solutions far beyond the period in which worldwide media attention focuses on the plight of the displaced.

Another worrying trend is the increase in proportion of civilian over military casualties of wars and conflicts. Although statistics are difficult to pin down, there is general agreement that there has been an enormous heightening in the proportion of civilian as opposed to military casualties of conflicts. Most worrisome, civilians are often the intended targets of hostilities, in absolute violation of the fundamental principles of international humanitarian law. Despite the promises made by governments and the UN following the failure to protect civilians in the 1990s in genocides that occurred in such places as Rwanda and Bosnia-Herzegovina, the failure of the international community to act decisively to protect civilians in armed conflict was made clear again in the first decade of the 21st century in places such as Darfur, Sudan, and the Democratic Republic of Congo (DRC).

What did develop, however, was so-called soft law, including the emergence of a new international security and human rights norm, the *Responsibility to Protect,* or "R2P." R2P is based on the principle that state sovereignty entails responsibilities, specifically to prevent the four mass atrocity crimes of genocide, war crimes, ethnic cleansing, and crimes against humanity. Both the UN General Assembly (in 2005) and the UN Security Council (UNSC; in 2006) formalized their support for R2P by adopting the following statement: "We are prepared to take collective action, in a timely and decisive manner...should peaceful means be inadequate and national authorities are manifestly failing to protect their populations from genocide, war crimes, ethnic cleansing, and crimes against humanity."

This conviction was borne out in March 2011 when NATO took military action against the Gaddafi regime in Libya under approval of the UNSC after it found Libyan authorities to have failed in their responsibility to protect their own population. This intervention proved controversial on legal and moral grounds, as did the apparent inconsistency highlighted by the lack of intervention in early 2012 by the international community in the bloody internal conflict in Syria.

An increasing number of natural disasters, too, have been reported in the past several decades, affecting an increasing number of people, according to the Center for Research in the Epidemiology of Disasters (CRED) in Belgium. Interestingly, while the number of people affected by natural disasters and the estimated financial cost of damages have increased over this time, the number of people reported killed by them has declined steadily.[16] Extreme poverty is among several factors that magnify human suffering in disasters. To better understand these factors, specialists separate out three aspects of disasters: The *hazard,* which is the physical or bio-physical event itself (e.g., flood, earthquake, tsunami); *exposure,* which is the degree to which people are in danger of falling in the path of a hazard (e.g., the number of people living in disaster-prone areas, how well built their houses are); and *vulnerability,* which is how susceptible people are to the event due to physical, social, economic, and environmental factors (Do people have the means to escape? Are warning systems in place? How well do medical systems function?). In addition to natural disasters, technological disasters such as industrial accidents affect a great number of people each year worldwide, although the trend has been decreasing over the past decade.[17]

PREPAREDNESS AND PREVENTION

Often preparedness and prevention are the last things international health workers think about when responding to a crisis. However, lightning often strikes twice, with populations affected by one disaster later experiencing another. In the United States, many of those who fled Hurricane Katrina in September 2005 were, several weeks later, displaced by Hurricane Rita. Here are just a few ways international aid workers may promote preparedness and prevention:

- Build the response capacity of local health agencies, hospitals, clinics, and caregivers
- Prioritize physical improvements for health facilities and other critical structures
- Promote safe housing solutions for displaced populations
- Educate the public about potential disaster threats and how to respond to them
- Build human bridges between conflict-affected areas, for example, by hiring staff from various sides of a conflict, bringing together health workers for training programs, and supporting ceasefires for vaccination campaigns

MEDICAL AND PUBLIC HEALTH PRIORITIES

Humanitarian assistance is both an ancient moral practice and an increasingly professional social scientific discipline. The failure of humanitarian agencies to avert widespread death and suffering among refugee populations in the 1990s (in particular among Rwandan refugees in what was then Zaire) led to calls for minimum standards in aid, increased qualifications of aid workers, and better research on what does and does not work to decrease morbidity and mortality in affected populations. A result of this work was the 1997 Sphere Project, which led to a widely used handbook of minimum standards in relief. Now in its third edition released in 2011, it covers water supply, sanitation and hygiene promotion, food security and nutrition, shelter, settlement and nonfood items, and health action.

Sphere is based on the idea that aid workers provide assistance not just out of their own desire to relieve human suffering, but also because disaster-affected populations have a right to human dignity and therefore to receive quality assistance. The goals of Sphere are stated in its Humanitarian Charter, which focuses on enhancing the quality of protection and assistance of those affected by disaster and promoting the accountability of aid workers to those they seek to help.

Groups that join Sphere agree to a common set of principles based on international law, including the right to life with dignity; the distinction between combatants and non-combatants; and the principle of non-refoulement (that refugees must not be forced to return to the country they fled if a danger still exists for them there). The groups also commit to minimizing the adverse effects that aid delivery has too often had in the past, such as paradoxically leaving civilians more vulnerable to attack or contributing to hostile activities.

Sphere is not without its critics, including members of MSF and some other organizations. They argue that technical proficiency is not the only means by which humanitarian action should be judged—humanitarians should be held equally accountable for showing compassion, promoting human solidarity, bearing witness to human suffering, and upholding justice.

Although previously lacking emphasis on physical protection, the latest edition of the Sphere handbook includes four "Protection Principles" to guide the work of humanitarians: "Avoid exposing people to further harm as a result of your actions"; "Ensure people's access to impartial assistance—in proportion to need and without discrimination"; "Protect people from physical and psychological harm arising from violence and coercion"; and "Assist people to claim their rights, access available remedies and recover from effects of abuse." Human rights groups have also emphasized the importance of measuring and assessing human rights violations in the context of emergencies.

Chief Causes of Morbidity and Mortality in Conflicts and Disasters

In recent years, epidemiologic surveillance and research have deepened understanding of the specific causes of morbidity and mortality in war and disaster-affected populations (Table15-3). The most robust data come from camp situations, which have proven to be ideal settings for epidemiologic research while at the same time often being dreadful living arrangements for displaced populations.

Major infectious threats with epidemic potential include diarrheal infections (particularly cholera), measles, respiratory infections, and malaria. Infectious disease outbreaks tend to be less common among populations displaced by natural disasters than by war. The preexisting health profile of a population affects its experience during displacement. For example, populations with poorer pre-disaster health status often have a higher proportion of problems due to infectious diseases, particularly vaccine-preventable diseases, and greater overall vulnerabilities if they are also malnourished.

Gathering Data: Assessment, Surveillance, and Monitoring

An aid agency hires you to respond to an earthquake. You arrive on the ground ready to act. First, though, you need some basic information. How many people were affected by this disaster? Moreover, what was the population's baseline health status and health infrastructure? What are the immunization rates and incidences of endemic diseases? Are there any major gender, ethnic, or tribal disparities in healthcare? How many health facilities and health workers were operating here before the catastrophe? You will also need to assess quickly if there is a potential for a food crisis,

Table 15-3. Frequent causes of morbidity and mortality in complex emergencies.

Infectious diseases
Traumatic injuries
Emotional distress
Malnutrition/micronutrient deficiencies
Exacerbations of chronic illnesses (often due to treatment interruption).

and if there will be populations in need of shelter, sanitation, and water supplies. It is also worthwhile to know whether livestock have been or will be affected. You will also want to know whether the logistics of your assistance will be adversely impacted by roads, airports, and weather. Most important, you'll want to visit the sites where people are gathered to rapidly assess their size, current health problems, and the health facilities and personnel now available to them. You'll talk with community leaders and health workers, and you'll examine health facility records to glean the population-based information you're seeking.

The key point here? An assessment is a way of saying to a community that you are there to provide what they need and want, not what you *think* they need, or what you readily have at your disposal to give. Generally, the more-foreign aid workers listen to, collaborate with, and involve affected communities in priority setting and relief provision, the more useful and sustainable their aid efforts will be. Table 15-4 lists some key aspects of an initial assessment.

It would waste time and put too much of a burden on the first responders and community leaders if everyone responding to an emergency conducted an in-person rapid assessment. So you'll want to share data with other agencies at meetings and through computer databases. You may be asked to fill out a standardized rapid assessment form. Digital data collection using handheld devices is proving superior to traditional paper-based methods in terms of speed, quality of data, and security, although electric power disruptions common in emergencies have limited their usefulness in the past.[18]

Joint multiagency assessments are also undertaken on occasion. Also, in this information age, take advantage of Geographic Information Systems, crowd sourcing platforms such as Ushahidi, and related mobile phone and Internet-based mapping technologies to help identify populations in need and select groups for assessment. The use of satellite imagery for monitoring population movements, as well as gathering evidence of human rights violations, as done in Sudan by the Satellite Sentinel Project, is a rapidly evolving technology in humanitarian assistance and protection.[19]

Once your agency has established itself and is aiding the survivors, there are some critical indicators you need to track.[7] One is the *crude mortality rate* (CMR), the number of deaths per 10,000 population per day. Health workers use it as a proxy for assessing the general health of a disaster-struck population and an ongoing measure to judge the effectiveness of relief work. Baseline CMR gives a sense of the preexisting health of the population. It typically falls well below 0.5 per 10,000 per day. During a humanitarian crisis, the CMR is used to monitor the situation. If the baseline CMR doubles or, in the absence of a reliable baseline, exceeds 1 per 10,000 per day (or more than 2 per 10,000 per day for children under 5 years), this is considered an emergency. A CMR greater than 2 per 10,000 per day in the general population (or more than 4 per 10,000 per day in the under-5 population) is considered a severe emergency. The nutritional status of children under age 5 is another sensitive indicator used to detect health stress on a population. Because mortality rates can fluctuate, they should be calculated over an extended period of time, from 1 week to 1 month.

Other important statistics that reflect preexisting health status include *maternal mortality rate*, typically expressed as number of maternal deaths per 100,000 live births; and *infant mortality rate*, the measure of the yearly rate of deaths in children less than 1 year of age, expressed as deaths per 1,000 live births in the same year.

Surveillance

In an emergency, the World Health Organization (WHO), NGOs, and governmental agencies frequently join forces to establish or enhance a health information system. Healthcare practitioners are asked to document and report the occurrence of key outbreak-potential illnesses, as well as perinatal deaths of mothers and babies, on a daily or weekly basis. Figure 15-3 shows a sample weekly surveillance form,

Table 15-4. Initial Rapid Emergency Assessment.

Location of the area assessed
Accessibility and supply and transportation lines
Security
Population data
Vulnerable groups present
Water supply
Sanitary facilities
Shelter and accommodations
Food and livestock availability; health of accompanying animals; local zoonoses
Health problems, including the main causes and rates of morbidity and mortality in children and adults
Availability of medicines, health workers and health facilities
Other needs of the affected community
Capacities of local government, civil society, and others providing aid
Obstacles to return of IDPs or refugees
Available infrastructure and storage capacity
Potential environmental impact of relief operations
Electricity supply
Goals, continuity plans, and exit strategy (knowing when the job is finished)

Sample Outpatient WEEKLY Surveillance Reporting Form
Morbidity (disease) and Mortality (death)

Province   District: Sub district:
Town/Village/Settlement/Camp: ……………………………..

Population size   < 5 years ………………   > = 5 years …………………..
Type of Health Facility: Fixed,
                            Mobile with fixed catchments
                            Mobile with varying catchments
Supporting agency: ………………………

Name and telephone number of reporting officer: …………………………………………..

Week from Monday: _____/_____/200_ to **Sunday**_____/_____/200_

	Report the number of CASES	MORBIDITY (cases)		MORTALITY (deaths)	
		<5 years	≥5 years	<5 years	≥5 years
A	TOTAL CONSULTATIONS				
B	TOTAL DEATHS				
C	Pregnancy-related death				
D	Neonatal deaths (<28 days)				
E	Acute watery diarrhea				
F	Bloody diarrhea				
G	Malaria conf by rapid test				
H	Other Fever >38.5°				
J	Suspected Measles				
K	Acute respiratory infection				
L	Acute jaundice syndrome				
M	Meningitis				

- Write 0 (zero) if you had no case or death during the week for one of the syndromes listed in the form.
- Deaths might have occurred in the health facility or might have been reported from the community.
- Be careful to report only the deaths that occurred during the week.
- Deaths should be reported only in the mortality section, NOT in the morbidity section.

Case definitions for surveillance are presented on the back.

OUTBREAK ALERT

At any time **you suspect** any of the following diseases, you should alert the Surveillance Coordination by sending an SMS or phone to _____, with maximum information on time, place and number of cases and deaths.

Acute watery diarrhea/Cholera		Bloody diarrhea	Measles	Increase in malaria
Typhoid	Tetanus	Hepatitis	Dengue fever	Meningitis

Figure 15-3. This Outpatient Weekly Surveillance Reporting Form was developed by the WHO and the Indonesian Ministry of Health and used by health workers after the December 2004 tsunami disaster in Aceh.

GENERAL OBSERVATION (e.g., water, sanitation)

WHO RECOMMENDED CASE DEFINITIONS

ACUTE WATERY DIARRHEA
Three or more abnormally loose or fluid stools in the past 24 hours with or without dehydration.

To suspect a case of cholera:
Person aged over 5 years with severe dehydration or death from acute watery diarrhea with or without vomiting.
Person aged over 2 years with acute watery diarrhea *in an area where there is a cholera outbreak.*

To confirm a case of cholera:
Isolation of *Vibrio cholerae* O1 or O139 from diarrheal stool sample.

ACUTE JAUNDICE SYNDROME
Illness with acute onset of jaundice **and** absence of any known precipitating factors **and/or** fever.

ACUTE LOWER RESPIRATORY TRACT INFECTION/PNEUMONIA IN CHILDREN <5 YEARS
Cough or difficult breathing.
        and
Breathing 50 or more times per minute for infants aged 2 months to 1 year.
Breathing 40 or more times per minute for children aged 1 to 5 years.
        and
No chest in drawing, no stridor, no general danger signs.

Note: **Severe pneumonia** = Cough or difficult breathing **+** any general danger sign (unable to drink or breastfeed, vomits everything, convulsions, lethargic or unconscious) or chest indrawing or stridor in a calm child.

BLOODY DIARRHEA
Acute diarrhea with visible blood in the stool.

To confirm case of epidemic bacillary dysentery:
Take stool specimen for culture and blood for serology. Isolation of *Shigella dysenteriae.*

MALARIA
Person with fever or history of fever within the last 48 hours (with or without other symptoms such as nausea, vomiting and diarrhea, headache, back pain, chills, myalgia) with positive laboratory test for malaria parasites [blood film (thick or thin smear) or rapid diagnostic test].

MEASLES
Fever **and** maculopapular rash (i.e., nonvesicular) **and** cough, coryza (i.e., runny nose) or conjunctivitis (i.e., red eyes).
        or
Any person in whom a clinical health worker suspects measles infection.

To confirm case:
Presence of measles-specific IgM antibodies.

MENINGITIS
Suspected case:
Sudden onset of fever (>38.5) with stiff neck.
In patients under one year of age, a suspected case of meningitis occurs when fever is accompanied by a bulging fontanelle.

Probable case of bacterial meningitis:
Suspected case of acute meningitis as defined above with turbid cerebrospinal fluid.

Probable case of meningococcal meningitis:
Suspected case of meningitis as defined above
With gram stain showing gram negative diplococcus
Or ongoing epidemic
Or petechial or purpura rash

Confirmed case:
Suspected or probable case as defined above
With either
Positive CSF antigen detection for *Neisseria meningitidis*
Or positive culture of CSF or blood with identification of *Neisseria meningitidis*

Figure 15-3. (Continued)

including case definitions of epidemic-potential infectious diseases. A more extensive surveillance form might include mental health problems, injuries, and chronic diseases.

Overworked local healthcare professionals sometimes view additional data collection and reporting as burdensome. They will appreciate help with the logistics of collecting and compiling forms and communicating results, and they will appreciate it if all agencies can agree on a single reporting form that complements existing health reporting systems. Cell phone and handheld computer-based reporting systems may help reduce the work involved.

The only reason to gather information is to use it! The goal of surveillance should be to guide programmatic decision making and healthcare. Toward that end, it is critical that results—such as regional surveillance reports—be fed back to the practitioners who collected the data and who will be responsible for implementing local interventions for the health of the population they serve.

Research

Large-scale population-based studies of nutrition and disease may be needed to truly understand the health problems and needs of the population. Academic researchers and epidemiologists from the US Centers for Disease Control and Prevention (CDC) often serve as consultants to humanitarian agencies conducting such studies. Because of the extensive resources required to do quality research, it is best to collaborate with other agencies and to work with and empower local and national research bodies.

Evaluation

You and your colleagues have been working tirelessly for weeks or months following a disaster. How are you doing? Real-time and periodic evaluations will help you assess the effectiveness of your organization's work and guide your future efforts. In fact, the donor agencies that give you the funding to do your work may require that you demonstrate your effectiveness. You will need to track two types of indicators. *Process indicators* reflect your actual activities, such as the number of patients seen in your clinic or the number of children you have vaccinated against measles. More important, *outcome indicators* reflect the result of those activities in a population, such as the number of children who contract measles or the number of deaths in a refugee camp. The Sphere Project identifies a number of *key indicators* to help humanitarian workers judge whether minimum standards of aid have been met. To establish whether a particular program is having an effect, you'll need to assess the *baseline* level of each indicator at the beginning of the program. Not all evaluations are quantitative—qualitative measures are important, too. Often agencies hire external evaluators to study their programs.

However, because evaluations can be costly, repetitive, and demanding on field staff trying to implement programs, collaboration is an option. Aid workers from 50 agencies set up the Tsunami Evaluation Coalition after the 2004 Indian Ocean earthquake and tsunami. It was designed to evaluate effectiveness in each humanitarian sector and to study the impact of humanitarian policies.

Key Public Health Interventions

Often aid workers think of the disaster response in phases, beginning with the immediate aftermath (hours to days), followed by an emergency phase (days to weeks), then the late/recovery phase (weeks to months), and finally the rehabilitation and rebuilding phase (months to years). Rather than distinct phases, however, typically a population's needs in the aftermath of a disaster or population displacement vary along a continuum. For some segments of the affected population, emergency needs may linger far into the rebuilding phase. Furthermore, in the context of certain conflicts, for example those involving siege or repeated population displacement, the emergency phase may last for years.

Conversely, some of the public health interventions that are typically conducted in the later phases of a disaster can and should be implemented much earlier if both the need and the capacity to do so exist. Humanitarian and development work have traditionally been funded and implemented separately. However, given that poverty and poor infrastructure contribute to vulnerability to disasters and conflicts, there is an increasing recognition that some rudimentary development work may be appropriate even in an emergency context. For example, the huge outpouring of generosity for tsunami survivors in Aceh, Indonesia, allowed some NGOs to rapidly begin training midwives. This was critical because of the alarming maternal mortality rate that existed even before the tsunami. Still, it is useful to consider the priorities that take precedence at various points in the disaster continuum.

What follows is a summary of key preventive public health interventions. Treatment guidelines for common medical conditions fall outside the scope of this chapter but can be readily accessed in the publications of the WHO, the CDC, and NGOs such as MSF.[20]

Immediate Aftermath

The immediate health priorities after an acute event include rescue, first aid, trauma care, and protection of the population from further exposure to harm.

Depending on the time it takes to organize an external response and move human and mechanical assets to affected areas, the local community will be in charge of providing the bulk of these services.

Triage[21]   *Triage* is a word once used by the French in reference to the sorting of coffee beans and applied to the battlefield by Napoleon's chief surgeon, Baron Dominique-Jean Larrey. Today triage is used when the number of injured exceeds available resources. Surprisingly, perhaps, there is no consensus on how best to do this. Typically, medical workers try to divide care to achieve the greatest good for the greatest number of people. There is an ongoing debate about how to do this and what the "greatest good" means. Is it the number of lives saved? Years of life saved? Best "quality" years of life saved? Or something else? Should age be a factor in prioritizing care? What about value to others in the emergency?

At least nine well-recognized triage systems exist. Most call for people with relatively minor injuries to wait while patients with the most acute needs are evacuated or treated. Some call for the inclusion of an additional category: patients who are seen as having little chance of survival given the resources on hand. That category is most commonly created during a devastating event like a war-zone truck bombing in which there are far more severely injured victims than ambulances or medics.

The decision that certain severely ill or injured victims should be treated or evacuated last has its risks. Predicting how a patient will fare is inexact and subject to biases. In one study of triage, experienced rescuers were asked to categorize the same patients and came up with widely different answers.[22] Also, patients' conditions can change; it should never be forgotten that more resources can become available to help those whose situations at first appeared hopeless. The importance of reassessing each person is easy to forget once a ranking is assigned.

Recent work on standards of care in slower-moving emergencies like pandemics has stressed the importance of ethical decision-making and engagement with the local community about how decisions are made to allocate medical resources.[23] Doing this helps maintain trust in the medical profession. Finally, the urge to be efficient and aid the most patients must be balanced with procedures that are just and fair.

Emergency

As the emergency phase continues, and help arrives from outside, top priorities include the provision of safe water in adequate quantities, safe shelter, food, and proper sanitation.

Local and regional medical structures often need support. The biggest emphasis of international medical assistance typically should be on primary healthcare, emergency healthcare, and preventive health services focusing on the major causes of morbidity and mortality in displaced populations, particularly communicable disease surveillance and control. In some populations, maintaining the treatment of chronic conditions such as diabetes, renal and cardiac disease, as well as HIV/AIDS and tuberculosis, are urgent priorities in situations of disaster or displacement.

The lack of water in adequate quantity and quality and ineffective sanitation and poor hygiene can result in epidemics of diarrheal illnesses, including cholera, which tend to be the greatest killers in refugee and displaced persons situations due to profound dehydration. Water needs vary, but in general a minimum of 15 liters per person per day is needed for drinking, cooking, and personal hygiene. Survival needs for drinking and food are 2.5 to 3 liters per day. When a choice needs to be made between quantity and quality, assuring an adequate quantity should take precedence. The *Sphere* handbook provides guidance on selecting water sources, recommended maximum queuing times, and the minimum number of water taps needed per population dependent on their flow rate. Water quality should be monitored at the point of use. Piped water and all water at risk for contamination or during diarrheal epidemics should be disinfected (e.g., with chlorine), as should water used in health centers, hospitals, and in feeding centers.

To prevent diarrheal outbreaks, good hygiene practices such as hand washing with soap (or, when unavailable, ash) and water should be promoted. In addition, latrines should be established downwind, downgrade, and at least 30 meters away from sources of groundwater and a minimum of 1.5 meters above the water table. A minimum of one latrine per 20 persons is recommended, but one per 50 is acceptable during the early emergency stage. Latrines must be well maintained, well lit, and kept clean.

Early availability and institution of rehydration therapy for diarrhea is critical because the vast majority of diarrhea-related deaths may be prevented with proper oral rehydration alone. Prevention of malnutrition in children with diarrhea is a key priority.

When large groups of people lack access to food or the means to buy it, aid agencies may introduce supplementary or therapeutic feeding programs to address threats ranging from anemia and micronutrient deficiency to acute global or severe protein-energy malnutrition (see Chapter 7). The decision to distribute food must be made carefully, based on assessments and with consideration of other more sustainable ways to promote "food security."

In the emergency phase of a disaster, at least 2,100 kilocalories per person per day should be assured, with 10% of energy from protein, 17% of energy from fat, and adequate micronutrients provided by fresh or fortified foods. Special supplementation may be needed for young children (nutritious, high-energy complementary foods), pregnant or breastfeeding women (additional nutrients and support), and those with AIDS and other diseases. The food provided to a population should be appropriate and acceptable according to cultural practices, religious beliefs, and practicality. Careful attention must be paid to food preparation needs.

To promote health and prevent diarrhea and dehydration in infants under 6 months, exclusive breast-feeding is recommended. International disasters are a magnet for large donations of baby formula; however, feeding formula to infants is to be discouraged in emergencies for several reasons, including the shortage of clean water with which to mix formula. UNICEF and other agencies have established guidelines and training modules for infant feeding in emergencies, which should be included in community health education activities.

If severe malnutrition reaches a certain threshold and distribution in the population, therapeutic feeding programs may be indicated. These involve both nutritional and medical treatment. Traditionally programs have been based at feeding centers; however, new protocols are allowing therapeutic feeding to take place in communities, which reduces the hardship on families.

Measles has been a top killer of children in some displaced populations. Rapid organization of a mass measles vaccination campaign for children aged 6 months to 15 years should be implemented if local vaccination coverage falls below 90% or is unknown, including the administration of vitamin A to children aged 6 to 59 months. Because it takes time for immunity to develop following vaccination, healthcare workers need to be alert to signs of measles, and be prepared to quarantine sick children, trace their contacts, and "ring vaccinate" those children who have been in close proximity.

Sudden-onset natural disasters are often associated with a large number of injuries and a relatively increased risk of tetanus. Although emergency mass vaccination against tetanus is not recommended, a tetanus toxoid booster is advised for those with contaminated wounds and those involved in rescue or cleanup operations that put them at risk. Patients with contaminated wounds who have never received a full course of vaccination should also receive a dose of tetanus immune globulin (TIG), followed by Td or Tdap. TIG should be administered for tetanus-prone wounds in patients infected with HIV, regardless of the history of tetanus immunizations. Wounds should be cleaned and debrided properly if dirt or necrotic tissue is present.

In addition to diarrhea and measles, acute respiratory infections are extremely common in displaced populations and can lead to significant levels of mortality and morbidity in very young children, the aged, and people of any age who suffer from other illnesses. Refugee populations are particularly susceptible because of close quarters, malnutrition with vitamin deficiency, exposure to smoke, and extremes of temperature. Pertussis (whooping cough) should be considered in populations with poor vaccination coverage. It is commonly misdiagnosed, very contagious, and can lead to apnea in infants and dehydration and malnutrition in children.

Closely packed living conditions and displacement to endemic areas also provide ideal conditions for malaria to become a major cause of preventable death, especially to pregnant women and children. Use of insecticide-treated bed nets dramatically reduces the incidence of malaria; therefore, bed net distribution and instruction are key public health measures following disasters in endemic areas. Insecticide-impregnated sleeping sheets, insecticide-treated plastic sheeting, and vector control (killing of mosquitoes) through spraying are also useful. Removal of standing water is essential to deprive mosquitoes of their breeding grounds. Healthcare workers should wear long sleeves and pants in the dawn and dusk hours of the day, apply insect repellents, and sleep under mosquito netting. Aid workers from non-malaria-endemic regions should consider taking chemoprophylaxis. In emergency situations there are protocols for the treatment and prevention of malaria established by the WHO and international agencies based on local conditions. These protocols use locally effective medications and should be strictly followed.

Plasmodium falciparum malaria can be rapidly fatal; cases must be detected and treated early. Because laboratories may be unavailable in emergencies, and malaria is often chloroquine resistant, rapid diagnostic tests are becoming the standard in field operations in malaria diagnosis as is treatment with artemisinin-based combination therapy (see Chapter 9). The Mentor Initiative has useful resources.[24]

Dengue is another mosquito-transmitted febrile illness common in tropical climates. Patients who develop hemorrhagic complications can die rapidly if not transferred or evacuated to a facility where they can receive intensive hemodynamic and hematologic support. The white-spotted *Aedes aegypti* mosquitoes that carry dengue feed during the day, so environmental and public health measures are needed to decrease populations of breeding mosquitoes. Bed nets are not sufficient to prevent infection.

Meningitis is a potentially severe health issue in some displaced populations. Eye infections and skin infections are also common acute health problems.

In the past, many of the infectious diseases resulted from overcrowded conditions and the inadequate provision of shelter. Facilitating better shelter options for catastrophe-affected populations should be a key priority for humanitarians. Even where camps are the only option, better planning can reduce the spread of endemic diseases and improve human security, for example, ensuring that women do not have to walk to remote latrines along dark pathways at night. Gender-based violence and rape often plague displaced and conflict-affected populations, and it is important for international health workers to be aware that their patients may be at risk.

To promote disease prevention, international health agencies often recruit and train local health outreach workers to help monitor for infectious disease outbreaks and other health threats, and to promote good hygiene awareness within their communities and healthy practices, such as breastfeeding rather than bottle feeding of infants. Ensuring access to health services among the affected population is critical. Many displaced persons are reluctant or unable to leave their families or their enclave to seek care.

Aid workers often provide medical supplies, medicines, and technical support to local health professionals providing curative services, particularly in health structures that are overburdened, looted, or cut off from usual pharmaceutical supply chains. Aid agencies often stockpile the *Interagency Emergency Health Kit 2011* (IEHK 2011), the fourth edition of the WHO's standardized set of essential medicines, supplies, and equipment, with instructions designed to meet the initial primary healthcare needs of a displaced population without health facilities.[25] Each kit serves approximately 10,000 people for 3 months. International suppliers such as the International Dispensary Association (IDA), MSF, and UN Children's Fund (UNICEF) maintain readily available stockpiles of standardized health kits made of high-quality medicines from approved pharmaceutical companies labeled and proportioned as appropriate for various emergency situations.

Some governments set guidelines for those who wish to make medical donations to their countries. These may be aligned with the WHO's Essential Medicines List. National health officials who know their supply and needs are in a good position to accept or to reject donations. They can specify and quantify based on project needs, avoid duplication, support supply chain management systems, and indicate special needs, such as pediatric formulations. Ideally, even in a disaster setting, maintaining and updating a central registry can assist a host nation in a quick prioritization and allocation of rapid and intermittent donations from abroad. Moreover, systems that can quickly inspect, confirm receipt, and store donations securely will serve the needs of the populations whose drug systems have been disrupted by conflict or natural disasters.

Table 15-5. Guidelines for drug donations.

Select drugs based on actual needs
Notify recipients in advance of donation arrival
Ensure that drugs are similar in presentation, strength, and formulation to those used by recipient health workers
Obtain drugs from sources that meet quality standards set by donor and recipient countries and are manufactured according to Good Manufacturing Practice (GMP)
Clearly label drugs in a language understood by local practitioners. Label with International Nonproprietary Name (INN) or generic name
Ensure at least one year of shelf life before expiration, except in extraordinary situations
Include detailed packing lists
Cover costs of transport, warehousing, and customs clearances

Unfortunately, disasters often attract inappropriate, useless, and expired medical donations that end up as a toxic medical waste problem at the exact time and place in which communities are least able to deal with them. (Sometimes these are well-meaning; other times they may be motivated by significant tax breaks for the donor hospital or drug company.) Guidelines for appropriate donations have been developed by the WHO and are summarized in Table 15-5.

There may also be a need to support higher-level medical services such as orthopedic and neurosurgery and intensive care. However, the importance of these types of services may quickly wane after the occurrence of a natural disaster such as an earthquake. Often, well-meaning nations make the public gesture of donating field hospitals or the use of navy hospital ships. When these arrive weeks or months after a disaster's occurrence, it is assumed that they will be appreciated by patients suffering from long-untreated medical conditions in countries with poor health infrastructure. However, much of their capacity may go unused, as was the case of the USNS *Mercy* during the 2004 tsunami in the Indian Ocean. It is important to support the rehabilitation, reconstruction, and staffing of existing health facilities, to improve patient care in the long term, and mitigate future disasters that may occur in the area. As with all services provided by international agencies, the emphasis should be on supporting and developing local capacity whenever possible.

In conflict situations, however, attacks on civilians may create an ongoing need for general surgeons capable of treating physical trauma. For example, during Sri Lanka's civil war between the military and the Liberation Tigers of Tamil Eelam, MSF supplied international surgeons and surgical support over the years to their facilities on the island country.

International surgeons from several organizations have also worked for long periods of time in recent conflicts in Liberia, Sudan, and the DRC, among others.

Psychosocial trauma is recognized as a major cause of suffering in emergencies.[26] Responding appropriately to it depends greatly on cultural context. For example, Western-style focus on debriefing and individual psychotherapy may not be particularly appropriate or helpful in many societies, especially where health-seeking behavior for psychological distress is limited. The most beneficial ways to promote mental health across a population often involve social interventions that help restore a sense of control, safety, and purposeful activity to a community. For children, this is especially important. Useful interventions include providing safe spaces for recreation and rapidly organizing the resumption of education. Adults benefit from playing an active role in assisting their families and communities, maintaining mourning customs and religious observances, being informed of and involved in plans for rehabilitation and rebuilding, and having opportunities for income generation and economic activity. For all, family reunification is a top priority, as is identification of the dead.

However, those with preexisting psychiatric illness, particularly those who depend on medication, often experience an exacerbation of their conditions. Emergency psychiatric care and psychiatric medicines should be made available. Access to basic mental healthcare should be facilitated in both the health system and in the community. All interventions should be designed in collaboration with mental health professionals from within the affected countries because they will have an understanding of the cultural context.

Many international relief agencies have also committed to rapidly implement the Minimum Initial Service Package (MISP), a set of actions designed to respond to reproductive health needs (including the risks of maternal and neonatal mortality, HIV, and sexual violence) in the midst of acute emergencies.[27] The MISP involves distributing standardized kits (appropriate for various levels of the health system from community midwives up to referral hospitals) that contain equipment, supplies, and drugs related to normal deliveries, basic obstetric emergencies, postrape management, contraception, universal precautions for infection control, and safe blood transfusions. Many factors associated with the transmission of HIV are heightened in a disaster, such as the displacement of people, social instability, worsening poverty due to income loss (which may lead to bartering of sex for food and other resources), sexual violence and rape, poor access to condoms, and the influx of new populations, including reconstruction and relief workers, soldiers, and transporters. The MISP addresses HIV prevention in two key ways: making condoms freely available and ensuring that medical equipment and blood for transfusion are free from infectious agents. In addition it is crucial to avoid treatment disruption for those with HIV and AIDS.

Later Phases of the Emergency

The MISP ideally forms the basis of reestablishing and ensuring comprehensive reproductive health services in later phases of the disaster response (see Chapter 4). Other important priorities in the disaster aftermath are described next.

Chronic Conditions These would include support for detection and treatment of tuberculosis, AIDS, chronic diseases, and psychological conditions. Tuberculosis is one of the greatest infectious disease killers in the world today,[28] and it is common among displaced populations. Given the need for long-term consistent therapy, tuberculosis treatment should be a high priority in the later phases of disaster response. Rehabilitation, physical therapy, and prosthetic and orthotic services should be made available for amputees, those with spinal cord injuries, and other survivors of physical trauma.

In 2011 at a high level meeting, the UN General Assembly stressed the importance of international action to combat noncommunicable diseases, including diabetes, heart and lung disease, and cancers. These diseases account for a high and increasing proportion of morbidity and mortality in nations of every income level, and many people displaced by war and disaster are likely to experience them or be at risk of developing them. Exposure to cigarette smoke is the major risk factor.

Child Health Priorities include reestablishment of the Expanded Program on Immunizations, Integrated Management of Childhood Illnesses, and ongoing nutritional interventions, such as mass deworming of children in populations with high levels of childhood anemia and parasitic infection.

Health Infrastructure The presence of foreign aid workers is only a temporary situation, but it is an important opportunity to offer training and specialized education to health workers who have had little chance to receive such knowledge or experience. This may lead to longer-term commitments to support formal health education opportunities in the affected country. In addition to medical training, aid workers can support drug supply management, health systems management (particularly where large numbers of health administrators have been killed or have left the area), and laboratory services.

Preparedness and Prevention Helping societies stave off future suffering is one of the most important contributions that can be made. Disaster prevention and preparedness are key as are, in the wake of violent conflict, national reconciliation, the reintegration of former soldiers, and the strengthening of civil institutions.

Agencies involved in the public health and medical response may not have the expertise or the mandate to carry out this work directly; however, these activities clearly merit greater emphasis and awareness than they have historically received from the humanitarian community.

SPECIAL CONSIDERATIONS IN CERTAIN CRISES

Some health threats are likely to be encountered in many types of crises. The following issues arise less commonly but also deserve attention.

Dealing with Human Remains

Survivors have a strong need to know what has happened to their loved ones—both for emotional well-being as well as for legal reasons (e.g., survivor benefits can be delayed for years if a survivor lacks a death certificate for a spouse). Therefore, it is important to manage the dead with dignity and in a way that facilitates their identification and allows family members to be kept involved and informed.

Typically, dead bodies in natural disasters pose little risk of causing epidemics, so rapid burial—unless dictated by religious need—should not take precedence over identification. The basic requirements for handling human remains include wearing gloves and boots, washing hands, and disinfecting clothing, equipment, and transport vehicles. It is also wise to avoid contact with body fluids such as blood and feces. Most infectious organisms do not survive beyond 2 days; however, HIV has been found six days postmortem. Toxic gases can build up in confined, unventilated spaces, so body recovery in these situations should be approached with caution.

In certain cases, human remains may indeed pose major risks to the living. These include epidemics of plague, cholera, typhoid, anthrax, and viral hemorrhagic fever (naturally occurring or as a result of biologic warfare or terrorism), and following chemical attacks where chemical residue may remain on bodies. In these cases, body handling should be left to specialists whenever possible.

In the case of epidemic diseases, chlorine solution or other medical disinfectants are the best choices for disinfection. Family members need to be made aware that traditional practices such as washing the dead and large funerals risk spreading the epidemic—it is best to bury or cremate the body quickly near the site of death with a limited number of people in attendance. Dealing with disposal of bodies in an Ebola virus or other hemorrhagic fever outbreak requires high levels of protection. In typhus and plague, protective clothing should be worn to avoid infestation with fleas or lice. Those who have contact with bodies in a cholera epidemic should carefully wash with soap and water. Victims who may have active pulmonary tuberculosis should have respiratory protection placed over the face prior to moving the body to protect the living from exposure to exhaled infectious material.

Collecting and identifying the deceased has not historically been the purview of humanitarian workers, but given the massive scale of recent disasters, knowledge of this field has become imperative. Identification errors occur frequently in mass disaster situations. When immediate visual identification by close contacts is not possible, rapid use of photography, forensic examination (including fingerprinting and dental examination), and the recording of basic and unique features and personal effects found on bodies should all be used to aid in identification. Bodies rapidly decompose in hot climates, so facial recognition can be difficult after 12 to 48 hours. If possible, bodies should be kept in body bags or wrapped in sheets and refrigerated or buried temporarily in well-organized graves. Waterproof labels with unique ID numbers should be securely attached to bodies, rather than writing on bodies or body bags, which is easily erased. DNA-matching technology has been used to identify thousands of people (e.g., in New York after the 2001 World Trade Center attack, and in Bosnia-Herzegovina after the 1992–1995 war), but it requires significant long-term financial commitments and community cooperation.

In Thailand, where a mass identification effort took place following the December 2004 tsunami, most of the bodies were identified in person or later through photographs, fingerprints, and dental records and only later confirmed with DNA. Sadly, forensic technology was applied inequitably. Soon after the tsunami disaster, victim identification teams raced to Thailand from more than two dozen countries and at first worked independently from Thai scientists to identify foreign tourists. The folly of this approach was soon revealed—within a few days, it was difficult to tell Asian bodies from white bodies. Only by working together and treating all bodies with equal respect could victims and their relatives be matched. In 2009, the Pan-American Health Association (PAHO) published the second edition of a field manual for managing dead bodies after disasters, which is available for download from their website.[29]

Chemical, Biologic, Radiologic, and Nuclear Threats

Threats from chemical, biologic, radiologic, and nuclear (CBRN) sources are an ever-present danger from industrial accidents, war, and terrorism. In the run-up to the Iraq war in 2003, several efforts were made to develop guidelines for international aid workers who might be called on to respond to such incidents or whose work might put them in danger.[30] The conclusion of many experts was that international aid workers were poorly prepared to respond to these threats, and few aid workers had much experience with them. The risk of exposure to CBRN agents and weapons during humanitarian action is currently considered low, but the March 2011 nuclear power accident following the massive Japanese earthquake and tsunami highlighted the possibility.[31]

Key principles in responding to CBRN events include:

- **Predeployment preparation:** Learn what CBRN threats exist in the environment in which you will be deployed. Consider smallpox vaccination for yourself and your team. It is wise to include disposable masks, coveralls, gloves, booties, and tape in the gear being taken to the field.
- **Emergency response plan:** Develop and disseminate the plan in advance, including evacuation procedures.
- **Surveillance:** In an environment where CBRN threats exist, appropriate indicators should be added to surveillance forms. Signs of dead animals (e.g., rodents, birds) or livestock with difficulty walking suggest the need for immediate evacuation. A single case of smallpox demands immediate action. Clinicians need to be aware of the threat and potential signs and symptoms so they can diagnose sentinel cases.
- **Exposure avoidance and decontamination:** A safe room, such as an entirely sealed inner room, may be useful to take shelter in during the time of the attack. In the case of radiation, take shelter underground or in the interior of a building with thick concrete walls until the cloud passes, if unable to flee in another direction. Only sealed water and food should be assumed to be safe. There will be a need for ample safe water and increased food security.
- **Treatment:** It is important to keep in mind that many of the medicines needed to treat CBRN incidents are not included in the WHO emergency health kit.
- **Coordination and information sharing:** Military in the area may have contamination sensors and equipment for decontamination and treatment of victims. Evacuation may be necessary and will need to be coordinated.

Chemical Threats

Chemical releases can cause health effects in minutes to hours, affect a large number of people, and persist in the environment. They also pose a risk of secondary contamination. Key principles are first to get away from the threat and then decontaminate. In the Tokyo subway attack using Sarin nerve gas, first responders were also affected. Nerve agents cause symptoms such as miosis (constriction of the pupils) and stumbling. Exposed patients must be treated immediately with atropine or they may die. Blister agents such as mustard gas cause tearing and swelling of the eyes and can cause burns with longer exposure. Decontamination is critical—aid workers can be put in danger by secondary spread. Other potential chemical threats include choking agents, blood agents, tearing agents, and incapacitating agents. Industrial risks include petroleum products, pesticides, and their precursors (such as methyl isocyanate, responsible for the Bhopal accident). Most of the latter are extremely irritating, and the instinct to get away from the source should be followed. Oil well fires can cause heavy smoke—placing a wet cloth over the nose and mouth can protect against some heavy particles. Useful protective clothing for chemical attacks includes disposable cloth masks, paper coveralls, gloves, and booties (taped to coveralls).

In chemical attacks, key treatment principles, in order of priority, include:

1. Removal from the site of exposure
2. Thorough decontamination, including removal of clothing, blotting of exposed skin, and washing entire body and hair with soap and water
3. Stabilizing and triaging patients

Biologic Threats

Biologic threats tend to come from naturally occurring infectious particles harnessed to produce widespread illness. The CDC maintains a list of high-priority biologic agents. Some of the most potentially threatening include smallpox, anthrax, plague, botulism, tularemia, and Ebola and other hemorrhagic infections. It is important that when these are a threat, international aid workers are trained to recognize and treat these illnesses. Many can be prevented and treated by antibiotics. Surveillance and the use of good infection control measures are critical.

Radiologic and Nuclear Threats

As the Great East Japan Earthquake and tsunami of 2011 showed, radiologic emergencies at nuclear power plants and waste storage or processing facilities can result from natural disasters and accidents, not only military attacks or terrorism. Dangers also come from nuclear bombs, including a number of suitcase-sized miniature nuclear devices that were reportedly stolen from depots in the former Soviet Union. There is also the potential of a so-called dirty bomb, an explosive device to disperse radiologic material, which may cause panic far beyond its physical effects. Removal from the source and shielding are key actions. Care for blast and burn injuries is typically the first priority, followed by decontamination. Most external contamination can be removed by disposing of clothing and washing with water and mild soap. Use universal precautions to minimize secondary exposure. The greatest long-term threat of radiologic exposure comes from inhalation of gamma particles from contaminated fallout. Respiratory protection is imperative because even one millionth of a gram of some radiologic compounds can cause lung cancer.

PARTICULAR NEEDS OF SPECIFIC POPULATIONS

Balanced with the desire to provide the greatest benefit for the greatest number of people, aid workers must keep in mind the particular needs of specific groups within the populations they serve.

Patients Requiring Medical Services Unavailable in the Immediate Area

Some patients require higher-level care than they can receive in the immediate area where they have taken shelter (such as a camp-based primary health clinic). Transfers to higher-level care frequently do not go smoothly. For example, in a country of asylum, national and local authorities may consider refugees an additional burden on an already overworked health system. The standard of care in tertiary care hospitals may be low, so it is important to remain involved in the care of the transferred patient and possibly support the receiving hospital with materials to compensate for the extra case load.

In these situations, the fully-equipped and staffed field hospitals that are donated in some emergencies can certainly be of use. Alternatively, sometimes foreign hospitals and doctors offer to treat patients if they can be evacuated. Medical evacuations, although potentially lifesaving, are almost always fraught with difficult logistical and ethical concerns. Medical workers become inundated with evacuation appeals from patients and their families, often for long-standing chronic conditions. Desperation for evacuation may lead to corruption and payoffs within the medical system. It makes sense for an experienced impartial outside organization, such as the International Organization for Migration (IOM), to take charge of screening, prioritization, and logistics (travel and repatriation, liaisons with receiving hospitals). Clear medical guidelines for evacuation need to be set and communicated to the community.

In some cases, a medical evacuation program has been paired with efforts to improve local and national capacity to provide specialized medical treatment—for example the Medical Evacuation and Health Rehabilitation Program for Iraq (MEHRPI)

coordinated by the IOM. From 2003 to 2004, it facilitated the treatment of 250 patients abroad while supporting advanced training for several Iraqi medical professionals. Tragically, the upsurge in violence against civilians and the deterioration of medical services in subsequent years necessitated the re-launch of a medical evacuation program for Iraq.

Case Study/Dilemma 3: Srebrenica Medical Evacuations[32]

In April 1994, the town of Srebrenica in eastern Bosnia-Herzegovina had been under siege by nationalist Serb forces for a year, and the town's population was desperate. As the first aid convoys reached the town, an attempt was made to evacuate seriously wounded women and children on returning trucks. Injured men could not be evacuated by road due to the likelihood that they would be taken away by soldiers at checkpoints.

An international doctor noted which patients were to be evacuated by referring to their hospital bed numbers, but the stronger patients forced the weak patients from their beds. Doctors took to marking patients' evacuation priorities with indelible ink on their foreheads. As the selected patients were being brought from the hospital, noninjured women and children surged onto the evacuation trucks, themselves desperate to leave the town. The trucks became so overcrowded that several people died on the hours-long journey. Local authorities accused the UN of aiding in the "ethnic cleansing" of the town.

Several weeks later, a ceasefire was established, and the UNSC designated Srebrenica a "safe area." After long negotiations, Serb forces agreed to a medical evacuation of injured men from Srebrenica by helicopter. Male amputees in the town staged a protest when they learned the criteria for evacuation did not include them (see Figure 15-4).

The first attempt at the evacuation had to be scrapped when the helicopter landing area was shelled, but the evacuation began again after firmer security guarantees were received. A senior ICRC worker and a UN relief worker were in charge of the mission. The Red Cross worker followed every procedure to the hilt, checking each patient, filling out paper work, and obtaining all required signatures before allowing patients onto helicopters. The UN relief worker had a different approach—he quickly loaded as many men as possible onto the helicopters, whatever their condition, sensing this would be the only chance for them to escape the besieged town.

Over the three-day course of the evacuation, nearly 500 men were airlifted to safety. The war continued for two more years with few other men ever able to leave the town. In July 1995, the forces surrounding Srebrenica launched an attack. In spite of the town's

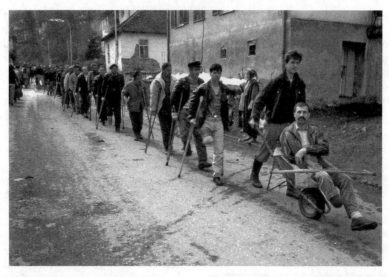

Figure 15-4. April 1993, Srebrenica, Bosnia, and Herzegovina: Wounded men, most of them amputees, march through the town of Srebrenica, protesting their exclusion from an aerial medical evacuation out of the besieged enclave overseen by UN and ICRC personnel. (*Photo by Philipp von Recklinghausen.*)

UN-protected status, the presence of a Dutch contingent of UN soldiers in the town, and an air support agreement with NATO, there was no international effort to counter the attacking forces militarily. Dutch military doctors in the town were forbidden by their commanding officer from treating injured civilians. During the attack, Serb forces ultimately captured the town and massacred an estimated 8,000 men and several women and boys, burying them in mass graves. Two international medical workers from MSF were present in Srebrenica. They managed to save the lives of their national staff by refusing to evacuate without them. The UN War Crimes Tribunal for the Former Yugoslavia and the International Court of Justice, both in the Hague, found that the crime of genocide was committed in Srebrenica.

What would you have done if you were in charge of the 1993 medical evacuations? What does this story say about the ability of international health workers to protect patients in a war zone?

Case Study/Dilemma 4: The Arab Spring[33]

Where does healthcare fit into a new political regime? Following civilian demonstrations in Tunisia and Egypt, Libyans began protesting in mid-February 2011 against the government led for 42 years by Col. Muammar Gaddafi. Unrest spread quickly, leading to armed conflict between Gaddafi loyalists and opponents. Refugees flowed into neighboring countries while internally displaced populations sought refuge in safe havens and temporary settlements. Many aid organizations, UN agencies, and foreign governments, including the United States provided humanitarian assistance. NATO conducted military operations following a UNSC resolution. By October, Gaddafi was captured and killed and his family fled. Within months, the United States and other countries recognized the opposition Transitional National Council (TNC) as the legitimate governing authority for Libya until an interim authority could be put in place.

A key consideration for the TNC and humanitarian workers was the proper healthcare and disposition of the war wounded. Estimates of those injured varied widely: from 500 to 1,000 to tens of thousands.[34] Some were evacuated via multinational efforts to hospitals and facilities in other countries in the Middle East, Europe, and the United States. However, the medical evacuation program was imperfectly designed. Although many war-wounded received excellent care abroad, some medical evacuees were disappointed in their experiences at foreign facilities for a variety of medically and nonmedically-related reasons. Moreover, Libyan health officials, focusing on long-term solutions, wanted international efforts to concentrate on rebuilding and upgrading healthcare facilities and healthcare professionals in Libya, not sending patients elsewhere.

The immediate challenge was how to help those war-wounded individuals who remained in Libya, including home-bound amputees in urban and rural areas who were unemployed, disenfranchised, and still armed. Some had been fighters; others, including children, were injured by unexploded ordnance, downed electrical wires, or the effects of detention and torture. Beyond prostheses and basic physical therapy, the country did not have the physical and psychosocial rehabilitative services to care for them. In addition, stigma was strongly associated with amputation and led to further marginalization.

Other Postconflict Health Issues? Long-term residents of Libya from other Sub-Saharan nations were persecuted under suspicion of being Gaddafi loyalists or African mercenaries. These "stranded migrants," as they were officially called, had fled their homes for IDP camps, living in crowded substandard conditions, and were periodically assisted by MSF and IOM. From the outside and sometimes within, the camp residents experienced intimidation, theft, and assaults, and women especially found it difficult to access healthcare.

A dearth of Libyan social workers and psychiatrists limited the outreach to those traumatized by war, including children and stigmatized female survivors of gender-based violence and war-associated rape.

After 7 months of fighting, abandoned and unexploded ordnance posed the risks of additional injuries and deaths. Uncontrolled flows and dispersion of small arms and light weapons among a population unused to such access resulted in misuse, deaths, and injuries from celebratory firing of weapons and unsafe storage of small arms within the home.

Motor vehicle accidents were a major cause of morbidity and mortality as free movement returned at a time of weakened rule of law. Chronic disease, such as diabetes, cardiovascular disease, stroke, and tobacco-related disease, continued to place a major burden on the healthcare system. Environmental health management was also an issue, including disposition of biomedical waste (tissue, blood, sharps), community waste, and abandoned weapon depots. The health hazards included risks to children and animals foraging in dumps.

Transition to Sustainability? A transitional government juggling multiple priorities could devote only so much attention to healthcare. The new health ministry emphasized the need for reestablishing the trust of Libyans in their own healthcare system. In almost every instance, hospital directors were newly elected or appointed, some of whom had little hospital administration and management skills. Reports of drug stock-outs and lab supply shortages reflected a broken supply chain, and the lack of a functioning information and inventory system.

Many nurses and allied health professionals were foreigners (often from the Philippines, Korea, or Ukraine) who left Libya during the war and only trickled back as the conflict died down and security

improved. Patient medical record systems, quality improvement and assurance, and information systems that collated data on disease burden, service statistics, and procurement all needed strengthening as did primary and preventive healthcare, long neglected.

Political, Ethnic, and Religious Minorities and Socially Marginalized Groups

Many recent wars and conflicts have targeted specific groups for displacement and even killing. Providing medical aid to members of these groups is in some sense a political act. As one US government aid official, who requested anonymity, once put it, "You're making a political statement when you say that someone should live when someone else doesn't want them to live." There are two mine fields here for aid workers. One is the danger that aid organizations will be steered away from these groups and might not notice their needs. Therefore, minority and marginalized groups need to be identified early and monitoring must be instituted to ensure equal access to aid.

However, another danger is that these groups will receive what appears to those around them as *preferential* treatment, thus heightening the risk of their further persecution or abuse. This is one reason why good communication and transparency are critical to the work of aid organizations. Explain to authorities and recipients why and how aid is being given, and that it is being given impartially and based on need (and, if true, to "their side," too). To get aid through to vulnerable populations, workers may have to decide when to privately negotiate, when to publicly denounce, and when to consider a proportion of aid stolen by paramilitary soldiers at a checkpoint as a price worth paying.

One of the dangers of committing to providing a high standard of aid to victims of disasters is that it can heighten existing tensions (or create new ones) between populations. For example, the disaster-affected subset of the population may receive more food or higher quality shelter than those around them who are at baseline living in much poorer circumstances. This problem of equity has not yet been resolved satisfactorily by the aid community.

Case Study/Dilemma 5: Aceh, Indonesia, 2004

Before the 2004 Indian Ocean earthquake and tsunami, the Indonesian province of Aceh was embroiled in a three-decade conflict between the rebel Free Aceh Movement and the government of Indonesia. Foreigners, including most aid workers, had been banned from working in the province. After the tsunami, the rebel group and the government concluded a peace agreement, and the conflict-affected interior

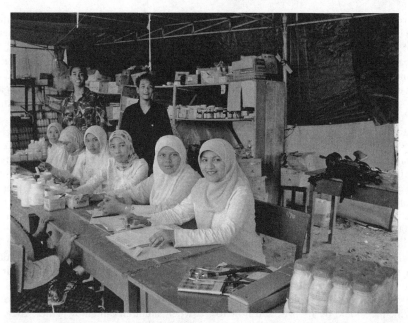

Figure 15-5. February 2005, Aceh Utara District, Nanggroe Aceh Darussalam, Indonesia: Indonesian nurses and doctors who survived the December 2004 tsunami work at an improvised health clinic in a tent camp for displaced persons. Local professionals typically provide the bulk of healthcare services following a disaster. A government of Indonesia soldier armed with an automatic weapon is present at the clinic—a common practice discouraged by many international aid organizations. (*Photo by Dr. Sheri Fink.*)

of the province was finally opened to aid workers, who were already amassed along the coastline responding to the tsunami (see Figure 15-5).

However, leaders of aid agencies were unsure whether they could legitimately use tsunami recovery donations to implement programs in areas that were instead primarily devastated by the conflict. Disparities in the provision of aid to coastal versus inland areas heightened tensions among residents of some of Aceh's conflict-affected districts.

The humanitarian principle of impartiality demands that aid be allotted without any standard other than need. Was it moral, with billions of dollars on the table, to distribute food to children along the coasts while allowing children in the mountains above to die of malnutrition? Is there any justification for rebuilding only tsunami-wrecked health centers but not war-damaged ones serving sicker children a few miles inland?

Children

UNICEF recently estimated that more than 1 billion children under the age of 18 were living in conflict-affected areas or areas emerging from war; many of those children were separated from their families and subsequently unaccompanied.[35] In a medical sense,

children are more vulnerable than adults to the stresses and deprivations of trauma and displacement. They are more prone to dehydration, malnutrition, micronutrient deficiencies, and fatigue compared with adults, and their immature immune systems can leave them more vulnerable to infections. Illnesses and malnutrition experienced early may continue to impact them throughout their lives—for example, studies have shown that malnutrition in childhood can have harmful long-term stunting effects on the brain and on behavioral development.

Exploitation of children, including child trafficking into labor or prostitution rings, other sexual abuse, and abduction by the military, may take place in camps and other situations of displacement. Child marriage of girls is also common in some cultures, and pressure for girls to marry may increase when many men have lost wives in a disaster. Some aid agencies, such as UNICEF, Save the Children, and IRC, often dispatch a child protection officer with their disaster response team to organize services for children and advocate for them. The 1989 Convention on the Rights of the Child and its two Optional Protocols (2000) as well as the Geneva Conventions and their two Additional Protocols, the Refugee Convention, the 1993 Vienna Declaration and Program of Action, the 1999 Convention Concerning the Prohibition and Immediate Action for the Elimination of the Worst Forms of Child Labor, and human rights law provide a legal basis for child protection work.

Unaccompanied children, children separated from their customary caregivers, orphans, and child-headed households are particularly vulnerable to exploitation, including trafficking. The Protocol to Prevent, Suppress and Punish Trafficking in Persons, Especially Women and Children, supplementing the UN Convention against Transnational Organized Crime (2003), and the UN Global Plan of Action to Combat Trafficking in Persons (2010) were developed to specifically tackle this growing global phenomenon. It is therefore crucial to make every effort to preserve family unity. The 2004 Interagency Guiding Principles on Unaccompanied and Separated Children provide further useful guidance.[36] The 2008 UNHCR Guidelines on Determining the Best Interests of the Child is also a practical resource on the international legal framework regarding the protection of children, how the Best Interests Principle should be applied, and how to support national child protection systems.[37]

Evacuations, including medical evacuations, can cause separation. If at all possible, children should be evacuated with their intact families, or at minimum one caregiver. If this is not possible, a file of personal and family information should travel with the child with copies retained by parents, governmental representatives, and monitoring agencies such as the ICRC's Central Tracing Agency. Evacuation should be to the closest possible location to home and family, and efforts should be made to allow the child to communicate with family members while separated from them.

Any disaster can lead to children being separated from their families. It is important for unaccompanied children to be rapidly identified, registered, photographed, and provided with documentation—all in a way that will not further endanger or stigmatize them or disrupt their community's efforts to care for them. Whenever possible (except, for example, where this could put a family in danger), a concerted search must be made for surviving family members. Typically, the ICRC or UNICEF works with governmental authorities and humanitarian agencies to register and trace separated family members.

Media coverage of suffering children always sparks offers of international adoption. However, many experts believe that children are better off staying with family members or community members. Many countries have instituted policies barring international adoption following disasters because it cuts children off from the chance of reuniting with families and maintaining links with their communities.

Likewise, committing these children to orphanages and other institutions should be avoided whenever possible. It is better to place the children with relatives, neighbors, or friends within their communities. Special attention should be paid to the proper healthcare and nutrition of these children (e.g., children under 6 months should be breastfed if possible by a lactating woman who tests HIV negative). Ensuring that birth registration takes place during a disaster also helps to protect children.

Psychological trauma is very real for children and can have long-term impact, but children are also highly resilient. It should not be assumed that children who experience war will be psychologically scarred. In fact, the vast majority are capable of going on to lead productive and happy lives. To facilitate this, it is important as quickly as possible to establish structures where children can experience normalcy. Resumption of education is particularly important—UNICEF offers "School -in-a-Box" kits that contain supplies and materials for a teacher and up to 40 children, designed for short-term temporary classrooms created in camp settings. Child recreation centers are sometimes created where children can enjoy games, safety, and counseling if needed.

Women

Security should always be an utmost priority because women are frequently victims of physical and sexual assault in unstable circumstances.[38] Contraceptive and prenatal care programs should be initiated to avoid long-term consequences of unintended pregnancies and premature births. The WHO and MSF have published numerous manuals providing guidelines on such healthcare operations. It is often helpful to involve local women in the provision of healthcare and health and hygiene education within the disaster or conflict-affected populations. This type of health outreach is important because many women are reluctant to leave their living quarters to seek medical care out of fear of being separated from children or putting them at risk during travel.

Men

Men are not typically considered a vulnerable group. Indeed, medical aid workers may not think much about the particular problems of men. However, military-aged men are often at risk of being killed by hostile forces or pressured into fighting. Men may also be less willing to seek help for physical and especially psychological problems.

Older and Chronically Ill People

Older people are defined by the UN as those over 60 years, and their numbers and proportions are growing throughout the world. The great value of older people to their communities in terms of knowledge, caregiving, and resilience should be kept in mind during emergencies. Tragically, they are often among the most vulnerable and poor, and they have often been neglected during humanitarian crises. Physical frailty and isolation exacerbate the vulnerability of older people during these times; in the Great East Japan Earthquake and tsunami of 2011, nearly 65% of deaths were reportedly among older people, about double their proportion in the population.[39]

Older people often depend on others to provide for their food, shelter, and basic needs, and thus they are prone to exploitation and neglect and in need of particular attention. Furthermore, in disasters they are commonly separated from their families and left alone. An effort should be made to identify older people who are incapable of caring for themselves, trace and reunite them with family members, and otherwise provide for their care.

In an emergency, providing care only to those who show up for it is not sufficient. No matter how busy medical professionals are, they must also take time to seek out people who may be lying helpless in a corner of a tent with a serious but treatable illness. Such people exist in every disaster—from the camps in Darfur, Sudan, to shelters following Hurricane Katrina and the Indian Ocean and Japanese tsunamis.

Older people often suffer from chronic diseases that require medicines and ongoing care. Their conditions may be exacerbated by the stress of the disaster or by running out of needed medications. In many recent conflicts and disasters, exacerbation of chronic diseases accounted for a great deal of morbidity and mortality, in particular from hypertension, diabetes, renal disease, cardiac disease, and stroke. The global burden of these diseases is rising. During the 2012 civil conflict in Syria, the WHO reported critical shortages of lifesaving medicines and supplies not only for trauma and surgical care, but also for noncommunicable and chronic diseases.

Insulin treatment may be difficult in places where refrigeration is a problem. Cold boxes are often needed. Renal dialysis-dependent patients require rapid transfer to facilities that have dialysis capabilities, or they will die. Although sophisticated cancer treatment is typically unavailable in conflict or disaster situations, cancer patients are often given low evacuation priority due to their poorer prognosis. Shamefully, humanitarian organizations have historically not done a good job of making drugs, available to treat their severe pain, such as narcotic analgesics. In many developing countries, essential drugs, including morphine are all but nonexistent even in normal times due to legal restrictions, regulations, and fears of misuse; many patients suffer and die with untreated pain. See treatthepain.com or the Global Access to Pain Relief Initiative (www.gapri.org).

People Living with HIV and AIDS

Those who are living with HIV and AIDS when disaster hits may experience problems coping with the physical stresses of displacement.[40] Their survival is at risk from infections and malnutrition, and it is important for them to have access to extra clean water for drinking and hygiene, and to nutritious foods to stay healthy (energy requirements may be increased, and micronutrients are important to maintain immune function). Often chronic diarrhea is a problem. When combined with weakness, this may make it difficult for those with AIDS to reach latrines. Simple inventions, such as a bucket fitted with a toilet seat and toilet lid, can help restore a sense of dignity and improve the quality of life for those with AIDS and those caring for them in difficult circumstances. Aid workers must make efforts to ensure that discrimination does not occur against people living with HIV and AIDS.

HIV prevention activities and information campaigns are important parts of aid programs. In addition, several aid agencies have demonstrated the feasibility of initiating highly active antiretroviral therapy in refugee settings. Increasingly, those affected by conflict and disaster may already be taking antiretroviral (ARV) treatment, and, due to the likelihood of resistance developing, it is critical that their treatment regimens not be interrupted as occurred during the post election violence and displacement in Kenya in 2008. Steps to ensure continuity include providing established patients with an increased supply of ARVs and the locations of other clinics during periods of instability; using radio, phone hotlines, other media, and direct outreach (e.g., through existing networks of people living with HIV) to inform and locate them in crises; and recording multiple ways of reaching them, including through family contacts. Be aware that HIV stigma still exists in some places, and patients may not be immediately forthcoming about HIV status and ARV use. In all cases, those living with AIDS should be afforded appropriate medical care to decrease their risk of acquiring opportunistic infections and to reduce mother-to-child transmission. Recommendations for HIV and AIDS treatment change rapidly, so it is important to consult updated guidelines.

People with Physical Challenges

It is important to ensure that people with limited mobility not be separated from needed equipment, such as wheelchairs or prosthetic limbs, during a disaster. They may also require additional assistance accessing food, shelter, or medical care. Disability should be considered in every aspect of camp and settlement creation, so that drinking water sources, bathing facilities, latrines, and other services (e.g., schools and health posts) are made accessible to all. Established settlements should be evaluated and remedied where necessary. Unfortunately, these considerations are typically overlooked, creating hazards for people with disabilities. The Convention on the Rights of Persons with Disabilities (2006) supports the rights of those with physical challenges under all other human rights treaties; Article 11 specifically refers to "the protection and safety of persons with disabilities in situations of risk, including situations of armed conflict, humanitarian emergencies and the occurrence of natural disasters."[41] In the United States, public agencies have been sued for failing to include people with disabilities in disaster planning. Handicap International (www.handicap-international.org) is an important agency with expertise in emergency situations.

Case Study/Dilemma 6: Kosovo-Macedonia Border 1999

During the Kosovo (or Kosova) war in 1999, many Kosovar Albanians were forced to flee. However, the Macedonian government at first closed its border with Kosovo, trapping roughly 100,000 people in a cold, muddy noman's-land beside the border crossing. Several NGOs and the Macedonian Red Cross created a tented medical treatment area. Two lines of Macedonian police in riot gear stood between the population and the medical area, and the police did not allow family members to accompany sick persons for care. This resulted in several dozen elderly, chronically ill, developmentally disabled, mentally ill, and paraplegic people ending up in the medical area with no family members to care for them. Medical workers were busy with acute medical cases, and they moved these people into a separate "respite" tent and all but forgot about them.

That miserable tent became known as "the tent of the damned." Those who could not walk soiled themselves and were not cleaned. They did not receive enough food or water. Some of them experienced pain and were not given pain killers or treatment. Aid workers made several appeals for help to the Macedonian health ministry, but authorities refused to take these vulnerable patients into care facilities. Several days later, the border area was evacuated. Representatives of the Organization for Security and Cooperation in Europe and UNHCR agreed to transfer the inhabitants of the "tent of the damned" to a local hospital, care facility, or camp. For unknown reasons they were left alone for another cold night in the tent with no nursing care before being transferred. An additional woman died.

People Affected by Mental Illness

Those individuals being treated for preexisting mental illnesses often run short of their medicines during disasters. In addition, the stressful situations can cause psychological distress or psychological disorders in a portion of the population. In some societies, a great deal of shame surrounds mental illness, and those affected may be hidden away or mistreated. In other cases, depression or a traumatic experience such as rape may decrease a person's motivation to seek medical assistance or even food. All of these problems highlight the need to conduct active "case finding" in emergency contexts. Furthermore, medical care givers must be sensitive to the fact that patients appearing at the clinic with physical complaints may also be experiencing psychological distress.[42]

People with Cognitive Impairments

Displacement can be particularly disorienting for people with cognitive impairments. They too may require additional assistance to ensure their basic needs are met and to protect them from danger.

A Vulnerable Group: Aid Workers

Providing humanitarian assistance is a risky business. Hundreds of aid workers have been killed on the job in recent years. They have often been intentionally targeted. Many more have been injured or subject to gender-based violence. Every aid worker has the responsibility to ensure that his or her agency provides adequate security training and has a solid security plan. Short courses on security in emergencies are available from organizations, including RedR (www.redr.org). The UN offers an online Basic Security in the Field (BSITF II) training module that is compulsory for all its staff.[43] In addition, the risks of infectious diseases, traffic accidents, and kidnapping may be greater where aid workers do their jobs than in their home countries.

Humanitarian work is often stressful, too. The temptation to work until exhaustion should be resisted because it can reduce effectiveness dramatically and lead to burnout. Aid workers also run the risk of encountering extremely disturbing situations that may leave a long-lasting psychological impact. Transition to life back home can be difficult. Many have found it helpful to seek professional counseling, which may be provided for free by the hiring agency.[31,44]

THE ROLES AND LIMITATIONS OF HEALTH PROFESSIONALS IN PHYSICAL PROTECTION AND CONFLICT MITIGATION

Humanitarians are often among the few outsiders present in situations of extreme violence. Their traditional role has been to both assist and protect the vulnerable. Although responsibility for ensuring the physical protection of civilians during wartime rests primarily with governments and militaries, humanitarians should also embrace this goal as central to their work. Most important is to examine activities regularly to assess whether they are contributing to or detracting from protection.

Some analysts argue that the mere presence of humanitarian aid workers provides a measure of protection to civilians. However, recent experience has suggested that humanitarian presence may also confer a false sense of protection to a population and may paradoxically represent an obstacle to effective military action aimed at neutralizing aggressive forces. In addition, the presence of desirable aid commodities may make a population more prone to attack. In these cases, thought should be paid to making aid less desirable to potential looters, for example by delivering aid in small family-size packages.

However, there are several ways that medical aid workers can promote protection by responding to human rights violations, remediating them, and building a positive environment for protection. This is known as the ICRC "egg" model of protection. Aid workers may worry that speaking out directly about human rights violations or war crimes will endanger their access to the people they are assisting. This is a very difficult decision for aid workers. The Active Learning Network for Accountability and Performance in Humanitarian Action (ALNAP; www.alnap.org) has published a Protection Guide that details five options for aid workers responding to protection problems:

1. Public denunciation of those committing atrocities or human rights violations
2. Direct persuasion of those involved to end the pattern of abuse
3. Mobilization or discreet information sharing with human rights advocates, journalists, peacekeeping monitors, or others who may have the ability to influence military or political leaders to conform to human rights standards and international humanitarian law
4. Substitution or providing aid to assist those at risk of disease, malnutrition, and death
5. Capacity building or offering support to others providing protection.

International health workers can also promote links between conflicting (or recently conflicting) populations. For example, they can facilitate cooperation between health workers on different sides of the frontlines, or hire staff from different religious or ethnic groups. Health workers have also been successful in coordinating humanitarian ceasefires to allow vaccinations to take place, a strategy often referred to as "Peace through Health."

Health workers have used their professional expertise to inform the wider public about the terrible health effects of certain weapons, such as landmines. Indeed,

medical professionals played an important part in the Nobel Peace Prize–winning International Campaign to Ban Landmines, which resulted in the 1997 Mine Ban Treaty. The treaty became international law in 1999.

In addition, health workers have documented the effects of torture and rape on asylum seekers and furnished evidence in war crimes prosecutions. Physicians, epidemiologists, and others with research expertise have also conducted epidemiologic-style studies of human rights violations that reveal strong evidence about patterns of abuses and can be used in criminal courts. Of course, those committing atrocities are increasingly aware that they may be held to account for their crimes and may try to hide evidence, avoid leaving survivors, or refuse health workers access to populations that have been targeted.

WORKING WITH REPORTERS AND COMMUNICATING WITH THE PUBLIC

Media coverage can shape crisis response by the public, politicians, and the donor community. It can expose violations of human rights and the laws of war that impact civilians and aid workers. Reporters also promote accountability in aid provision, helping uncover unethical, harmful practices and catalyze improvements.

Journalists and communications specialists have related, but different roles. Reporters must seek and report the truth, translating what is happening into stories for various segments of the public. Public relations specialists represent the humanitarian agencies that employ them and help disseminate information about their work. They often inform reporters, arrange interviews, or transmit messages or stories from the agency directly to the public through meetings, radio, Internet, social media, and other outlets.

There are many areas of potential synergy between reporters and aid workers. For instance, reporters can achieve access and security in a crisis zone by traveling with humanitarians. Aid organizations, in return, may increase public understanding and support by cooperating with journalists and inviting them to cover their work. Independence is a key journalistic value, and the journalist must report what he or she finds to be true from a variety of sources rather than what an aid worker or government official wants the "message" to be.

Some rules of thumb for humanitarians communicating with reporters and the public: Use clear language and not jargon or acronyms that a nonexpert would not understand. If you wish to provide information but not be quoted as a source, be clear about the ground rules with the reporter before you share the information. Reporters are ethically allowed to use what you tell them unless you have come to an agreement beforehand. Additionally, reporters from a range of countries and media outlets may adhere to different sets of journalistic values, making it important to assess trustworthiness as the working relationship deepens. (These days anyone with a smartphone, not only a traditional reporter, has the potential to share information with a broad audience.) Some reporters and communications professionals have medical or public health training or experience in the field of public health crisis reporting. Others do not.

Make time to understand the political and historical context of the place in which you are working. Be cognizant of politics, lines of authority, hidden agendas, and sensitivities that could lead your words to be misinterpreted or cause unintended offense to some audiences. This may be particularly important in tense military situations or for those aid workers who are affiliated with governments or come from countries that are involved in a conflict. There may be rare occasions where something you say or that a journalist wants to cover might endanger your beneficiaries or the larger relief effort. In these cases, you may wish to discuss these fears frankly with the reporter working on the story, first making sure that he or she agrees that what you are about to discuss will not be quoted.

If your team lacks a designated public relations representative, it may be helpful to choose someone as the media go-to person to receive and transmit data, stories, and updates from everyone else. If there is something you or others in your organization feel is important to get across, make sure that the reporter understands this. Repeating those key facts or perspectives may be necessary.

Keeping composed under pressure, making sure you understand the questions, and offering objective, reliable data and regular updates on the situation help make you a trustworthy source to a reporter. Do not compromise the science in the messaging because you want the reporter to take you seriously. If the reporter has the facts wrong, gently correct him or her for the record. In addition, where possible, being predictably available to the media (at the very beginning or end of the day, for example) is an efficient way of getting basic information to numerous media outlets, leaving you open to grant special access and interviews to reporters working on more unique or in-depth stories.

Offer to quickly research any answers that are not known; do not appear to be passing the buck or being evasive about information. Yet if you cannot divulge something, state that clearly. Lastly, remember that journalists are never off duty, and casual conversations can still be picked up and reported.

SUMMARY

The job of an international aid worker is one of great challenge, responsibility, and potentially great rewards. It requires excellent medical skills and a solid understanding of medical ethics and international law. Relief workers often gain a deeper understanding of current events, persistent international health problems, and the human implications of political and military decisions. The work often gives its practitioners a deep sense of purpose. The dedication and humanity of colleagues, particularly those who come from the affected society, is inspiring. At times, however, when dispensing a pill, vaccinating a child, or even documenting an atrocity seems almost purposeless amid the overwhelming violence and destruction, the most important gifts an international health worker can give to those affected are kindness, solidarity, and hope.

STUDY QUESTIONS

1. You are an aid worker faced with a disaster involving a large displaced population. List at least 10 medical and public health interventions you would consider applying in the short (hours to days), medium (days to weeks), and long-term (weeks to months) situation. List at least three factors you will need to weigh in choosing your priorities, and describe how these factors will influence your choices.

2. Some NGOs rely heavily on government funding to support their lifesaving work. Reread the Iraq case study. If a NGO is offered money from a government that is party to a conflict, do you think the NGO should accept the funds to serve the population in need, or should it turn them down to avoid undermining the agency's independence? What practical, ethical, or other factors influence your decision? What other solutions might be possible?

3. In every disaster and war there is a subset of highly vulnerable people who are at risk of suffering more than others. Reread the case study about the "the tent of the damned" during the Kosovo war. If you were an aid worker on the Kosovo border, what other ways might you have approached the situation? List at least three interventions that might have improved the lives and protected the health of the vulnerable patients.

KEY RESOURCES

Books And Articles

1. Amundson D, Dadekian G, Etienne M, et al. Practicing internal medicine onboard the USNS *Comfort* in the aftermath of the Haitian earthquake. *Ann Intern Med* 2010;152(11):733–737.
2. *Humanitarian Charter and Minimum Standards in Disaster Response.* Geneva: Sphere Project, 2011. http://www.sphere-project.org/handbook/.

3. Médecins Sans Frontières. *Clinical Guidelines: Diagnosis and Treatment Manual.* 8th ed. Paris: Médecins Sans Frontières, 2010. http://www.refbooks.msf.org/.

4. Médecins Sans Frontières. *Refugee Health: An Approach to Emergency Situations.* London: Macmillan, 1997. http://www.refbooks.msf.org/.

5. Moss WJ, Ramakrishnan M, et al. *Child Health in Complex Emergencies.* Washington, DC: The National Academies Press, 2006. www.nap.edu/catalog.php?record_id=11527.

Documents

1. Inter-Agency Standing Committee (IASC). *Guidelines for Addressing HIV in Humanitarian Settings,* 2010. http://www.unhcr.org/4b603d1e9.html.

2. Inter-Agency Standing Committee (IASC). *Humanitarian Action and Older Persons: An Essential Brief for Humanitarian Actors,* 2008. http://www.unhcr.org/refworld/docid/490b0c102.html.

3. UNHCR. *Managing the Stress of Humanitarian Emergencies.* Geneva, July 2001. http://www.the-ecentre.net/resources/e_library/doc/managingStress.pdf.

4. World Health Organization. *25 Questions and Answers on Health and Human Rights* (via WHO Webpage). Health and Human Rights Publication Series, no. 1. Geneva: WHO, July 2002.http://www.who.int/hhr/activities/publications/en/.

5. World Health Organization. *Guidelines for Medicine Donations—Revised 2010.* Geneva: WHO, 2011. http://whqlibdoc.who.int/publications/2011/9789241501989_eng.pdf.

6. World Health Organization. *Mental Health in Emergencies: Psychological and Social Aspects of Health of Populations Exposed to Extreme Stressors.* Geneva: WHO, 2003. www.who.int/mental_health/media/en/640.pdf.

Websites

1. Advanced Training Program on Humanitarian Action (ATHA). Online multi-media training program in humanitarian action. http://www.atha.se/.

2. AlertNet. Disaster and conflict news. http://www.trust.org/alertnet/.

3. ALNAP. Active Learning Network for Accountability and Performance in Humanitarian Action. http://www.alnap.org.

4. EM-DAT. The International Disaster Database of the Center for Research on the Epidemiology of Disasters. http://www.emdat.be/.

5. Enhancing Learning and Research for Humanitarian Action (ELRHA). A collaborative network dedicated to supporting partnerships between higher education institutions and humanitarian organizations and partners around the world. http://www.elrha.org/.

6. Forced Migration Online. Links to full-text versions of many documents related to health in disasters and humanitarian emergencies. http://www.forcedmigration.org/sphere/health.htm.

7. Harvard Humanitarian Initiative. A Harvard-wide program dedicated to advancing the science and practice of humanitarian response worldwide, including through crisis mapping projects. http://hhi.harvard.edu.

8. Humanitarian Practice Network. The Humanitarian Policy Group with publications, events, and resources for humanitarian work. www.odihpn.org.

9. IRIN: Humanitarian News and Analysis. An editorially independent news service covering around 70 countries delivering unique stories and unheard voices, run out of UN OCHA. http://www.irinnews.org.

10. Professionals in Humanitarian Action and Protection (PHAP). International association committed to professional development and networking opportunities among individuals deployed in the context of humanitarian crises. http://phap.org/.

11. Program on Humanitarian Policy and Conflict Research (HPCR). A Harvard-based academic initiative providing technical assistance and information support for international organizations engaged in humanitarian action and conflict transformation. http://www.hpcrresearch.org/.

12. Reliefweb. Up-to-date information on individual disasters and complex emergencies. Job listings for aid workers. http://reliefweb.int/.

13. The Responsibility to Protect. Resources from the Office of the United Nations Special Adviser on the Prevention of Genocide. http://www.un.org/en/preventgenocide/adviser/responsibility.shtml.

14. The Sphere Project. Humanitarian charter and minimum standards in disaster response. http://www.sphereproject.org.

15. Ushahidi. A nonprofit tech company that develops open source software for information collection and sharing. http://ushahidi.com/.

16. World Health Organization. Technical Guidelines for Humanitarian Health Action in Crises. http://www.who.int/hac/techguidance/en/.

17. World Health Organization/Pan-American Health Association. *Health Library for Disasters.* Geneva: WHO/PAHO, 2007. http://helid.desastres.net/?e=d-000who--000--1-0--010---4-----0--0-10l--11es-5000---50-packa-0---01131-001-110utfZz-8-0-0&cl=CL1.2&d=Js2912s.10&az=A%3E=0&gc=&ihs=0%3E=2.

Journals and Newsletters

Disaster Medicine and Public Health Preparedness, American Medical Association. http://dmphp.org/.

Disasters: The Journal of Disaster Studies, Policy and Management, Overseas Development Institute. http://old.library.georgetown.edu/newjour/d/msg02569.html.

Humanitarian Practice Exchange. Humanitarian Practice Network. http://www.odihpn.org/.

Prehospital and Disaster Medicine. World Association for Disaster and Emergency Medicine. http://pdm.medicine.wisc.edu/.

REFERENCES

1. Dunant H. *A Memory of Solferino.* Geneva: International Committee of the Red Cross, 1986.

2. Introduced via the Third Additional Protocol (Protocol III) to the Geneva Conventions in 2005. http://www.icrc.org/ihl.nsf/FULL/615?OpenDocument.

3. Sistenich V. *Briefing Note: UN Integration & Humanitarian Coordination: Policy Considerations towards Protection of the Humanitarian Space.* Program on Humanitarian Policy and Conflict Research, Harvard University, 2012. http://hpcrresearch.org/blog/vera-sistenich/2012-07-06/briefing-note-un-integration-humanitarian-coordination-policy-conside.

4. Metcalfe V, Giffen A, Elhawary S. *UN Integration and Humanitarian Space. An Independent Study Commissioned by the UN Integration Steering Group.* Humanitarian Policy Group (HPG) & Stimson Center, 2011. http://www.stimson.org/images/uploads/research-pdfs/Integration_final.pdf.

5. Stoddard A, Harmer A, Haver K, Salomons D, Wheeler V. *Cluster approach evaluation final.* OCHA Evaluation and Studies Section, 2007. www.humanitarianoutcomes.org/pdf/ClusterApproachEvaluation.pdf.

6. Code of Conduct for the International Red Cross and Red Crescent Movement and NGOs in Disaster Relief. IFRC. http://www.ifrc.org/publicat/conduct/index.asp.

7. *Humanitarian Charter and Minimum Standards in Disaster Response.* Geneva: Sphere Project, 2011. www.sphereproject.org/handbook/index.htm.

8. Amundson D, Dadekian G, Etienne M et al. Practicing internal medicine onboard the USNS *Comfort* in the aftermath of the Haitian earthquake. *Ann of Intern Med* 2010; 152(11): 733-737.

9. Statistics for the USNS *Comfort*'s Haiti earthquake deployment are drawn from an analysis of all patients evaluated and treated between January 19 and February 27, 2010, as recorded in medical charts in the ship's database: Walk R, Safford S, Donahue T et al. Haitian Earthquake Relief: Disaster Response Aboard the USNS *Comfort. Disaster Medicine and Public Health Preparedness* 2012;6(4):370-377.

10. Etienne M, Powell C, Amundson D. Healthcare ethics: the experience after the Haitian earthquake. *American Journal of Dis Med* 2010;5 (3):141-147.

11. Etienne M, Powell C, Faux B. Disaster relief in Haiti: a perspective from the neurologists on the USNS COMFORT. *Lancet Neurol* 2010;9:461-463.

12. Fink S. "Haitians under US treatment are often separated from families." *ProPublica,* February 2, 2010. http://www.propublica.org/article/haitians-under-u.s.-treatment-are-often-separated-from-families.

13. Fink S. Haiti loses its lifeboat. *ProPublica/The Daily Beast,* March 13, 2010.

14. Egeland J, Harmer A, Stoddard A. To stay and deliver: Good practice for humanitarians in complex security environments. Office for the Coordination of Humanitarian Affairs (OCHA), 2011. http://ochanet.unocha.org/p/Documents/Stay_and_Deliver.pdf

15. International Humanitarian Law: Answers to your Questions. International Committee of the Red Cross, 2002. http://www.icrc.org/eng/assets/files/other/icrc_002_0703.pdf

16. EM-DAT, The International Disaster Database. *Natural Disaster Trends.* Centre for Research on the Epidemiology of Disasters—CRED, 2011. http://www.emdat.be/natural-disasters-trends.

17. EM-DAT, The International Disaster Database. *Technological Disasters Trends.* Centre for Research on the Epidemiology of Disasters—CRED, 2011. http://www.emdat.be/technological-disasters-trends.

18. The KoBo Toolbox is an open-source, sophisticated but user-friendly suite of applications designed to support in-field digital data management. http://www.kobotoolbox.org/.

19. For example, http://hhi.harvard.edu/programs-and-research/crisis-mapping-and-early-warning/satellite-sentinel-projectandhttp://satsentinel.org/

20. Médecins Sans Frontières. *Clinical Guidelines: Diagnosis and Treatment Manual.* Paris: MSF, 2010. http://www.refbooks.msf.org/.

21. Fink S. The Deadly Choices at Memorial. *The New York Times/ProPublica,* 2009.

22. Navin M, Waddell B 2nd. Triage is Broken. *Emerg Med Serv* 2005;34(8):138-142.

23. Committee on Guidance Crisis Standards of Care for Use in Disaster Situations; for Establishing Institute of Medicine. In: Hanfling D, Altevogt B, Viswanathan K, Gostin L., Eds. *Crisis standards of care: A systems framework for catastrophic disaster response.* Washington DC: The National Academies Press, 2012.

24. The MENTOR Initiative. http://thementorinitiative.org/.

25. *The Interagency Emergency Health Kit 2011: Medicines and medical devices for 10,000 people for approximately three months.* Geneva: The World Health Organization, 2010. http://www.who.int/medicines/publications/emergencyhealthkit2011/en/index.html.

26. World Health Organization. *Psychological First Aid: Guide for Field Workers.* Geneva: WHO, 2011. http://whqlibdoc.who.int/publications/2011/9789241548205_eng.pdf.

27. For more information on the MISP, see: http://misp.rhrc.org/.

28. World Health Organization. *The Top 10 Causes of Death: Fact Sheet Number 310,* Updated June 2011. http://www.who.int/mediacentre/factsheets/fs310/en/index.html.

29. *Management of Dead Bodies after Disasters: A Field Manual for First Responders.* PAHO, 2009. http://www.paho.org/english/dd/ped/DeadBodiesFieldManual.pdf.

30. *Chemical, Biological, and Radiation Threats: A Guide for Aid Workers* is a training CD-ROM produced by the International Medical Corps (IMC) and the Center for International Emergency Medicine at UCLA in 2003. http://pdf.usaid.gov/pdf_docs/PNACU009.pdf.

31. Roberts D. *Staying Alive: Safety and Security Guidelines for Humanitarian Volunteers in Conflict Areas.* Geneva: ICRC, 2005. http://www.icrc.org/eng/assets/files/other/icrc_002_0717.pdf.

32. For a more complete story of war-time Srebrenica, see Fink S. *War Hospital: A True Story of Surgery and Survival.* New York: Public Affairs, 2003.

33. This case study is based on first hand observations by author Clydette Powell.

34. Personal communication to author Clydette Powell from representatives of the Ministry of War Wounded, Transitional National Council, Tripoli, Libya, December 2011.

35. *Machel study 10-year Strategic Review: Children and Conflict in a Changing World.* New York: United Nations Children's Fund (UNICEF), 2009. www.unicef.org/publications/files/Machel_Study_10_Year_Strategic_Review_EN_030909.pdf.

36. *Inter-agency guiding principles on unaccompanied and separated children.* Geneva: International Committee of the Red Cross Central Tracing Agency and Protection Division, 2004. http://www.unicef.org/violencestudy/pdf/IAG_UASCs.pdf.

37. UN High Commissioner for Refugees, *UNHCR Guidelines on Determining the Best Interests of the Child.* Geneva: UNHCR, 2008. http://www.unhcr.org/refworld/docid/48480c342.html.

38. The Task Force on Gender of the Inter-Agency Standing Committee (IASC). *Guidelines for Gender-Based Violence Interventions in Humanitarian Settings: Focusing on Prevention of and Response to Sexual Violence in Emergencies.* Geneva: UNHCR, 2005. http://www.unhcr.org/refworld/docid/439474c74.html.

39. Sawai M. *Who is vulnerable during tsunamis? Experiences from the Great East Japan earthquake 2011 and the Indian Ocean tsunami 2004.* Working paper, United Nations Economic and

Social Commission for Asia and the Pacific (ESCAP). Tokyo: 2011. http://www.unescap.org/idd/working%20papers/IDD-DRS-who-is-vulnerable-during-tsunamis.pdf.

40. Inter-Agency Standing Committee. *Guidelines for Addressing HIV in Humanitarian Settings*. Geneva: UNHCR, 2009. http://www.unhcr.org/4b603d1e9.html.

41. *The Convention on the Rights of Persons with Disabilities*. Geneva: UNHCR, 2007. http://www2.ohchr.org/english/law/disabilities-convention.htm.

42. *Mental Health in Emergencies*. Geneva: WHO, 2003. http://www.who.int/mental_health/media/en/640.pdf.

43. Basic Security in the Field (BSITF) II. UNDSS, 2012. https://dss.un.org/dssweb/Resources/BasicSecuritybrIntheFieldBSIT-FII.aspx.

44. *Humanitarian action and armed conflict: Coping with stress*. Geneva: ICRC, 2001. http://www.icrc.org/eng/resources/documents/publication/p0576.htm.

Aging Populations and Chronic Illness

16

Wayne A. Hale, Jané D. Joubert, and Sebastiana Kalula

LEARNING OBJECTIVES

- *Develop an overview of the demography and societal effects of global aging and its relationship to noncommunicable diseases (NCDs)*
- *Understand the increasing contribution of NCDs to the global burden of disease, especially in less developed countries*
- *Develop a perspective on the rank order of chronic diseases, risk factors, and causes of death when disability effects are included*
- *Recognize the increasing contributions of development-related risk factors to the expansion of NCDs*
- *Become aware of institutional and governmental responses to the challenges of managing increasing numbers of older persons and chronically ill patients*

INTRODUCTION

As countries become more developed, changes occur in their populations that alter the types of problems faced by their health care systems and providers. Successful reduction of deaths at younger and adult ages eventually shifts the age distributions so that older persons become an increasingly larger portion of populations. Reductions in deaths related to childbirth, undernutrition, infectious diseases, and injuries allow people to live longer and become more vulnerable to chronic diseases. Although these diseases, as classified in the Global Burden of Disease framework[1] may be secondary to group 1 (infectious diseases,

perinatal, and nutrition related) conditions or group 3 (injuries), this chapter focuses on the increasingly prevalent group 2 conditions (noncommunicable diseases [NCDs]).

Developing as a nation increases access to the products of global markets. As consumers, people often respond to convenience and marketing influences by changing their lifestyle. Generally, as an economy develops, its citizens utilize less exertion to meet the demands of life, at the same time that they experience increased access to food calories from nontraditional sources. The resulting increase in overweight and obesity with associated comorbidities, combined with the adverse effects of increased tobacco and substance abuse, contribute to increased incidence and the younger onset of many chronic diseases. Although the less developed countries often find it difficult to respond to the double burden of communicable and noncommunicable disease, the more developed countries meet the challenges of chronic NCDs by devoting more resources, including labor. Skilled health care workers are recruited from less developed parts of the world to meet these needs. Initially chronic diseases can be managed medically utilizing these expensive resources, but with time even these resources are unable to prevent functional decline and death.

Chronic diseases have recently become the predominant worldwide causes of death and disability in most countries, and that burden is being carried more and more by the developing areas of the world. Institutions and governments are increasingly focusing on the challenges that this transition in the global burden of disease will present to efforts to improve world health. Age is widely acknowledged to strongly influence the pattern and extent of ill health at both the individual and population level. This makes it important to consider demographic and epidemiologic change in populations, as well as their health systems' responses to both individual and population aging.

GLOBAL AGING THROUGH DEMOGRAPHIC CHANGE

Defining Population Aging

Whereas *individual aging* refers to the aging process in a person, *population aging*, in simplistic terms, refers to the process by which older persons, here defined as persons 60 years and older, become a proportionally larger part of a country's or region's total population.[2] This process, also referred to as *demographic aging*, leads to changes in the age structure of a population and a higher median age.

Demographic Drivers of Population Aging

Over the last century, changes in three principal population factors (fertility, mortality, and migration) contributed to global population aging. It was primarily declining fertility and longer life expectancy that reshaped age structures in most countries of the world by shifting relative weight from younger to older segments of a population while international migration played a much less important role.[3] Although one intuitively thinks of changes in longevity when considering why populations age, falling levels of fertility have been the most prominent historical determinant in global population aging.[2,4,5]

Fertility

Although *declining* fertility is the most prominent driver of population aging, fertility-related factors play a multipart role in the aging process. For example, persistently lowered fertility brings about a decline in the proportion of children, which accordingly increases the proportion of older persons. This effect is referred to as aging from the base of the population structure.[6] However, past fertility decline, such as the lowered fertility experienced in some countries during the Great Depression and World War II, has also led to a fall in the growth rate of the older population as the smaller birth cohorts over time reach older ages. However, past fertility increase as experienced in some countries after World War II, has contributed to an increase in the growth rate of the older population. From around 2008 until about 2018, these postwar baby boom cohorts will have been augmenting the numbers of older persons significantly.[4]

Although global fertility is estimated to have been persistently high during the 1700s and 1800s at a total fertility rate (TFR) of around 6.0 children per woman, the second half of the 1900s saw a dramatic decline in global TFR levels, declining from 5.0 for the period 1950–1955 to 2.5 for 2005–2010. As a result of the sustained fertility decline during the 1900s, all 45 developed countries were at or below the replacement level of 2.1 for 2005–2010 with the median 1.5. Highest TFRs for developed countries in 2005–2010 were found in New Zealand, Iceland, Ireland, and the United States at 2.1, and lowest in Bosnia and Herzegovina, Slovakia, Poland, and Japan at 1.2 to 1.3.[7] Fertility decline in the developing countries commenced later but has proceeded at a faster pace. Total fertility fell from 5.4 for 1970–1975 to 2.7 for 2005–2010 with a median TFR of 2.7 children per woman. The TFR for the least developed countries has fallen more slowly, with many of these countries still having TFRs above 5.0. Figure 16.1 illustrates the difference among the development regions. Large disparities also exist among nations within development regions. For example, Hong Kong SAR, China, has the lowest rate among the less developed nations at 0.99 and Niger the highest at 7.2. For the world's two most populous nations, China had an estimated TFR of 1.64 in 2010 and India's was 2.73.[7]

Although there continue to be numerous developing nations with high levels of fertility and relatively low proportions of older persons, it is important to acknowledge that fertility decline in the less developed regions generally has been much more rapid than experienced in the more developed regions, that the decline is expected to continue, and that a particularly sharp reduction is expected for the least developed countries.[7] These countries are therefore expected to age at a more rapid pace than has happened in the developed nations, leaving them with a much shorter time to prepare the policies, infrastructure, health, and other resources to meet the needs associated with rapidly changing demographic and epidemiologic profiles.[4]

Mortality and Life Expectancy

It is intuitive to think that, once mortality is reduced in a population, it will automatically lead to aging of that population. However, mortality reduction influences population dynamics in particular ways according to whether such mortality reductions happen in younger or older ages. Infant and child mortality rates usually are reduced in a population before reduction of adult mortality rates. This means that more infants and children survive in that population; therefore it is common to argue that mortality declines in a population usually first lead to a rejuvenation of that population. In general, countries' demographic histories have shown that such improvements in infant and child mortality, preceded by fertility declines, improved chances of survival for adults to older ages and became a more important factor in population aging.[2–5] It is

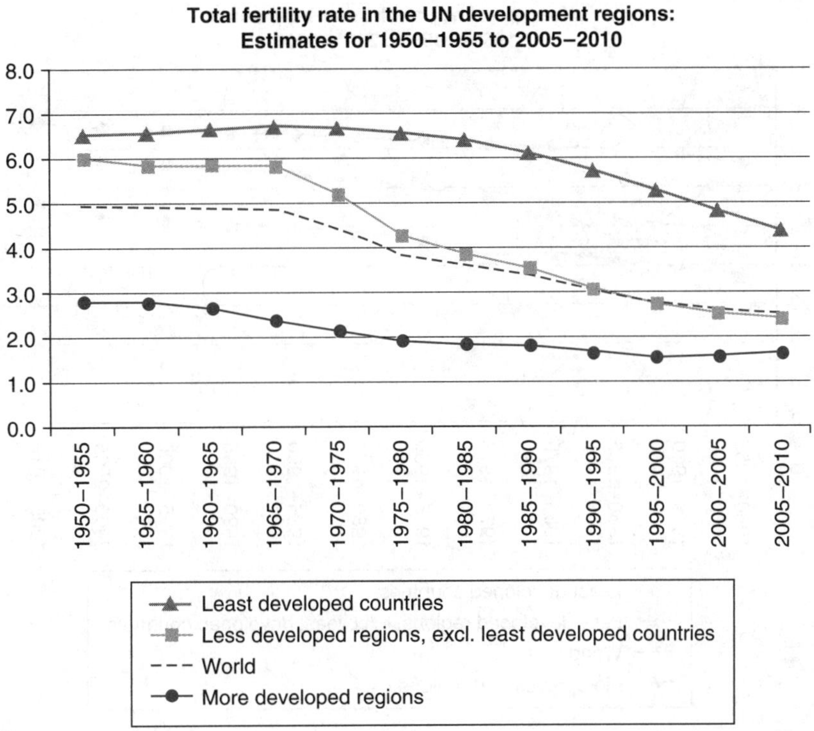

Total fertility rate in the UN development regions:
Estimates for 1950–1955 to 2005–2010

Figure 16-1. Estimated total fertility rate in the United Nations development regions, 1950–1955 to 2005–2010. (Data extracted from United Nations, Department of Economic and Social Affairs, Population Division (2011). *World Population Prospects: The 2010 Revision*, CD-ROM Edition.)

therefore usually at a later stage that declines in adult mortality contribute to population aging.

Since the middle of the previous century, life expectancy at birth increased globally by 20 years, from 47.7 to 67.9 years.[7] Great variations exist between more and less developed regions as shown in Figure 16-2. For example, life expectancy reached 70 years for more developed countries during the late 1960s, whereas this mark has not yet been reached by the populations in less developed countries. Even greater variations exist among nations within the less developed regions, but differences are expected to decrease and more people to survive to older ages. Given current mortality levels, almost 75% of newborns in the world will survive to age 60, and about 33% to age 80. These proportions, respectively, are projected to increase to about 88% and over 50% by the middle of this century. Moreover, gains in life expectancy are expected to be higher at older than younger ages. This means that, not only are more persons surviving to old age, but also that once they reach old age, they tend to live longer[2] (Figure 16-2).

In many of the more developed countries, the numbers of persons of extreme old age are of growing importance. Despite the problems with obtaining accurate age data on oldest old persons, researchers in Europe estimated that the number of persons over age 100 in Europe and Japan increased by 7% annually.[5] The UN Department of Economic and Social Affairs in 2007 estimated that the population of centenarians was about 270,000 as of 2005 and will reach 2.3 million by 2040.[4]

According to UN projections, increases in life expectancy at birth began in the mid-1800s, continued during the 1900s, and will continue to increase in all regions of the world to 2050.[2] Despite global gains in life expectancy at birth being the norm, changes in the sociopolitical and epidemiologic status quo of some countries have been shown to challenge this historical pattern with particular consequences for the process of population aging. In Eastern Europe and the former Soviet Union, for example, the rate of increase in life expectancy had decelerated sharply by the mid-1960s, and male life expectancy declined during the 1970s and 1980s. In some countries, the decline continued into the 1990s. Although causal mechanisms are not clearly understood, the increases in adult male mortality are attributed to a

Life expectancy at birth for both sexes
1950–1955 to 2005–2010

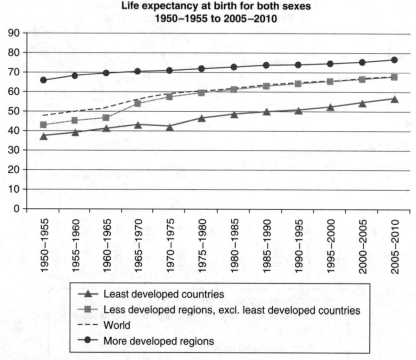

Figure 16-2. Estimates of life expectancy at birth in the UN development regions, 1950–1955 to 2005–2010. (Data extracted from United Nations, Department of Economic and Social Affairs, Population Division (2011). *World Population Prospects: The 2010 Revision,* CD-ROM Edition.)

combination of factors, including poor diet, increased accident and homicide rates, environmental and workplace degradation, but are predominantly due to excessive alcohol consumption.[8]

In other countries, particularly in sub-Saharan Africa, the HIV/AIDS epidemic has had a devastating effect on life expectancy. Because mortality from AIDS usually is concentrated in infant, childhood, and early and middle adult ages, the impact on life expectancy at birth has been shown to be substantial in countries such as Botswana, South Africa, Swaziland, Uganda, and Zimbabwe. Careful analyses of South African mortality data of the 1990s, for example, show marked increases in age-specific death rates in infants and children with a severe increase in young adult mortality. The year 2000 Burden of Disease analysis for South Africa estimated that HIV/AIDS was the cause of almost 40% of premature mortality measured as years of life lost in that year, and would account for as much as 75% of premature mortality by 2010 depending on the efficacy of interventions.[9] The nadir of South African life expectancy was estimated to have occurred in 2005 with life expectancy at birth of 49.6 years for men and 53.8 years for women.[10]

Migration

International migration's role in changing the age distribution of national populations has been far less important compared with fertility and mortality.[2,4] A UN-facilitated assessment of the likely impact of migration as a counterbalance to aging led to the conclusion that, unless the migration flows are of a very large magnitude, inflows of migrants will not be able to rejuvenate national populations. However, there is some evidence that population aging can be influenced in smaller nations, as has been the case in certain Caribbean populations. There the emigration of working-age adults, immigration of foreign retirees, and return-migration of former worker-emigrants contribute to the aging of these populations.[4]

Urbanization of the Older Population

Internal migration also affects the distribution of a country's older population. By 2005, half of the world's older people were living in urban areas, as was half of the total world population by 2007. The delay in urbanization of the total world population reflects the larger, younger, and more rural populations in the developing world. Whereas Latin America has joined

North America, Europe, and Oceania in this urbanization, Africa and Asia remain largely rural populations. Even though the people moving to urban areas tend to be in the young adult ages, available data show that population aging is occurring in all urban and rural populations, except in rural Africa. Due to the lower fertility and mortality characteristics that commonly occur in cities, this population shift is expected to accelerate the transition to an older world population.[11,12]

In spite of the increasing urbanization of today's older populations, most nations continue to have higher percentages of older persons in their rural areas. This is largely the result of rural-to-urban migration of younger people in search of employment with a small contribution by return migration of older persons from urban to rural areas. Regional differences exist, and although older persons in Africa are more likely to live in rural areas than are older persons of other regions, the proportion of urbanized older persons in Latin America and the Caribbean is very similar to the average proportions found in the more developed countries. A marked exception is the Oceania region, which is dominated by the populations of Australia and New Zealand, where the elderly predominantly live in cities.[3] In fact, there is great variability in the percentage of urban people over age 65 compared with the percentage of aged in the total population of the country when cities around the world are compared.[4] Increasing attention is being turned to promoting healthy environments for older urban residents.[5]

Global Extent of Population Aging

Most, if not all nations, at some time in their history had a youthful age structure, but nearly all nations are now experiencing growth in the numbers of their older populations.[4] In 1950–1955, the average annual growth rate of the number of persons older than 60 years at 1.7% was similar to that of the total global population at 1.8%. For 2005–2010, the 60-plus growth rate at 2.6% was more than twice that of the total population at 1.2%. By 2045–2050, the growth rate of the 60-plus population is expected to decline to 1.8%; however, it will still be more than five times that of the total population at 0.3%.[3] In 1950, older persons made up 8% (200 million) of the world population, in 2000, 10% (600 million), and by 2050, the proportion is projected to increase to 22% (2 billion).[13] These numbers indicate a tripling of the population 60-plus over each of the two consecutive 50-year periods,[13] implying that the global older population is projected to increase by an average of 28 million persons per year, or approximately 78,000 per day between 2000 and 2050. Increasing numbers hold both opportunities and challenges for countries, in particular for those five countries projected to have more than 50 million people older than 60 years by 2050: China (440 million), India (316 million), United States (111 million), Indonesia (72 million), and Brazil (64 million).[3]

Rectangularization of Population Age Structures

These demographic changes lead to changes in the balance between age groups. The population pyramid is a frequently used way to graphically represent the age and sex distributions of a population. Historically the shape has been pyramidal due to the preponderance of people in younger age groups, with smaller proportions in the older age groups. As the adult age group becomes proportionally larger, the pyramid shape commonly changes to a dome shape, after which it rectangularizes, as shown in Figure 16-3.[7]

Extent and Rate of Population Aging in the More and Less Developed Regions

In general, the more developed countries are in a more advanced stage of their demographic transitions to lower fertility and mortality, and already by 1950, developed countries as a group had a higher proportion of population ages 60 and older (12%) compared with developing countries (6%). Developed countries continue having a larger proportion at 21% compared with 8% in developing countries.[3] Among the world's major regions, Europe has had the highest proportion of older persons for many decades, and it is projected to remain as such for the next five decades. Except for Japan, the world's 25 demographically oldest countries were all in Europe. Among the oldest in 2012 by percentage of population 60 years and older, were Japan (32%), Italy (27%), Germany (27%), Finland (26%), Greece (25%), Sweden (25%), and Belgium (24%). The North America and Oceania regions have somewhat lower, but still relatively high percentages, with Canada and the United States, respectively, at 21% and 19%, and Australia and New Zealand, respectively, at 20% and 19%, in 2012. Altogether, 22% of persons living in the more developed regions were 60 years and older in the year 2012. This number is expected to grow to 32% by 2050.[5] Before the middle of the current century, some of these countries may have more grandparents than children under age 18.[4]

In contrast, 9% of the population of developing countries was 60 years and older in 2012. Of the UN-classified major areas, Africa (6%) housed the smallest proportions of older persons globally. Some less developed countries were further advanced in demographic change and had higher proportions

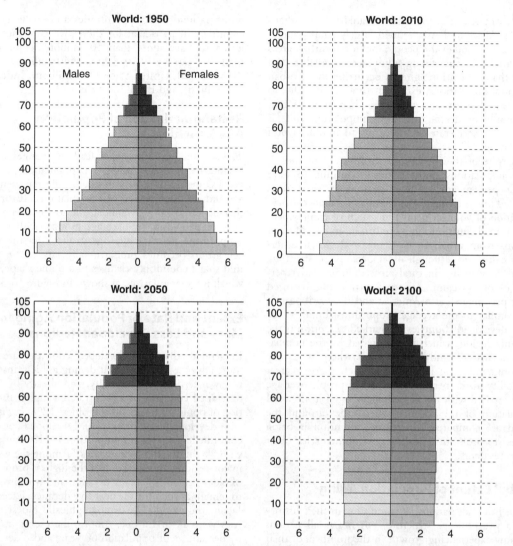

Figure 16-3. World population by age groups and sex: percentage of the total population in 1950, 2010, 2050, and 2100, respectively. (Data extracted from United Nations, Department of Economic and Social Affairs, Population Division (2011). *World Population Prospects: The 2010 Revision.*)

in 2012, including Tunisia (10%), Singapore (15%), Israel (15%), Argentina (15%), Cuba (18%), and Uruguay (19%). These were still below the average 22% of the more developed countries.[5] By 2050 it is projected that, although Japan will still lead with 42% of its population over age 60, Bosnia and Herzegovina (40%), Cuba (39%), and the Republic of Korea (39%) will have entered the top 10 list.[14]

Proportions by themselves, however, do not give a real sense of the aging momentum in the world's countries. Of larger public health concern is the total number of older persons and the annual growth rate of the older population. Compared with the relatively slow process of population aging experienced so far by most developed countries, population aging in most developing countries is occurring at a faster pace and, as such, over a shorter period. Furthermore, many developing countries have large populations, and large numbers of older persons live in those countries despite comprising relatively low proportions of the total population.[3] In contrast to 1950–1955 when the number of persons 60+ was growing slightly more rapidly in the more developed (1.9% per year) than less developed regions (1.6% per year), the current average annual growth rate is 1.9% in the more developed regions and 3.0% in the less developed regions. By the middle of this century, the growth rate of the 60+ population in the less developed regions (2.1%) is projected to be over five times that in the more developed regions (0.4%), and the growth rate of the 60+ population in the least developed countries (3.5%), about nine times that in the more developed regions.[3]

With such growth rates, the concentration of persons 60+ in the less developed world will intensify, and many individual developing countries can expect large increases in their numbers of older persons. Over half (54%) of the world's older persons lived in less developed regions in 1950. This proportion rose to 64% in 2009 and is projected to rise to nearly 80% by 2050. Drastic increases in the older population are expected in several developing countries, spanning a wide range of development levels. For the period 2011–2050, particularly large percentage increases are expected for the United Arab Emirates (35%), Bahrain (29%), Iran (26%), and Oman (25%).[5]

SOCIOECONOMIC EFFECTS OF AGING ON POPULATIONS

Dependency Ratios

Dependency ratios, a commonly used measure of potential social support needs, are a way of describing how the gradual rectangularization of age group distributions will produce socioeconomic effects. These ratios compare the part of the population expected to be in some sense dependent to that part that is likely to be economically productive. This likelihood is estimated using age groupings because aggregate data about individual productivity is not available. Those under age 15 and over age 64 are considered to be unproductive in economic terms, and those aged 15 to 64 are presumed to provide direct or indirect support to those in the dependent ages. It can be argued that these assumptions are not accurate for many populations. For example, in developed countries educational requirements can defer productivity until age 20+, and many adults are economically active until 70 or longer. Additionally, in some developing countries with high unemployment levels, productivity in the working age population is not optimal, and large proportions do not provide direct or indirect support. Also disability in people ages 15 to 64 may remove them and often a caregiver from the working population. In the future, more accurate measures of the number of workers and dependents will be needed for economic projections, but this measure will be used as an approximation of the burden of dependency for the purposes of this chapter (Figure 16-4a and 16-4b).

Child, old-age, and total dependency ratios for the world population, and for the more, less, and least developed nations are shown in Figure 16-4a, and the composition of the total dependency ratio for the development regions and the world population are illustrated in Figure 16-4b.

Due to the large size of their populations, the less developed regions have ratios that are much closer to the world's ratios compared with those of the more developed regions. The total dependency ratio of the world population decreased from the 1970s and is projected to continue declining to around 2015 as those born in years of high birth rates have aged into the productive age groups and as fewer children were produced in succeeding generations. Around 2020 the total dependency ratio is projected to begin to increase due to the rapidly growing older age groups. In the more developed regions, the old-age share of the total dependency ratio was already large by 2010 (49%) and is projected to increase to over 60% by 2050. Figure 16-4b illustrates very small increases in the old-age component in less developed nations until about 2015 after which the increase is projected to become larger. Less than half of their dependents are projected to be older persons by 2050 (41%); however, this is a large increase from the approximate 10% that older persons accounted for in 1950. In the least developed countries, the old-age share has increased very slowly since 1950, is expected to increase more rapidly around 2025, and will constitute about 20% of the total dependency by 2050.[7]

Delayed Demographic Transition as Productivity Opportunity

Almost all of the increase (from 2.8 to 4.1 billion people) in the world population's working age group will occur in the less developed regions. In contrast, this age group in the developed regions began declining in 2005 and will be 15% smaller in 2050. These demographic trends have been said to present an opportunity for the less developed regions to utilize their higher proportion of productive workers to improve economic conditions in their countries. It is, however, important to note that the benefits associated herewith are not automatic but depend on sound macroeconomic policies that increase employment opportunity, promote productive investment, and ensure a stable socioeconomic environment.[11]

Living Arrangements of Older Persons

A 2005 UN study found that one of seven older persons live alone, and most of these are women. In developing regions, 7% of the older persons live alone, whereas 25% of those in developed regions do so. The trend in many developed countries for older people to more often live alone has started to

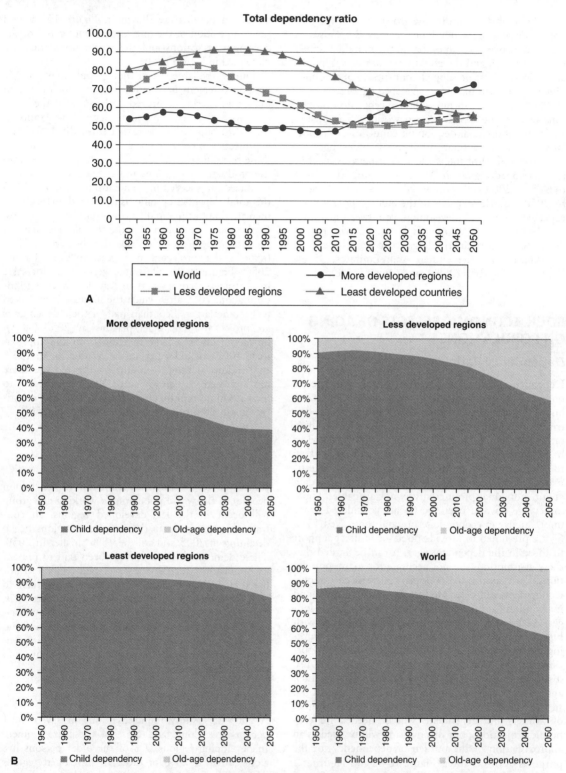

Figure 16-4. (a) Total dependency ratio: world and development regions, 1950–2050. (b) Composition of the total dependency ratio: development regions and world, 1950–2050.

decline in some countries, perhaps due to factors such as an increase in the age when children leave home, and possibly also due to greater survival to oldest-old ages where a greater need exists for live-in assistance or institutionalization. As people become very old, they have increasing functional disability and eventually need assistance with basic activities of daily living. In some societies, these needs can be managed as three- and even four-generation households become more common. In some developing countries this happens more in families with higher socioeconomic status (SES). In a number of countries, labor migration of adult children has been known as a reason for skipped-generation households, but recent research has found that such households are becoming more common in countries where children live with grandparents due to loss of their parents to HIV infection. Older women are more likely than older men to live in such living arrangements. In more developed economies, the perceived demand for family income is pushing more family members into the workforce, leaving fewer caregivers in the home. Ultimately, greater demands are placed on institutions to assist family caregivers. In poor economies, analogous situations of greater labor force participation and fewer caregivers in the home exist, but little is known about how older persons cope where no institutions, formal homecare, or assisted-living options exist to help care for dependent older persons.[12]

CHALLENGES OF POPULATION AGING

Shifting Age Structures

The shifts in age structures associated with population aging hold important implications for a broad range of economic, political, and social conditions. The older population is growing faster than the total population in both more and less developed nations, and huge increases continue to be experienced in the numbers of older persons. More persons are surviving to older age, and once they reach older age, they tend to live longer. As more persons live longer, retirement, retirement funds, social grants, and other social benefits tend to extend over longer periods of time, necessitating changes in social security systems.[5] Having more people who live longer, results in rising demands for health services and increasing medical costs. In general, health conditions decline and frailty and disability increase with advancing age, so the growth in the numbers of this oldest-old age group is of particular concern. The increase in this group suggests an increase in the demand for chronic care, rehabilitative care, palliative care, and other types of long-term care.[5,15] These, in turn, promote growing institutional populations and an increased demand for

appropriately trained health care staff where institutions are affordable, as well as an increased demand for informal caregivers where institutions are not an option.

Shifting Fertility, Mortality, and Migration Patterns

An outcome of persistent fertility decline, likely to be of more importance in the less developed nations, relates to the progressive decline in the availability of kin on whom future cohorts of older persons can rely for support.[2] Fewer family members are available to provide assistance with activities of daily living and disability, life management, financial and subsistence support, and informal long-term care in frailty and severe illness.

As more people live longer through changes in mortality in most of the world's nations, various socioeconomic challenges are posed at the societal level. In affected nations, AIDS-specific mortality diminishes a crucial support base (income-generating and/or care giving children), producing thereby socioeconomic challenges at societal, community, and individual levels. Older persons are commonly involved with the living and care giving arrangements of AIDS-sick persons and their dependents in many affected countries. Although it is a common phenomenon in some of these countries that many older persons, in particular those in multigenerational households, assist in raising their grandchildren, the AIDS epidemic has brought added responsibilities, concerns, and stressors to many affected older persons. These include care giving for a relatively unknown disease; a greater burden of housework tasks; dealing with the stigmatization of the disease and those living with the disease; the risk of HIV infection through care giving activities; extra demands on older caregivers' financial resources to cover health care costs related to AIDS-ill children, costs related to raising and nurturing the dependents of AIDS-ill children, and funeral costs; as well as the loss of current and future financial support from the ill child.[16,17]

Although international migration usually does not play a major role in population aging, internal migration may pose challenges to the aging of local populations within country boundaries. At the familial or household level, internal migration in the form of rural-to-urban movement in some countries may be disadvantageous to older persons who lose their traditional care giving base (in some communities the only local support base) as children emigrate. At the community and local level, older persons may be negatively affected through a weakened local workforce resulting in a diminished pooling of taxpayers' resources, in turn effectuating lesser access to health, welfare, or recreation infrastructure and resources in the form of health centers, health personnel, social welfare centers, social workers, and social and cultural events.[18] Lack of amenities, services and infrastructure, and harsh living conditions in many rural areas pose difficulties for older persons. The provision of health, social welfare, and other support services to ill, disabled, and frail older persons in rural areas continue to present particular challenges to many governments around the world.[4] Also, the provision of services to older persons is likely to present challenges in both urban and rural areas where youthful age structures stimulate an emphasis on infant/child and reproductive health. These challenges related to fertility, mortality, and migration will be more of a concern in less developed countries with limited resources and less preparedness for an aging population than is the case in more developed countries.

Increasing Female Share

Due to their greater life expectancy, women constitute a large majority of the 60+ population in most countries. The female share increases with age, and women's survival advantages are anticipated to continue so that by 2050 only 38% of the 80+ population will be men. This increasing female share is relevant to public policy because older women are more likely to be widowed; dependent on social support; and to have less education. They also usually have less work experience and access to income-generating opportunities, assets, and private income sources. The latter socioeconomic characteristics may stem from lifelong gender disadvantages in formal market opportunities, and women's greater burden of providing care for the sick, frail, and disabled. These issues have implications for social support and public planning.[2–5]

Increasing Prevalence of Chronic Disease and Disability

It is clear that the world is facing unprecedented magnitudes and speed of population aging. The timing and rapidity of population aging are being experienced differently in developed and developing nations, and as the relative size of the youth, working-age, and older-age components of populations change, the shifting weights of these broad age groups are likely to increase social, economic, and political pressures on societies. Population aging has become a well-publicized phenomenon and public concern in most developed nations, but there is much less awareness and public concern in developing nations. This is despite the fact that many developing countries are aging at a much faster rate than countries in the developed world, and that the numbers of older persons in developing

countries exceed those in developed nations. The rapidity and compressed time frame within which these changes are happening in the developing world, and the fact that it is occurring on relatively larger population bases than in the developed world, pose particular challenges to social and economic institutions in nations with scarce resources.[15]

As individual longevity increases, frailty, chronic disease, and disability rise while physical, mental, and cognitive capacities decline.[5] At the societal level, the demographic aging of populations is directly related to fundamental changes in the health and disease patterns within a population as epidemiologic change progresses from the predominance of infectious, parasitic, and nutritional disease to the predominance of NCDs.[18]

THE EPIDEMIOLOGIC TRANSITION TO NONCOMMUNICABLE DISEASES

Historically, the health status and disease profile of human societies were linked to their level of social and economic development. With industrialization, the major causes of death and disability in more developed societies shifted from a predominance of nutritional deficiency related and infectious (group 1) diseases to diseases classified as NCDs (group 2), such as cardiovascular disease, cancer, and diabetes. This epidemiologic transition can occur within organ-specific diseases as well as between different disease categories, with childhood infections and malnutrition being substituted by adult chronic diseases and rheumatic heart disease by coronary heart disease.[15,19,20]

Trends in Communicable and Noncommunicable Diseases

Whereas communicable diseases were previously the main cause of death, improvement in living conditions, the management of infections, and the advent of vaccinations caused NCDs to proliferate, especially in Western countries. NCDs (cardiovascular disease, diabetes, cancer, chronic pulmonary disease, and mental illness) have increased the demand for health care in these countries. By the turn of the 21st century, NCDs were present across the globe and showed an increase even in developing countries. However, developing countries must still deal with the challenges of the double burden of NCDs and communicable diseases because the latter have not been eliminated.[15] In the latter part of the 20th century, the leading causes of the disease burden were communicable diseases and perinatal conditions resulting from malnutrition, poor sanitation and hygiene, and unsafe water (Table 16-1).

In 2008, of the estimated 57 million global deaths, 36 million (63%) were attributed to NCDs. Whereas infectious disease deaths are expected to decline, the

Table 16-1. Evolution of Noncommunicable Diseases (NCDs) in Developing Countries (in millions and percentage distribution 1990-2020) (Boutayeb, 2005).

	Non-communicable Disease	Communicable Disease + Maternal + Perinatal + Nutritional	Injuries	Total
1990	18.7 (47%)	16.6 (42%)	4.2 (11%)	39.5 (100%)
2000	25.0 (56%)	14.6 (33%)	5.0 (11%)	45.0 (100%)
2020	36.6 (69%)	9.0 (17%)	7.4 (14%)	53.0 (100%)

From: Boutayeb A, Boutayeb S. The burden of noncommunicable disease in developing countries. *Int J for Equity in Health* 2005; 4(2). http://www.equityhealthj.com/content/4/1/2

annual NCD deaths are projected to reach 55 million by 2030. Close to 29 million, 80% of all NCD deaths in 2008, happened in low- and middle-income countries. Nearly half (48%) of NCD deaths in low- and middle-income countries occur under age 70, compared with 25% in high-income countries and with the global average of 44%.[15]

Africa is the only region to still have more deaths from infectious diseases than from NCDs, but that will change because it is one of the fastest growing regions for NCD death prevalence. The change will be greatest in sub-Saharan Africa where NCDs will cause 46% of all deaths by 2030, compared with 28% in 2008. South Asia will see the portion of deaths caused by NCDs increase from 51% to 72% over the same period.[20]

Risk factors and disease patterns in these regions differ substantially. In low-income countries, underweight, unsafe water, poor sanitation and hygiene, unsafe sex, suboptimal breastfeeding, and indoor smoke from solid fuels are the leading risk factors causing disability-related life years (DALYs). The top four diseases causing DALYs continue to be infectious diseases.[21] Of the total 7.6 million children who died before 5 years of age in 2010, 4.4 million (58%) died of infectious diseases. In sub-Saharan Africa, malaria was still a major killer causing about 15% of under-5 deaths in the region[22] (Table 16-2).

For middle-income countries, alcohol use, high blood pressure, tobacco use, overweight/obesity, and high blood glucose are the leading risk factors, and depression, ischemic heart disease, cerebrovascular disease, and road traffic accidents lead the diseases or injuries causing DALYs. Lower respiratory infections are the highest infectious cause, in fifth place (Table 16-3).

In the high-income countries, tobacco is definitely the leading risk factor, with alcohol use, overweight/obesity, high blood pressure, and high blood glucose completing the top five.[21] As in the middle-income countries, unipolar depression leads the causes of

Table 16-2. Major burden of disease: leading 10 selected risk factors and leading 10 diseases in low-income countries, 2004.

Risk factors	% DALYs	Disease or injury	% DALYs
Childhood underweight	9.9	Lower respiratory infections	9.3
Unsafe water, sanitation, hygiene	6.3	Diarrheal diseases	7.2
Unsafe sex	6.2	HIV/AIDS	5.2
Suboptimal breast feeding	4.1	Malaria	4.0
Indoor smoke from solid fuel	4.0	Prematurity and low birth weight	3.9
Vitamin A deficiency	2.4	Neonatal infections and other	3.8
High blood pressure	2.2	Birth asphyxia and birth trauma	3.6
Alcohol use	2.1	Unipolar depressive disorder	3.2
High blood glucose	1.9	Ischemic heart disease	3.1
Zinc deficiency	1.7	Tuberculosis	2.7

HIV /AIDS, human immunodeficiency/acquired immunodeficiency syndrome
Sources: World Health Organization. *Global health risk. Mortality and burden of disease attributable to selected major risks.* Geneva: World Health Organization, 2009. http://www.who.int/healthinfo/global_burden_disease/GlobalHealthRisks_report_full.pdf & World Health Organization. *The Global Burden of Disease: 2004 Update.* Geneva: World Health Organization, 2008. http://www.who.int/healthinfo/global_burden_disease/GBD_report_2004update_full.pdf

Table 16-3. Major burden of disease: leading 10 selected risk factors and leading 10 diseases and injuries, middle-income countries.

Risk factors	% DALYs	Disease or injury	% DALYs
Alcohol use	7.6	Unipolar depressive disorders	5.1
High blood pressure	5.4	Ischemic heart disease	5.0
Tobacco use	5.4	Cerebrovascular disease	4.8
Overweight and obesity	3.6	Road traffic accidents	3.7
High blood glucose	3.4	Lower respiratory infections	2.8
Unsafe sex	3.0	COPD	2.8
Physical inactivity	2.7	HIV/AIDS	2.6
High cholesterol	2.5	Alcohol use disorders	2.6
Occupational risks	2.3	Refractive errors	2.4
Unsafe water, sanitation, hygiene	2.0	Diarrheal diseases	2.3

COPD, Chronic Obstructive Pulmonary Disease
Sources: World Health Organization. *Global health risk. Mortality and burden of disease attributable to selected major risks.* Geneva: World Health Organization, 2009 http://www.who.int/healthinfo/global_burden_disease/GlobalHealthRisks_report_full.pdf & World Health Organization. *The Global Burden of Disease: 2004 Update.* Geneva: World Health Organization, 2008. http://www.who.int/healthinfo/global_burden_disease/GBD_report_2004update_full.pdf

disease or injury-related DALYs with dementia in fourth place following ischemic heart disease and cerebrovascular disease (Table 16-4).

The tables use DALYs for the measure of global burden of disease. DALYs is a metric that combines years of life lost due to premature death and years lived with disability (YLDs) based on severity and duration of nonfatal outcomes. Thus one DALY is viewed as one year of "healthy" life lost, and the measured burden of disease is the gap between a

population's health and that of a normative global reference population with high life expectancy lived in full health. See Chapter 2 for a more detailed description of these measures.

Global trends show a declining communicable disease burden, but HIV/AIDS was the second leading cause of mortality and morbidity among adults age 15 to 59 years in 2004[23] (Table 16-5). In 2007, sub-Saharan Africa, with 11% to 12% of the world's population, had 67% of the people living with

Table 16-4. Major burden of disease: leading 10 selected risk factors and leading 10 diseases and injuries, high income countries, 2004.

Risk factors	% DALYs	Disease or injury	% DALYs
Tobacco use	10.7	Unipolar depressive disorders	8.2
Alcohol use	6.7	Ischemic heart disease	6.3
Overweight and obesity	6.5	Cerebrovascular disease	3.9
High blood pressure	6.1	Alzheimer's and other dementias	3.6
High blood glucose	4.9	Alcohol use disorders	3.4
Physical inactivity	4.1	Hearing loss adult onset	3.4
High cholesterol	3.4	COPD	3.0
Illicit drugs	2.1	Diabetes mellitus	3.0
Occupational risks	1.5	Trachea, bronchus, lung cancers	3.0
Low fruit and vegetable intake	1.3	Road traffic accidents	2.6

COPD, Chronic Obstructive Pulmonary Disease
Sources: World Health Organization. *Global health risk. Mortality and burden of disease attributable to selected major risks.* Geneva: World Health Organization, 2009 http://www.who.int/healthinfo/global_burden_disease/GlobalHealthRisks_report_full.pdf & World Health Organization. *The Global Burden of Disease: 2004 Update.* Geneva: World Health Organization, 2008. http://www.who.int/healthinfo/global_burden_disease/GBD_report_2004update_full.pdf

Table 16-5. Leading disease burden (DALYs) among adults (15-59 years) worldwide, 2004.

Rank	Cause	DALYs (000)
1	Unipolar depressive disorders	56,532
2	HIV/AIDS	47,514
3	Road traffic injuries	30,240
4	Ischemic heart disease	30,204
5	Tuberculosis	27,556
6	Alcohol use disorders	22,392
7	Hearing loss (adult onset)	20,589
8	Cerebrovascular disease	19,689
9	Violence	19,374
10	Self-inflicted injuries	17,345

HIV/AIDS, human immunodeficiency/acquired immunodeficiency syndrome
Source: World Health Organization. *The global burden of disease*: 2004 update. Geneva: World Health Organization, 2008. http://www.who.int/healthinfo/global_burden_disease/GBD_report_2004update_full.pdf

Table 16-6. Leading disease burden (DALYs) among adults over age 60 worldwide, 2004.

Rank	Cause	DALYs (000)
1	Ischemic heart disease	32,025
2	Cerebrovascular disease	26,081
3	Chronic obstructive pulmonary disease	15,994
4	Alzheimer's and other dementias	9,244
5	Lower respiratory infections	7,902
6	Refractive error	7,737
7	Diabetes mellitus	6,901
8	Hearing loss, adult onset	6,768
9	Trachea, bronchus, lung cancers	6,164
10	Cataract	5,585

Source: World Health Organization. *The global burden of disease: 2004 update*. Geneva: World Health Organization, 2008. http://www.who.int/healthinfo/global_burden_disease/GBD_report_2004update_full.pdf

HIV/AIDS, 70% of new HIV infections, and 75% of AIDS-related deaths. In South Africa, it is estimated that over 5 million persons (a fifth of adults) are living with HIV infection. HIV/AIDS has reversed previous gains in life expectancy in these countries.[24] In 2006, Mathers and Loncar recalculated the global mortality and burden of disease projections, and HIV/AIDS was projected to become the number one cause of DALYs lost in all world age groups at 12.1% of total lost in 2030. It was predicted to be the top cause in middle- and low-income countries by that year, but to not be in the top 10% of total DALYs in high-income countries.[25] Fortunately, the number of AIDS-related deaths globally peaked at 2.2 million in 2005 and decreased to an estimated 1.8 million in 2010. Increased availability of antiretroviral therapy and public health measures may bend the curve downward significantly in future 2030 projections.[26]

In contrast to the younger age group, the burden of NCDs is much greater in the older population (Table 16-6). Population aging and an increase in the prevalence of risk factors have accelerated the epidemic of NCDs in many developing countries. With a large proportion of the world's population living in developing countries, where morbidity rates and risk factor levels are high and death occurs at a relatively younger age, the absolute number of DALYs attributable to each risk factor is greater in these countries than that in developed countries. Table 16-7 uses 2004 data to estimate the prevalence of moderate and severe disability caused by the most common disabling ailments for ages 0 to 59 and 60+ in high-income countries versus low- and middle-income countries.[23]

Case Study of Utility of the DALY Measure

At age 56, Mrs. Brown is hospitalized after a stroke paralyzed one side of her body. She is a widow and has been disabled for 2 years due to depression and complications of diabetes. Her daughter had to quit working 2 years ago to provide care after Mrs. Brown had a below-knee amputation. Their financial resources are exhausted, and government assistance is being sought to cover the costs of a nursing home for Mrs. Brown. Her institutionalization is likely to be long term since her daughter must return to work.

This case study demonstrates how the DALY better represents the total costs to society compared with simply listing patients' diseases and functional limitations. The lost earnings of Mrs. Brown's daughter and the balance of that loss with the costs of long-term nursing home care are much more difficult to capture. In the United States in 2008, the aggregate of lost wages, pension, and Social Security benefits for caregivers of parents was estimated to be nearly $3 trillion.[27] In some nations, incentives to keep working-age people in the workforce may lead to increased institutionalization of older and disabled people.

Global Estimates of Disability Prevalence

The two primary sources of estimates of global disability are the World Health Survey (WHS) and the Global Burden of Disease Study (GBD). The WHS is based on a household survey of people over 18 using

Table 16-7. Estimated prevalence of moderate and severe disability (millions) for leading disabling conditions by age, for high-income and low- and middle-income countries, 2004

	High-income countries				Low- and middle-income countries			
	Disabling condition	0-59 years	Disabling condition	60-years and over	Disabling condition	0-59 years	Disabling condition	60 years and over
1	Depression	15.8	Hearing loss	18.5	Depression	77.6	Hearing loss	43.9
2	Refractive errors	7.7	Osteoarthritis	8.1	Refractive errors	68.1	Refractive errors	39.8
3	Hearing loss	7.4	Refractive errors	6.4	Hearing loss	54.3	Cataracts	31.4
4	Alcohol dependence and problem use	7.3	Alzheimer's and other dementias	6.2	Unintentional injuries	35.4	Osteoarthritis	19.4
5	Drug dependence and problem use	3.7	Macular degeneration	6.0	Infertility due to unsafe abortion and maternal sepsis	32.5	Macular degeneration	15.1
6	Bipolar disorder	3.3	Chronic obstructive pulmonary disease	4.5	Alcohol dependence and problem use	31.0	Ischemic heart disease	11.9
7	Asthma	2.9	Ischemic heart disease	2.2	Cataract	20.8	Chronic obstructive pulmonary disease	8.0
8	Unintentional injuries	2.8	Cerebrovascular disease	2.2	Bipolar disorders	17.6	Glaucoma	7.9
9	Schizophrenia	2.2	Rheumatoid arthritis	1.7	Asthma	15.1	Alzheimer's and other dementias	7.0
10	Osteoarthritis	1.9	Glaucoma	1.5	Osteoarthritis	14.1	Unintentional injuries	5.7
11	Panic disorder	1.9	Cataract & Unintentional injuries	1.1 1.1	Schizophrenia	13.1	Cerebrovascular disease	4.9

Source: World Health Organization. The global burden of disease: 2004 update. Geneva: World Health Organization, 2008. http://www.who.int/healthinfo/global_burden_disease/GBD_report_2004update_full.pdf.

data from 59 countries obtained during 2002–2004. It indicated that 2.2% (92 million people) had very significant difficulties and 15.6% (650 million) had significant difficulties with everyday functions. Significant difficulty prevalence ranged from 11.8% in higher income countries to 18% in lower income countries. For people over age 60, the prevalence of disability was 43.4% in lower income countries compared with 29.5% in higher income countries. Analysis of the GBD data from 2004 estimated that 15.3% of the world population had "moderate or severe disability" and 2.9% had "severe disability."

Extrapolating the data to include everyone over age 15 and using 2010 population estimates, there were between approximately 785 million (15.6% using WHS data) and 875 million (19.4% using GBD data) people living with disability at that time. Large increases in NCD-related YLDs are expected in the rapidly developing regions of the world.[28]

Predominant Noncommunicable Diseases

Cardiovascular Disease

Cardiovascular diseases (CVDs) are a group of disorders of the heart and blood vessels, and they include hypertension, coronary heart disease, peripheral vascular disease, and cerebrovascular disease. These diseases predominate among the NCDs as causes of death (Table 2-6). The World Health Organization (WHO) estimates of the top 10 causes of death for all age groups in 2008 maintain ischemic heart disease (12.8%) and stroke and cerebrovascular disease (10.8%) as the top two causes, and project that to continue until 2030.[23]

Changes in lifestyle brought about by industrialization, urbanization, and globalization of food supplies have led to a rapid increase in CVDs in developing countries. Tobacco use, alcohol, physical inactivity, and an unhealthy diet are all risk factors for CVDs. By 2010, CVDs had become the leading cause of death in almost all developing countries with the exception of Africa. Nearly 80% of cardiovascular deaths are occurring in low- and middle-income countries, and they are occurring at a younger age than in high-income countries.[29,30] Projections based on 2002 data for 2030 maintain them in the top two positions, except in the low-income countries where HIV/AIDS pushes cerebrovascular disease into third place.[25]

Diabetes

Diabetes is among the top ten causes of disease and deaths worldwide. The number of people with diabetes in the world is expected to increase from 171 million in 2000 to 336 million in 2030.[31] In contrast to developed countries, diabetes in developing countries often affects a much younger age group. Complications of diabetes such as retinopathy, foot ulceration and amputation, nephropathy, and heart disease exacerbate the burden. Diabetes and its complications are costly to manage and impose great challenges to health care systems of developing countries. Globally, expenditures on diabetes are expected to total $US 376 billion and to reach $US 490 billion by 2030. In 2010, 12% of all world health expenditures were expected to be for treatment for diabetes-related illness.[32]

Cancer

Cancer becomes more common with age and thus is a growing cause of mortality throughout the world. An estimated 12.7 million new cases and 7.6 million cancer deaths (4.8 million in economically developing countries) occurred worldwide in 2008. This burden is expected to grow to 21.4 million new cancer cases and 13.2 million cancer deaths by 2030.[33] From 2008 until 2030, the cancer increase is projected to be 82% in low- and 70% in lower- and middle-income countries compared with 58% in upper-middle- and 40% in high-income countries, largely as a result of an increase in the number of older adults, an increase in tobacco consumption, and changes in lifestyle.[29] Lung cancer is currently the most common cancer and the most deadly, causing 1.38 million deaths in 2008, or 18.2% of total cancer deaths.[34] Its prevalence increases directly with increasing tobacco consumption. Oral cavity, pharynx, and esophageal cancer types are correlated to alcohol and tobacco use as well as micronutrient deficiency.

Colorectal cancer is in the top five causes of cancer death in both developed and developing countries, and has a two to three times higher incidence and mortality rate in the developed countries. Probably the greatest factor for that difference is that developed countries have more aged populations, but dietary and lifestyle factors have also been associated. Breast cancer has over twice the incidence per 100,000 in developed countries (66.4) compared with developing countries (27.3), but only 50% greater mortality. Most cases in developing countries are only detected at an advanced stage, and even if detected early, treatment is often unaffordable.[33]

Currently about 15% of new cancer diagnoses are attributable to infectious causes, but the prevalence is much higher in developing countries (26%) than in developed countries (8%). The most common of these, cancers of the stomach, liver, and cervix, are partially preventable with treatment or immunization against an infecting agent. Cervical cancer is the second most common cause of new cancer cases and deaths for women in developing countries. Effective screening programs and early detection have led to a marked decline in cervical cancer incidence and mortality in developed countries. The prevalence is increasing in low- and middle-income countries owing to their limited health care resources and a lack of preventive strategies within their health systems.[33]

Chronic Respiratory Disease

It was estimated that chronic obstructive pulmonary disease caused 3.0% of the disease- or injury-related DALYs in 2004 (Table 16-4). Worldwide in 2011, the WHO estimated that 235 million people suffer from asthma and that it is the most common chronic disease in children.[35] In 2004, an estimated 64 million people worldwide suffered from chronic obstructive pulmonary disease (COPD) or related diseases. Three million deaths were attributed to these diseases in 2005. Overall, 90% of deaths are occurring in low- and middle-income countries. Primarily caused by tobacco smoke, other risk factors for COPD are indoor and outdoor air pollution, including occupational dusts and chemicals and frequent lower respiratory infections during childhood. By 2030, COPD is expected to become the third most common cause of mortality in the world.[36] In most developing countries, death from respiratory diseases such as COPD and asthma occurs at a younger age because of poverty and its associated increase in respiratory infections, and poor access to health services.

Neuropsychiatric Conditions

The WHO's global status report on NCDs for 2011 listed mental health conditions as the leading cause of DALYs for the world's population, accounting for 37% of healthy years lost to NCDs. Unipolar depressive disorders cause nearly a third of mental health DALYs with alcohol use disorders (11.9%), schizophrenia (8.4%), and bipolar affective disorder (7.2%) also causing significant proportions. Over the next 20 years, mental health illnesses are projected to cost the world economy US$ 16.1 trillion.[37] The burden of depression is significantly higher for women than for men, and women have a higher burden of anxiety disorders, migraine, and late-onset dementias. In addition, a large proportion of people with chronic physical diseases such as diabetes, hypertension, malignancies, and HIV/AIDS experience concurrent depression, which significantly interferes with their adherence to health care regimens.

Mental illnesses have such a large effect on DALY losses due to their early age of onset. As these disorders and other chronic diseases are better managed and more people live to an advanced age, dementia will become a far greater contributor to disability and death. In 2008, Alzheimer's and other dementias were estimated at 5.6% of the world's mental health DALYs.[37] Traditional risk factors for CVD have been associated with increased risk of both Alzheimer's disease and vascular dementia. A 2005 study showed that the presence of smoking, hypertension, high cholesterol, and diabetes at midlife was associated with a 20% to 40% increase in the risk of late-life dementia. This risk increased exponentially with an increase in the number of risk factors.[38] It was estimated in 2010 that there were 35.6 million people worldwide with dementia, which was expected to almost double to 65.7 million by 2030. Most of this increase will occur in low- and middle-income countries, increasing from 58% of the world's demented people living there to 71% in 2050.[39]

Other Causes of Disability

Perinatal and infectious diseases to which children are most susceptible currently are the leading causes of DALYs for low-income countries. The main reason that more developed regions (excluding Eastern Europe) have much higher death rates from NCDs compared with other regions is their more aged populations. This obscures the fact that that there is greater risk of dying from NCDs acquired in low-income countries with younger populations.[19]

Risk Factors

In developing countries, urbanization and globalization lead to change from a diet rich in fruit, vegetables, and fiber to a diet high in saturated fat, sugar, and salt. The latter diet, combined with lowered levels of physical activity, alcohol abuse, and tobacco use, is a risk factor for many NCDs.

Tobacco Use

Although tobacco consumption is on the decrease in most developed countries, it is increasing in developing countries. A total of 80% of the 1 billion smokers worldwide live in low- and middle-income countries. Tobacco use increases the risk of lung cancer 20- to 30-fold and the risk of dying from coronary heart disease by 2- to 3-fold. Tobacco is a causative factor of between 80% and 90% of esophageal, laryngeal, and oral cavity cancers and exacerbates chronic respiratory diseases such as COPD and asthma. It is estimated to kill close to 6 million people annually, a tenth of whom are nonsmokers exposed to secondhand smoke. By 2030, the rate will be 8 million people worldwide annually, and 80% of these deaths will occur in low- and middle-income countries. Tobacco is an avoidable risk factor for NCDs against which the WHO is developing a Tobacco Free Initiative and has held a WHO Framework Convention on Tobacco Control.[29] Powerful economic interests continue to market tobacco products, but legal decisions are increasingly favoring public health measures that limit the public's exposure.

Alcohol Use

Alcohol use has increased globally, with major increases occurring in developing countries. Alcohol use is estimated to have been responsible for nearly 2.5 million deaths in 2004, representing 3.8% of global deaths and 4.5% of total DALYs. Worldwide, in the 15 to 29 years age group, 9% of deaths are alcohol related. [40]

Lifestyle

Overall, estimates are that, of modifiable behavioral risk factors in 2008, insufficient physical activity caused 3.2 million deaths and 2.1% of total DALYs, unhealthy diet caused 1.7 million deaths and 1.0% of total DALYs, high cholesterol caused 2.6 million deaths annually and 2.0% of total DALYs, elevated blood pressure 7.5 million deaths and 3.7% of total DALYs, and overweight/obesity 2.8 million deaths and 2.3% of total DALYs. Adequate intake of fruit and vegetables decreases the risk for CVDs, stomach cancer, and colorectal cancer. High salt intake, more than 5 grams daily, is associated with elevated blood pressure and overall cardiovascular risk. Saturated and trans-fat in the diet increase the risk of coronary artery disease and the development of type 2 diabetes. [29]

Changes in living and working conditions worldwide have led to less physical activity and physical labor. Moderate physical activity for 150 minutes weekly is estimated to decrease the risk of ischemic heart disease by 30%, diabetes by 27%, and breast and colon cancer by 21% to 25%. Participation in physical activity decreases the risk of hypertension, stroke, and depression and also reduces obesity. [29]

Overweight/Obesity

The dietary changes and decreased exercise that accompany increasing development appear to be major causes of the obesity epidemic and its associated illnesses. Overweight (body mass index [BMI] 25 kg/m^2 to 29.9 kg/m^2) and obesity (BMI 30 kg/m^2 or higher) lead to metabolic changes such as insulin resistance and increasing blood pressure, cholesterol, and triglyceride levels. Between 1980 and 2008, the global prevalence of obesity almost doubled. Worldwide, of all adults over age 20, 1.4 billion were overweight and 500 million were obese. Globally, over 2.8 million adults die annually from being overweight or obese. An additional 44% of the diabetes burden, 23% of the ischemic heart disease burden, and 7% to 41% of the burden due to certain cancers are attributed to overweight and obesity. The risks of cancer of the breast, colon/rectum, endometrium, kidney, esophagus, and pancreas increase as BMI rises. Because obesity becomes common beginning in childhood, many chronic diseases are occurring at an earlier age.

In 2010, of the over 40 million children under 5 who were overweight, nearly 35 million were living in developing countries. [29]

Obesity in Developed and in Developing Countries

Overweight and obesity are becoming epidemic in both developing and developed countries. The countries leading in economic development have also been the leaders in developing obese populations. In the United States, the 2009–2010 National Health and Nutrition Examination survey of adults 20 years and older estimated the prevalence of obesity at 35.7% with another 33% of the population being overweight. [41] The prevalence is nearly as high in other developed countries and higher in some developing countries. Overweight/obesity and malnutrition are found side by side in most low- and middle-income countries. In the least developed countries, overweight and obesity remain low. Obesity is below 10% in sub-Saharan Africa and in Haiti, the poorest country in the Western Hemisphere. [15]

A review of the studies of the relationship between SES and obesity in adults living in developing countries found a pattern for women but not for men. In most studies in low-income countries, the risk of obesity was highest in the most educated women but shifted to be higher in the lower SES groups as the country's gross national product increased. [42] In the United States in 1974, the lowest and middle SES groups of women had obesity prevalence, respectively, three times and twice that of the highest women's SES group, 7.3%, but obesity has increased most rapidly in the latter group. By 2005–2008, the prevalence ranged from 42% in the lowest SES group to 34.5 in the middle and 29% in the highest. A similar trend has occurred in men, although the middle SES group has been the heaviest having a prevalence of 34.6% in 2005–2008 compared with 29.2% in the lowest and 32.6% in the highest SES. All three levels of men's SES increased in weight from the 2000 survey with the highest SES group increasing 7 percentage points. [43] In the United States, as in increasing numbers of other regions of the world, being more educated and economically well off appears to have been only transiently protective against "obesogenic environments." [42]

Those countries that have the resources to treat chronic illness and stave off mortal results from one organ failure are finding that these patients then live long enough to develop multiple organ failures. Continued maintenance of these patients requires dependence on externally powered technological treatments and skilled caregivers. Interruptions of technology, such as natural disasters, will place these patients at risk of death if the people, power, and supplies for these support systems suddenly become unavailable. Even where these technological supports are available, there is evidence that life expectancies are declining in some populations.[44] Functional dependency in the young-old (60 to 70 years) may become more common and reverse earlier progress toward compression of morbidity into the latter years of life. Population-wide public health measures to encourage increased physical activity and decreased daily calories should be put in place in concert with research mechanisms able to document their efficacy and lack of perverse incentives.

RESPONSES TO THE DEMOGRAPHIC AND EPIDEMIOLOGIC CHALLENGES

International Responses

Various international entities have responded at different levels in various formats to demographic aging, including the International Association of Gerontology (IAG), the International Federation on Aging (IFA), the International Monetary Fund, the Population Council, the Population Reference Bureau, the United Nations (UN), the World Bank, and the WHO. This section and Table 16-8 focus briefly on selected responses from the UN and the WHO. These initiatives often

work in conjunction with more general international instruments such as the UN Universal Declaration of Human Rights[45] and the UN Declaration on the Right to Development[46] that aim to promote fundamental freedoms, care, protection, fair treatment, and development of all citizens. Various initiatives aiming to guide thinking and the formulation of policies and programs on aging have been initiated by the Programme on Aging of the United Nations, including some of those listed in Table 16-8. The Second World Assembly on Aging and the resultant Madrid International Plan of Action on Aging are remarkable initiatives devoted to a response to the growing global concern about the speed and magnitude of population aging, and continued promotion of the concept of a "society for all ages." Covering the three priority directions of older persons and development, advancing health and well-being into old age, and ensuring enabling and supportive environments, the International Plan provides planners and policymakers with a set of 117 recommendations, tailored to suit both more and less developed country needs (Table 16-8).

Within the WHO's Noncommunicable Diseases and Mental Health Cluster, the response of the Ageing and Life Course Programme to aging includes a number of online publications at http://www.who.int/ageing/publications/active/en/index.html, focusing on topics that are pertinent to population and individual aging.

Table 16-8. Selected international responses to population aging and increase in noncommunicable diseases.

Year	Selected international initiatives
1982	First World Assembly on Aging, and its International Plan of Action on Aging (UN)
1991	United Nations Principles for Older Persons (UN)
1999	International Year of Older Persons 1999 (UN)
1999	WHO Minimum Data Set on Aging and Older Persons (WHO)
2002	Madrid International Plan of Action on Aging (UN)
2002	Political Declaration adopted at the Second World Assembly on Aging (UN)
2002	Research Agenda on Aging for the 21st Century (UN and IAG)
2002	Active Aging: A Policy Framework (WHO)
2002	WHO Study on Global Aging and Adult Health (SAGE) Wave 0 baseline cohort from WHS 2002-04 http://www.who.int/healthinfo/systems/sage/en/index.html
2004	Towards Age-friendly Primary Health Care (WHO) http://libdoc.who.int/publications/2004/9241592184.pdf
2005	Valetta Declaration (Help the Aged and UN International Institute on Aging)
2005	The Framework for Monitoring, Review and Appraisal of the Madrid International Plan of Action on Aging (UN)
2007	Beginning of the Global Burden of Diseases, Injuries, and Risk Factors 2010 Study by Institute for Health Metrics and Evaluation.
2011	High Level Meeting of the General Assembly on the Prevention and Control of Non-communicable Diseases http://www.who.int/nmh/events/un_ncd_summit2011/political_declaration_en.pdf
2012	WHO Study on global Aging and adult health (SAGE) Wave 4 http://www.who.int/healthinfo/systems/sage/en/index.html

One of these publications, *Active Ageing: A Policy Framework,* conceptualizes "active aging" as a goal for policy and program formulation, and it provides a policy framework for active aging and suggestions for key policy proposals that include the prevention and reduction of the burden of excess disabilities, chronic disease, premature mortality, and risk factors.[47]

The WHO has endorsed the need for universal health insurance coverage for all of the world's population if the burden of chronic disease management is to be effectively and efficiently managed by the nations of the developing world.[48]

International Organizations' Strategies Related to Aging Populations and Chronic Diseases

SAGE, the WHO Study on global aging and adult health, began wave one in 2002 and began wave four in 2012, as a survey program to compile comprehensive longitudinal information on the health and well-being of adult populations and the aging process. The core SAGE collects data on respondents ages 18+ years, with an emphasis on populations ages 50+ years, from nationally representative samples in six countries (China, Ghana, India, Mexico, Russian Federation, and South Africa). Household and individual level data on persons ages 50+ years are available from 20 countries as part of the core SAGE, the World Health Survey Plus (WHS+), COURAGE, and SAGE-INDEPTH.[49]

Global Burden of Disease Studies and the Disease Control Priorities Project

Through World Bank and WHO collaborations, two large projects have served as major international responses toward enhancing global health. These are the Global Burden of Disease Studies that provide descriptive information about demographic and epidemiologic changes and challenges in the world, and the Disease Control Priorities Project, which suggests cost-effective interventions in low- and middle-income countries. These projects include publications with chapters on NCDs, risk factors for disease and injury, as well as demographic change.

In 2008, the WHO presented its 2008–2013 Action Plan for the Global Strategy for the Prevention and Control of Noncommunicable Diseases. In brief, its six objectives for prevention and control of NCDs are to promote:

1. Increased global and national awareness of these diseases and integration of action plans into all government departments,
2. Fully developed national policies and plans,
3. Interventions for the main modifiable risk factors,
4. Relevant research,
5. Pertinent partnerships, and
6. Monitoring of NCDs and their determinants to evaluate progress at all levels.

Initiatives in Collaboration with the Food Industry

In 2003, the WHO began dialogues with the international food and beverage industry regarding positive roles that the private sector could play in promoting good diet and physical activity. The Global Strategy on Diet, Physical Activity and Health was endorsed by the May 2004 World Health Assembly (WHA) of the WHO. They recognized that supermarkets increasingly dominate retail sales, and that five multinational companies control 50% to 80% of the global markets. Due to the power of food industry advertising, the assembly recommended that governments work with that industry to stimulate the production and marketing of healthier foods. Governments were also encouraged to use mass media to publicize health initiatives such as environmental changes that promote increased levels of physical activity in communities.[50]

Risk Factor Control Measures

Countries are urged by the WHO and other agencies to develop efficient preventive measures to halt the growing trend of NCDs through control of risk factors. An example of this is the WHO Framework Convention on Tobacco Control (WHO FCTC) that was negotiated under the auspices of the WHO and entered into force in February 2005. The WHO FCTC was developed in response to globalization of the tobacco epidemic. It asserts the importance of demand reduction strategies as well as supply issues and liability. Member states that have signed the convention indicate that they will show a political commitment not to undermine the objectives outlined in it. For further information on the convention, see www.who.int/tobacco/framework/en/. Prohibiting smoking in public areas has been adopted in only a few countries that include South Africa, Brazil, Thailand, Poland, Bangladesh, and Canada. This together with increases in tobacco product prices and government tobacco taxes would produce significant health benefits at a very low cost. Promoting physical activity, healthy diet, and controlling alcohol abuse is necessary but not actively implemented in many countries.

Although many developed nations have focused considerable efforts on addressing NCDs, the rising burden of chronic disease in developing countries has received inadequate attention. Improving primary health care for prevention, screening, and early detection of chronic disease may be hampered by inadequate financing, and lack of labor, but very substantial health gains can be made with relatively modest health expenditure. There are additional factors limiting the control of NCDs. Some of these factors are the emphasis of health care systems on acute care and decision makers' lack of understanding of economic factors that influence chronic disease risks, information on the burden of chronic disease, and goodwill. In the absence of early detection, many people are diagnosed at advanced stages of cancer, CVD, and diabetes complications. Without further action it is estimated that in 2020 the disease burden attributed to tobacco will be nearly double its current level, and there will be a one-third increase in the loss of healthy life as a result of overweight and obesity. For the effective control of the burden of NCDs, a balanced approach to prevention and management is needed at government, community, and individual levels.[51]

National Responses to Aging and Noncommunicable Disease

South Africa's Response to Population Aging

Table 16-9 shows certain governmental initiatives undertaken in South Africa to address the concerns and needs of older persons. In 2011, South Africa's population ages 60 years and older constituted 7.7% of the total population[10] This proportion is similar to that in Brazil (7.8%), Mexico (6.9%), Samoa (6.8%), and Vietnam (7.5%).

The South African government's commitment to caring for older persons is evident in various legislative and policy initiatives that contain provisions of either direct or indirect relevance to older persons. For example, the supreme law of the country, the Constitution of 1996, which includes a Bill of Rights, states under Section 9, "Equality," that no person or the state may unfairly discriminate directly or indirectly against anyone on the ground of age.[52]

Table 16-9. Selected governmental responses to population aging and a growing number of older persons in South Africa.

Year	Selected responses
1996	Constitution of the Republic of South Africa http://www.info.gov.za/documents/constitution/index.htm http://www.info.gov.za/documents/constitution/1996/a108-96.pdf
1998	The Domestic Violence Act http://www.info.gov.za/view/DownloadFileAction?id=70651
1999	National Guideline on the Prevention of Falls in Older Persons http://www.westerncape.gov.za/Text/2003/falls.pdf
2000	National Guideline on the Prevention, Early Detection and Intervention of Physical Abuse of Older Persons at Primary Level http://sgdatabase.unwomen.org/uploads/National%20guideline%20on%20prevention%20of%20physical%20abuse%20of%20elderly%20persons.pdf
2000	Guideline for the Promotion of Active Ageing in Older Adults at Primary Level http://www.westerncape.gov.za/Text/2003/ageing.pdf
2001	National Guideline on the Management of Osteoporosis at Hospital Level and Preventative Measures at Primary Level http://www.westerncape.gov.za/eng/your_life/4483
2002	National Guideline on the Prevention of Blindness in South Africa http://www.westerncape.gov.za/Text/2003/blindness.pdf
2003	Older Persons Bill 2003 http://www.info.gov.za/gazette/bills/2003/b68-03.pdf. Was repealed when the Older Persons Act no 13 of 2006 came into effect in 2010
2004	The Social Assistance Act http://www.info.gov.za/view/DownloadFileAction?id=131972
2006	The Aged Persons Amendment Act http://www.info.gov.za/view/DownloadFileAction?id=67839 The 1998 Act was repealed when the Older Persons Act no 13 of 2006 came into effect in 2010
2010	Older Persons' Charter (2010) (available at: http://www.saopf.org.za/your-rights/older-persons-charter)

Other Policy and Legislative Developments Include:
Protocol guidelines for the management of Chronic health conditions. (Available at: Chronic illness. http://www.westerncape.gov.za/eng/your_life/4483.

The Older Persons Act No. 13 of 2006, which came into effect in 2010, superseded the Aged Persons Amendment Act of 1998. The aim of the 2006 act is to deal effectively with the plight of older persons by establishing a framework within which to empower and protect them. The framework provides specifically for the promotion and maintenance of older persons' status, rights, well-being, safety, and security in an enabling environment that the state should create.[53]

The initiatives listed in Table 16-9, combined with broad perspectives in local instruments such as the White Paper for the Transformation of the Health System in South Africa,[54] the National Health Act,[55] and the White Paper for Social Welfare,[56] are aimed at fostering the economic, social, and physical protection of older persons; enhancement of their health and well-being; and promotion of their access to and the affordability of health care. In addition, the government is committed to tenets that emanated from the 1999 International Year for Older Persons; is a signatory to the Political Declaration that commits countries to implement the 2002 Madrid International Plan of Action on Ageing; and has shown remarkable support to various international responses by integrating their aims and objectives into the different drafts of the South African policy for older persons that culminated in the Older Persons Bill in 2003.[57]

A salutary response to the needs of poor older persons, who are the majority, is the government's Social Security program, which transfers a monthly noncontributory, but means-tested social pension to beneficiaries who are eligible for one based on income and age. Sixty years is the age of eligibility for a social pension. The near universality and generosity of the wealth transfer is unique in developing countries and on a level with the pension program in Brazil.[58] The value of the South African social old age pension is R1200 at present (approximately US$144). Although the amount may be small, it represents a safety net for each beneficiary. South Africa currently has a high poverty level and a high unemployment rate, and through pension sharing, the grant benefits entire families and households in which a beneficiary resides.

In addition, the government subsidizes services for older persons through the Ministry of Social Development, which are delivered by nongovernmental organizations (NGOs). These services include social work services, such as the organization of community and intersectoral programs, and community-based care to support older persons in the community. Regarding health care for older persons, the government has established a directorate of Chronic Diseases, Geriatrics and Disability, which produces and disseminates guidelines on the management of various health syndromes in older persons.[59]

The initiatives listed in the table demonstrate that at a policy and legislative level, South Africa is responding to population aging and the growing number of older persons. It shows a commitment moreover to contributing to older persons' well-being. However a gap remains between policy formulation and program implementation, and most of the initiatives are yet to be put into practice. Guidelines on the management of health syndromes in older persons, for example, are not well known and are underutilized by health professionals for whom they are developed.

Case Studies of National Responses to Cardiovascular Disease

Forty years ago, Finland had the highest death rate from CVD. Between 1972 and 2006, utilizing interventions including tobacco advertising bans, incentives to lower the fat content of dairy products, and rewards to communities lowering citizens' cholesterol levels, the country reduced heart disease death rates by 85% and also decreased cancer death rates. During that period of time, life expectancy for men was extended by 7 years and for women by 6 years.[60] Participants in a study in Finland also decreased their incidence of type 2 diabetes by 60% by improving diet and increasing physical activity. They had lower levels of glucose, cholesterol, triglycerides, and blood pressure after a year and continued the improvement through the 6 years of the study.[61]

In 1996, the State Secretariat of Health of São Paulo, Brazil, initiated the Agita program to increase public awareness of the importance of physical activity for health with a goal to increase activity levels by 20% over 10 years. This program was promoted through mass media, promotional giveaways, megaevents, access to sporting facilities, improving physical environments, and health professionals' prescriptions of physical activity. Between 2002 and 2008, public awareness of the program increased from 37% to 60%. During the same period, the proportion of residents with no physical activity fell from nearly 10% to less than 3%, and the proportion of residents with less than 150 minutes of exercise weekly fell from 43.7% to 11.6%.[62]

SUMMARY FROM A GLOBAL PERSPECTIVE

1. Demographic change has ensured that the number of older people is increasing rapidly throughout the world.
2. Demographic, epidemiologic, dietary, and social changes have contributed to chronic diseases being reported as the predominant challenge for medical care throughout the world.

3. Developing countries will be most challenged due to insufficient resources and ill-equipped health care systems.

4. As the average age of death increases, the disability effects of disease generally become more significant for a nation's productivity than the death rate. The most recent Global Burden of Disease study has reinforced the importance of including nonfatal outcomes in assessing population health.

5. An economy's success at increasing availability of food, transportation, and discretionary money to buy products such as tobacco often has adverse effects on the health of its population.

6. Medical care can manage the ill effects of risk factors, but it must utilize expensive diagnostic and treatment methods to do so. These methods are often not an option to low-income countries, and creative intervention approaches within a prevention paradigm may prove more cost effective.

7. Companies marketing their products globally and utilizing mass media to promote "desirable" ways of living must consider the health effects on targeted populations.

8. Governments can promote healthier diets and lifestyles by changing incentives.

9. To enhance decision making and planning for better health, all governments should take responsibility for population health by promoting regular, comprehensive, and consistent descriptions of their country's demography, their burden of disease and injury, and the associated risk factors.

10. Large contributions to global loss of healthy life are associated with a small number of major risk factors. Several risks are relatively prominent in regions at all stages of development. Relatively inexpensive multiple risk factor interventions can make rapid and significant improvements in the ill effects of NCDs.

STUDY QUESTIONS

1. How would you allocate funds for health care if you were directing your country's budget and $100 million in new money became available annually?

2. What measures might be effective in a developed country whose population is aging to effectively care for a burgeoning retired population while maintaining a workforce capable of growing the economy?

3. What methods have been shown effective to help a population growing in affluence make discretionary choices in lifestyle, diet, and habits that promote health?

4. "As the proportion of the world's population in the older ages continues to increase, the need for improved information and analysis of demographic aging increases."[2] Critically argue whether knowledge generation is an important priority in the aging discourse in developed and developing nations.

5. Epidemiologic knowledge led to Omran's 1971 Epidemiological Transition Theory, which implies that, as countries become more developed, their disease profile changes from one of infectious and other pretransitional conditions to a predominance of NCDs.[63] However, different countries experience different trends in mortality, morbidity, and disability, and more theories of health change have been generated to accommodate such differences. How applicable are these theories to your country's health situation? Demonstrate how demographic and epidemiologic changes interact to allow for changing theories.

6. Breslow's classic 1952 paper recognized that weight control is a "major public health problem today" among Americans.[64] Eighty years ago, individuals were charged higher premiums on insurance because of overweight (Dublin and Marks, 1951, as quoted in Breslow, 1952).[64] The WHO describes obesity as one of the most blatantly visible public health problems.[65] However, health problems associated with overweight and overnourishment have gained global recognition only during the past 15 years.[66] What factors are responsible for this lag in global recognition of a leading risk factor for chronic disease and disability, and how should health agents, such as health ministries, respond to remedy the situation?

REFERENCES

1. Lopez AD, Mathers CD, Ezzati M, Jamison DT, Murray CJL. Global and regional burden of disease and risk factors, 2001: systematic analysis of population health data. *Lancet* 2006;367:1747–1757.

2. United Nations. *World Population 1950–2050.* New York: UN, 2002:1–34. http://www.un.org/esa/population/publications/worldageing19502050/.

3. United Nations. *World Population Ageing 2009.* New York: UN, 2009. http://www.un.org/esa/population/publications/WPA2009/WPA2009_WorkingPaper.pdf.

4. Kinsella K, Wan He. *An aging world: 2008.* International Population Reports. Series P95/01-1. Washington, DC: US Department of Commerce, 2009:19–31. http://www.census.gov/prod/2009pubs/p95-09-1.pdf.

5. Beard J, Biggs S, Bloom D, et al. *Global Population Ageing: Peril or Promise.* Geneva: World Economic Forum, Program on the Global Demography of Aging, 2011:3–5. http://www3.

weforum.org/docs/WEF_GAC_GlobalPopulationAgeing_Report_2012.pdf.

6. Pressat R. *Demographic Analysis: Methods, Results, Applications.* London: Edward Arnold, 1972.

7. United Nations, Department of Economic and Social Affairs, Population Division. *World Population Prospects: The 2010 Revision.* New York: UN, 2011. CD-ROM edition.

8. Rehm J, Sulkowska U, Manczuk M, et al. Alcohol accounts for a high proportion of premature mortality in central and eastern Europe. *Int J Epidemiol* 2007;36:458–467.

9. Bradshaw D, Groenewald P, Laubscher R, et al. Initial burden of disease estimates for South Africa, 2000. *South Afr Med J* 2003;93:682–688.

10. Statistics South Africa, Mid-year population estimates, 2011. http://www.statssa.gov.za/publications/P0302/P03022011.pdf.

11. Population Division of the Department of Economic and Social Affairs of the United Nations Secretariat. *The Diversity of Changing Population Age Structures in the World.* New York: United Nations, 2005. http://www.un.org/esa/population/meetings/EGMPopAge/1_UNPD_Trends.pdf.

12. United Nations, Department of Economic and Social Affairs, Population Division. *World Urbanization Prospects: The 2011 Revision.* New York: UN, 2011.

13. Population Division, Department of Economic and Social Affairs, United Nations Secretariat. *World Population Prospects: The 2010 Revision.* New York: United Nations, 2011.http://esa.un.org/unpd/wpp/index.htm.

14. Bloom D, Boersch-Supan A, McGee P, et al. *Population Aging: Facts, Challenges, and Responses.* Boston: Program on the Global Demography of Aging: Working Paper Series, 2011: 1–2. http://www.hsph.harvard.edu/pgda/WorkingPapers/ 2011/PGDA_WP_71.pdf.

15. World Health Organization. *World Health Statistics 2012.* Geneva: WHO, 2012. http://www.who.int/healthinfo/EN_WHS2012_Full.pdf.

16. World Health Organization. *Impact of AIDS on Older People in Africa: Zimbabwe Case Study.* Geneva: WHO, 2002.

17. Kautz T, Bendavid E, Bhattacharya J, et al. AEDS and declining support for dependent elderly people in Africa: retrospective analysis using demographic and health surveys. *BMJ* 2010;340c2841.

18. Joubert JD, Bradshaw D. Population aging and its health challenges in South Africa. In: Steyn K, Fourie J, Temple N, eds. *Non-Communicable Disease in South Africa, 2005.* Cape Town: South African Medical Research Council, 2006:204–219.

19. Population Facts. *Population Ageing and the Non-Communicable Diseases.* New York: United Nations, 2012.

20. Human Development Network. *The Growing Danger of Non-Communicable Diseases: Acting Now to Reverse Course.* Washington, DC: The World Bank, 2011:1–14.

21. World Health Organization. *Global Health Risk: Mortality and Burden of Disease Attributable to Selected Major Risks.* Geneva: WHO, 2009.

22. World Health Organization, Global Health Observatory. *Causes of Child Mortality for the Year 2010.* Geneva: WHO, 2010. http://www.who.int/gho/child_health/mortality/mortality_causes_text/en/index.html.

23. World Health Organization. *The Burden of Disease: 2004 Update.* Geneva: WHO, 2008.

24. Henry J. Kaiser Family Foundation. *HIV/AIDS Policy Fact Sheet.* Menlo Park, CA: Henry J. Kaiser Family Foundation, 2008. http://www.kff.org/hivaids/upload/7391-071.pdf.

25. Mathers C, Loncar D. Projections of global mortality and burden of disease from 2002 to 2030. *PLoS Med* 2006;3(11):e442.

26. World Health Organization. *Key Facts on Global HIV Epidemic and Progress in 2010.* Based on Progress Report 2011: Global HIV/AIDS response. Geneva: WHO, UNAIDS, UNICEF, 2011.

27. MetLife Mature Market Institute. *Caregiving Costs to Working Caregivers. Double Jeopardy for Baby Boomers Caring for Their Parents.* New York: MetLife, June 15, 2011.

28. World Health Organization. *World Report of Disability.* Geneva: WHO, 2011.

29. World Health Organization. *Global Status Report on Non-Communicable Diseases.* Geneva:WHO, 2011.

30. Gersh B, Sliwa K, Mayosi B, et al. The epidemic of cardiovascular disease in the developing world: global implications. *Eur Heart J* 2010;31:642–648.

31. Wild S, Gojka R, Anders G, et al. Global prevalence of diabetes. Estimates for the year 2000 and projections for 2030. *Diabetic Care* 2004;27:1047–1053.

32. Zhang P, Zhang X, Brown J, et al. Global healthcare expenditures on diabetes for 2010 and 2030. *Diabetes Res Clin Pract* 2010:92(2):301.

33. American Cancer Society. *Global Cancer Facts and Figures.* 2nd ed. Atlanta: American Cancer Society, 2011:1–5.

34. GLOBOCAN 2008. *Lung Cancer Incidence and Mortality Worldwide in 2008.* Geneva: International Agency for Research on Cancer, World Health Organization, 2008.

35. World Health Organization. *Asthma, Fact Sheet #307.* Geneva: WHO, 2011. http://www.who.int/mediacentre/factsheets/fs307/en/index.html.

36. World Health Organization. *Chronic Obstructive Pulmonary Diseases (COPD), Fact Sheet #315.* Geneva: WHO, 2011.

37. Bloom DE, Cafiero ET, Jané-Llopis E, et al. *The Global Economic Burden of Non-Communicable Diseases.* Geneva: World Economic Forum, 2011.

38. Whitmer RA, Sidney S, Selby J, et al. Mid-life cardiovascular risk factors and risk of dementia in late life. *Neurology* 2005;64(2):277–281.

39. World Alzheimer's Report 2010. *The Global Economic Impact of Dementia.* London: Alzheimer's Disease International, 2010.

40. World Health Organization. *Global Strategy to Reduce the Harmful Use of Alcohol.* Geneva: WHO, 2010.

41. Fryar CD, Carroll MD, Ogden CL. *Prevalence of Overweight, Obesity, and Extreme Obesity Among Adults: United States, Trends 1960–1962 Through 2009–2010.* Atlanta: Centers for Disease Control and Prevention, 2012.

42. McLaren L. Socioeconomic status and obesity. *Epidemiol Rev* 2007;29:29–48.

43. Ogden CL, Lamb MM, Carroll MD. *Obesity and Socioeconomic Status in Adults: United States 2005–2008.* National Center for Health Statistics. Atlanta: Centers for Disease Control and Prevention, 2010.

44. Olshansky SJ. A potential decline in life expectancy in the United States in the 21st century. *N Engl J Med* 2005; 352:1138–1145.

45. United Nations. *Universal Declaration of Human Rights.* Resolution 217 A (III) of December 10, 1948, adopted and proclaimed by the General Assembly of the United Nations. New York: UN, 1948.

46. United Nations. *Declaration on the Right to Development.* Resolution 41/128 of December 4, 1986, adopted by the General

Assembly of the United Nations. New York: UN, 1986. http://www.un.org/documents/ga/res/41/a41r128.htm.

47. World Health Organization. *Active Aging: A Policy Framework.* Geneva: WHO, 2002. http://whqlibdoc.who.int/hq/2002/WHO_NMH_NPH_02.8.pdf.

48. World Health Organization. *Health Systems Financing: The Path to Universal Coverage.* Geneva: WHO, 2010. http://www.who.int/whr/2010/10_summary_en.pdf.

49. He W, Muenchrath MN, Kowal P. *Shades of Gray: A Cross-Country Study of Health and Well-Being of the Older Populations in SAGE Countries 2007–2010.* Washington, DC: International Population Reports, US Census Bureau, 2012. http://www.census.gov/prod/2012pubs/p95-12-01.pdf.

50. World Health Organization. *Global Strategy on Diet, Physical Activity and Health.* Geneva: WHO, 2004. http://www.who.int/dietphysicalactivity/strategy/eb11344/strategy_english_web.pdf.

51. Yach D, Hawkers C, Gould CL, et al. The global burden of chronic diseases. Overcoming impediments to prevention and control. *JAMA* 2004;291:2616–2622.

52. Republic of South Africa. *Constitution of the Republic of South Africa, Act No. 108 of 1996.* Pretoria: Republic of South Africa, 1996. http://www.info.gov.za/documents/constitution/index.htm.

53. Republic of South Africa. *Older Persons Bill. Act No 13 of 2006.* Pretoria: Republic of South Africa, 2006. http://www.info.gov.za/view/DownloadFileAction?id=67839.

54. Ministry of Health. *White Paper for the Transformation of the Health System in South Africa.* Pretoria: Ministry of Health, 1997. http://www.doh.gov.za/docs/policy/white_paper/healthsys97_01.html.

55. Republic of South Africa. *National Health Act, Act No. 61 of 2003.* Pretoria: Republic of South Africa, 2004. http://www.info.gov.za/speeches/2004/04081914451006.htm.

56. Department of Welfare. *White Paper for Social Development.* Pretoria: Department of Welfare, 1997.

57. Republic of South Africa. *Older Persons Bill, Bill No. 68 of 2003.* Pretoria: Republic of South Africa, 2003. http://www.pmg.org.za/bills/040803b68-03.pdf.

58. Institute of Development and Policy Management (IDPM) and HelpAge International. *Non-Contributory Pensions and Poverty Prevention: A Comparative Study of Brazil and South Africa.* London: IDPM & HelpAge International, 2003.

59. Western Cape Government. *Chronic Illness.* South Africa: Western Cape Government, 2012. http://www.westerncape.gov.za/eng/your_life/4483.

60. Puska P. Successful prevention of non-communicable diseases. 25 year experiences with North Karelia project in Finland. *Public Health Med* 2002;4(1):5–7.

61. Tuomilehto J, Lindstrom J, Eriksson JG, et al. Prevention of type 2 diabetes with changes in lifestyle among subjects with impaired glucose tolerance. *N Engl J Med* 1994;308:367–372.

62. Fioravanti C. Brazilian fitness programme registers health benefits. *Lancet* 2012;380:206.

63. Omran A. The epidemiological transition: a theory of the epidemiology of population change. *Milbank Mem Fund Q* 1971;49:509–538.

64. Breslow L. Public health aspects of weight control. Am J Public *Health Nations Health* 1952;42:1116–1120. (Reprinted in *Int* J Epidemiol 2006;35:10–12.)

65. World Health Organization. *Obesity: Preventing and Managing the global epidemic.* WHO Technical Report Series, No. 894. Geneva: WHO, 2000.

66. Haslam DW, James WPT. Obesity. *Lancet* 2005;366:1197–1209.

Global Mental Health: The World Mental Health Surveys Perspective

17

Jordi Alonso, Somnath Chatterji, Yanling He, Philip S. Wang, and Ronald C. Kessler

LEARNING OBJECTIVES

- *Recognize the public relevance of mental disorders worldwide*
- *Understand indicators of the frequency, the impact and the use of services in relation to mental disorders*
- *Stimulate the search for additional information and knowledge about solutions needed to diminish the global burden of mental disorders*

INTRODUCTION

As health care spending continues to rise, treatment resource allocation decisions will need to be based increasingly on information about the prevalence and societal burden of illness. Interest in societal burden has increased dramatically over the past decade based on this recognition and as part of a larger movement to rationalize the allocation of treatment resources and maximize benefit in relation to cost. Much of the current interest in mental disorders among health policy makers is based on the fact that these disorders have consistently been found in studies of disease burden to be both among the most burdensome health problems in the world[1] and also to be among the disorders with the lowest ratio of investments in treatment to disease burdens.[2]

A number of factors account for the high burden of mental disorders. They are commonly occurring, often begin at an early age, often are quite persistent throughout the life course, and often have substantial adverse effects on functioning. The low investments in treatment are more difficult to explain but presumably are due at least partly to failure of health policy-makers to recognize the high prevalence and burden of mental disorders.

Data are here presented from the World Health Organization (WHO) World Mental Health (WMH) surveys initiative.[3] This initiative was launched to diminish the information gap regarding the high prevalence and burden of mental disorders, with the specific objectives of assessing the prevalence, severity, and comparative societal burden of mental disorders throughout the world. Although the WMH is still a work in progress, enough useful information has been produced to warrant a review of data produced by WMH up to now on the global epidemiology of common mental disorders.

THE WORLD HEALTH ORGANIZATION WORLD MENTAL HEALTH SURVEYS INITIATIVE

WMH includes a series of geographically representative mental health surveys carried out in all major regions of the world. A key aim of the surveys is to help countries that would not otherwise have the expertise or infrastructure to implement high-quality community epidemiologic surveys that can be used for health policy planning purposes by providing centralized instrument development, training, and data analysis (www.hcp.med.harvard.edu/wmh). Twenty-eight countries have so far completed WMH surveys. The vast majority of these surveys are nationally representative, although a few are representative of only a single region (e.g., the São Paolo metropolitan area in Brazil) or regions (e.g., six metropolitan areas in Japan). The details about sampling in the countries that have been analyzed for the present analyses are shown in Table 17-1.

All WMH surveys use the same diagnostic interview, the WHO Composite International Diagnostic Interview (CIDI).[4] The CIDI is a state-of-the-art fully structured research diagnostic interview designed to be used by trained lay interviewers who do not have any clinical experience to diagnose mood disorders, anxiety disorders, behavior disorders, and substance use disorders. Consistent interviewer training materials, training programs, and quality control monitoring procedures are used to guarantee comparability across all WMH surveys. Consistent WHO translation, back translation, and harmonization procedures for the interview text and training materials are also used across countries. Methodological studies have documented good concordance between diagnoses based on the CIDI and blinded clinical diagnoses.[5]

The CIDI was designed to go well beyond the mere assessment of mental disorders to include a wide range of measures about important correlates of these disorders. For purposes of this report, two of these extensions are of special importance. One is that the CIDI includes disorder-specific measures of role impairment that are administered in exactly the same fashion for each mental disorder in the surveys as well as for each of a wide variety of chronic physical disorders assessed for comparison purposes in the surveys. These measures, a modified version of the Sheehan Disability Scales (SDS), assess condition-specific role impairments in four role domains: home management, work, social life, and personal relationships. Previous methodological studies have documented good internal consistency reliability across the SDS domains,[6,7] a result that was replicated in the WMH data both in developed and developing countries.[1]

Second, the CIDI assesses not only disorder prevalence but also disorder *severity*. This is important in light of the finding in previous epidemiologic surveys that quite a high proportion of the general population in many countries meets criteria for a *Diagnostic and Statistical Manual of Mental Disorders* (DSM) or *International Classification of Diseases* mental disorder.[8–10] Faced with this high prevalence, mental health policy planning efforts need to consider disorder severity for treatment planning purposes because the simple presence of a diagnosis may not indicate need for services. All WMH respondents who were classified as meeting criteria for one or more mental disorders at some time in the 12 months before the interview were consequently classified either as serious, moderate, or mild cases. *Serious* cases were defined as those with nonaffective psychosis, bipolar I

disorder, or substance dependence with a physiologic dependence syndrome; those who made a serious suicide attempt (i.e., not merely a suicide gesture); those that reported severe role impairment due to their mental illness in at least two areas of functioning measured by the SDS; and those having overall functional impairment due to their mental illness consistent with a Global Assessment of Functioning (GAF)[11] score of 50 or less. Disorders not classified serious were classified as *moderate* if they included substance dependence without a physiologic dependence syndrome; or at least moderate interference on the SDS in at least one disorder-specific scale of role impairment. All other disorders were classified as *mild*.

A comment is required about diagnostic coverage before turning to results. Almost all previous community epidemiologic surveys of common mental disorders focused on mood disorders (major depression, dysthymia, bipolar disorder), anxiety disorders (generalized anxiety disorder [GAD], panic disorder, phobia, obsessive-compulsive disorder, posttraumatic stress disorder [PTSD]), and substance use disorders (alcohol and drug abuse and dependence). The WMH surveys expanded this list to include disruptive behavior disorders (attention-deficit/hyperactivity disorder, conduct disorder, oppositional-defiant disorder, and intermittent explosive disorder). Nonaffective psychoses (NAP) including, for example, schizophrenia, schizophreniform disorder, schizoaffective disorder, delusional disorder and brief psychotic reaction have also been included in a number of community epidemiologic surveys (e.g., Kessler et al, 2005; Ochoa et al, 2008; Gureje et al, 2010),[12–14] but the sensitivity of survey measures of NAP is so low that great caution is needed in interpreting results. Data on NAP are consequently not reviewed here, although a screen for NAP was included in many of the WMH surveys. Excellent reviews of the literature on the epidemiology of NAP are available elsewhere.[15,16] In addition, Axis II personality disorders have generally not been included in community epidemiologic surveys of mental disorders. Although some preliminary data exist on the epidemiology of these disorders[17] and a number of WMH surveys included screens for personality disorders,[18] these data are not reviewed here because they are so sparse.

Prevalence of Common Mental Disorders in the WMH Surveys

The WMH surveys that have been completed so far (which are only a subset of the 28 in the initiative) show clearly that the mental disorders assessed in the CIDI are quite common in all the countries studied. 12-month prevalence estimates, that is estimates of the proportion of respondents who met criteria for

Table 17-1. Sampling characteristics by country income level: the WMH surveys.[a]

Income level	Survey[b]	Sample characteristics[c]	Field dates	Age range	Sample size Part I 121,899	Part II[d] 63,678	Response rate[e] 72.0
I. All countries							
II. Low/lower-middle income countries							
Colombia	NSMH	All urban areas of the country (approximately 73% of the total national population).	2003	18–65	4,426	2,381	87.7
India: Pondicherry	WMHI	Pondicherry region.	2003–5	18–97	2,992	1,373	98.8
Iraq	IMHS	Nationally representative.	2006–7	18–96	4,332	4,332	95.2
Nigeria	NSMHW	21 of the 36 states in the country, representing 57% of the national population. The surveys were conducted in Yoruba, Igbo, Hausa, and Efik languages.	2002–3	18–100	6,752	2,143	79.3
PRC[f]: Beijing/Shanghai	B-WMH S-WMH	Beijing and Shanghai metropolitan areas.	2002–3	18–70	5,201	1,628	74.7
PRC[f]: Shenzhen[g]	Shenzhen	Shenzhen metropolitan area. Included temporary residents as well as household residents.	2006–7	18–88	7,132	2,475	80.0
Ukraine[g]	CMDPSD	Nationally representative.	2002	18–91	4,724	1,719	78.3
Total					35,559	16,051	
III. Upper-middle income countries							
Brazil: São Paulo	São Paulo Megacity	São Paulo metropolitan area.	2005–7	18–93	5,037	2,942	81.3
Bulgaria	NSHS	Nationally representative.	2003–7	18–98	5,318	2,233	72.0
Lebanon	LEBANON	Nationally representative.	2002–3	18–94	2,857	1,031	70.0
Mexico	M-NCS	All urban areas of the country (approximately 75% of the total national population).	2001–2	18–65	5,782	2,362	76.6
Romania	RMHS	Nationally representative.	2005–6	18–96	2,357	2,357	70.9
South Africa[g]	SASH	Nationally representative.	2003–4	18–92	4,315	4,315	87.1
Total					25,666	15,240	
IV. High-income countries							
Belgium	ESEMeD	Nationally representative. The sample was selected from a national register of Belgium residents.	2001–2	18–95	2,419	1,043	50.6
France	ESEMeD	Nationally representative. The sample was selected from a national list of households with listed telephone numbers.	2001–2	18–97	2,894	1,436	45.9
Germany	ESEMeD	Nationally representative.	2002–3	18–95	3,555	1,323	57.8
Israel	NHS	Nationally representative.	2002–4	21–98	4,859	4,859	72.6
Italy	ESEMeD	Nationally representative. The sample was selected from municipality resident registries.	2001–2	18–100	4,712	1,779	71.3

(Continued)

389

Table 17-1. Sampling characteristics by country income level: the WMH surveys.[a] (Continued)

Income level	Survey[b]	Sample characteristics[c]	Field dates	Age range	Sample size	Response rate[e]
Japan	WMHJ2002–2006	Eleven metropolitan areas.	2002–6	20–98	4,129	1,682	55.1
The Netherlands	ESEMeD	Nationally representative. The sample was selected from municipal postal registries.	2002–3	18–95	2,372	1,094	56.4
New Zealand[g]	NZMHS	Nationally representative.	2003–4	18–98	12,790	7,312	73.3
Northern Ireland	NISHS	Nationally representative.	2004–7	18–97	4,340	1,986	68.4
Portugal	NMHS	Nationally representative.	2008–9	18–81	3,849	2,060	57.3
Spain	ESEMeD	Nationally representative.	2001–2	18–98	5,473	2,121	78.6
United States	NCS-R	Nationally representative.	2002–3	18–99	9,282	5,692	70.9
Total					60,674	32,387	70.9

[a]The World Bank (2008). Data and Statistics. Accessed May 12, 2009 at http://go.worldbank.org/D7SN0B8YU0

[b]NSMH (The Colombian National Study of Mental Health); WMHI (World Mental Health India); IMHS (Iraq Mental Health Survey); NSMHW (The Nigerian Survey of Mental Health and Wellbeing); B-WMH (The Beijing World Mental Health Survey); S-WMH (The Shanghai World Mental Health Survey); CMDPSD (Comorbid Mental Disorders during Periods of Social Disruption); NSHS (Bulgaria National Survey of Health and Stress); LEBANON (Lebanese Evaluation of the Burden of Ailments and Needs of the Nation); M-NCS (The Mexico National Comorbidity Survey); RMHS (Romania Mental Health Survey); SASH (South Africa Health Survey); ESEMeD (The European Study of the Epidemiology of Mental Disorders); NHS (Israel National Health Survey); WMHJ2002–2006 (World Mental Health Japan Survey); NZMHS (New Zealand Mental Health Survey); NISHS (Northern Ireland Study of Health and Stress); NMHS (Portugal National Mental Health Survey); NCS-R (The US National Comorbidity Survey Replication).

[c]Most WMH surveys are based on stratified multistage clustered area probability household samples in which samples of areas equivalent to counties or municipalities in the United States were selected in the first stage followed by one or more subsequent stages of geographic sampling (e.g., towns within counties, blocks within towns, households within blocks) to arrive at a sample of households, in each of which a listing of household members was created and one or two people were selected from this listing to be interviewed. No substitution was allowed when the originally sampled household resident could not be interviewed. These household samples were selected from census area data in all countries other than France (where telephone directories were used to select households) and the Netherlands (where postal registries were used to select households). Several WMH surveys (Belgium, Germany, Italy) used municipal resident registries to select respondents without listing households. The Japanese sample is the only totally unclustered sample, with households randomly selected in each of the 11 metropolitan areas and one random respondent selected in each sample household. Overall, 17 of the 25 surveys are based on nationally representative household samples.

[d]See the text of the chapter for a discussion of the difference between Part I and Part II samples. Only 62,971 Part 2 respondents were asked questions about chronic conditions due to these questions being omitted inadvertently for 429 respondents in Lebanon and 278 in Northern Ireland.

[e]The response rate is calculated as the ratio of the number of households in which an interview was completed to the number of households originally sampled, excluding from the denominator households known not to be eligible either because of being vacant at the time of initial contact or because the residents were unable to speak the designated languages of the survey. The weighted average response rate is 72.0%.

[f]People's Republic of China.

[g]For the purposes of cross-national comparisons, we limit the sample to those 18+.

(Adapted, with permission, from Alonso J, et al. Mol Psychiatr 2011;16:1359–4184/11. Table 1, pp. 1236–1237.)

one or more of the mental disorders assessed in the surveys at some time in the year prior to the interview, are presented here. The 12-month prevalence estimates average 9.7% for any anxiety disorder with an interquartile range (IQR) (25th to 75th percentiles) across countries of 6.6 to 13.7 (Table 17-2). Mood disorders are generally found to be the next most prevalent class of disorders, with 12-month prevalence estimates for any mood disorder in the WMH surveys averaging 5.5%, with an IQR of 3.4 to 7.0. Prevalence estimates of anxiety and mood disorders are generally higher in Western developed countries than in developing countries.

The 12-month prevalence estimates for substance disorders (0.2% to 6.4%; IQR: 1.2% to 3.5%) and disruptive behavior disorders (0.1% to 10.5%; IQR: 1.1% to 3.5%) are consistently lower than for anxiety or mood disorders. It is noteworthy, though, that some WMH surveys did not assess illicit drug abuse or dependence, possibly leading to artificially low prevalence estimates compared with other countries. Substance dependence was also assessed only in the presence of abuse, possibly further reducing estimated prevalence.[19]

Noticeable international variation exists in the 12-month prevalence of the mental disorders assessed in the WMH surveys. The lowest prevalence estimates are in Nigeria (6%), Beijing/Shanghai metropolitan area (7.1%), and Japan (7.4%); the highest are in São Paulo (29.6%), the United States (27%), and Northern Ireland (23.1%). In general, countries/regions with low prevalences show lower frequencies of all types of disorders. Explanations of international variations in the prevalence of mental disorders have long been discussed.[20] Among several issues, cultural relevance of mental diagnoses and severity of cases have been raised as possible explanations for cross-national variation in prevalence estimates. These issues are addressed in the next section.

Severity of Mental Disorders

Many previous epidemiologic surveys estimated disorder prevalence, but the WMH surveys are the first ones to generate systematic estimates of disorder severity. As mentioned earlier, in the WMH analyses the severity of mental disorders is categorized as serious, moderate, and mild, taking into account information on the type of disorder, the degree of impairment, and the presence of suicide ideation. The proportions of respondents with a constellation of 12-month DSM-IV/CIDI disorders classified as either serious (7.2% to 36.8%; IQR: 18.5% to 25.7%) or moderate (12.5% to 50.6%; IQR: 33.0% to 42.3%) in the first set of completed WMH surveys, using the definitions of those terms described earlier, are generally smaller

than the proportions with mild disorders (Table 17-3). The severity distribution among cases varies significantly across countries ($p < 0.001$), with severity not strongly related either to region or to development status. The unconditional 12-month prevalence estimate of serious mental illness in the WMH surveys is in the range of 4.0% to 6.8% for half the surveys, 2.3% to 3.6% for another quarter, and 0.8% to 1.9% for the final quarter.

There are substantial positive associations across surveys between overall prevalence of any disorder and both the proportion of cases classified as serious (Pearson $r = 0.40$, $p < 0.005$) and the proportion of cases classified as either serious or moderate (Pearson $r = 0.50$, $p < 0.001$). These positive associations are important because they address an issue that has been raised in the methodological literature regarding the possibility of biased prevalence estimates. Two separate research groups found a pattern opposite the one found in the WMH surveys, leading them to argue that prevalence estimates are biased in some epidemiologic surveys. One of these groups, based in Korea, compared results from their Korean Epidemiologic Catchment Area (KECA) Study[21] with results from a parallel survey in the United States and argued that the lower estimated prevalence of major depression in the KECA than the US survey was due, at least in part, to a higher threshold for reporting depression among people in the Korean population than in the United States. In support of this assertion, the investigators showed that Koreans diagnosed as depressed with an earlier version of the CIDI, which was the diagnostic instrument used in the KECA survey, had considerably higher levels of role impairment than respondents diagnosed as depressed using the same instrument in the United States. The second group that reported a similar finding was the group of collaborators in the WHO Collaborative Study on Psychological Problems in General Health Care (PPG). In that study, nearly 26,000 primary care patients in 14 countries were assessed using an earlier version of the CIDI that included an evaluation of current symptoms of depression. As in the WMH surveys, substantial cross-national variation was found in the prevalence of major depression. However, the investigators found that the average amount of impairment associated with depression across countries was inversely proportional to the estimated prevalence of depression in those countries.[21,22] The investigators suggested that this result is consistent with the possibility that the substantial differences in estimated prevalence of depression in the PPG study might be due, at least in part, to cross-national differences in diagnostic thresholds.

The WMH finding of a positive association between prevalence and the proportion of cases classified severe

Table 17-2. The 12-month prevalence estimates of common DSM-IV/CIDI mental disorders in the WMH surveys.[1,2]

	Any anxiety disorder		Any mood disorder		Any impulse control disorder		Any substance disorder		Any disorder	
	%	(SE)	%	(SE)	%	(SE)	%	(SE)	%	(SE)
I. Low/lower-middle income countries										
Colombia	14.4	(1.0)	7.0	(0.5)	4.4	(0.4)	2.8	(0.4)	21.0	(1.0)
India: Pondicherry	10.5	(0.8)	4.8	(0.4)	4.3	(0.7)[9]	5.3	(0.6)	20.0	(1.1)
Iraq	10.4	(0.7)[3]	4.1	(0.4)	1.5	(0.2)[8,9]	0.2	(0.1)	13.6	(0.8)
Nigeria	4.2	(0.5)	1.1	(0.2)	0.1	(0.0)[7,9]	0.9	(0.2)	6.0	(0.6)
PRC[11]: Shenzhen	6.6	(0.4)[3,13]	4.5	(0.3)	2.4	(0.3)[9]	–	–	10.6	(0.5)
PRC: Beijing/Shanghai	3.0	(0.5)	1.9	(0.3)	3.1	(0.7)[7,9]	1.6	(0.4)	7.1	(0.9)
Ukraine	6.8	(0.7)[3,4]	9.0	(0.6)[5]	5.7	(1.0)[7,9]	6.4	(0.8)	21.4	(1.3)
II. Upper-middle income countries										
Brazil: São Paulo	19.9	(0.8)	11.0	(0.6)	4.3	(0.4)	3.6	(0.4)	29.6	(1.0)
Bulgaria	7.6	(0.7)[12]	2.8	(0.3)	0.8	(0.3)[7,9]	1.2	(0.3)	11.2	(0.8)
Lebanon	12.2	(1.2)	6.8	(0.7)	2.6	(0.7)[9]	1.3	(0.8)	17.9	(1.7)
Mexico	8.4	(0.6)	4.7	(0.3)	1.6	(0.3)[6]	2.3	(0.3)	13.4	(0.9)
Romania	4.9	(0.5)	2.3	(0.3)	1.4	(0.3)	1.0	(0.2)	8.2	(0.7)
South Africa	8.2	(0.6)[3,4]	4.9	(0.4)[5]	1.9	(0.3)[7,8,9]	5.8	(0.5)	16.7	(1.0)
III. High-income countries										
Belgium	8.4	(1.4)	5.4	(0.5)[5]	1.7	(1.0)[6]	1.8	(0.4)[10]	13.2	(1.5)
France	13.7	(1.1)	6.5	(0.6)[5]	2.4	(0.6)[6]	1.3	(0.3)[10]	18.9	(1.4)
Germany	8.3	(1.1)	3.3	(0.3)[5]	0.6	(0.3)[6]	1.2	(0.2)[10]	11.0	(1.3)
Israel	3.6	(0.3)[3,4]	6.4	(0.4)	–	–[6,7,8,9]	1.3	(0.2)	10.0	(0.5)
Italy	6.5	(0.6)	3.4	(0.3)[5]	0.4	(0.2)[6]	0.2	(0.1)[10]	8.8	(0.7)
Japan	4.2	(0.6)[3]	2.5	(0.4)	0.2	(0.1)[7,8,9]	1.2	(0.4)	7.4	(0.9)
Netherlands	8.9	(1.0)	5.1	(0.5)[5]	1.9	(0.7)[6]	1.9	(0.3)[10]	13.6	(1.0)
New Zealand	15.0	(0.5)[3]	8.0	(0.4)	–	–[6,7,8,9]	3.5	(0.2)	20.7	(0.6)
Northern Ireland	14.6	(1.0)	9.6	(0.8)	3.4	(0.6)	3.5	(0.5)	23.1	(1.4)
Portugal	16.5	(1.0)	7.9	(0.6)	3.5	(0.4)	1.6	(0.3)	22.9	(1.0)
Spain	6.6	(0.9)	4.4	(0.3)[5]	0.5	(0.2)[6]	0.7	(0.2)[10]	9.7	(0.8)
United States	19.0	(0.7)	9.7	(0.4)	10.5	(0.7)	3.8	(0.4)	27.0	(0.9)

SE, standard error.

[1]See the chapter text for a listing of the disorders included in each entry.
[2]Impulse disorders restricted to age ≤39 (China, Ukraine, Nigeria) or to age ≤44 (all other countries).
[3]Adult separation anxiety disorder was not assessed.
[4]Specific phobia was not assessed.
[5]Bipolar disorders were not assessed.
[6]Intermittent explosive disorder was not assessed.
[7]Attention-deficit/hyperactivity disorder was not assessed.
[8]Conduct disorder was not assessed.
[9]Oppositional-defiant disorder was not assessed.
[10]Only alcohol abuse with or without dependence was assessed. No assessment was made of other drug abuse with or without dependence.
[11]People's Republic of China.
[12]Obsessive-compulsive disorder was not assessed.
[13]Posttraumatic stress disorder was not assessed.
(*Adapted, with permission, from: Kessler RC, et al. Global Mental Health Epidemiology, 2011. Table 2, p. 42.*)

Table 17-3. The 12-month prevalence of common DSM-IV/CIDI mental disorders by severity in the WMH surveys.[a]

	Serious		Moderate		Mild	
	%	(SE)	%	(SE)	%	(SE)
I. Low/lower-middle income countries						
Colombia	23.1	(2.1)	41.0	(2.6)	35.9	(2.1)
India: Pondicherry	21.7	(1.6)	39.0	(3.1)	39.3	(2.8)
Iraq	21.9	(2.3)	36.0	(2.6)	42.1	(2.9)
Nigeria	12.8	(3.8)	12.5	(2.6)	74.7	(4.2)
PRC: Beijing/Shanghai	13.8	(3.7)	32.2	(4.9)	54.0	(4.6)
PRC: Shenzhen	7.2	(1.4)	37.9	(2.3)	55.0	(2.8)
Ukraine	22.9	(1.8)	39.4	(2.9)	37.7	(3.5)
II. Upper-middle income countries						
Brazil: São Paulo	33.9	(1.4)	33.0	(1.8)	33.2	(1.4)
Bulgaria	20.3	(2.7)	32.0	(3.5)	47.7	(2.7)
Lebanon	22.4	(3.1)	42.6	(4.7)	35.0	(5.5)
Mexico	25.7	(2.4)	33.9	(2.2)	40.5	(2.6)
Romania	28.1	(3.5)	28.7	(3.7)	43.2	(3.5)
South Africa	25.7	(1.8)	31.5	(2.2)	42.8	(2.2)
II. High-income countries						
Belgium	31.8	(4.2)	37.8	(3.3)	30.4	(4.8)
France	18.5	(2.5)	42.7	(3.0)	38.8	(3.6)
Germany	21.3	(2.5)	42.6	(4.6)	36.1	(4.3)
Israel	36.8	(2.4)	35.2	(2.3)	28.0	(2.1)
Italy	15.9	(2.7)	47.6	(3.8)	36.5	(3.9)
Japan	13.2	(3.1)	45.5	(5.3)	41.3	(4.6)
Netherlands	30.7	(3.4)	31.0	(3.7)	38.3	(4.6)
New Zealand	25.3	(1.0)	40.8	(1.4)	33.9	(1.2)
Northern Ireland	28.8	(3.0)	33.4	(2.6)	37.8	(3.3)
Portugal	17.5	(1.5)	50.6	(2.0)	31.9	(1.9)
Spain	19.3	(2.4)	42.3	(4.0)	38.4	(4.7)
United States	25.2	(1.4)	39.2	(1.2)	35.7	(1.4)

SE, standard error.
[a]See the chapter text for a description of the coding rules used to define the severity levels.
(*Adapted, with permission, from Kessler RC, et al. Global Mental Health Epidemiology, 2011. Table 3, p. 43.*)

is striking in relation to these earlier studies. The countries with the highest prevalence estimates of the DSM-IV disorders in the WMH surveys also have the highest reported levels of impairment associated with those disorders (data not shown here). It is not entirely clear why this consistent WMH pattern should differ so dramatically from the pattern in the two earlier studies, but one possibility is that the WMH surveys used special probing procedures to encourage complete and accurate reporting of mental disorders so that less severe cases were reported more completely than in the earlier studies.

Another possibility worth considering is that the prevalence in some countries might have been underestimated because the DSM categories are less relevant to symptom expression in some countries than others. This possibility was not investigated in the WMH surveys but rather it was assumed that DSM-IV categories apply equally well to all countries. A sophisticated analysis of the possibility that DSM categories might not apply equally to all countries was carried out as part of the PPG. In that study, an analysis of cross-national variation in the structure of depressive symptoms was carried out using item response theory methods.[22] The results showed clearly that both the latent structure of depressive symptoms and the associations between specific depressive symptoms and this latent structure were very similar across the countries studied. These results argue against the suggestion that the large cross-national variation in estimated prevalence of depression found in the WMH surveys is due to cross-national differences in the nature of depression. Comparable psychometric analyses have not yet been completed for other disorders though, so it remains possible that cross-national differences exist in latent structure that might play a part in explaining the substantial differences in prevalence estimates of other disorders in the WMH surveys.

At the same time, it is noteworthy that the countries with the lowest disorder prevalence estimates in the WMH series also have the highest proportions of treated cases classified as "subthreshold," that is, as not meeting criteria for any of the DSM-IV/CIDI disorders assessed in the WMH interview. This finding at least indirectly raises the possibility that the assessments in the CIDI are less adequate in capturing the psychopathologic syndromes common in all the WMH countries. In particular, the syndromes associated with treatment in low-prevalence countries are not well characterized by the CIDI because a high proportion of the people who report being in treatment for emotional problems fail to meet criteria for any of the disorders assessed in the CIDI. Additional WMH clinical reappraisal studies using flexible and culturally sensitive assessments of psychopathology are currently underway in both developed and developing countries aimed at exploring the implications of this finding empirically.

Mental Disorders and Use of Services

Indicators Used in the WMH Surveys

Making cross-national assessments of the mental health services in the WMH countries requires careful consideration of the highly variable nature of mental health treatments, both within and between countries. Patients can receive treatments for mental disorders from both general medical doctors (e.g., family practice, internal medicine) and mental health specialists (psychiatrists and neurologists). The specific treatments received from these physicians may also differ depending on their specialization and training (e.g., medications, psychotherapies). However, what makes the treatment of mental disorders considerably more variable than the treatment of most general medical conditions is that a wide range of other personnel provide treatment for emotional problems, including mental health specialists (e.g., psychologists, marriage and family counselors, psychiatric social workers), human services professionals (e.g., religious and spiritual advisors), and complementary and alternative medicine providers (e.g., traditional healers, acupuncturists, self-help group moderators). To truly understand the mental health services used nationally and cross-nationally, the WMH surveys had to capture systematically this breadth of information on potential treatments for mental disorders from respondents.

In addition to assessing respondents' use of a wide range of services, the WMH surveys contain sufficient detail to begin comparing respondents' actual treatment regimens with those recommended in evidence-based practice guidelines. Such information is crucial to begin breaking down the problem of unmet need for effective treatment into its component parts, such as failure to receive any treatment, receiving treatment but only after long delays, or receiving treatment that is inadequate in relation to published treatment guidelines and therefore unlikely to be effective. All these issues have been covered previously for a selected number of WMH countries.[23] Two of these issues are addressed here. The first is the use of any services for mental health in the prior year taking into consideration the adequacy of treatment received among those with any prior use of services. The second is the adequacy of this treatment.

Use of Services and Mental Disorder Severity

The prevalence of using any mental health services in the year prior to the survey varied significantly across surveys, ranging from 1.6% in Nigeria to 17.9% in the United States ($p < 0.0001$). In general, lower proportions of respondents used treatments in lower than in higher income countries (Table 17-4). Statistically significant relationships existed between disorder severity and service use in all WMH countries with the exception of the People's Republic of China metropolitan areas. Lower service use was generally observed for developing versus developed countries in all severity categories. Although this could be interpreted to mean that mental health care is being allocated rationally in most countries based on the availability of resources, it is important to point out that only between 5.0% (in Shenzhen metropolitan area) and 62.1% (in Belgium) of serious cases received any 12-month services. In general, lower proportions of moderate and mild cases received services. Although only small proportions (between 1.0% in Nigeria to 9.7% in the United States) of respondents that did not meet criteria for 12-month disorders used treatments, these could still be potentially meaningful given that people without disorders make up the large majority of the general population. However, further analysis of these respondents who did not meet criteria for disorders, but were using services, revealed that many had lifetime disorders in partial remission or subthreshold syndromes associated with meaningful role impairment and were probably using treatments appropriately.[24]

Adequacy of Treatment

Those respondents who received minimally adequate treatment according to evidence-based guidelines were identified.[25–27] Minimally adequate treatment was defined as receiving either pharmacotherapy (1 month or longer of a medication, plus four or more visits to any type of medical doctor) or psychotherapy

Table 17-4. Percentages using 12-month services by severity of DSM-IV/CIDI mental disorders in the WMH surveys.[1]

Columns under "Severity of mental disorders": Severe, Moderate, Mild. "No 12-month mental disorders" and "Test of difference in probability of treatment by severity" are separate groupings.

	Any treatment			Severe			Moderate			Mild			No 12-month mental disorders			Test of difference in probability of treatment by severity	
	N	%[2]	SE	n	%[2]	SE	n	%[2]	SE	N	%[2]	SE	n	%[2]	SE	X^2[3]	(p value)
I. Low/lower-middle income countries																	
Colombia	217	5.5	0.6	54	27.8	4.8	47	10.3	2.0	30	7.8	1.6	86	3.4	0.6	96.1*	(<0.001)
India: Pondicherry	103	1.4	0.2		9.8	2.9	19	6.7	1.2	12	5.1	1.7	45	0.2	0.1		
Iraq	57	2.2	0.4	27	23.7	6.2	19	9.2	3.2		5.3	2.5	29	0.9	0.2	18.7*	0.001
Nigeria	57	1.6	0.6	8	21.3	11.9	6	13.8	7.4	14	10.0	3.0	29	1.0	0.3	27.7*	(<0.001)
PRC: Beijing/Shanghai	74	3.4	0.6	5	11.0	5.4	11	23.5	10.9	3	1.7	1.2	55	2.9	0.6	16.1*	(0.001)
PRC: Shenzhen		1.7	0.2		5.2	2.0		10.3	2.8		6.4	1.4		1.0	0.2		
Ukraine	212	7.2	0.8	49	25.7	3.2	68	21.2	3.6	19	7.6	2.6	76	4.4	0.8	81.2*	(<0.001)
II. Upper-middle income countries																	
Brazil: São Paulo		8.7	0.4		32.8	2.4		20.0	2.7		12.7	2.1		3.6	0.3		
Bulgaria		3.5	0.3		30.7	5.0		21.9	3.3		14.1	3.0		1.8	0.2		
Lebanon	77	4.4	0.6	22	20.1	5.2	19	11.6	3.1	7	4.0	1.6	29	3.0	0.7	34.9*	(<0.001)
Mexico	240	5.1	0.5	52	25.8	4.3	53	17.9	2.9	33	11.9	2.3	102	3.2	0.4	132.9*	(<0.001)
Romania		3.4	0.4		36.4	7.3		17.9	6.4		14.8	4.5		1.8	0.4		
South Africa	675	15.4	1.0	45	26.2	3.6	66	26.6	3.9	67	23.1	3.2	497	13.4	0.9	41.0*	(<0.001)
III. High income countries																	
Belgium	187	10.9	1.4	46	62.1	9.2	30	38.4	8.3	13	12.7	4.6	98	6.8	1.1	227.1*	(<0.001)
France	272	11.3	1.0	56	48.0	6.4	70	29.4	4.0	43	22.4	3.4	103	7.0	1.1	82.6*	(<0.001)
Germany	183	8.1	0.8	30	40.6	8.9	39	23.9	4.7	27	20.5	5.2	87	5.9	0.9	54.5*	(<0.001)
Israel	421	8.8	0.4	81	53.9	4.0	54	32.6	3.7	19	14.4	3.2	267	6.0	0.4	368.1*	(<0.001)
Italy	141	4.3	0.4	29	51.6	6.5	38	25.9	4.2	21	17.8	4.5	53	2.2	0.4	192.7*	(<0.001)
Japan	92	5.6	0.9	10	24.2	5.0	16	24.2	5.0	9	12.8	4.4	57	4.5	0.9	44.5*	(<0.001)
Netherlands	202	10.9	1.2	57	49.2	6.6	36	31.3	7.2	15	16.1	6.0	94	7.7	1.3	66.8*	(<0.001)
New Zealand	1592	13.8	0.5	458	56.6	2.2	421	39.8	1.9	184	22.2	1.9	529	7.3	0.5	664.8*	(<0.001)
Northern Ireland		14.8	1.0		77.1	4.8		35.2	4.3		19.3	4.3		6.8	0.8		
Portugal		15.0	0.8		66.4	4.6		35.1	2.5		18.2	2.9		9.0	0.8		
Spain	375	6.8	0.5	79	58.7	4.9	93	37.4	5.0	35	17.3	4.3	168	3.9	0.5	446.1*	(<0.001)
United States	1477	17.9	0.7	385	59.7	2.4	394	39.9	1.3	219	26.2	1.7	479	9.7	0.6	668.5*	(<0.001)
X^2_{16}[4]	764.6* (<0.001)			186.9* (<0.001)			145.6* (<0.001)			104.1* (<0.001)			330.0* (<0.001)			(<0.001)	

SE, standard error.

*Significant at the 0.05 level, two-sided test.

[1] Percentages are based on entire Part II samples.

[2] 'Percentages' are based on respondents using any services within each level of severity.

[3] Severe and moderate cases were combined into one category for Japan and the percentage using services was displayed in both columns. The X^2 test was two degrees of freedom for this country.

[4] X^2_{16} is from a model predicting any 12-month service use among respondents within each level of severity.

(Adapted, with permission, from Wang et al., Mental Health Service, 2010, Table 6.17, pp. 151–152.)

(eight or more visits with any professional). The decision to have four or more physician visits for pharmacotherapy was based on the fact that for medication assessment, initiation, and monitoring, four or more visits are generally recommended during the acute and continuation phases of treatment.[25–27] At least eight sessions were needed for psychotherapy because clinical trials showing efficacy have generally included eight or more visits.[25–27] Any respondent in continuing treatment was regarded as having met this definition.

Due to insufficient numbers, only data of 14 countries are presented (Table 17-5). The proportions of respondents using services who received treatments that met the definition for being minimally adequate ranged between 10.4% (Nigeria) and 42.3% (France). Lower income countries generally had smaller proportions, although the small proportion observed in the United States (18.1%) was a notable exception. The relationships between disorder severity and probability of receiving minimally adequate treatment were significant in only five countries. Again, there were meaningful proportions of both severe cases using services that did not receive minimally adequate treatment and apparent noncases using services that did.

Burden of Common Mental Disorders

Indicators Used in WMH Surveys

Among other important personal variables, two outcomes of interest were foci for the WMH surveys: educational attainment and role functioning. These indicators can provide insight on potential personal achievement as well as the productivity and degree of fulfillment of the individual. To assess educational attainment, respondents were asked how many years of education they had completed. Because countries varied by the age of starting school and the duration of each stage of schooling, the stage of education was standardized within country by years of education. An orderly academic progression was assumed and four educational milestones were defined as follows: finishing primary education after 8 years of education, finishing secondary education after 12 years of education, entry to tertiary education after 13 years of education, and graduation from tertiary education (such as university or other higher levels of education after secondary education) after a total of 16 years of education. The standardization of these educational stages was done for all the countries studied (higher, middle, and lower income levels) with the help of researchers from the participating countries.

As an approximation to the impact of common mental disorders on productivity and functioning, the WMH surveys assessed, among other outcomes, the number of days each respondent was totally out of their main role due to illness in the 30 days before the interview. A modified version of the WHO Disability Assessment Schedule[28] was used to ask respondents the number of days in the 30 days before interview (i.e., beginning the day before the interview and going back 30 days) that they were totally unable to work or carry out their normal activities because of problems with physical health, mental health, or the use of alcohol or drugs. In addition, questions on "partial disability" asked about the number of days in which respondents had to (1) cut down on what they did (hereafter referred to as "cut-down days"), (2) cut back on the quality of what they did, and (c) make an extreme effort to perform as usual. Partial disability was expressed in full-day equivalents to allow for the variation in the number of disability hours per day. Good concordance of these reports has been documented both with payroll records of employed people[29] and with prospective daily diary reports.[30]

Impact of Early Mental Disorders on Educational Achievement

Education is a basic asset for individuals to realize a productive and healthy life. Premature termination of education puts individuals at clear risk of lower productivity, health, and self-realization during adulthood.[31] WMH data that assessed lifetime prevalence of mental disorders and dated age-of-onset of each disorder were analyzed to examine retrospectively reported associations between disorders that had onsets at earlier ages than the age of completing education and the subsequent early termination of education. Results suggest that early mental disorders are associated with significantly elevated odds of premature termination of education (Table 17-6).

The associations (odds ratios [ORs] and 95% confidence intervals [CIs]) of mental disorders with early termination of education are strongest and most consistent during secondary school in upper-middle and high-income countries. Particularly, in the upper-middle income countries, mood (OR: 1.5; 95% CI, 1.2 to 2.0) and disruptive behavior disorders (OR: 1.3; 95% CI, 1.0 to 1.6) are significantly associated with termination of secondary education, but, interestingly, substance use disorders are not. A steady increase in the risk of termination of secondary education with increasing comorbidity was not observed in these countries. In the high-income countries, all four categories of disorder are significantly associated with termination of secondary school, with the magnitude of the association lowest for anxiety disorders (OR: 1.3) and strongest for substance use disorders (OR: 2.8).

Having just one disorder is associated with a higher likelihood of termination in this group of countries, and the likelihood of termination increases

Table 17-5. Percentages receiving minimally adequate treatment among respondents using services in the WMH surveys.[1]

	Any severity			Severe			Moderate			Mild			No 12-month mental disorders			Test of difference in probability of minimally adequate treatment by severity X² (p value)[5]	
	n	%[2]	SE	n	%[3]	SE	n	%[3]	SE	n	%[3]	SE	n	%[3]	SE	(1, 2, or 3 df)[5]	
I. Low/lower-middle income countries																	
Colombia	33	14.7	3.4	11	23.1	8.5	7	21.7	10.5	3	6.3	4.6	12	10.1	3.5	4.7	(0.20)
Nigeria	1	10.4	9.8	0	—[4]	—[4]	0	—[4]	—[4]	0	12.4	11.8	1	12.4	11.8		
PRC: Beijing/ Shanghai	19	24.1	7.0	0	—[4]	—[4]	3	—[4]	—[4]	2	20.1	5.9	14	20.1	5.9	0.8	(0.36)
II. Upper-middle income countries																	
Lebanon	18	24.5	7.1	5	24.0	6.2	3	24.0	6.2	3	24.8	10.7	7	24.8	10.7	0.0	(0.95)
Mexico	42	15.2	2.7	8	11.3	4.5	13	28.6	6.3	6	19.8	5.8	15	11.3	4.0	10.5*	(0.014)
III. High income countries																	
Belgium	78	33.6	5.2	23	42.5	8.5	12	35.5	12.6	5	—[4]	—[4]	38	29.4	6.2	1.7	(0.63)
France	113	42.3	5.4	29	57.9	8.5	28	36.5	6.6	15	41.5	9.7	41	40.2	8.3	3.4	(0.34)
Germany	91	42.0	6.1	21	67.3	10.7	21	53.3	8.4	14	—[4]	—[4]	35	35.4	8.8	6.1	(0.11)
Israel	148	35.1	2.5	28	34.4	5.4	21	40.3	6.8	6	—[4]	—[4]	93	34.3	3.1	0.7	(0.87)
Italy	45	33.0	5.1	12	—[4]	—[4]	11	35.7	9.4	6	—[4]	—[4]	16	29.9	7.4	3.5	(0.32)
Japan	35	31.8	6.8	6	—[4]	—[4]	6	—[4]	—[4]	5	27.9	7.0	18	27.9	7.0	4.4*	(0.037)
Netherlands	98	34.4	5.0	37	65.7	9.2	19	34.1	10.2	10	—[4]	—[4]	32	21.9	5.2	23.2*	(<0.001)
Spain	152	37.3	3.3	41	47.5	7.5	37	43.6	5.6	20	44.8	9.9	54	30.1	4.4	8.5*	(0.037)
United States	302	18.1	1.1	160	41.8	3.2	101	24.8	2.1	41	4.9	0.8	—	—	—	114.0*	(<0.001)
X²_{16}[6]	117.0*	(<0.001)		41.0*	(<0.001)		31.2*	(0.002)		25.9*	(0.011)		96.7*	(<0.001)			

*Significant at the 0.05 level, two-sided test.

[1]Minimally adequate treatment was defined as receiving eight or more visits to any service sector, or four or more visits and at least one month of medication, or being in ongoing treatment at interview.

[2]Percentages based on entire Part 2 samples.

[3]Percentages are those receiving minimally adequate treatment among those in treatment within each level of severity.

[4]Percentages not reported if the number of cases with any treatment in a level of severity <30.

[5]The test was not performed for Lebanon, Japan, and People's Republic of China, where combined severe and moderate was compared against combined mild and none category. One degree of freedom chi-square tests were performed for Nigeria because there was only one (unweighted) case with adequate treatment. Two degree of freedom test was performed for the United States, where the mild and none categories were collapsed. Three degree of freedom tests were performed for all other countries.

[6]X13 is from a model predicting minimally adequate treatment among respondents in each level of severity that used any 12-month services.

(Adapted, with permission, from: Wang et al. Mental Health Service 2010. Table 6.20, pp. 158–159)

Table 17-6. Mental disorders as predictors of noncompletion of four educational milestones by country income level: the WMH surveys.

Income level	Noncompletion of primary school			Noncompletion of secondary education			Nonentry into tertiary education			Noncompletion of tertiary education		
	OR	(95% CI)	χ^2	OR	(95% CI)	χ^2	OR	(95% CI)	χ^2	OR	(95% CI)	χ^2
I. Low/lower-middle income countries												
Mood disorders	1.5	(0.4–6.2)	0.3	0.9	(0.5–1.4)	0.4	0.7	(0.5–1.2)	1.3	0.9	(0.6–1.4)	0.11
Anxiety disorders	0.9	(0.6–1.5)	0.1	1.0	(0.8–1.2)	0.0	0.6*	(0.4–0.9)	6.9	0.9	(0.7–1.3)	0.4
Disruptive behavior disorders	1.7*	(1.0–3.1)	3.8	1.2	(1.0–1.5)	3.5	1.0	(0.7–1.3)	0.1	0.9	(0.6–1.1)	1.0
Substance disorders	2.0	(0.7–6.1)	1.5	1.7	(1.0–3.1)	3.5	0.5*	(0.3–0.9)	5.4	1.1	(0.7–1.9)	0.2
Any 1 disorder	1.1	(0.8–1.4)	0.5	1.0	(0.8–1.1)	0.3	1.0	(0.8–1.2)	0.1	1.1	(0.9–1.3)	0.5
Any 2 disorders	1.2	(0.7–2.1)	0.3	1.4*	(1.0–1.9)	3.9	0.9	(0.6–1.4)	0.2	0.9	(0.7–1.3)	0.4
3+ disorders	0.1*	(0.0–0.6)	7.3	1.5	(1.0–2.4)	3.1	1.1	(0.6–1.8)	0.1	1.0	(0.6–1.7)	0.0
II. Upper-middle income countries												
Mood disorders	1.5	(0.9–2.6)	2.8	1.5*	(1.2–2.0)	9.1	1.0	(0.7–1.6)	0.0	1.0	(0.6–1.7)	0.0
Anxiety disorders	1.0	(0.8–1.2)	0.1	1.2	(1.0–1.4)	3.6	1.2	(0.8–1.6)	0.8	1.0	(0.7–1.5)	0.0
Disruptive behavior disorders	1.1	(0.8–1.5)	0.3	1.3*	(1.0–1.6)	5.2	1.1	(0.7–1.6)	0.1	1.3	(0.8–2.0)	1.0
Substance disorders	1.7	(0.6–4.4)	1.1	1.2	(0.9–1.7)	1.4	1.0	(0.7–1.5)	0.0	1.1	(0.7–1.6)	0.2
Any 1 disorder	1.0	(0.8–1.2)	0.0	1.0	(0.9–1.1)	0.3	1.0	(0.8–1.2)	0.0	1.3	(1.0–1.7)	2.6
Any 2 disorders	1.2	(0.8–1.6)	0.8	1.1	(0.9–1.3)	0.5	1.0	(0.7–1.4)	0.0	1.3	(0.9–1.9)	2.3
3+ disorders	1.8*	(1.1–3.0)	6.2	1.8*	(1.3–2.5)	13.8	1.4	(0.9–2.4)	2.0	1.1	(0.6–2.2)	0.1
III. High income countries												
Mood disorders	2.0*	(1.3–3.1)	11.2	1.5*	(1.3–1.7)	25.4	1.0	(0.9–1.2)	0.1	1.1	(1.0–1.3)	1.7
Anxiety disorders	1.0	(0.8–1.3)	0.1	1.3*	(1.2–1.4)	26.1	1.1	(0.9–1.2)	0.8	1.1	(1.0–1.3)	3.4
Disruptive behavior disorders	1.2	(0.8–1.8)	0.6	1.8*	(1.5–2.1)	39.6	1.1	(0.9–1.3)	0.5	1.4*	(1.2–1.7)	16.9
Substance disorders	12.8*	(5.5–29.7)	35.5	2.8*	(2.3–3.3)	134.8	1.4*	(1.2–1.6)	17.3	1.4*	(1.2–1.6)	17.4
Any 1 disorder	0.9	(0.7–1.1)	1.1	1.2*	(1.1–1.3)	12.8	1.1	(1.0–1.2)	3.5	1.0	(0.9–1.2)	0.4
Any 2 disorders	1.2	(0.8–1.8)	0.6	1.6*	(1.4–1.8)	45.6	1.0	(0.9–1.2)	0.0	1.2*	(1.0–1.4)	6.0
3+ disorders	1.6	(1.0–2.5)	3.4	2.2*	(1.9–2.6)	115.6	1.2*	(1.1–1.4)	7.2	1.3*	(1.1–1.5)	10.3

CI, confidence interval; OR, odds ratio.
*Significant at the 0.05 level.
Adapted, with permission, from: Lee S et al. B J Psych 2009; 411-417 Table 2, pp. 414.

with higher numbers of comorbid disorders. Rather, the association of disorder with termination was observed only among those with relatively high levels of comorbidity, suggesting there may be synergistic interactions among co-occurring disorders. In the low- and lower-middle income countries, none of the disorder categories is individually associated with termination of secondary education, but termination is more common among those with two or more disorders, again suggesting synergistic interactions between disorders. For both of the postsecondary educational milestones, college entry and college graduation, there were stronger associations of mental disorders with early termination of education in the high-income countries than in the other two groups of countries. In the high-income countries, substance use disorders are associated with early termination at both of these milestones, with ORs of 1.4 in both, and disruptive behavior disorders are associated only with termination of college prior to graduation (OR: 1.4; 95% CI, 1.2 to 1.7); increasing comorbidity is associated with a higher likelihood of termination. This pattern is not observed for the other country groups.

In the low- and lower-middle income countries, only two of the associations are statistically significant and both are negative, indicating that people with these disorders (anxiety and substance disorders) are less likely to terminate their postsecondary education than people who do not have these disorders. In the upper-middle income countries, none of the associations reach statistical significance for either of the postsecondary educational milestones, suggesting that among those who reach this level of educational attainment, mental disorders are not important determinants of academic progression. It is striking that in this large sample there was no statistically significant elevation in the likelihood of early termination of education associated with high levels of comorbidity, that is, three or more mental disorders, in either the low- and lower-middle income countries or the upper-middle income countries.

The overall pattern showed that the percentage change of people failing at educational milestones attributable to prior mental disorders was generally larger in developed countries than in developing countries. Among all educational milestones, the change of probability between those with mental disorder and those without was largest for the stage of completing secondary education in both developed and developing countries.

Role Limitation Associated with Mental Disorders

Previous studies have suggested that a substantial proportion of the total societal costs of mental disorders are due to productivity losses (including work absenteeism and low work performance while on the job, and early retirement) caused by mental disorders.[32,33] The WMH results are consistent with these claims.

Table 17-7 shows the associations of common mental and physical disorders with days totally out of role in the WMH surveys. Although, as noted earlier, information on days out of role was obtained for the 30 days before the interview, estimates are projected to a full year for each disorder. Two indicators are used: additional days or "individual-level effects" and population attributable risk proportions (PARPS), considered "societal effects"). All estimates were adjusted by age, gender, marital status, and employment, as well as the number and type of comorbid disorders. Additional days are estimated for individuals with a particular disorder, taking into account all other coexisting disorders as well as the total number of comorbid disorders when compared with a hypothetical individual with the same morbidity pattern except for the disorder of interest. The estimate is the additional number of days totally out of role due to the particular disorder, and it is considered its "individual-level" effect. Individual-level coefficients do not take into consideration how common the predictor disorders are in the population and consequently can be used only to describe the relative importance of predictor disorders from the perspective of the individual.

PARPs were used to evaluate the expected effects of either preventing or successfully treating one or more of the mental disorders included as predictors in the regression equations. To obtain the PARPs, the estimated individual-level effects for a particular disorder was multiplied by its prevalence. The PARP can be interpreted as the proportion of all days out of role in the general population that would be prevented if the effects of a given disorder on days totally out of role were prevented.

Mental disorders are associated with a higher level of disability measured by the additional days totally out of role (more than 40 for panic disorder, PTSD, and bipolar disorders). Rank correlations of individual effects of the conditions were low across country type (from 0.12 to 0.26). Interactions were found to be subadditive for most disorders in all three income groups (i.e., the incremental increase in days out of role is smaller when a disorder occurs comorbidly compared with when the same disorder occurs in isolation). This may imply that for preventing disability more effectively, as many as possible of the coexisting disorders should be addressed together. Addressing only one disorder will render a less effective outcome.[34]

In addition to those days of totally limited functioning due to their health, respondents had days

Table 17-7. Days totally out of role due to common mental and physical disorders. Additional days out of role ("individual-level effects") and population attributable risk proportions ("societal effects") by country income level: the WMH surveys.

	Income level															
	All countries				Low/lower-middle				Upper-middle				High			
	Additional days		PARP		Additional days		PARP		Additional days		PARP		Additional days		PARP	
	Mean	(SE)	%	(SE)	Mean	(SE)	%	(SE)	Mean	(SE)	%	(SE)	Mean	(SE)	%	(SE)
I. Mental disorders																
Alcohol abuse	1.9	(3.2)	0.3	(0.5)	−2.8	(7.2)	−0.5	(1.3)	8.2	(5.0)	1.9	(1.2)	−0.3	(4.5)	0.0	(0.6)
Bipolar disorder	17.3	(4.9)	1.4	(0.4)	36.5	(15.0)	1.6	(0.7)	23.2	(9.6)	1.7	(0.7)	9.6	(5.8)	1.0	(0.6)
Drug abuse	2.5	(4.0)	0.1	(0.2)	14.7	(13.9)	0.3	(0.3)	3.9	(12.2)	0.2	(0.6)	1.2	(5.5)	0.1	(0.3)
Generalized anxiety	7.7	(3.6)	1.0	(0.5)	13.5	(9.1)	1.4	(1.0)	24.6	(8.4)	3.4	(1.1)	7.6	(4.9)	1.2	(0.7)
Major depressive disorder	9.0	(2.5)	5.1	(1.4)	13.1	(5.0)	8.1	(3.1)	14.7	(4.1)	9.7	(2.5)	4.1	(3.2)	2.2	(1.7)
Panic and/or agoraphobia	14.3	(3.5)	2.6	(0.6)	24.3	(12.9)	3.3	(1.8)	17.7	(5.5)	4.9	(1.4)	11.7	(4.1)	2.2	(0.8)
Posttraumatic stress	15.2	(3.5)	2.2	(0.5)	15.3	(11.3)	1.2	(0.9)	−1.1	(9.5)	−0.1	(1.0)	16.2	(4.0)	3.1	(0.8)
Social phobia	7.3	(2.8)	1.7	(0.6)	5.7	(10.0)	0.6	(1.1)	9.0	(8.4)	1.9	(1.9)	7.5	(2.9)	2.2	(0.9)
Specific phobia	3.9	(2.5)	1.8	(1.2)	−6.6	(5.2)	−2.6	(2.1)	4.2	(4.7)	2.2	(2.3)	6.7	(3.3)	3.4	(1.6)
II. Physical disorders																
Arthritis	2.7	(1.8)	2.7	(1.8)	6.1	(4.4)	6.5	(5.0)	0.8	(5.0)	0.9	(5.6)	1.8	(2.4)	1.7	(2.3)
Cancer	5.5	(3.5)	0.7	(0.5)	19.4	(17.9)	0.7	(0.7)	−4.2	(12.9)	−0.3	(0.9)	6.9	(3.6)	1.4	(0.7)
Cardiovascular	5.7	(2.1)	6.3	(2.3)	2.7	(6.7)	2.5	(6.2)	1.0	(3.6)	1.7	(6.0)	7.3	(2.7)	7.6	(2.8)
Chronic pain	14.3	(1.5)	21.5	(2.3)	0.9	(3.1)	1.6	(5.5)	11.0	(2.5)	21.8	(5.2)	19.6	(2.1)	25.7	(2.9)
Diabetes	8.6	(2.8)	2.3	(0.7)	4.0	(6.4)	0.8	(1.2)	0.5	(5.6)	0.2	(2.2)	9.6	(3.8)	2.6	(1.0)
Digestive	7.6	(3.0)	1.8	(0.7)	−4.3	(4.8)	−1.5	(1.8)	−0.4	(4.0)	−0.2	(1.5)	16.6	(4.8)	2.6	(0.7)
Headache/migraine	7.1	(1.5)	6.9	(1.5)	10.4	(3.6)	11.7	(3.8)	6.5	(3.3)	10.7	(5.5)	4.5	(2.1)	3.3	(1.5)
Insomnia	7.9	(2.7)	3.0	(1.0)	5.7	(5.3)	2.2	(2.1)	4.6	(5.4)	2.0	(2.2)	9.4	(3.2)	3.5	(1.2)
Neurologic	17.4	(5.8)	1.5	(0.5)	33.7	(23.0)	2.5	(1.6)	18.6	(7.0)	2.4	(0.9)	15.3	(7.4)	1.2	(0.6)
Respiratory	2.6	(1.3)	2.9	(1.4)	10.7	(3.0)	9.2	(2.9)	−1.1	(2.6)	−1.2	(2.7)	0.9	(1.4)	1.1	(1.7)
All mental	11.9	(1.4)	16.5	(1.8)	10.5	(3.1)	13.7	(4.3)	12.8	(2.3)	20.7	(3.1)	11.3	(1.7)	16.0	(2.2)
All physical	14.1	(0.8)	47.6	(2.7)	12.6	(3.1)	42.7	(8.3)	9.3	(1.9)	39.9	(7.9)	16.3	(1.0)	52.7	(3.4)
All disorders	16.5	(0.7)	62.2	(2.1)	15.3	(1.9)	58.1	(5.7)	12.5	(1.7)	59.2	(7.2)	18.4	(0.8)	66.6	(2.6)

PARP, population attributable risk proportions; SE, standard error.
(Adapted, with permission, from Alonso J, et al. Mol Psychiatr 2011; 16: 1359–4184/11. Table 5, p. 1242.)

where their health partially affected their functioning. The number of additional disability days varied considerably by type of disorder, but was in the 2.30 to 4.19 range for physical disorders (median: 3.09 days) and in the 2.32 to 5.26 range for mental disorders (median: 4.04 days). Respondents with PTSD (5.26 days), GAD (4.52 days), and bipolar disorder (4.22 days) reported the highest number of partial disability days. Generally, respondents with mental disorders systematically reported 15% to 28% more partial disability days than respondents with physical disorders.

Other Adverse Effects of Mental Disorders

The results reported here about adverse effects of mental disorders on educational attainment and days out of role are merely illustrative of a much wider range of adverse effects of mental disorders on role incumbency (e.g., unemployment, marital stability), role performance (e.g., marital quality, quality of work performance), and morbidity (physical health problems either caused or exacerbated by preexisting mental disorders). Many of these other adverse effects have been investigated in the WMH surveys and are discussed in depth elsewhere.[35]

IMPLICATIONS AND FUTURE RESEARCH

The WMH data reviewed in this chapter document that mental disorders are commonly occurring in the general population and often are associated with significant adverse societal costs. Yet only a small minority of people with even seriously impairing mental disorders receive treatment in most countries, and even fewer receive adequate treatment. This situation needs to change.

Evidence indicates that some of the burdens of mental disorders can be reversed with best practices treatment. An implication of the WMH survey results regarding the adverse effects of mental disorders is that an expansion of treatment might be a human capital investment opportunity from employer or societal perspectives. Ongoing WMH analyses will continue to refine the naturalistic analyses of the adverse effects of mental disorders in an effort to target experimental interventions that can demonstrate the value of expanded treatment to address the enormous global burden of mental disorders.

SUMMARY

This chapter presents an overview of evidence on the descriptive epidemiology of mental disorders from the World Health Organization (WHO) World Mental Health (WMH) Surveys. WMH is the largest cross-national series of community epidemiologic surveys of mental disorders ever carried out, with over 150,000 respondents surveyed across 28 different countries. WMH surveys evaluate the prevalence, correlates, and the burdens of a wide range of mental disorders along with information about patterns of treatment for these disorders. This chapter has reviewed WMH data on prevalence, treatment, and adverse consequences of the four broad classes of disorder assessed in the WMH surveys: anxiety disorders, mood disorders, behavioral disorders, and substance disorders. The results clearly document that these disorders are commonly occurring and have many adverse consequences for the people who experience them throughout the world. The WMH data also show that only a minority of people who experience these disorders receive treatment and that the quality of treatment is often low. This is especially true in lower income countries and among people in disadvantaged segments of society. The enormous societal burdens of mental disorders, not only for the individuals who experience these disorders but also for their families and communities, make it critically important to expand high-quality treatment.

STUDY QUESTIONS

1. How would you describe (indicators, sources of information) the burden of mental disorders in a given region (e.g., your country)?
2. Take one aspect of mental health (frequency, impact, or care) and expand on its causes and possible corrective actions.
3. Identify and discuss some generic causes of the international variation of the prevalence of mental disorders.

ACKNOWLEDGMENTS

This chapter was prepared with support from the World Health Organization World Mental Health (WMH) Survey Initiative. A complete list of WMH publications can be found at http://www.hcp.med.harvard.edu/wmh. Core WMH activities are supported by the National Institute of Mental Health (R01 MH070884), the John D. and Catherine T. MacArthur Foundation, the Pfizer Foundation, the US Public Health Service (R13-MH066849, R01-MH069864, and R01 DA016558), the Fogarty International Center (FIRCA R03-TW006481), the Pan American Health Organization, Eli Lilly and Company, Ortho-McNeil Pharmaceutical, Inc., GlaxoSmithKline, and Bristol-Myers Squibb. The Chinese World Mental Health Survey Initiative is supported by the Pfizer Foundation. The Colombian National Study of Mental Health (NSMH) is supported by the Ministry of Social Protection. The ESEMeD project is funded by the European Commission (Contracts QLG5-1999-01042; SANCO 2004123, EAHC 20081308), the Piedmont Region (Italy), Fondo de Investigación Sanitaria, Instituto de Salud Carlos III, Spain (FIS 00/0028), Ministerio de Ciencia y Tecnología, Spain (SAF 2000-158-CE), Departament de Salut, Generalitat de talunya, Spain, Instituto de Salud Carlos III (CIBER CB06/02/0046, RETICS RD06/0011 REM-TAP), and other local agencies and by an unrestricted educational grant from GlaxoSmithKline. The Israel National Health Survey is funded by the Ministry of Health with support from the Israel National Institute for Health Policy and Health Services Research and the National Insurance Institute of Israel. The World Mental Health Japan (WMHJ) Survey is supported by the Grant for Research on Psychiatric and Neurological Diseases and Mental Health (H13-SHOGAI-023, H14-TOKUBETSU-026, H16-KOKORO-013) from the Japan Ministry of Health, Labour and Welfare. The Lebanese National Mental Health Survey (LEBANON) is supported by the Lebanese Ministry of Public Health, the WHO (Lebanon), Fogarty International, Act for Lebanon, anonymous private donations to IDRAAC, Lebanon, and unrestricted grants from Janssen Cilag, Eli Lilly, GlaxoSmithKline, Roche, and Novartis. The Mexican National Comorbidity Survey (MNCS) is supported by the National Institute of Psychiatry Ramon de la Fuente (INPRFMDIES 4280) and by the National Council on Science and Technology (CONACyT-G30544- H), with supplemental support from the Pan-American Health Organization (PAHO). Te Rau Hinengaro: The New Zealand Mental Health Survey (NZMHS) is supported by the New Zealand Ministry of Health, Alcohol Advisory Council, and the Health Research Council. The Nigerian Survey of Mental Health and Wellbeing (NSMHW) is supported by the WHO (Geneva), the WHO (Nigeria), and the Federal Ministry of Health, Abuja, Nigeria. The South Africa Stress and Health Study (SASH) is supported by the US National Institute of Mental Health (R01-MH059575) and National Institute of Drug Abuse with supplemental funding from the South African Department of Health and the University of Michigan. The Ukraine Comorbid Mental Disorders during Periods of Social Disruption (CMDPSD) study is funded by the US National Institute of Mental Health (RO1-MH61905). The US National Comorbidity Survey Replication (NCS-R) is supported by the National Institute of Mental Health (NIMH; U01-MH60220) with supplemental support from the National Institute of Drug Abuse (NIDA), the Substance Abuse and Mental Health Services Administration (SAMHSA), the Robert Wood Johnson Foundation (RWJF; Grant 044708), and the John W. Alden Trust.

REFERENCES

1. Ormel J, Petukhova M, Chatterji S, et al. Disability and treatment of specific mental and physical disorders across the world. *Br J Psychiatry* 2008;192:368–375.

2. Druss BG, Marcus SC, Olfson M, Pincus HA. The most expensive medical conditions in America. *Health Aff (Millwood)* 2002;21(4):105–111.

3. Kessler RC, Ustun TB. *The WHO World Mental Health Surveys: Global Perspectives on the Epidemiology of Mental Disorders.* New York: Cambridge University Press, 2008.

4. Kessler RC, Ustun TB. The World Mental Health (WMH) Survey Initiative Version of the World Health Organization (WHO) Composite International Diagnostic Interview (CIDI). *Int J Methods Psychiatr Res* 2004;13(2):93–121.

5. Haro JM, Arbabzadeh-Bouchez S, Brugha TS, et al. Concordance of the Composite International Diagnostic Interview Version 3.0 (CIDI 3.0) with standardized clinical assessments in the WHO World Mental Health surveys. *Int J Methods Psychiatr Res* 2006;15(4):167–180.

6. Hambrick JP, Turk CL, Heimberg RG, Schneier FR, Liebowitz MR. Psychometric properties of disability measures among patients with social anxiety disorder. *J Anxiety Disord* 2004;18(6): 825–839.

7. Leon AC, Olfson M, Portera L, Farber L, Sheehan DV. Assessing psychiatric impairment in primary care with the Sheehan Disability Scale. *Int J Psychiatry Med* 1997;27(2):93–105.

8. Somers JM, Goldner EM, Waraich P, Hsu L. Prevalence and incidence studies of anxiety disorders: a systematic review of the literature. *Can J Psychiatry* 2006;51(2):100–113.

9. Waraich P, Goldner EM, Somers JM, Hsu L. Prevalence and incidence studies of mood disorders: a systematic review of the literature. *Can J Psychiatry* 2004;49(2):124–138.

10. Wittchen HU, Jacobi F. Size and burden of mental disorders in Europe—a critical review and appraisal of 27 studies. *Eur Neuropsychopharmacol* 2005;15(4):357–376.

11. Endicott J, Spitzer RL, Fleiss JL, Cohen J. The global assessment scale. A procedure for measuring overall severity of psychiatric disturbance. *Arch Gen Psychiatry* 1976;33(6):766–771.

12. Gureje O, Olowosegun O, Adebayo K, Stein DJ. The prevalence and profile of non-affective psychosis in the Nigerian Survey of Mental Health and Wellbeing. *World Psychiatry* 2010; 9(1):50–55.

13. Kessler RC, Birnbaum H, Demler O, et al. The prevalence and correlates of nonaffective psychosis in the National Comorbidity Survey Replication (NCS-R). *Biol Psychiatry* 2005;58(8):668–676.

14. Ochoa S, Haro JM, Torres JV, et al. What is the relative importance of self reported psychotic symptoms in epidemiological studies? Results from the ESEMeD-Catalonia Study. *Schizophr Res* 2008;102(1–3):261–269.

15. McGrath JJ, Susser ES. New directions in the epidemiology of schizophrenia. *Med J Aust* 2009;190(4 Suppl):S7–S9.

16. Saha S, Chant D, Welham J, McGrath J. A systematic review of the prevalence of schizophrenia. *PLoS Med* 2005;2(5):e141.

17. Lenzenweger MF. DSM-IR personality disorders in the National Comorbidity Survey Replication. *Biol Psychiatry* 2007;62: 553–564.

18. Huang Y, Kotov R, de Girolamo G, et al. DSM-IV personality disorders in the WHO World Mental Health Surveys. *Br J Psychiatry* 2009;195(1):46–53.

19. Hasin DS, Grant BF. The co-occurrence of DSM-IV alcohol abuse in DSM-IV alcohol dependence: results of the National Epidemiologic Survey on Alcohol and Related Conditions on heterogeneity that differ by population subgroup. *Arch Gen Psychiatry*;61(9):891–896.

20. Weissman MM, Bland RC, Canino GJ, et al. Cross-national epidemiology of major depression and bipolar disorder. *JAMA* 1996;276(4):293–299.

21. Chang SM, Hahm BJ, Lee JY, et al. Cross-national difference in the prevalence of depression caused by the diagnostic threshold. *J Affect Disord* 2008;106(1–2):159–167.

22. Simon GE, Goldberg DP, Von KM, Ustun TB. Understanding cross-national differences in depression prevalence. *Psychol Med* 2002;32(4):585–594.

23. Wang PS, Aguilar-Gaxiola S, Alonso J, et al. Delay and failure in treatment seeking after first onset of mental disorders in the World Mental Health Survey Initiative. In: Ronald CK, ed. *The WHO World Mental Health Surveys: Global Perspectives on the Epidemiology of Mental Disorders. New York*: Cambridge University Press, 2008: 522–533.

24. Druss BG, Wang PS, Sampson NA, et al. Understanding mental health treatment in persons without mental diagnoses: results from the National Comorbidity Survey Replication. *Arch Gen Psychiatry* 2007;64(10):1196–1203.

25. Agency for Health Care Policy and Research (AHCPR). *Depression Guideline Panel: Vol 2, Treatment of Major Depression, Clinical Practice Guideline, No. 5.* Rockville, MD: Department of Health and Human Services, Public Health Service, Agency for Health Care Policy and Research; 1993.

26. Lehman AF, Steinwachs DM. Translating research into practice: the Schizophrenia Patient Outcomes Research Team (PORT) treatment recommendations. *Schizophr Bull* 1998;24(1):1–10.

27. American Psychiatric Association. *Practice Guidelines for Treatment of Psychiatric Disorders: Compendium 2006.* Arlington, VA: American Psychiatric Association Press, 2006.

28. Von Korff M, Crane PK, Alonso J, et al. Modified WHODAS-II provides valid measure of global disability but filter items increased skewness. *J Clin Epidemiol* 2008;61(11):1132–1143.

29. Kessler RC, Ormel J, Demler O, Stang PE. Comorbid mental disorders account for the role impairment of commonly occurring chronic physical disorders: results from the National Comorbidity Survey. *J Occup Environ Med* 2003;45(12): 1257–1266.

30. Gureje O. The pattern and nature of mental-physical comorbidity: specific or general? In: Von Korff MR, Scott KM, Gureje O, eds. *Global Perspectives on Mental-Physical Comorbidity in the WHO World Mental Health Surveys.* Cambridge, MA: Cambridge University Press, 2009: 51–83.

31. Lee S, Tsang A, Breslau J, et al. Mental disorders and termination of education in high-income and low- and middle-income countries: epidemiological study. *Br J Psychiatry* 2009;194(5): 411–417.

32. Kawakami N, Abdulghani EA, Alonso A, et al. Early-life mental disorders and adult household income in the WHO World Mental Health Surveys. *Biol Psychiatry* 2012;72(3):228–237.

33. Gustavsson A, Svensson M, Jacobi F, et al. Cost of disorders of the brain in Europe 2010. *Eur Neuropsychopharmacol* 2011; 21(10):718–779.

34. Alonso J, Petukhova M, Vilagut G, et al. Days out of role due to common physical and mental conditions: results from the WHO World Mental Health surveys. *Mol Psychiatry* 2011;16(12):1234–1246.

35. Alonso J, Chatterji S, He Y, (eds). *The Burdens of Mental Disorders in the WHO World Mental Health Surveys.* Vol 4. New York: Cambridge University Press, 2012.

Global Health Communications, Social Marketing, and Emerging Communication Technologies

18

Gary Snyder

LEARNING OBJECTIVES

- *Understand how health communications research and campaigns impact the wellness of individuals and communities globally*

- *Describe the role of news media, social media, trusted community members, participatory communication, and "edutainment" in health promotion and education*

- *Define common barriers to health communications research and delivery, particularly in developing countries and with underserved minority populations worldwide*

- *Explain the principles of social marketing to deliver health information and services and to change behaviors*

- *Show how mobile phones and other information communication technologies can accelerate access to knowledge, spur innovation, and improve health*

INTRODUCTION

One significant driver of improvements in public health globally over the past 40 years has been the increased understanding and employment of health communication research, campaigns, and technologies, as well as social marketing strategies.

Health communications research provides a picture of the knowledge, attitudes, and behaviors of individuals and communities. Health communications and social marketing campaigns use multiple channels to raise awareness and provide culturally appropriate messages about disease, environmental conditions, nutrition, safety, literacy, and a host of other issues. The communicators must understand individual and community needs and wants, as well as the social and political pressures and competitive forces. They will then be able to inform the people of the community in a manner they trust. This process should help the community be more open to receiving the communication and can lead to motivating them to change behavior and, ultimately, to improving their health and productivity.

Interventions to advance global health have centered typically on clinical and research endeavors, but that has been changing over the past three decades. An important missing piece of the prevention-treatment puzzle was the strategic use of health communication and marketing tools that can empower communities with the knowledge, motivation, and incentive to improve their environment and wellness, and in return, their social and economic potential and sustainability.

Many examples of health communications and social marketing success in changing behaviors and improving health now exist. Effective global health practitioners, particularly those working in developing countries, understand the importance of using communications and marketing at all stages of behavior change. To impact entrenched beliefs and practices, as well as open up access to new knowledge, health communications and marketing must continue to be an essential piece of community-driven global health strategies.

This chapter explores:

- Health communications research and program development
- Applying a social marketing process to improve and sustain healthier behaviors
- Partnering with media to promote and inform

- Tapping into the latest communication technologies to empower individuals and communities with new health knowledge and increased ways to stay connected, share their stories, and sustain lasting positive behavior changes

HEALTH COMMUNICATIONS AND PROMOTION

Eliminating or diminishing the burden brought on by the overwhelming diseases of our day calls for aggressive clinical prevention, treatment, and research, but also connecting meaningfully with individuals and communities to promote healthy behavior change. Human behavior plays a significant role in the leading causes of disease, disability, and death. By itself or with other strategies, health communications can inform and influence individuals and groups to quit smoking, use contraceptives, sleep under insecticide-treated bednets, fortify with iron the foods they produce, get an annual mammogram, make their own oral rehydration therapies, filter their water, stay compliant with medications, properly fund immunization programs, exercise regularly, refute myths, or begin to change long-held destructive cultural practices.

Health communications has been defined many ways, but essentially it is the use of communications planning, research, strategy, tactics, and evaluation to increase knowledge and motivate action that improves health. Combined with adequate health

services, technological advances, necessary infrastructure, and responsive policies, it can bring about sustained changes that transform individual, community, and global health status for the better.

Early use of health communications relied on one-way messages such as "Don't pollute!" or "Don't do drugs" that spoke only to the action the researcher or program leader wanted to bring about. By not taking into account what motivated the related action, what kind of need it fulfilled, what social or economic pressures the individual faced, the one-message campaigns had limited impact. But increasingly, health communication professionals have learned that to achieve the desired outcome of improved health, solid research and evaluation must be employed. Program development and delivery must reflect the needs, wants, and cultural values of the community (rather than a "top-down," Western mindset approach). Program developers must tap creatively into channels of communication that are easily accessed—or can be driven—by the target audience. Because communication and marketing efforts aim to motivate an individual or group to take some type of action based on their needs and wants, it is useful to understand what may influence an individual within their "social and health ecosystem."

A well-known model involving motivation is Maslow's hierarchy of needs shown in Figure 18-1.[1] Maslow constructed this theory based on individual behavior and needs, described in the form of a pyramid. As the basic physiologic needs of food, water, shelter, and security are addressed, individuals seek

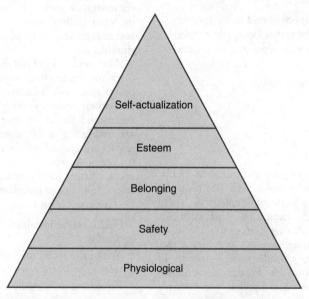

Figure 18-1. Maslow's hierarchy of needs.

to attain successively "higher needs" such as the social elements of friendship, family, belonging, and love, and then they may be motivated by self-esteem, ego, achievement, and respect of others. At the top of the pyramid is the need for self-actualization and fulfillment. Maslow championed this as reaching one's full potential, with motivation not centered on the self, but rather understanding and helping to solve problems of the wider community.

Applied to global health, Maslow's hierarchy of needs can be particularly useful in understanding where the greatest needs are of the individual and community, and how to best position messages, materials, and programs to that level or a higher aspired-to level so they have the most meaning and relevance. If a core set of youth aspire to become leaders in their community, communications and marketing can be directed at their "stepping up" and being recognized for taking action that benefits the entire community. They could help develop the message, advertising, and campaign and be featured in it, which could add credibility. Examples include their choosing to be tested for human immunodeficiency virus (HIV), or the effective "Truth" stop smoking campaign, designed and developed by US teenagers who describe the reality of why they choose not to smoke.

The values realized at self-actualization (acceptance of other views and traditions, lack of prejudice, using creativity and spontaneity, pursuing solutions to broader problems) parallel the qualities needed by global health communications professionals to effectively change behavior and improve health conditions. Maslow also exhibited a worldview when, in explaining self-actualization, he defined it as when one transcends cultural conditioning and becomes a world citizen.

Connecting Communications to Levels of Influence

Many levels of influence affect a group or individual's behavior, and health communications professionals must take these into account when designing effective strategies. These include individual, interpersonal, institutional, community, and public policy factors.[2]

Health communications, sometimes referred to as "behavior change communications," can affect *individual* knowledge, attitudes, practices, skills, and dedication related to the desired change. Information and programs aimed at informal *interpersonal* relationships present with family, coworkers, barbers, bus drivers, health professionals, and so on, can be effective because they come from known respected sources. Targeted health messages and calls to action to formal *institutional* groups of like-minded individuals can influence behavior. Organizations can reinforce

health information and support programming for their members that promote screenings and expectations of healthier living. Knowing the norms and standards, and gaining the support of trusted *community* leaders, elders, and key peer groups can go a long way toward advancing and sustaining a behavioral change communications process.

Finally, efforts to impact public policy and societal views and laws can be realized through a comprehensive health communications approach that educates, personalizes, and motivates the public, industry, and government to change the norm and take action for the greater good. Examples include work related to transportation and public safety: increasing the wearing of seatbelts in the United States and reducing the number of passengers allowed by law riding in Kenyan public mini-buses or *matatus*.

Behavior Change Communications: Theories, Models, and Frameworks

Effective health communications should start with the use of single or multiple theories and frameworks to build appropriate goals, structure, implementation, impact evaluation, and sustainability with various audiences. Each individual, community, or country presents special challenges and opportunities, and the global health communications professional may combine various theories to understand and influence behavior change related to the problem(s) faced.

Theories and models do not take the place of quality planning and targeted community-driven research. However, they can serve as a foundation during the formative stage of planning health communication initiatives and provide insight as to what may motivate and resonate with the audience when the program is rolled out. They can also highlight some of the outcomes that should be considered when evaluating programs or campaigns.

For a summary of some of the most commonly used health communications frameworks, theories and models, see Table 18-1.

Steps for Carrying Out Effective Health Communication Programs

Improving the health of individuals and communities through communications starts with understanding the needs, strengths, and perceptions of the population, and exploring whether the program or desired behavior changes can be successfully adopted. Will the individual, community, organization, or policymaker agree that the *benefits* to making the change outweigh the *costs*? What are the barriers to getting a clear picture of the capabilities of those you want to inform and influence? Have programs worked in the

Table 18-1. Behavior-change theories used in health communications.

Level	Theory/Model/Framework	Description
Individual	Stages of change model	Focuses on individuals' readiness to change or attempt to adopt healthy behaviors. Behavior change is a process not an event, and individuals are at different levels of motivation to change.
	Health belief model	Centers around: perception of risk of acquiring a health condition; the severity of the consequences; the perceived benefits of adopting the behavior; the barriers and cues to action that may hinder or spur the change. Also factoring into individuals' decisions: are they capable of making the change and sustaining it? Demographic issues and knowledge level play a role.
	Behavioral intentions theory	Suggests that the likelihood of intended audiences' adopting a behavior can be predicted by researching their attitudes toward the behavior's benefits, in addition to how their peers will view their behavior.
Interpersonal	Social learning theory	Explains behavior as a three-way "triadic reciprocal" relationship in which environmental issues, personal factors, and behavior interact and shape each other.
Community	Community mobilization theory	With roots in social networks, it emphasizes active participation and community development where the community helps identify, plan, implement, and solve problems with coordination from outside practitioners. Capacity building and addressing social injustices for the oppressed are hallmarks.
	Organizational change theory	Involves processes and strategies for increasing the likelihood of a formal organization adopting healthy policies and programs.
	Diffusions of innovation theory	Addresses how new ideas, products, and social practices spread within a society or from one society to another. Examines the innovation, the channels, and the social networks involved.
Individual, interpersonal, and community	Social marketing framework	Centers on applying proven marketing technologies and research for developing, executing, and evaluating programs that influence voluntary behavior change to improve individual welfare and the society they live in. Focuses on research, the customer, and changing behaviors, rather than attitudes/knowledge.

Source: Adapted from United States National Cancer Institute.[7]

past? If not, why? What tools or channels are available to communicate the information in a convincing and credible way? Are the resources available to impact awareness, provide incentives, and motivate sustainable change over time? Who are the trusted individuals that can help carry the messages and bring about the change in behavior?

As seen in Figure 18-2, several basic stages are involved in developing a successful health communications program. The process is fluid, with steps overlapping, but these represent the basic ingredients:

- Starting with a perceived problem and the desired change to bring about
- Using existing or conducting new research, and setting strategies
- Working with the community closely in the development and testing of messages and materials
- Implementing the program

- Assessing its impact on the goals and success
- Planning with the community for sustaining the program and the healthier behavior changes

Successful strategic behavior change campaigns are also benefit oriented, can be expanded to scale, and are cost effective.

Let us take a closer look at what needs to be considered and done at these different stages for behavior change communications to work in the global health setting.

ANALYZING PROBLEMS, CREATING INTERVENTIONS, IMPROVING LIVES: A HOPI STORY

You could take several approaches to discerning the initial core problem you want to address through health communications and marketing, implementing

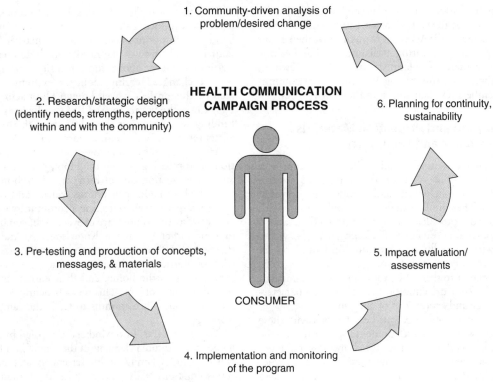

Figure 18-2. Health communication campaign process.

and evaluating the program, and sustaining the behavior change. The approach you choose will depend on your health field, experience, affiliated organization's focus, and familiarity with the region/community you are working in.

Because good communication tells a good story, let us put this in terms of a story.

You are part of a clinical team that wants to understand why health providers in a rural Indian Health Service clinic keep seeing female patients come in with the same condition of malnourishment and iron deficiency, even though they were provided written instructions on how to prevent it. The 3-minute clinic exchange between the Ivy League–trained doctor and the Hopi mother does not provide either party much opportunity for communication or discussion about underlying issues and barriers to her maintaining good nutritional health.

So you, as a health communications researcher, know research must be done within the community to get at the core problem. You find out who the respected women leaders of the village are and arrange to conduct several interviews with them in their homes, a place where they feel comfortable and more confident. After multiple group discussions, a common theme surfaces related to the issue: it is culturally inappropriate for a Hopi mother to focus on her own nutritional needs until her children and husband have plenty to eat. Because nutritious food is not abundant, you find she often goes without, skipping meals or not having access to fruits and vegetables after she takes care of the others.

Armed with that knowledge, you start to design a communications campaign, with the help of the women, that involves the entire family and community, and which supports the message that the mother's health matters much to the health of the family and to the wider community. The strategy will use multiple channels—from social media to radio to entertainment—to inform and influence, and you will involve traditional healers giving their blessing that an iron supplement will be safe to add to Hopi meals.

You identify women who are leaders to step forth to educate other women and families, and local lay health promoters agree to work with the Western physicians to increase their cultural awareness. A local youth group volunteers to incorporate the "good nutrition for mother" themes into a new play they will perform at the community's Hopi Corn Festival.

As part of your strategy, you enlist the aid of radio stations on the reservation to air future public service announcements (PSAs) from women to women about the importance of eating well and staying healthy. Similar content is planned for use on Twitter, YouTube, and a storytelling Website where community members tell their stories in their own voices.

Developing and Pretesting Materials for Relevance and Credibility

Since you received your public health training at a university in Ohio, you ask the university's creative services team to help write and produce the campaign materials. They produce high-quality publications with content you provide, a script for the PSAs, and a short video for YouTube. Slick posters, ads, video, new Twitter account, and brochures in hand, you are understandably excited as you go to the Hopi community center to share the prototypes of the campaign materials. Your presentation is met with uncharacteristic silence and expressions of chagrin.

After some prodding, you hear reasons why these materials will not work. Some Hopis consider the centipede symbol on the brochure cover taboo. The sepia tone photo of the traditional kiva structure inside depicts a ceremonial home where women were only allowed in to serve food and clean. There are only photos of individuals by themselves, which certainly does not express the positive Hopi concept of "Naya," which means people working together for a common good. The music provided for the PSA and video is Tibetan, not traditional or modern Hopi. Finally, the glossy paper stock is not made from recycled materials—not appropriate given the sacred value Hopis place on the environment and their emphasis on recycling and reusing.

This is an example of why pretesting of materials, health messages, and calls to action with the community for the community are so vital. Sometimes tens or hundreds of thousands of dollars are spent on a campaign by well-intentioned but culturally out-of-touch communications professionals who bypass pretesting and then do not understand why the communications campaign failed so miserably to change behavior and improve health.

Implementing, Evaluating, and Sustaining

You dig deeper and find right in the Hopi community creative writers, illustrators, designers, student actors, and a printer who understand the Hopi traditions, and redo the materials so they reflect the Hopi experience and will hopefully better resonate with the audience. The health messages must be developed in the Hopi context.

You meet a fledgling young Hopi filmmaker who agrees to produce a short video aimed at young husbands, an important segment of the market because your research showed the need to include men if the traditional views about food security and mothers were to change. Hearing about the excitement generated by this project, a well-known Hopi actor volunteers to do the vocals for the PSAs and agrees to raise funding for sustaining the effort through the online entrepreneurial Website, kickstarter.com.

Having taken the time to learn about the rich tradition of storytelling among the Hopi, you work to create a Hopi section on cowbird.com, a Website where individuals can add their photos, videos, and words to create a larger mosaic reflecting a community's story.

Knowing the importance of evaluation, you included in your earlier research a Knowledge, Attitudes, and Practices (KAP) survey of community members' knowledge of nutrition and family health, attitudes about gender roles in the home, and their current behaviors related to the problem. This sets a benchmark you can measure against in 6 months to see if the campaign is working.

You kickoff the "Iron Mothers" campaign by making it one of the featured elements of the Hopi Corn Festival, which includes family health screenings and nutrition counseling from Native American health promoters. The nonnative clinic physicians assist with the screenings and passing out multivitamins with iron. The local creators of the campaign materials are honored for their contributions to strengthening the Hopi community.

The PSAs air every day, a nutrition health column is written weekly for the local newspaper and placed on the new Website created for the campaign, and the culturally relevant publications connecting the health of the mother to the well-being of the Hopi community are distributed to homes and businesses. A comic book for kids written in both Hopi and English tells the story of a child who becomes a superhero by keeping his mother healthy and strong. Kids dressed as superheroes help lead a march through a retail section of town, raising social pressure for more affordable access to vitamins and nutrients. The story continues online via the Native American, youth-focused Website, "wernative.org," and user-generated content from the community grows.

To sustain the program's momentum, monthly community events weave in the health message and materials. The high school football team premiers the 5-minute video at halftime on the scoreboard. The theater group debuts its nutrition-inspired production, "Food Fight," and the strong, energetic mother character becomes a favorite of the packed house. Students at the local community college create a free mobile application for smartphones that helps families track nutrition and diet, and find healthy, affordable foods close to home. Pharmacists and discount stores in the area announce an unprecedented cooperative buying strategy to purchase multivitamins and iron supplements in bulk and sell them at a heavy discount to women in the "Iron Mothers" program. Mothers and their spouses and children begin coming to the clinic together each month for screenings and checkups with the physician and a newly hired Hopi nutritionist. Finally, after much advocacy from many groups and individuals, the tribal government passes legislation to use a percentage of the grocery tax to consistently fund low-cost vitamin supplements for families in need.

After 6 months, the clinical results look good: 80% of the women enrolled in the program now show normal iron levels compared with only 35% before, and the levels for other women outside the program coming to the clinic have risen as well. You conduct another KAP survey with the families, showing more support from men for helping to keep their wives, sisters, and mothers healthy, and a marked increase in children's understanding of why their mothers need to have fruits, vegetables, and vitamins too. Women overall are missing fewer days of work, a positive result that benefits both the family and the community.

By all accounts, the "Iron Mothers" health communications and marketing campaign was making a real difference—with individual and community health, but also capacity building. Thanks to the social, community, and business networks built to support it, the tapping of Hopi community talent to help produce it, and the pride of knowing the mothers, families, and the Hopi community were growing stronger because of it, the possibility of sustaining the effort and making it part of everyday life appears high.

This hypothetical campaign worked because it followed the framework for researching, designing, testing, implementing, and evaluating a health communications effort. But it also engaged the community to lend its knowledge, talent, and passion in developing creative ways to keep attention on this problem and to bring about the desired behavior change and health improvement. The program, grounded in the values of the Hopi tribe, employed research to study the problem and measure success, as well as various communication technologies to deliver the messages. Finally, it always stayed focused on the *consumer* (the mother) and the *benefits* to her, the family, and community.

CROSS-CULTURAL HEALTH AND COMMUNICATIONS

Health providers, educators, and media wanting to improve their communications and health care outcomes with underserved minority communities such

as the Hopi must understand the value and belief systems they bring with them, and link the program's benefits to the deeper values held. An example is the Latino population, which is growing rapidly in the United States, whose core values and beliefs often include:

- *Familismo* (significance of the family to the individual)
- *Collectivismo* (importance of friends, extended family)
- *Simpatia* (need for positive, relaxed relationships)
- *Personalismo* (preference for friendly relations with members of their same ethnic group)
- *Fatalismo* (little belief or experience with prevention—there is little an individual can do to change his or her destiny)
- *Respeto* (deferential treatment to those based on age and position)[3]

Of all of these beliefs, *fatalismo* is perhaps the one that keeps Latinos from taking prevention measures for their health or being motivated to manage a chronic health condition like diabetes. Some feel they cannot do anything about a condition like diabetes, most think insulin is harmful, and many avoid health screenings because of the belief that if you do not know you have the disease, it must not be real.[4]

Many Latinos believe that "stress, fear, and anger" bring on diabetes. Although "stress, fear, and anger" are not direct causes of diabetes, it is not surprising that Latinos would view them as so, given their cultural values and the need to keep life in *simpatia* or harmony to maintain good health. Regarding what motivates them to exercise more may point to the need for health communications researchers, community health providers, and policymakers to consider the Latino belief system centered around *collectivismo*, or the importance of family and friends working together collectively toward a shared goal or interest.

This was borne out in a Columbus, Ohio, survey of new Latino immigrants' knowledge, attitudes, and practice about health and media use. In response to a question about what would help them exercise more, many responded "if friends or family were involved," and "if there were free programs at a park or organization near where the family lives."[5]

Health promotion and communications campaigns can dispel misconceptions about the causes of disease and build on strengths in communities, such as *collectivismo* and *simpatia* with Latinos, in designing and implementing health marketing that motivates and changes behavior in a positive way.

Belief systems play an important role in how diseases are perceived in other cultures as well. Some Native Americans believe that if they are ill, they brought it on themselves. African Americans are often tested for conditions such as HIV or diabetes later than other groups, sometimes referred to as "last to test." This view may be akin to the Latino *fatalismo* belief that knowing one has a condition may not matter either way, so why confirm it.

With this cultural lens in mind, the US Centers for Disease Control and Prevention's "Testing Makes Us Stronger" national campaign targets men who have sex with men (MSMs) in the African American community. The message? Knowing one's HIV status is important and empowering information. The campaign—developed by an expert panel of black gay and bisexual community leaders working with the CDC—features bold, strong messages and images in digital, print, Web, outdoor, and transit ads.

The "Testing Makes Us Stronger" campaign shows men taking responsibility for their bodies and their HIV status, thereby making themselves, their partners, and their community stronger. The campaign runs in select cities experiencing high levels of HIV infection in African American gay and bisexual men (HIV rates can be three times higher among black MSMs in the United States than white MSMs). More than 400 black men in five US cities helped refine the messages used in the campaign, a strong testament to the need for health communications campaigns to be driven by the core community where the hoped-for changes would take place.[6]

The stigma surrounding conditions in certain cultures, communities, and societies can be a particularly intractable barrier to overcome—for both the individual and for health communications practitioners.

Those living with mental illnesses, for example, face societal prejudices borne out of a lack of information or a prevailing stereotype. The result is that a soldier returning home from conflict may not seek needed treatment for posttraumatic stress disorder, or a mother experiencing a deep depression is not comfortable discussing it with her family or receiving treatment from her doctor.

Successful health outcomes may require a strategy that delivers multiple communications to the audiences that, when combined, influence whether the change can be made. For example, to increase the number of women receiving mammograms, a successful campaign will need to communicate different messages to doctors and women, as well as help push for change in health policy to provide needed resources and technology (see Figure 18-3).

Messages, Methods, and Channels for Health Communications

Health communications professionals possess many outlets and strategies for making sure key messages are relevant, accepted, and acted on. Some of the methods for designing effective campaigns include the following:[7]

- **Media literacy:** Instructs audiences on how to understand media messages to identify the sponsor's motives, and how to compose messages targeted effectively to the intended audience's point of view

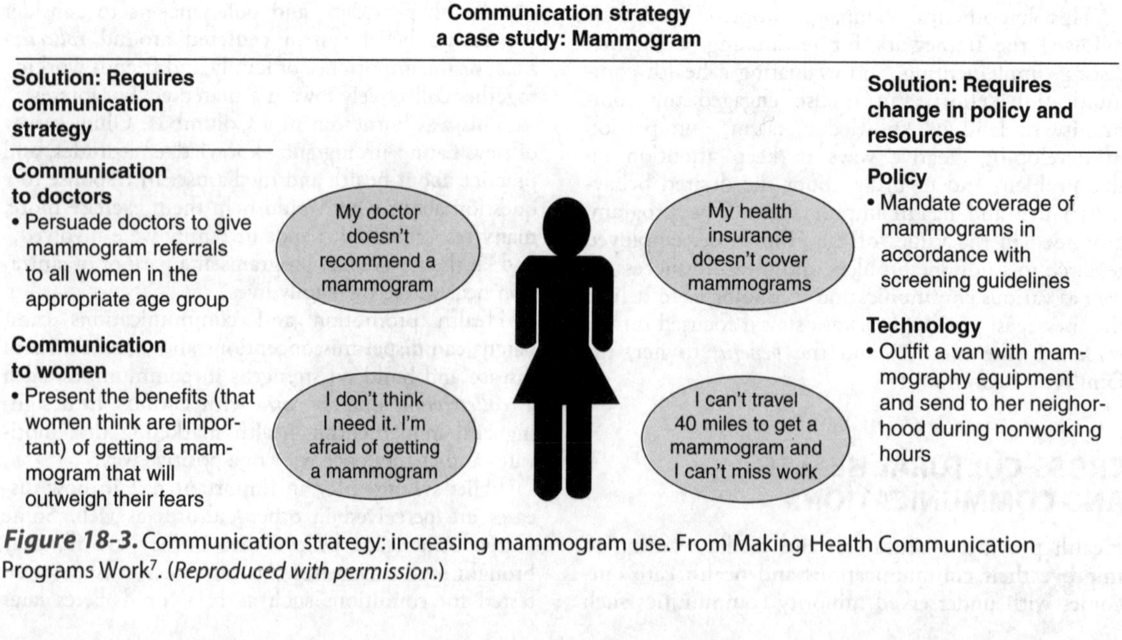

**Communication strategy
a case study: Mammogram**

Solution: Requires communication strategy

Communication to doctors
- Persuade doctors to give mammogram referrals to all women in the appropriate age group

Communication to women
- Present the benefits (that women think are important) of getting a mammogram that will outweigh their fears

My doctor doesn't recommend a mammogram

I don't think I need it. I'm afraid of getting a mammogram

My health insurance doesn't cover mammograms

I can't travel 40 miles to get a mammogram and I can't miss work

Solution: Requires change in policy and resources

Policy
- Mandate coverage of mammograms in accordance with screening guidelines

Technology
- Outfit a van with mammography equipment and send to her neighborhood during nonworking hours

Figure 18-3. Communication strategy: increasing mammogram use. From Making Health Communication Programs Work[7]. (*Reproduced with permission.*)

- **Traditional and new media advocacy:** Seeks to change the social and political environment in which decisions are made by influencing print, digital, and social media's selection of stories and by shaping the debate about those subjects
- **Public relations:** Advances certain messages about a health issue or behavior to the media or other influencers to raise knowledge and increase attention around the topic
- **Advertising:** Places paid or public service messages in the media or public spaces to increase visibility and support for a product, service, or behavior
- **Education entertainment:** Often called "edutainment," it seeks to integrate health-promoting messages and storylines into popular culture entertainment and news programs; also seeks entertainment industry support for a health issue to multiply the effect
- **Individual and group instruction:** Influences, guides, and provides skills and incentives to support positive behaviors
- **Partnership development/advocacy:** Deepens support for a program or issue by attracting the influence, credibility, and resources of profit, nonprofit, or governmental policymakers

According to McGuire's "Communications for Persuasion," to communicate the message successfully, these five communication elements all must work:

- Credibility of the message source
- Message design
- Delivery channel
- Intended audience
- Intended behavior[8]

Pitfalls and Possibilities with Health Communications

In all areas, but particularly in developing countries, several challenges to effective communication programs may exist. These include:

- Developing trust within the community and the culture
- Low literacy rates of the audience you want to address
- Lack of existing quality baseline information and research on the subject
- Environmental disruptions such as floods and earthquakes, and armed conflict can affect roads, telecommunications, transportation, and access to accurate information
- Corruption—funds for a program at the local level may never see the local community

- Long-held cultural and spiritual beliefs; traditions that run counter to fact
- Values imposition (by researcher or funding organization)
- Too much top-down "grass-tops" approach to implementation; not enough community or grassroots talent driving the program
- Multiple languages and dialects in region; lack of quality interpreters in the health care setting
- Lack of existing mediums and channels to reach intended community
- Censorship and other factors restricting access to digital communications platforms, such as smartphones, Web, and social media.
- Insufficient resources—funding and people—to maintain a sustained presence
- Literal translation of images and visuals

The meaning applied by community members to words and pictures can be a barrier to raising awareness of a health condition or attempting to receive feedback about the prevalence of a problem. In its research on HIV/AIDS media reporting, the Kaiser Family Foundation found that the word *prostitute* had a negative connotation but discovered that *sex worker* was more acceptable in some cultures because it more accurately described situations where a woman had no other economic opportunity.[9]

In rural villages of Ecuador, researchers from Ohio University's Tropical Disease Institute carried a placard with them that had an enlarged 5-inch photo of the triatomine "kissing bug," the vector for the parasite *Trypanosoma cruzi,* which causes Chagas disease. As they went to each village conducting surveillance, they pointed to the bug on the poster and asked the residents if they had seen it in their homes or community (see Figure 18-4). In each village, the answer was "no," they had never seen a bug like that, which surprised the researchers.

Clearly, the kissing bug and Chagas disease clinical symptoms were present, but the villagers denied ever seeing the bug. Was it because the bug only attacks humans at night while villagers slept? Finally, after further discussion, they realized the community members looked at the size of the bug on the placard literally, and with that cultural prism, understandably responded that they had never seen a 5-inch kissing bug in their village.

The researchers went back and immediately produced publications with photos depicting the literal sizes of the young and adult triatomines (see Figure 18-5). Resurveying the same villagers with the new material, they heard "oh yes, of course we've seen *those* bugs . . . they're everywhere!"

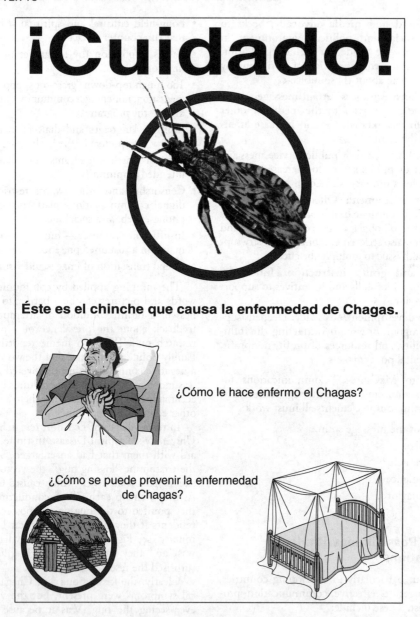

Figure 18-4. Chagas poster, literal size. Ecuadorian villagers had a literal interpretation of the size of this triatomine bug, shown in this poster as 5 inches long, and told researchers they had never seen it in their community.

SOCIAL MARKETING

A major development in health communications—social marketing—began to take shape as a discipline in the 1970s with the idea that the same marketing principles being used to sell products to consumers could be used to "sell" ideas, attitudes, and behaviors that could benefit the individual, community, and society. As defined by Andreasen, social marketing "seeks to influence social behaviors, not to benefit the marketer, but to benefit the target audience and the general society"[10]

Social marketing aims to change behaviors, first and foremost. Social marketers place a high value on conducting market research to "listen" and determine

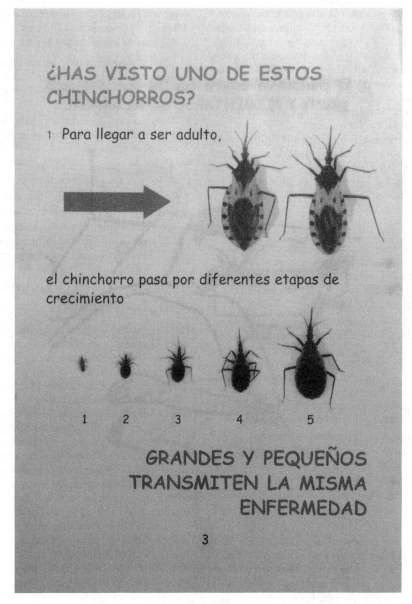

Figure 18-5. Chagas triatomines, "book" actual sizes. Ohio University Tropical Disease Institute researchers then designed a booklet with the actual sizes of the bugs and showed it to the community. "Oh yes, we've seen *that* bug, that's the chinchero!" From Ohio University Tropical Disease Institute. (*Reproduced with permission.*)

the needs, wants, and perceptions of the "customer." They recognize that behavioral change will only come about if the researcher focuses the work on where the customer is now. When possible, researchers carefully segment audiences rather than treating them as one mass group, and competing forces that detract from

the desired behavior change are addressed by diminishing their appeal and reinforcing the benefits and ease of accessibility of the new "product."

The social marketing process has been used extensively in global health programs for contraceptive use; oral rehydration therapy; literacy; multidrug-resistant tuberculosis (TB); and HIV/AIDS prevention, treatment, and education. Social marketing can be seen in campaigns to reduce drug abuse, increase condom use, encourage stewardship of the environment, exercise more frequently, motivate more people to donate their organs, and stop smoking cigarettes. This framework or mindset centers on determining and delivering the benefits the consumer desires and ensuring the *benefits* to them outweigh the *costs*.

Based on marketing principles, but dealing with more complex issues involving behavioral change, social marketing applies the traditionally commercial concepts of the "four P's" of product, price, place, and promotion, and adds a fifth: positioning. When applied to social marketing, these elements become:

- **Product:** The behavior or health idea that the campaign planners would like the consumers to adopt. The product can be an action (e.g., performing breast self-examinations regularly) or material (e.g., fat-free dairy products).

- **Price:** The costs associated with "buying" or adopting the product. Costs can involve sacrifices related to psychological well-being (e.g., increased anxiety), sociality (e.g., possibility of ostracism or stigma), economics (e.g., financial sacrifice), or time (e.g., inconvenience). Price can be offset by benefits, whether in the form of monetary incentive or improved outcomes, such as increased productivity.

- **Place:** The distribution channels used to make the product available in an easily obtainable way. The consumer must be informed of where, when, and how he or she can obtain the product.

- **Promotion:** The efforts taken to ensure the priority audience is aware of the campaign, the benefits, and how peers are adopting it.

- **Positioning:** The product must be positioned in a way that maximizes benefits and minimizes costs. "Positioning" is a psychological construct that involves the location of the product relative to other products and activities with which it competes. For instance, physical activity could be repositioned as a form of relaxation, not exercise.[11] Or the benefits of exercise on preventing dementia could be positioned as a positive for families, caregivers, and communities who want to keep seniors independent and healthy as long as possible.

Social marketers working to bring about healthier behaviors will conduct an analysis of the individual, community, or organization's environment. This can involve doing a strengths, weaknesses, opportunities, and threats (SWOT) analysis to examine the audience's strengths and weaknesses, as well as the economic, competitive, regulatory/laws/customs, social, and technological opportunities and threats.

Questions asked during this exploration could be:

- What strengths, skills, and accomplishments does this individual or community have that could be tapped into and built on during a health social marketing campaign?

- What cultural traditions, beliefs, laws, or biases are present that may support or impede the hoped-for behavioral change?

- What's the economic, educational, and social capacity for embracing the change?

- Can the benefits of the proposed change win out over competing desires, habits, and interests?

- Are there sufficient communication channels and resources available to inform and motivate the individual(s) to make the change and sustain it?

SEGMENTING, RESEARCHING, AND SUSTAINING

Effective social marketing health programs tap into other elements of marketing to achieve success. These include differential advantage, audience segmentation, and research.

The *differential advantage* of a product, service, or behavior change is that feature or benefit that makes it more desirable to adopt than the alternative choices. You may see your differential advantage in a stop smoking campaign to be that it will save the smoker's life. However, focusing on the short-term benefits and advantages, such as better breath, not smelling like smoke, appearing more attractive, or saving money, may be more relevant to the smoker now and have a better chance of success for both the consumer and the social marketer.

Segmenting a population means defining the subgroups based on their common characteristics and traits. Because populations are different, segmentation helps you develop materials, messages, and channels for delivery that are tailored to those you want to inform and motivate, and who may be most at risk yet ready for the change. Segmentation also helps you figure out the individuals or groups who can help you bring about the program and change.

You can segment a population into a priority audience by using the following characteristics to define them:

- **Behavioral:** Health-related activities or choices, degree of readiness to change, technology early adopter, information-seeking behavior, media use, and lifestyle characteristics

- **Cultural:** Language proficiency and preferences, religion, ethnicity, generational status, family structure, degree of acculturation, and lifestyle factors (e.g., special foods, activities)

- **Sociodemographic:** Age, gender, occupation, income, educational attainment, family situation, and places of residence and work
- **Physical:** Type and degree of exposure to health risks, medical condition, disorders and illnesses, and family health history
- **Psychographic:** Attitudes, outlook on life and health, self-image, opinions, beliefs, values, self-efficacy, life stage, social class, and personality traits[7]
- **Cohort:** Looks at individuals bound together in history by a series of events. The events may have been the technological upheavals, wars, political crises, and major sociological changes that form and shape an individual's attitudes and beliefs regarding health, prevention, practices. Depending on the timeframe they came of age, these groups can be characterized as worrying about financial security, very accepting of authority, conforming to norms, having great trust in institutions, questioning everything, cynical, conservative, idealistic team players, always been connected digitally, achieving, and community serving.[12]

Research is at the heart of all successful social marketing programs. In defining the intended audience, their knowledge, attitudes, practices, and sociodemographics, the needed intervention, and the outcome goals, market researchers may apply primary and secondary data. Primary data, information collected by observing individuals or asking them questions, address a specific research question. Secondary data were collected previously for another purpose such as the US census or media access habits, but can be helpful in building a social marketing program.

Observational research is one way to study individual or community behavior. Gender roles within a village could be observed, or how patients of each gender are treated when they first enter a health care facility. This research can show what happens but cannot describe why it happens.

Another common method used is survey research. Surveys can be administered through telephone interviews, personal in-depth interviews, focus groups, mail, software on smartphones, and Web-based applications. Depending on their structure and the skill of the researcher, surveys can yield much about an individual's knowledge, attitudes, and practices related to health. See Figures 18-6 and 18-7 for examples of community-based health surveys conducted in an impoverished community in Lima, Peru, and in the Dadaab refugee camp in Kenya.

Similar to other health communications, those using a social marketing approach to increase health literacy and produce healthier behaviors employ several channels to send their messages. These channels may be:

- Interpersonal (patient counseling)
- Organizational/community (town hall meetings, workplace campaigns)
- Mass media (newspaper, radio and TV ads, news, letters to editor, opinion pieces, talk shows, and education entertainment)
- Digital communications (Internet and Intranet Websites, e-mail, newsgroups, Website ads, topic or campaign blogs, podcasts, and various digital social media and activist networks online)

Fiscal Incentives to Improve Behaviors and Lower Costs

Health communication practitioners should plan for the "price" or cost perceived to be associated with a positive behavior change. Another important consideration or tactic within this sphere is the potential benefit that offsets any costs brought on with the change. This could be the benefit of living longer and being able to enjoy more time with one's grandchildren. Or it could be a financial benefit or incentive paid to the individual for taking measurable action that prevents illness and improves health.

Direct financial incentives can help drive consumer behavior to improve an individual's or group's health. Examples include:

- Employers paying employees to adopt healthier habits, such as a $200 discount off a fitness membership if the employee exercises a set number of times, or providing a $100 credit on health insurance premiums if an employee is a nonsmoker.
- The Ecuadorian government paying $240 per month to patients living with multidrug-resistant TB to increase the likelihood that they will stay compliant with and finish their treatment schedule. Preliminary results of the national program show that the financial support has resulted in a dramatic reduction in the percentage of patients who abandon their treatment program.[13]

One of the most comprehensive studies that examined the effects of financial incentives on consumer health behavior involved a multinational company based in the United States and attempts to encourage employees who were smokers to quit. Researchers provided information about smoking-cessation programs to 442 employees; a separate set of 436 employees received the same information plus financial incentives. The financial incentives were $100 for completion of a smoking-cessation program, $250 for cessation of smoking within 6 months after study enrollment, as confirmed by a biochemical test,

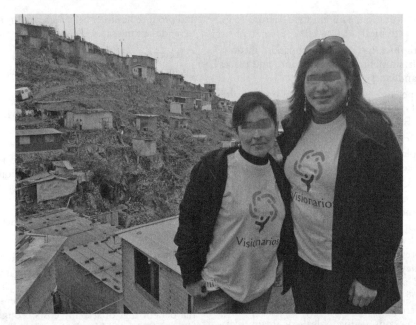

Figure 18-6. Two public health community leaders from Los Visionarios NGO in Peru, working in the impoverished Alto del Arenal community of Villa Maria del Triunfo in Lima. Visionarios is conducting the first survey of residents living in the highest section of the shanty town, which is also the poorest and most underserved. Dartmouth's Geisel School of Medicine is partnering with the NGO and the government of Peru to improve education, research, and health care delivery. (*Courtesy of Gary Snyder, Dartmouth Geisel School of Medicine.*)

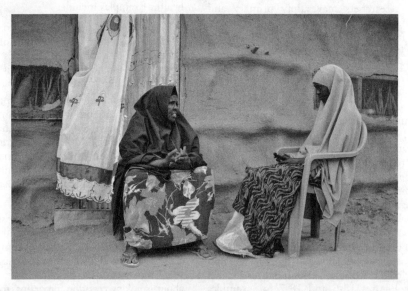

Figure 18-7. Kowsar Mohamed Warsame uses a smartphone to survey Hawa Musa Farah, from Mogadishu, Somalia, at her home in Dagahaley refugee camp in Dadaab, Kenya, in August 2011. An Internews-led assessment team conducted an extensive survey among refugees in the three main Dadaab refugee camps aimed at understanding the information needs of refugees in Dadaab and exploring ways to improve the flow of communication between refugees, aid agencies, and host communities. (*Courtesy of Quintanilla J, Goodfriend L. When Information Saves Lives: 2011 Annual Report, Internews Humanitarian Information Projects. Internews, 2011. Photo credit: Meridith Kohut.*)

and $400 for abstinence for an additional 6 months after the initial cessation, as confirmed by a biochemical test.

Results showed that the financial incentive group had significantly higher rates of smoking cessation than did the information-only group 1 year after enrollment. Employees were more than three times as likely to quit smoking if they were given $750 in incentives, compared with those who were merely encouraged to quit but offered no cash.[14]

Health Promoters and "Edutainment" Take Center Stage

An essential part of any health communications program involves finding out who in the community are the most trusted sources to help deliver information and encourage behavior change. In many cultures, lay health promoters serve this role because of their knowledge and their respected place in the family or community.

A broader group called cultural "brokers" can help connect the researcher, educator, or organization to the community as well. These individuals may range from nurses, lay health promoters, and shamans to school counselors, social workers, and youth leaders. By recruiting individuals within the community as leaders, the programs will be more relevant, be communicated by known individuals, and stand a better chance

of producing improved health outcomes. Health promoters and brokers within the community often bring more credibility and increase the likelihood of sustained change, particularly because groups or individuals from outside the community may be perceived as having only temporary, more selfish motivations.

Latino *promotoras*, trusted professional or lay health workers in the Latino community, have proven to be effective for delivering culturally sensitive health information and increasing knowledge about breast and cervical cancer. Researchers found that having *promotoras* conduct the programs improved participants' cancer knowledge and changed their perceptions of the barriers to cancer screening.[15]

Bilingual cultural brokers bridge the gap between the educator or health organization and certain communities, particularly those "hard to reach" because of language, culture, or other differences. They can make the difference whether communications and programming are accepted and believed by the community or not (see Figure 18-8).

Research has shown that *edutainment*, the practice of using mass entertainment to deliver public health messages, raises awareness of issues and motivates action and behavior change. Developing powerful human interest storylines through popular characters that are woven into *telenovellas* (Spanish language

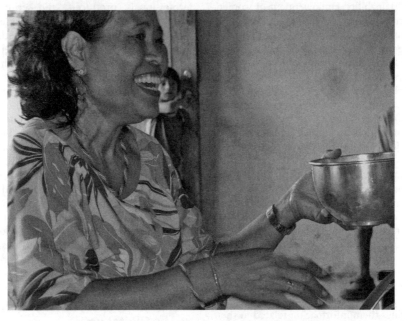

Figure 18-8. Health promoter with community drink. Trusted health educators bridge the gap between researchers and the community's culture. Here a health promoter in a rural Ecuadorian village shares a traditional drink with the community before talking with them about good nutrition and safe water practices. (*Courtesy of Gary Snyder, Dartmouth Geisel School of Medicine.*)

soap opera dramas), radio dramas, community theater, or other media and shows can have a profound impact on reader, listener, and viewer understanding of health issues and behavior.

One of the earliest examples of how mixing social change content into popular entertainment affects behavior was the Peruvian telenovela *Simplemente Maria*. The central character, Maria Ramos, was a rural-to-urban migrant who moved from the Andes to Lima. She worked as a maid during the day and struggled economically because she was illiterate. She also became a single mother. Her fortunes changed, though, when she decided to start attending adult literacy classes at night and also learned how to become a seamstress. Empowered by her ability to read and her growing seamstress business, she started her own fashion business that became a great success, with Maria becoming known all the way to Paris. Most importantly, during this storyline, enrollment in adult literacy classes in Peru skyrocketed in the 1970s, and rural-to-urban migration accelerated.[16]

Another example of the innovative use of media to reach the audience with human development stories is *Story Story,* a successful radio drama broadcast that reaches millions in Nigeria and on the BBC Network. It combines a storyline with discussion of issues raised during the week's shows, centers around everyday people—poor, rich, farmers, teachers, market traders—and covers topics like violence, HIV/AIDS, corruption, environmental sustainability, empowerment of women, education, and citizenship.[17]

Radio, because of its low-cost accessibility and lower literacy demands, has great potential for reaching populations in developing countries with consistent health stories and messages.

In "The Digital World of the US Hispanic II" study, Cheskin found that radio is highly accessed and "culturally relevant" to Latinos. The study showed that Latinos listen to about 15 hours of radio per week, with just more than half of that being to Spanish radio.[18] Radio listening is part of a tradition in Latin America, which has more than 4,000 radio stations (zonalatina.com).[19] Korzenny points out that in the United States, Latinos tend to be concentrated in the service and labor areas of the economy (construction, transportation, agriculture, food service, hospitality), jobs that lend themselves to listening to the radio. Latino radio reminds the listener of home and being "culturally connected . . . in a way English radio cannot." The most effective programming entertains people with humor, music, and storytelling, and brings them information related to their jobs, immigration issues, and education.[20]

A United Nations Acquired Immunodeficiency Syndrome (UNAIDS) effort in India is using television-based programming to address HIV/AIDS-related social stigma. The education-entertainment telecast called "Kalyani," meaning "the one who provides welfare," is an effort to encourage positive health attitudes and behaviors. It addresses HIV-related stigma, discrimination, and treatment through short spots, folk songs, and informative segments with experts. "Kalyani" airs in the capital cities of eight highly populated Indian states, reaching nearly 50% of the country's population. The program is reinforced by follow-up action in the form of visits to rural areas in which experts and actors from the show interact with intended audiences. Among the storylines has been a young man who contracted the disease while migrating to a village looking for work. The village initially shuns him, but after being educated through a visit by the actors about how HIV is transmitted and how there should be no stigma, the HIV-positive man is accepted and then becomes a champion for HIV prevention in the area.[21]

According to a Porter Novelli Health Styles survey, more than 60% of regular primetime and daytime telenovela drama viewers reported that they learned something about a disease or how to prevent it from a TV show. Nearly half of regular viewers said they took some action after hearing about a health issue or disease on a TV show.[22]

In light of the growing potential entertainment channels hold for social change, there have been increased efforts to link public health communication professionals, producers, and scriptwriters together. One initiative, the Hollywood, Health & Society project at the University of Southern California, works with the CDC to provide entertainment industry professionals with accurate and timely information for health storylines.[23]

"Participatory communication" reflects the reality (both strengths and challenges) of communities in delivering health information through entertainment, sports celebrities, radio, TV, periodicals, theater, stories told through photographs (photo-novellas), folk entertainment, music, oral storytelling, emerging digital communications, and trusted community members. The essential elements needed to inform and influence must be a community-grounded approach to the content, real characters that the audience can relate to, vivid storylines that evoke emotion, and information delivered as part of the story but in such a way that motivates the audience members to take action to improve their health.

Community Storytelling Platforms in the Digital Age

Researchers today have many tools to help facilitate positive behavior change within the communities they are working with. Perhaps the most useful growth in this area has been the increased creative and technical capabilities of the Internet and smartphones, digital photography, video and audio, user-generated content and management, social media, and content-sharing platforms.

An excellent example of researchers joining with the community to develop a long-term initiative for good sustained change and using communications to help tell the story is the Healthy Environments project, created by two College of Social Work faculty members at the University of South Carolina.[24] The 3-year program's goal was to help residents of two low-income neighborhoods in Columbia, South Carolina, identify their concerns and strengths, become more involved and build trust with each other, and help create healthy spaces in their own neighborhoods.

The researchers kicked off the first year of the project by launching a program called Photovoice. With Photovoice, researchers select members of the community to participate, and they provide them with digital cameras and training on both how to compose and technically shoot images. The participants—teens and adults—then documented their everyday lives and environment by taking photos that showed their world through their eyes. The community members then wrote captions describing their photos and then told their accompanying stories as part of an exhibit of their work at a university art museum (http://ces4health.info/find-products/view-product.aspx?code=RBKP8RZS) (see Figures 18-9 and 18-10).

The Photovoice project ensured that the stories and issues being raised were authentic and driven from the perspectives of the community. A set of strengths and concerns surfaced because of the Photovoice project, which led into the second year and the creation of a Community Empowerment Center, along with training of individuals on how to write grant applications for supporting the improvements. The community then agreed on the three needs, and spent the third year focused on launching those community-driven ideas: creating a food pantry nearby to improve access to healthy foods; training eight residents to be certified exercise instructors who will lead weekly classes for children and adults; and developing a newsletter to keep residents up-to-date regarding health and safety issues.

Social media, photo and multimedia sharing Websites have multiplied over the past few years. An example, though, of a platform built completely around the art of storytelling and the empowerment of the individual and community's voice is cowbird.com. Aaron Huey, a photojournalist for *National Geographic,* among other media, created a photo essay of life on the Pine Ridge Oglala Lakota Native-American Reservation in South Dakota. The finished product, in the eyes of some from inside and outside the Pine Ridge communities, did not portray a balanced look and was too focused on the darker images and stories of life on the reservation. Huey also felt that a limited number of photos on pages constrained the complexities of the community's full picture.

After taking the response to heart, Huey set out in 2012 to find a way to have the Pine Ridge stories told through the experience and the lens of the people themselves, rather than his third-party, outside-looking-in perspective. Huey partnered with cowbird.com, a participatory and storytelling Website, so that the people of Pine Ridge could tell their own story, unedited. *National Geographic* agreed to embed the Pine Ridge Community Storytelling Project on its Website: http://ngm.nationalgeographic.com/2012/08/pine-ridge/community-project. There have been nearly 300 submitted photo stories from the Pine Ridge community, many accompanied by an audio recording from the photographer-storyteller (http://cowbird.com/huey/collection/pineridge/stories/).[25]

Cowbird.com describes its philosophy and platform as "a global community of storytellers, interested in telling deeper, longer-lasting, more nourishing stories than you're likely to find anywhere else on the Web." The site aims to strengthen communities "by building a public library of human experience."

MEDIA

Reporters, editors, and publishers can be powerful allies in the push to motivate individuals and communities to adopt healthy practices. This section briefly explores how to work with the media to get coverage of health issues, what is done to train the media about certain health issues and conditions so they more accurately report on them, and the emerging trend toward more grassroots, community-, or citizen-based journalism.

Attracting Media Coverage of Your Issue or Work

Whether you're a public health practitioner in Nebraska, a student volunteer with a women's health nongovernmental organization (NGO) in China, or a trauma counselor in Kenya, understanding the media and partnering with them can help greatly to advance your work and improve health outcomes for the communities you are working in.

Too often, individuals and organizations make the mistake of thinking media are just waiting to tell their story. They do not take the time to understand the editorial interests or focus of the newspaper, radio, or TV station, their capacity (personnel and knowledge

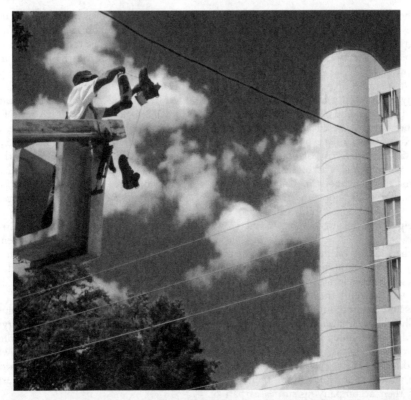

Figure 18-9. University of South Carolina social work researchers used the Photovoice community-based participatory research (CBPR) method to help surface needs and strengths, and bring positive changes within a public housing community. This photo, titled "Power Line," taken by Photovoice community participant Tanjenique Paulin-Anderson, shows a worker removing sneakers dangling from an overhead power line. Anderson's photo caption read *"Gang members throw up their shoes in my neighborhood./It's something crazy that I've never understood./ It kind of bothers me that they wear the colors and talk in code./But I know them; they are not always in 'gangsta mode.'/ When I saw this display I couldn't pretend it was fine. I called the front office and the POleese,/That's my Power line."* (*Courtesy of Tanjenique Paulin-Anderson; Columbia, South Carolina.*)

level, or resources) to adequately cover a story, or the political-social pressures they may need to consider on certain topics. When working with the media, be sure to:

- **Take time to examine what issues or topics are covered most in newspaper or broadcast programs.** Do they cover mainly local or regional news? Is there a health section or segment? If they cover a good deal of business news, can you tie in the economic effects of health problems? What are the trends or issues most important to them and their audience? Do they have the personnel to go out into the field, research, and cover stories, or will they run stories you put together? What is the culture or political situation in their circulation area? Are they independent, government run, or owned by a corporation? What are the technological capabilities for receiving information and using content? Who are their readers, listeners, or viewers? What digital formats are available?

- **Develop a relationship with key reporters by showing them you understand their needs, goals, audiences, and constraints.** Appreciate that they have deadlines, and return their calls and e-mails promptly. Foster goodwill by being a consistent, reliable, and accurate source of information for them. Contact or send them only press releases that have newsworthiness to their audiences. If you do not know an answer, say, "I do not know." Remember, there's no such privilege as "off the record." If you do not want a comment printed or broadcast, do not say it.

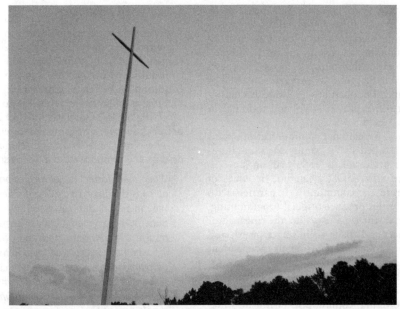

Figure 18-10. Photovoice project participant, Floyd Cutner, snapped this photo of a cross and a crescent moon during a visit to the Columbia, South Carolina, city cemetery where his son, who was killed by gang violence, is buried. Cutner wrote in his photo caption: *"A visit to the cemetery to see those who have gone from here, especially my son who tried to avoid the streets and gangs but unfortunately he didn't see the trouble ahead of him. It's up to all of us to realize the trouble around us and be aware we have to stay one step ahead. One day all of us will be together again, if we have faith. The tiny speck in the sky is a half moon. At that moment, I knew half my life was gone, but with faith, life everlasting is only the beginning."* (Courtesy of Floyd Cutner.)

- **Position yourself and others in your organization as experts in their fields and valuable sources to the media.** Train others in your organization on how to be responsive to the media, how to conduct an effective interview, and how to get your information out concisely, plainly, and clearly. Explore creating a media relations database on your Website, so media can easily search by name or expertise area.

- **Create a Google Alerts account to monitor news stories and Web content daily related to your field, company or work.** This will help you keep abreast of the latest news and trends, as well as the media covering them.

Educating Media About Key Health Issues

Media, particularly in developing countries, play an important part in getting accurate information about serious diseases and problems to the public. Many people and policymakers form their views of diseases and conditions based on how they are presented via the media. Unfortunately, most reporters do not have

a health, medical, or science background, may not take cultural or social issues into consideration in their coverage, and may devote minimal time to health issues because of scarce resources. This is sometimes the case with reporting on the complex and sensitive condition of HIV/AIDS. Some communities and countries remain misinformed about AIDS. The role of journalists and communicators is also central to containing this health care burden in places like Africa and India.

Journalists must continue to be educated about the basics of the disease, how it is prevented and transmitted, what the cultural stigmas are, what treatment is available, and what misconceptions and myths still linger about HIV/AIDS. Training sessions are essential to increase clinical knowledge among journalists about conditions such as HIV/AIDS and malaria, and how to report accurately, ethically, and with clarity.

To make it relevant to the media's growing focus on economic issues, global health communicators should connect the impact of disease, and issues like environmental disruption, to the economic effects. How many days of work were lost? What's the cost when a high percentage of a country's most productive age group is dying from HIV/AIDS complications? What's the cost to ecotourism or agriculture when war or disaster scars the environment? How does environmental degradation impact poverty and foster disease?

Several international groups, such as Internews and UNAIDS "on the ground" programs, as well as the Kaiser Family Foundation's globalhealth.kff.org Website, provide in-depth resources and training for media across the world.

Internews, an international communications nonprofit that has worked in 70 countries, trains thousands of media professionals each year on how to cover issues like HIV/AIDS, avian flu, or issues of greatest concern to the community. It partners with local media and helps produce original programming, build media infrastructure, provide the means for people to connect and make their voices heard, and advance laws and policies supporting an independent open media that serves as a "watchdog" to government and industry (see Figure 18-11). Considered to be one of the gold standard organizations for training reporters, empowering communities with information, and responding quickly to help fill a communications void after disasters, Internews also informs its work and helps increase sustainability by developing community-based journalists and reporters, even in challenging environments (see Figure 18-12).

Community Media

Local communities giving voice to their own needs, strengths, and challenges by developing their own content that tells *their* story and that will run in community-owned media can be empowering for education and change. Community radio, for example, makes radio more accessible to all, with content reflecting the local interests, be they economic, health, political, social, environmental, or entertainment.

The World Association of Community Broadcasters, describes community radio as follows:

> When radio fosters the participation of citizens and defends their interests; when it reflects the tastes of the majority and makes good humor and hope its main purpose; when it truly informs; when it helps resolve the thousand and one problems of daily life; when all ideas are debated in its programs and all opinions are respected; when cultural diversity is stimulated over commercial homogeneity; when women are main players in communication and not simply a pretty voice or a publicity gimmick; when no type of dictatorship is tolerated, not even the musical dictatorship of the big recording studios; when everyone's words fly without discrimination or censorship, that is community radio.

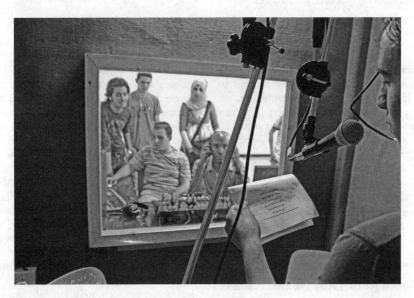

Figure 18-11. Internews in Libya. A group of friends launched Shabab Libya FM 101.1 in Benghazi in April 2012. "We are all still learning," said founder Yazid Ettaib. "Most of us are engineers, or accountants, and we have no idea about media." In the picture, the team records a short news announcement. Internews trains local voices to cover key needs in the community, and to empower an open democratic media. (*Courtesy of Quintanilla J, Goodfriend L. When Information Saves Lives: 2011 Annual Report, Internews Humanitarian Information Projects. Internews, 2011. Photo credit: Benedict Moran.*)

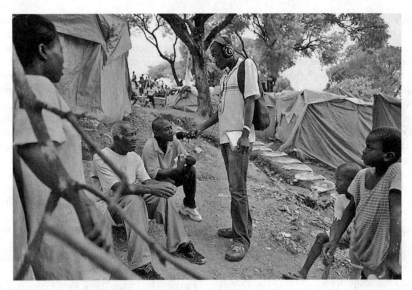

Figure 18-12. Internews during Haiti earthquake recovery. A local reporter from ENDK interviews camp residents in Port-au-Prince, Haiti, after the devastating earthquake in Haiti. Field work and community voices are at the core of Internews' humanitarian work around the world.(*Courtesy of Quintanilla J, Goodfriend L. When Information Saves Lives: 2011 Annual Report, Internews Humanitarian Information Projects. Internews, 2011. Photo credit: Eckert.*)

A key strategy in some community-based health communications programs is the use of "behavioral journalism," in which you identify people from the community who have made the desired behavioral change and who can be featured as role models in the media materials and outreach. Having role models within the community helping lead the campaign makes the messages understandable, relevant, and credible. Plus, the community sees proof that change is possible and desirable.

Citizen Journalists, User-Generated Content, and Activism

With the recent surge in mobile phone access, development of applications, and new digital platforms for creating and sharing content, a corresponding phenomenon has been a rapid rise in individuals generating content, distributing it in near real time on their Websites or on social media, and advocating for some type of action.

This user-generated content takes many shapes, including individuals shooting video on their phone of a hurricane or tsunami's destruction and uploading it to CNN via their iReports feature. Or citizens documenting abuse by leaders and what is happening "on the ground" during the Arab Spring conflicts and transitions of power by posting it directly to YouTube or Twitter, thereby avoiding censorship and getting it out to the world.

Another example is activists using text messaging or social media to educate others about some immediate need or cause and trying to motivate them to address it by taking action and giving financial donations online or via texting on their mobile phone. The most popular platform for online charitable giving is Network for Good, which facilitates more digital giving than any other medium. In their 10-year history, they have processed nearly $700 million for more than 80,000 nonprofits.[26]

INFORMATION COMMUNICATION TECHNOLOGIES

Over the past three decades, we have learned much about how health communications programs can be designed to educate and motivate human behavior toward healthy change globally. One of the most vital tools to generate knowledge and awareness is information communication technologies (ICTs). Advancements in this area are showing great promise at increasing access to information for individuals and communities.

The speed at which the information revolution is occurring is remarkable. Since 1975 the speed and memory of computers has increased a million-fold and prices have plummeted. A $2,000 PC is equivalent to a $10 million supercomputer in 1975. *The Economist* magazine in 1996 pointed out that if automobile technology improved as rapidly as information technology, a car would speed along at 100,000 miles per hour, get 200,000 miles per gallon of gas, and cost $5.

This communication technologies explosion over the past decade transformed entire communities and countries, some previously shut off from most communications, and allowed developing countries to leapfrog some costly and time-consuming stages of technology such as the building of telephone land lines or installation of physical broadband fiber. The changes have increased access to and sharing of information that benefits communities in many ways, but also have brought increased costs to individuals and communities as they "keep up" with technology.

Examples of Communication Technology Growth and Use

For many years, access to the Internet was largely enjoyed by individuals living in North America, Europe, and Australia. But that has changed. As of June 2012, North American residents had the most access to the Internet (nearly 80% of the population) and Asia had the most Internet users, but the greatest growth in Internet use over the previous 12 years occurred in Africa (3,606%), the Middle East (2,640%), and Latin America/Caribbean (1,311%).[27] Clearly, the rapid expansion of access to the Internet in developing regions will have a great impact on how health information is shared and what individuals, governments, and societies do with the new knowledge.

Among the many information communication technologies available—Internet, digital social media, computers, broadcast media, telecenters, tablets—one of the most significant developments worldwide has been the advent and adoption of mobile phones.

Mobile Phones: Journalism, Commerce, mHealth , and Empowerment

Perhaps no recent technological advancement has been more quickly embraced and life changing in the world than the mobile phone. For much of the globe, it empowers and connects people. It has become irreplaceable to many, particularly in the developing world, where it is helping to fuel economic and social change.

According to a report from the World Bank, "*Information and Communications for Development 2012: Maximizing Mobile,*"[28] around three quarters of the world's inhabitants now have access to a mobile phone. The number of mobile subscriptions in use worldwide has grown from fewer than 1 billion in 2000 to more than 6 billion in 2012, with nearly 5 billion of those accounts found in developing countries. Ownership of multiple subscriptions continues to accelerate, suggesting that their number will soon exceed that of the human population.

The report states that, "more than 30 billion mobile applications, or 'apps,' were downloaded in 2011, software that extends the capabilities of phones, for instance to become mobile wallets, navigational aids, or price comparison tools. In developing countries, citizens are increasingly using mobile phones to create new livelihoods and enhance their lifestyles, while governments are using them to improve service delivery and citizen feedback and engagement mechanisms."[28]

Mobile phones have emerged as a catalyst for development in many countries. They allow access to market information for farmers in India so they know where they can get the best price for their crops and can eliminate long, unnecessary trips to the city if not needed. In China, low-income farmers use text messages to learn about weather forecasts or ways to control pests. For those individuals who cannot afford their own phone, mobile phones in villages are rented out by the minute to callers to make them accessible.

The 2012 report from the World Bank illustrated that farmers and traders using mobile application technologies saw their incomes rise: 19% for potato farmers in India, 29% for Nigerian grain traders, and 36% for Ugandan banana farmers.

As a key tool of digital commerce, mobile phones are revolutionizing how consumers in African cities conduct financial transactions. With a few presses of the keypad, they can transfer money to merchants or to their bank to pay for supplies or services. Internet access, ATMs, and credit cards may be tough to find in some developing countries, so services have emerged such as Celpay and M-Pesa, companies that feature Internet banking through mobile phones.

Celpay customers in East Africa can transfer funds through the system and pay bills from their phones, and they also make deposits into their Celpay accounts at a number of stations in the country.[29] This is particularly significant to the poor who may have never been able to open up traditional bank accounts because they had no credit history and were seen as high risk.

M-Pesa (*M* for mobile, pesa for money in Kiswahili) is a mobile phone–based money transfer and microfinancing service in Kenya, Tanzania, Afghanistan, South Africa, and India. M-Pesa allows users with a national ID card or passport to deposit, withdraw, and transfer money without a bank account via a text message on a mobile device. More than 50% of the adult population in Kenya use M-Pesa to send money to relatives far away, to pay for shopping, utility bills, or a taxi ride home after a night out. Another benefit is increased security. Business owners in Kenya are not as vulnerable to being physically robbed while carrying cash to their banks, which could be hours away.[30]

A boon for conducting business, the accessibility and relative affordability of mobile phones have provided families and communities with a sense of security and connectedness to health services that was not available before. In rural areas, disconnected at night from neighbors or health care services, a child with a potentially fatal disease such as cholera or malaria could die before receiving treatment the next day at a clinic several hours away. With the mobile phone, a mother can summon help and transportation, or perhaps get advice from health care workers many miles away. Healthcare staff at remote clinics can call for ambulances using the cell phone, and fishers on African lakes can call for emergency help if they are threatened by bandits at sea.

Phones now have a global positioning system (GPS) chip that can be activated to locate wayward hikers, rural accident victims, or displaced people after disasters. GPS-enabled mobile phones can also be used by fishers to track coming storms or by farmers or disaster relief agencies to detect climate changes that may bring on drought and, subsequently, famine.

Migrant workers living in cities or rural areas several hundred or thousands of miles from home can stay connected with family and friends regularly via their mobile phones. This helps lessen the sense of isolation, and it may help workers away from their social support systems be less vulnerable to making unhealthy behavioral decisions.

Mobile phones are transforming the way news coverage happens—both in its immediacy and in the increased involvement of "citizen journalists." Sometimes referred to as "participatory social media," emerging technologies allow the public to contribute to telling the story and getting the facts out. They also improve communications during natural disasters and give an eyewitness account to the world about atrocities and injustice.

Mobile healthcare (mHealth) is another area being transformed by mobile technologies. For example, a remote medical facility in Botswana uses mobile phones and tablets equipped with cameras to send photos of patients for diagnosis and consultation with medical specialists.

In South Africa, a text message service alerts HIV patients when medications are due. Other applications allow diabetic patients to use their mobile phones to monitor their diabetes and send medical data to health professionals via cloud computing for accurate diagnosis.

Mobile phones are also changing how we search the Internet for information. Research data regarding user behavior on the US Health and Human Services AIDS.gov Website has shown that when individuals search the site from mobile phones, the searches are much more specific than they are from nonmobile platforms.

HARDSHIP INNOVATION, MOBILE PHONE GENDER GAP, AND "BASE OF THE PYRAMID"

Throughout the world, the digital revolution continues to spark innovation among entrepreneurs, companies, health agencies, universities, governments, and communities. A major outcome reinforced as part of this rapid growth has been the innovative ideas and expansion of existing products being generated from low-income creative individuals and businesses, particularly in so-called developing countries. This phenomenon of "hardship innovation" has, of course, always been present as limited-means individuals ingeniously modify products or create their own based on their needs within their communities or countries.

In health care, one example is the inexpensive quality prosthesis innovation of Dr. Therdchai Jivacate and the Prosthesis Foundation in Thailand. They have designed, built, and provided thousands of quality, free artificial legs for amputees in remote areas of Thailand and surrounding countries. Each prosthetic leg costs about $30 to make, a low cost made possible because it is constructed partly of recyclable items such as beer cans and aluminum pots that people donate. In the United States, an artificial leg costs about $10,000.[31]

The meteoric growth of mobile phone access and new opportunities from the "bottom up" in East Africa has helped fuel an increase in community-driven startup ventures, including iHub, an innovation tech incubator in Nairobi, Kenya, with a focus "on young entrepreneurs, Web and mobile phone programmers, designers and researchers. IHub is part open community workspace, part vector for investors and venture capitalists, and part business incubator."

Although four of five mobile connections are in developing countries, women—particularly those found at the so-called base of the pyramid, or BoP, meaning those living on less than $2.50 per day—are not benefiting from mobile technology in an equal manner to men, according to research by the GSMA and the Cherie Blair Foundation for Women. The research showed that a woman in a low- to middle-income country is 21% less likely to own a mobile phone than a man. This mobile phone gender gap represents 300 million women in the developing world who do not have access to this important technology. Benefits from access to mobile technologies include "improved women's literacy and girls' education, advancing access to health and education, supporting women's civic participation and activism, an increased sense of security and independence for women, and increasing economic opportunities and incomes."[32]

Mobile phones have become so essential to East Africans that according to a November 2012 report commissioned by the World Bank's infoDev, one in five Kenyans at the BoP forgo a usual expense, such as food or a bus pass, to afford mobile phone access and maintain their phone credit. The report, conducted by the Kenyan tech innovation incubator iHub, suggests that spending by the poor in Kenya is now influenced greatly by their expenditure on mobile phones. This trend could be worrisome in the future because limited incomes may go increasingly toward phone use expenses and not toward basic nutrition or prevention of disease or injury.[33]

Like any technology, mobile phones can be abused as well. They have been used for triggering explosive devices remotely, by government officials who force companies to give them free minutes on their cell phones as bribes, and by rebel armies coordinating their movements.

On the flip side, the World Bank started a peaceful disarmament program in the Congo where men and women fighters could turn in their weapons and then be notified through the mobile phone service that they are entitled to job training and a few hundred dollars over the course of a year.

ICTS: FILLING THE COMMUNICATION VOID CAUSED BY DISASTERS, GEOGRAPHY, AND POVERTY

ICTs can save lives through early warning systems and can alleviate hardship and trauma after a disaster strikes by providing accurate information as widely as possible. Media, digital, and mobile technology plays a large role in the response to disasters and conflicts by communicating with survivors and helping to rebuild communications and communities.

The cyclone preparedness program (CPP), created by the International Federation of Red Cross and Red Crescent Societies in the early 1970s, is credited with saving millions of lives over the past three decades. Its early warning system taps into Asia's largest radio network, and emerging storms tracked by satellite are relayed by radio to 33,000 well-trained volunteers in villages. The volunteers spread the warning to communities that will be affected by using hand-operated sirens or shouting through megaphones from motorbikes. The CPP can alert about 8 million people across the coastal region.[34]

One of the greatest challenges following disasters is filling the huge void of communications created when communities and physical spaces are ripped apart. In the race to get supplies to address some of the physical needs, the information response is often neglected. Vulnerable survivors need to know about the status of their loved ones. Logistics about when to expect food and clothing from aid agencies, and when electricity and clean water may be restored, must be shared.

Myths that grow out of ignorance or poor information in refugee camps also must be debunked quickly. Rumors that surfaced after recent disasters, some resulting in fatalities, included:

- Survivors of the Pakistan earthquake coated the inside of their tents with kerosene because they heard it would repel malaria-carrying insects, causing tents to catch fire, resulting in the deaths of a dozen people.
- Rural villagers in Pakistan, seeing bottled water for the first time, refused to drink it, thinking it was unsafe. Instead, they used it for washing and drank polluted river water.
- After the tsunami in Indonesia, survivors heard that dead bodies spread disease, so they immediately tossed the dead bodies into mass graves, causing more distress for families searching for their loved ones.

Internews, the international NGO that specializes in "humanitarian reporting" in post disaster/conflict environments as part of its mission, helped identify and correct some of these myths by broadcasting interviews with experts and getting the information dispersed. The group also rebuilds media infrastructure and gets accurate, culturally relevant communications out to survivors or loved ones as soon as possible through portable windup radios given to survivors and suitcase radio transmitters. Much of the news is created and reported by local individuals, who are trained in the art of humanitarian reporting. (See Box 18-1, a case study of how Internews helped rebuild lives and communications after the 2010 earthquake in Haiti.)

Some other emerging digital technologies and approaches that can make significant contributions to improving access to both knowledge and health outcomes in the coming years are:

- **The government of India, wanting to bridge the digital divide and get affordable tablet computers in the hands of millions of students**, partnered with Datawind in 2012 to produce the Aakash II tablet. The government is covering half of the price of the $40 tablet, the lowest priced tablet with a capacitive screen. Datawind's CEO said at the launch: "We wish to use technology to fight poverty with a passion. Access to computers and internet will help deliver a better quality education and level the playing field for all Indians." http://www.ubislate.com/
- **Google Person Finder helps people reconnect with friends and loved ones in the aftermath of natural and humanitarian disasters.** It provides a registry and message board for survivors, family, and loved ones to post and search for information about each other's status and whereabouts. It was created by volunteer Google engineers in response to the 2010 Haiti earthquake and has been used since in the aftermath of the 2011 Japan earthquake and tsunami, where it was live within an hour, and the

---

BOX 18-1. INTERNEWS: REBUILDING LIVES AND COMMUNICATIONS POST-DISASTER

Problem and Local Context

A devastating earthquake in 2010 centered just outside Haiti's capital left hundreds of thousands dead and more than a million displaced. Survivors were in immediate need of accurate information about the safety of loved ones, relief services, and, over time, recovery efforts. Some local radio stations remained operational or returned to the airwaves quickly, but local media had suffered its own setbacks and could not adequately fill the information void.

Solution

With a team of local reporters, Internews began production of Enfomasyon Nou Dwe Konnen (News You Can Use) (ENDK), a daily humanitarian news broadcast, and set up a distribution network of local radio stations, eventually airing on nearly 40 stations, reaching 70% of Haitians. Local journalists received training in humanitarian reporting and produced the daily show, reporting from displaced persons' camps, fielding questions from residents, seeking answers from the government and aid community, and investigating issues of concern.

Results

One month after ENDK's launch, 80% of surveyed focus group members were familiar with the program. By July, 100% were, and they could identify key pieces of information that they had integrated into their daily lives, such as how to prevent malaria by getting rid of standing water and how to prevent diarrheal diseases by washing hands regularly.

In a survey of 11,000 Haitians, 81% said they trusted radio as a source of information, second only to churches and religious communities. Overall, 57% of the population surveyed had radios; 72% had cell phones, which often had radio capabilities. Text messaging was a critical way for listeners to interact with ENDK, which fielded 50 to 100 text messages a day from listeners, seeking information that ENDK investigated and responded to on air.

"The creation of ENDK was vital to ensuring affected populations had access to timely and essential information to help them survive the aftermath of the earthquake. More recently, as priorities have shifted from emergency to reconstruction, ENDK has taken steps to keep up with listener needs, based on Internews research results, and begun to provide information more relevant to the recovery process" (Independent evaluation for USAID's Office of Transition Initiatives in Haiti).

Source: www.internews.org/what-we-do/case-studies/haiti.

---

flooding in the Philippines in 2012. http://google .org/personfinder

- **The Fletcher Lab at the University of California, Berkeley, has turned a standard mobile phone into a diagnostic-quality microscope** with a magnification of ×5–60. Mobile-phone microscopy—called cell scope—enables visualization of samples, followed by capture, organization, and transmission of images critical for diagnosis. This technology can be applied to a range of applications beyond diagnostic medicine. http://cellscope.berkeley.edu/

- **The Relationship Information Tracking System (RITS) allows coffee cooperatives from Peru to Tanzania to trace every step of the supply chain process**, starting from the grower. Using a cloud-based application, the coffee co-op manager is able to record individual coffee farmer deliveries, track the certification status of each delivery, process farmer payment, record quality-related information, bulk coffee deliveries according to quality, and generate reports on farm productivity, payments, and samples. This process could be fitted to other industries, including health care delivery and costs, particularly in developing countries. http://www.sustainableharvest.com/ RITS

- **The Health eVillages initiative equips healthcare professionals with mobile phones preloaded with** drug guides, medical alerts, journal summaries, and medical references, ensuring that healthcare workers even in remote locations have the latest medical information at their disposal. http://www .healthevillages.org/

- **Internews' Speak Safe: Media Workers' Toolkit for Safer Online and Mobile Practices** introduces reporters, journalists, bloggers, and media workers to simple yet effective practices to maintain control of important information and communications in any country or culture. The toolkit helps users "understand the interests and technological capabilities of those who want to limit the public's access to information and are taking decisive steps to curtail it." http://www.speaksafe.internews.org/

- **GEO (Global Emergency Overview) is an app launched in late 2012 for smartphones and tablet computers** designed to improve access to information and analysis on crisis impact, and contribute toward creating shared situation awareness at the early stage of a disaster. Focus is on improving the effectiveness of humanitarian operations, including addressing the information needs of disaster-affected communities. http://geo.acaps.org/

- **Mobile phones, social media, and the Internet have become important tools for public health HIV/AIDS outreach specialists and researchers around the world.** Public health practitioners working on HIV/AIDS education have turned to these digital media platforms to get their message out about the importance of prevention, testing, and HIV status notification, particularly for trying to reach MSMs who increasingly meet through "hook-up" or relationship sites on the Internet. The social phenomenon of meeting partners easily online or through location applications on the mobile phone, paired with growing evidence that use of the Internet increases the risk of HIV infection for MSMs, makes this a critical emerging area of HIV prevention interventions. http://www.ncbi.nlm.nih.gov/pmc/articles/PMC3345812/

- **Digital Green partners with villages and farmers to produce videos every month about improving agricultural processes and yields.** The 8- to 10-minute videos, shot with pocket video cameras, include testimonials from the farmers and demonstrations of improved production techniques, market links, and government plans. Because the Internet is often not available, the videos are distributed on memory cards for playback on battery-operated pico projectors in each village. The program now reaches more than 900 villages and 60,000 farmers in India, and it is being extended to parts of sub-Saharan Africa and South Asia. Digital Green has been found to be 10 times as effective, per dollar spent, in converting farmers to better farming practices than traditional approaches to agriculture extension. http://www.digitalgreen.org/

- **Dartmouth's Geisel School of Medicine and Thayer School of Engineering worked with the software company, Global Emergency Resources (GER),** to test and develop a handheld product that helps manage hospital and clinic databases, providing near real-time monitoring and mapping of healthcare systems during both emergencies and everyday healthcare operations. Results have shown significant improvements in emergency response, triage, and patient tracking. http://www.ger911.com

SUMMARY

1. An important missing piece of the prevention-treatment puzzle had been the strategic use of health communication and marketing tools that can empower communities with the knowledge and motivation to improve their environment and wellness, and in return, their social and economic potential and sustainability.

2. Social marketing seeks to influence social behaviors, not to benefit the marketer, but to benefit the target audience and the general society. Social marketers place a high value on conducting market research to "listen" and determine the needs, wants, and perceptions of the "customer."

3. Other marketing elements used are environment analysis, differential advantage, audience segmentation, and sustainability.

4. Based on marketing principles but dealing with more complex issues involving behavioral change, social marketing applies the traditionally commercial concepts of the "four P's" of product, price, place, and promotion, and adds a fifth, positioning.

5. Surveys can be delivered through telephone interviews; personal in-depth interviews; focus groups; and mail, mobile phone applications, and Web-based communications. Depending on their structure and the skill of the researcher, surveys can yield much information about an individual's knowledge, attitudes, and practices related to health.

6. Radio, because of its low-cost accessibility and lower literacy demands, has great potential for reaching populations in developing countries with consistent health stories and messages.

7. Research has shown edutainment, the practice of using mass entertainment to deliver public health messages, raises awareness of issues and motivates action and behavior change.

8. Media, particularly in developing countries, play an important part in getting accurate information about serious diseases and problems to the public. Many people and policymakers form their views of diseases and conditions based on how they are presented via the media.

9. The explosion of digital technologies and social media provides unprecedented tools for individuals, communities, and health communications professionals to connect, share information, and bring about positive behavioral change.

10. Mobile phones are transforming the way news coverage happens, both in its immediacy and

in the increased involvement of "citizen journalists." Phones with video and text capacity allow the public to contribute to telling the story and getting the facts out, improve communications during natural disasters, and offer eyewitness accounts to the world about atrocities and injustice.

11. The accessibility and relative affordability of the mobile phone has revolutionized commerce, health information access, "hardship innovation," and connectivity within communities and countries, particularly in developing nations.

12. To make it relevant to the media's focus on economic issues, global health communicators should connect the impact of disease, and issues like environmental disruption, to the economic effects.

13. To be successful, health communications programs should include community-based cultural brokers and health promoters, and empower the community to help shape, implement, evaluate, drive, and sustain the program.

14. One of the greatest challenges following disasters is filling the huge void of communications created when communities and physical spaces are ripped apart.

15. Emerging information communication technologies such as software that maps and tracks individuals during emergencies and disasters, mobile phone microscopy, and low-cost tablet computers can help make health knowledge and communications more accessible for all.

STUDY QUESTIONS

1. You are a public health researcher and have agreed to help lead a research and education team from the United States to the Dadaab Refugee Camp in Kenya to examine how refugees are receiving and understanding their health information. What barriers might you run into while pursuing this work?

2. Social marketing applies marketing principles and methods to motivate an individual or group to change behavior and improve health. Describe how the five P's would take shape in a campaign centered on motivating seniors to exercise regularly.

3. In the case study involving the Hopi, how would you work to sustain the educational campaign and the improvements in women's health? What other challenges might you confront in trying to maintain the momentum of the campaign?

4. You are a journalist with an NGO that specializes in humanitarian reporting. You are the first reporter from your agency to arrive at the scene of an earthquake in Peru. The media infrastructure has been destroyed, with minimal personnel and equipment left. Thousands of survivors need information immediately. Describe some of the community-based health communication approaches and the technologies and media mentioned in this chapter you would use to get accurate information out and help improve conditions.

5. As a health professional working in East Africa, you need to better connect with MSMs to deliver accurate information about HIV/AIDS prevention, testing, and treatment. Given the stigma these individuals may face in their communities, particularly those in rural villages, what digital communications tools and platforms might you use to safely reach this at-risk community and improve their health?

REFERENCES

1. Maslow A. Motivation and personality. *Psychol Rev* 1943;50(4): 370–396.

2. National Cancer Institute. *Theory at a Glance: A Guide for Health Promotion.* 2nd ed. Bethesda, MD: US Department of Health and Human Services, 2005.

3. National Heart, Lung and Blood Institute. *Salud Para Su Corazon, Bringing Heart Health to Latinos: A Guide for Building Community Programs.* Washington, DC: National Institutes of Health, No. 98-3796, 1998.

4. Interview with Hugo Melgar-Quinonez, assistant professor, Ohio State University Department of Human Nutrition, with Gary Snyder, May 24, 2005.

5. Snyder G. *Knowledge, attitudes and practices of central Ohio immigrant Latinos concerning health and information access.* Paper presented at: Global Health Education Consortium and Latin American and Caribbean Congress on Global Health; April 10, 2010;Instituto Nacional de Salud Pública, Cuernavaca, Mexico.

6. US Centers for Disease Control and Prevention. "Testing Makes Us Stronger" Campaign, Act Against AIDS. http://hivtest .cdc.gov/stronger/index.html.

7. National Cancer Institute. *Making Health Communication Programs Work.* Bethesda, MD: NIH Publication No. 04-5145, August 2004. http://www.nci.nih.gov/pinkbook/.

8. McGuire WJ. Public communication as a strategy for inducing health-promoting behavioral change. *Pre Med* 1984;13(3): 299–313.

9. *HIV/AIDS Reporting Manual.* Menlo Park, CA: Kaiser Family Foundation, 2011. http://globalhealth.kff.org/Journalists.aspx.

10. Andreasen A. *Marketing Social Change: Changing Behavior to Promote Health, Social Development, and the Environment.* San Francisco: Jossey-Bass, 1995.

11. Alcalay R, Bell RA. *Promoting Nutrition and Physical Activity Through Social Marketing: Current Practices and Recommendations.* Davis, CA: Center for Advanced Studies in Nutrition and Social Marketing, University of California, 2000.

12. Berkowitz E. *Essentials of Health Care Marketing.* Sudbury, MA: Jones and Bartlett, 2006.

13. Interview with Jaime Bayona, assistant professor, Dartmouth Geisel School of Medicine, with Gary Snyder, November 5, 2012.

14. Volpp KG, Troxel AB, Pauly MV, et al. A randomized, controlled trial of financial incentives for smoking cessation. *N Engl J Med* 2009;360(7):699–709.

15. Encarnacion-Garcia H. Promotoras de Salud: A Culturally-Sensitive Community Intervention Model for Cancer Prevention Among Hispanic/Latino women [dissertation].Bloomington: Indiana University, 2004.

16. Andaló P. Love, Tears, Betrayal . . . and Health Messages. *Perspectives in Health Magazine, The Magazine of the Pan American Health Organization* 2003;8(2).

17. UK Department for International Development. Tell Me a Story. *Developments*, 2005. http://developments.org.uk/data/issue32/tell-story.htm.

18. Cheskin Marketing. *The Digital World of the US Hispanic II.* Redwood Shores, CA: Cheskin, 2001.

19. Zona Latina. http://www.zonalatina.com/Radio.htm.

20. Korzenny F, Korzenny BA. *Hispanic Marketing.* Burlington, MA: Elsevier, Butterworth-Heinemann, 2005.

21. UNAIDS. India: Changing Lives through TV Programming, 2006. http://www.unaids.org/en/resources/presscentre/feature-stories/2006/april/20060424India/.

22. Beck V, Huang GC, Pollard WE, et al. Telenovela viewers and health information. Paper presented at: American Public Health Association 131st Annual Meeting and Exposition, San Francisco, CA; 2003.

23. Hollywood, Health & Society Project. University of Southern California, 2011 http://www.learcenter.org/html/projects/?cm=hhs.

24. Freeman D, Pitner R, Powers M, Paulin-Anderson T. Using Photovoice to develop a grounded theory of socio-environmental attributes influencing the health of community environments. *Br J Social Work,* November 11, 2012, 10.1093/bjsw/bcs173.

25. Huey A. Pine Ridge Reservation/Cowbird Storytelling Project. http://cowbird.com/huey/collection/pineridge/stories.

26. Network for Good. Washington, DC, 2012. http://www1.networkforgood.org.

27. Internet World Stats, June 2012. http://www.internetworldstats.com/.

28. The World Bank. *Information and Communications for Development 2012: Maximizing Mobile.* July 17, 2012. http://www.worldbank.org/en/news/2012/07/17/mobile-phone-access-reaches-three-quarters-planets-population.

29. Sullivan K. In war-torn Congo, going wireless to reach home. *Washington Post,* July 9, 2006:A01. http://pqasb.pqarchiver.com/washingtonpost/access/1073868531.html?FMT=ABS&FMTS=ABS:FT&date=Jul+9%2C+2006&author=Kevin+Sullivan+-+Washington+Post+Foreign+Service&desc=In+—War-Torn+Congo%2C+Going+Wireless+to+Reach+Home%3B+For+Poor%2C+Cellphones+Bridge+Digital+Divide.

30. Graham F. M-Pesa: Kenya's mobile wallet revolution. BBC News, November 22, 2010. http://www.bbc.co.uk/news/business-11793290.

31. Saletan W. Body Parts from Trash. Slate: Human Nature, February 2, 2009. http://www.slate.com/blogs/humannature/2009/02/02/body_parts_from_trash.html.

32. mWomen Newsletter. Why Women and Mobile for Development. http://www.mwomen.org/Wiki/Why_Women_and_Mobile_for_Development.

33. Crandall A. How the Kenyan Base of the Pyramid Uses Their Mobile Phone. iHUB, October 24, 2012. http://www.ihub.co.ke/blog/2012/10/how-the-kenyan-base-of-the-pyramid-uses-their-mobile-phone/.

34. UK Department for International Development. What on earth is happening? *Developments*, 2005.

Economics and Global Health   19

Kevin Chan

LEARNING OBJECTIVES

- *Understand the dual relationship between economics and health: how poverty can affect health and how health problems can result in poverty*
- *Comprehend the possible linkages between wealth and health and how both absolute and relative wealth have an impact on health*
- *Describe four key mechanisms by which health can affect wealth*
- *Show the interrelationships between health and economics looking at three key diseases (malaria, tuberculosis, and HIV/AIDS)*
- *Outline and describe four key factors in choosing the type of health care financing system*
- *Outline and describe five major financing methods for health care*
- *Describe and define risk pooling, risk aversion, adverse selection, and moral hazard*

INTRODUCTION TO ECONOMICS AND HEALTH

Peter Chirwa is a 4-year-old boy in northern Malawi. His family grows their food on their farm to provide subsistence for the year. When harvests are good, he and his five brothers and sisters eat well throughout the year, but when the harvests are bad, as they have been over the past 3 years, his brothers and sisters become malnourished and sick. Over the past year, two younger siblings died from malnutrition and pneumonia. Unfortunately, Peter's family is poor and cannot afford to buy food in the market. His family survives on less than 50 cents per person per day, far below the global absolute poverty line of $1.

Peter's uncle lives five houses down. Gaunt and thin and dying from AIDS, he gazes from his bed to his visitors. He has spent all his money trying to buy the lifesaving drugs but can no longer afford the prices. He will probably die in a few months. His family sits by the bedside caring for him, knowing that their future holds nothing but utter destitution. Just down the road, the devastation from poor health can impoverish families and leave them with no income, opportunity, or hope.

For a long time, it has been recognized that there is a relationship between health and wealth.[1] Three possible different pathways may explain this relationship:

1. Increased wealth leads to health.
2. Improved health leads to wealth.
3. The relationship is caused by a third unknown factor.[2]

Rising incomes increase government and private spending on goods that directly (e.g., purchasing health care and better nutrition) and indirectly (e.g., better housing, water, and sanitation facilities) improve health[3] (see Figure 19-1.)

In the past decade, there has been increasing recognition that poor health can lead to poverty.[4] These interrelationships are linked with political, demographic, and social pressures.

The first part of this chapter analyzes the growing evidence between "wealthier is healthier"[5] and the counterclaim "healthier is wealthier."[4]

The second part of this chapter focuses on the evidence that the relationship between health systems through their organization, financing, and behavior

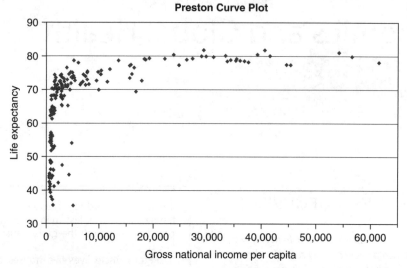

Figure 19-1. Health to wealth correlations. The figures provided are for the year 2004 or the latest year for 179 countries. *(From World Development Indicators 2006.*[67]*)* World Bank. World Development Indicators 2006. Washington DC: World Bank, 2006.

has an impact on health and economic outcomes. How health systems are financed influences the behaviors of consumers, producers, and intermediaries. It is important to understand how these structures are created, which may in turn have significant impacts on health and economic outcomes.

THE MECHANISMS FROM WEALTH TO HEALTH

In general, wealthier nations are healthier nations. Higher incomes provide the ability to purchase many of the goods and services that promote better health, including more calories and higher quality food products, access to cleaner water, safe sanitation, and higher quality and more complete health services both at a societal and individual level. Furthermore, more wealth can lead to better education and training.

Preston[1] noted a strong relationship between health and wealth, and suggested that there is a significant gain in health (as measured by life expectancy) with wealth up to $1,000 per capita. However, Preston noted that after exceeding $1,000 per capita, additional wealth did not lead to significant increases in life expectancy. His classic paper found that between 1940 and 1970, half of the rise in life expectancy was due to improvements in the level of income.

Furthermore, Pritchett and Summers[5] in their paper "Wealthier Is Healthier" found that 40% of cross-country differences in mortality can be explained

by differences in income growth rates. They estimated a 1% increase in world income would lead to a reduction of 33,000 infant and 55,000 child deaths.

On a countrywide basis at the microeconomic level, Case[6] examined the impact of a sudden increase in income from South African old-age pensions on household wealth. She found that the income protected all household members when the old-age pension was put into the overall family income, but when the old-age pension was not put into the family income pot, the income only benefited the individual pensioners. She outlined possible reasons for this advantage to be seen in pooled family incomes, including the ability to purchase more help, better sanitation, improved nutrition, and decreased household psychological stress.

Just as important a finding is that income inequality may lead to poor health. In the Whitehall Study of 10,000 British civil servants, age-adjusted mortality rates were 3.5 times higher for lower grade workers compared with senior administrators.[7-9] This suggests that income differentiation of wealth can make a major impact on countrywide health outcomes. A number of other studies support this finding. Wilkinson[10] in his study of the Organisation for Economic Co-operation and Development countries, a group of the wealthiest countries in the world, showed that although greater absolute incomes lead to higher life expectancy, greater inequality had a negative impact on average life expectancy. This relative income inequality holds at the individual level, suggesting that people who make lower levels of income than their peers have a worse health outcome.[11,12]

Wealth can also increase health via indirect mechanisms like education. The World Development Report in 1993, "Investing in Health," stated that one of the most effective ways to improve health is to provide primary education to young girls.[13]

THE MECHANISMS FROM HEALTH TO WEALTH

Four major mechanisms link health to increased wealth.[14] These four mechanisms are improved productivity, more investment in education (human capital), more investment in physical capital, and utilizing the demographic dividend.

The Role of Health in Impacting Productivity

Healthier individuals are more likely to be productive because they are more energetic and less likely to miss work due to illness. Furthermore, healthier families need less time off work to care for ill individuals.

A difficulty in looking at health impacts and its role in affecting productivity is the need to separate out the fixed genetic and socially acquired human capital components to health.[15] There is very little to do to change our genetic makeup, leaving us to concentrate on behavioral aspects to improve our health capital.

Strauss[16] believed productivity of labor increases when individuals receive more calories. Because increased labor productivity may have had a reverse effect in leading to more food consumption, he used community variation in the price of food as a control variable. A number of subsequent articles have confirmed that nutrition does increase labor productivity.[17-19] Strauss and Thomas[20] in a later work showed that these effects tend to diminish as the daily intake reaches approximately 2,000 kcal.

Thomas and Strauss[21] highlight two key conceptual links from health to productivity relevant to developing countries. First, the impact of predominantly communicable diseases in developing countries affects individuals throughout their lifetimes; noncommunicable diseases in more developed countries predominantly affect the elderly. Second, because developing countries tend to be labor intensive, poor health reduces income disproportionately since a higher percentage of the work force is employed in labor-intensive industries.[22] Bhargava et al[23] confirmed that higher adult survival rates lead to higher growth rates of income in low-income groups.

Schultz, in a series of papers, looked at the direct impact of health on wages.[15,24,25] He found that "an increase in BMI of one unit was associated with a 9% increase in wages for men in Ghana and Cote d'Ivoire, and a 7% increase in wages for women in Ghana and a 15% increase in Cote d'Ivoire."[15] Similarly, a 1 centimeter gain in height was associated with a 5% increase in wages in Brazil in men and a 7% increase in women.[15] Bloom, Canning, and Sevilla[22] showed that a 1-year increase in life expectancy at birth results in a 4% increase in economic output. In summary, better health does lead directly to better wages and overall, macroeconomic output.

When looking at the American South at the beginning of the 20th century, Bleakley[26] found that the eradication of hookworm led to an improvement in wages by 45%, and half the wage gap difference between the American North and American South was due to disease factors.

A number of economic studies[27-29] have shown that longer life expectancy and lower rates of mortality lead to higher incomes and better economic performance.

Similarly, much work has been done to look at the role of maternal health and nutrition as important determinants of future chronic health problems in children, otherwise known as the "Barker hypothesis."[30,31] Poor health does not just have productivity effects in the short term; it may have intergenerational effects that contribute to a country's long-standing poor labor productivity.

Increased Investment in Human Capital

Poor health conditions decrease life expectancy and reduce the amount of human capital investment because individuals have shorter time horizons to regain the costs of the human capital investment. Furthermore, health may directly decrease human capital investments because children may be sick or have less energy to go to school.

Health plays a fundamental role in developing learning capacity. Damages occur in two specific phases:

1. **In utero:** During the time the child is inside the mother's womb, a number of prenatal insults can occur, including poor genetics, alcohol, smoking, drugs, poor nutrition, infections, and hypertension that lead to poor brain development.

2. **Postnatal:** A number of problems after birth lead to poor development including, diseases such as meningitis, diarrhea, HIV/AIDS, and pneumonia, and other problems such as head injuries, malnutrition, poor maternal education, inadequate childhood stimulation, and poverty. Any of these insults may lead to poor intellectual development.

Leslie and Jamison[32] state that three general educational issues may occur with poor health:

1. Children may not start school at the typical age.
2. Children may have poor learning capacity once school starts.
3. There may be a gross gender imbalance with a decreased number of female children participating in school.

So poor schooling has what implications? Mincer[33] showed that an additional year of schooling appears to increase earnings by 10% in the United States and suggested that increasing an average level of schooling should increase economic growth. Bloom, Canning, and Chan[34] showed that increasing educational levels may significantly increase sub-Saharan African growth and help Africa escape its poverty trap. In particular, investing in higher education may have a benefit in improving the overall economic growth of Africa.

Therefore, poor health may lead to an underinvestment in health capital and subsequently have a large effect on wages and overall economic development.

Increased Investment in Physical Capital

Like human capital, short life expectancy will reduce the amount of investment in physical capital because of the reduction in time to recuperate investment costs. However, a consequential advantage of longer life is that individuals need to save for retirement, and hence increase the investment in physical capital with the hope of future return.

Disease has a disproportionate effect on poor rural households. As stated previously, there may be a significant reduction in individual productivity. Second, there may be spending to prevent, diagnose, and treat the disease. Third, Nur[35] showed that malaria decreases household savings as families increasingly spend money to hire labor to compensate for productivity losses from individuals infected with malaria. Therefore, there is less money available to invest in physical capital.

Even the threat of ill health may have an enormous impact. For example, severe acute respiratory syndrome was estimated to cost the city of Toronto $1.5 billion in lost tourism and investment in the city, even though it led to only 44 deaths.[36]

Capturing the Benefits from the Demographic Dividend

The final mechanism for how health improvements could affect economic growth is through the "demographic dividend." The theory is that health improvements trigger a decline in mortality rates, followed by a decline in fertility rates years later. This leads to a large population bulge. This group eventually proceeds through productive working years and produces a large working-age population relative to the young and old-age dependent populations. This large working-age to dependent-age population ratio gives a window of opportunity for economic growth but does not guarantee it. It requires appropriate country-wide conditions (stable politics, good macroeconomic policies, openness to trade, and good health status) to maximize the gains.

Bloom and Williamson[28] suggest a third to half of the East Asian miracle from 1965 to 1990 can be explained by the demographic dividend. Similarly, Bloom and Canning[37] highlight the importance of contraception in reducing fertility and triggering a demographic dividend, leading to the Irish economic boom in the 1980s and 1990s.

ECONOMIC IMPACTS OF THREE KEY DISEASES

Malaria, tuberculosis (TB), and HIV/AIDS are examples of diseases that have significant economic impacts on populations.

Malaria

Each year there are over 200 million new cases of malaria and about 600,000 to 1 million deaths, mostly children and pregnant women.[38,39] As Gallup and Sachs[40] reveal, countries where a high proportion of the population lived in regions of *Plasmodium falciparum* malaria transmission had annual growth rates 1.3% lower than other countries from 1965 to 1990, even after controlling for other standard growth determinants. They conclude that this effect cumulated over time and would reduce the gross national product level to half the amount of a nonmalarial country. In sub-Saharan Africa, malaria does not seem to have a significant class difference.[41]

There are various ways by which malaria could reduce economic productivity. First, there are the private and public medical costs to preventing, diagnosing, and treating malaria. Second, there are the costs due to lost days at work and for taking care of family members who are ill with malaria. Third, malaria has a longer-term consequence because it can lead to forgone earnings from premature death, decreased labor productivity, and in school-age children, reduced performance in school.[42,43] Sachs and Malaney[38] highlight that, more importantly, malaria can cause significant social costs on school, demography, migration, and savings. Furthermore, the macroeconomic effects may extend to trade, tourism, and foreign direct investment.

Historically, there has been a significant reduction in trade between malaria and nonmalaria zones. For example, in the 1950s, when the countries of southern Europe such as Greece, Portugal, and Spain began to eradicate malaria, foreign direct investment from Northern Europe increased rapidly to spur economic growth.[40] Therefore, control of malaria has historically been associated with economic well-being.

Tuberculosis

TB infects 8.7 million people and causes 1.4 million deaths per year, with 13% of patients having a coinfection with HIV.[44] Over 95% of cases occur in developing countries.[45] TB predominantly affects working-age populations between the ages of 15 and 54.[46] On average, 3 to 4 months of work is lost (resulting in a 20% to 30% loss of annual household income).[47] There is also a significant loss of income if a TB patient dies, equivalent to 15 years loss of income over a lifetime.[47]

Without a proper course of treatment, approximately 50% to 60% of those infected will die.[46] Yet, with proper treatment, the life expectancy of an otherwise healthy person would increase by an average of 25 to 30 years.[48]

TB and poverty are interlinked. Crowded conditions more likely allow the spread of TB. Yet TB can also lead to poverty. The presence of TB may lead to a significant sale of assets to pay for drugs, reducing food intake in children due to poverty, and decreasing educational opportunities. Therefore, TB is a classic example of the poverty and poor health dyad.[49]

HIV/AIDS

In 2010, 34 million people were living with HIV infection. There were 2.7 million new cases and 1.8 million deaths.[50] HIV/AIDS has a large impact on development because it targets people in prime working ages, accounting for approximately 65% of deaths.[51] Studies suggest that HIV/AIDS preferentially affects urban high-income skilled men and their partners.[52]

Ainsworth and Over[52] list four key reasons why HIV/AIDS is different from other infectious diseases:

1. HIV/AIDS has no cure.
2. HIV/AIDS affects working-age individuals, mostly through heterosexual intercourse.
3. HIV/AIDS decimates social fabrics of care for the young and old and slows down macroeconomic growth.
4. HIV/AIDS has not spared the economic and intellectual elites.

Bloom et al[53] highlight that HIV/AIDS has reduced the capacity to invest in human capital, which in turn leads to a further inability to identify and treat HIV/AIDS.

This reduced capacity leads to a downward "death spiral," resulting in the inability to deal with the consequences of the HIV/AIDS epidemic.

HIV/AIDS has a large impact in sub-Saharan African development. As just explained, HIV/AIDS decreases the working age to dependent age ratios leading to a higher dependency ratio on a smaller workforce. Furthermore, with an increasing loss of parents and an increase in HIV/AIDS orphans, there is a disproportionate burden on women and working-age populations to support the orphans. HIV/AIDS and related disease spending is a third of total health care costs and over half of total public health spending in many countries.[51]

There is evidence that HIV/AIDS is directly affecting companies. Aventin and Huard[54] examined three companies in Côte d'Ivoire and found that a 10% increase in the prevalence of HIV/AIDS results in an increase in cost of 6.8% to 10.0%. These effects can also be seen at a countrywide level. Arndt and Lewis,[55,56] Bonnel,[57] and ING Barings[58] all report that by 2010, South African gross domestic product (GDP) per capita will decrease by approximately 8% due to HIV/AIDS.

HIV/AIDS remains one of the great global health challenges, not just because of the enormous health implications around the world, but also due to its ability to stem economic development. Finding solutions to deliver services, drugs, and prevent disease remain paramount in this struggle.

THE IMPACT OF HEALTH CARE ON THE ECONOMY

One of the largest budgetary items in any government is health care spending. Health care spending accounts for 8% of global GDP[59] but rises to as much as 16% of GDP in the United States.[60] In this section, we concentrate on the importance of financing health care and describe the payment systems that help distribute this financing.

FINANCING HEALTH CARE

Every finance and health minister must decide how to finance their country's health care system. Five major methods are used: general revenue, social insurance, community insurance, private insurance, and direct purchaser payment.

Most countries use a combination of these different methods. How do we decide which methods to use? Four key factors determine each country's capacity to finance health successfully:

1. Financial resources
2. Stage of economic development

438 / CHAPTER 19

3. Ability to administer financial services
4. Political will and structure[61]

Financial Resources

The ability to generate revenues may determine a government's ability to use certain methods to finance health care. For example, in many developing countries, general taxation may not be feasible when over half the population works in the informal sector and weak enforcement mechanisms are in place. Health care is also just one of many competing departments in the general budget. There may be more emphasis on defense, infrastructure building, and education.

Social insurance requires an administrative structure that allows for the capture of contributions from companies. Very small businesses often find it difficult to separate out personal profits from wage earnings. In theory, social insurance should be based only on wage earnings, but this is extremely difficult to delineate. If there is significant social structure and well-being, a social insurance scheme should have a broad reach.

Community insurance refers to the pooling of risks to provide basic health services for a community. This often requires good social cooperation and tends to be geared toward poorer segments of the population.

Private insurance can occur when people with enough income want to buy more health care services and/or higher quality services. This often leads to two-tiering of the health care system between those that have private insurance that cover more services and those that do not.

Direct purchaser payment systems (user fees and out-of-pocket payment) are used in many developing countries in the world that include payments for drugs, supplies, and services provided when a patient

becomes ill or sick. Thus, because the payments tend to be acute in nature, they tend to be higher and may directly cause poverty.

Stage of Economic Development

The stage of economic development is an important factor in determining which financing method to use. Depending on a country's economic well-being, individuals may be able to pay more for health care, and likewise, the country is likely to face increased demand for health care. In general, as income increases per capita, there is an increase in spending per capita on health, especially within the public sector (see Table 19-1).

The implication of a lower level of spending in developing countries is that there is less health capital (beds, hospitals, clinics), service providers (physicians, nurses, and allied professionals), and hospital visits (both inpatient and outpatient). There is also concern that lower income countries have less "fair" access to health care. One of the arguments to improve economic development is that increased wealth can directly lead to better health care systems.

Ability to Administer Financial Services

One of the challenges governments face is the ability to administer health services. Medical records must be kept, financial tracking and auditing established, and other administrative services developed. These services depend on a country or locale's ability to set up and monitor the system, and effectively enforce health care regulation and legislation.

For example, many developing countries may not have the human resources and tracking systems to enforce tax collection. Furthermore, it may be

Table 19-1. Health expenditures by income group and region (2002).[a]

Income Group	Total Health Expenditure as % of GNP	Total Expenditures (Across Countries in Group)	Public Sector (% of GDP)	Private Sector (% of GDP)
World	10.2	588	5.9	4.3
Low-income	4.6	30	1.3	3.3
Middle-income	6.0	116	2.5	3.5
High-income	11.2	3449	6.7	4.5
East Asia and Pacific	5.0	64	1.9	3.1
Europe and Central Asia	6.5	194	4.5	2.0
Latin America and Carribean	6.8	222	3.3	3.5
Middle East and North Africa	5.6	92	2.7	2.9
South Asia	4.4	24	1.1	3.3
Sub-Saharan Africa	6.1	36	2.4	3.7

[a]From World Bank. World Development Indicators 2006. Table 2.14.[65]

extremely difficult to capture revenues from informal sector employment. These challenges lessen the number of formal workers increased from economic development. However, without these revenues, it may be difficult to develop a strong social insurance or general taxation method to finance health care.

In other countries there may be difficulties in gaining public acceptance of tax collection because of concerns over government corruption and concerns over service delivery. These challenges require a strong trusted monitoring system to ensure transparency of the financial structure and ensure services are provided.

Political Will and Structure

Another consideration is the importance of health care inside the government structure. Competing interests with other sectors such as defense may lead to different priorities. Often, health may be a primary interest (e.g., in Cuba and Canada), but in other countries, health care may take a far less important role (e.g., many developing countries). How government structures health care financing may help determine its priority and importance versus other segments of government.

FINANCING SYSTEMS

We now examine the major financing systems in use around the world today. However, first we must look at some basic definitions in financing health care.

Risk Pooling

Risk pooling refers to grouping a large number of people together to decrease the variance in health outcomes on an individual basis, and thereby spreading the financial risk of an adverse event. A health insurance company can help spread an individual's risk by grouping them with people at a similar risk level and spreading the costs between them. For example, if someone has a 1 in 100 chance of getting an illness, and it costs $5,000 to treat it, 100 individuals may be willing to put $50 into a joint pool to cope with this illness. Furthermore, this spreading of risk allows for greater precision at the individual level about the possibilities of financial loss.

Risk Aversion

Another aspect that favors the development of health insurance is that, in general, people prefer certainty over uncertainty. Thus people would rather know that they are paying a small amount every month than one giant lump sum of money when they get ill. Risk aversion is an important concept because it leads to more equivalent payments for health services, rather than lump-sum payments when adverse events occur.

Adverse Selection

Adverse selection refers to the practice of insurers choosing healthier people over sick people for the same insurance because this minimizes the expected costs to be paid. Conversely, sick individuals prefer to purchase insurance over healthier individuals at the same cost.

Moral Hazard

Moral hazard is one of the barriers to the implementation of health care insurance. Moral hazard occurs when individuals use services more frequently than they would normally because they have an insurance policy in place.

Direct Purchaser Payment (User Fees, Fee for Service, Out-of Pocket Payments)

The most basic system relied on to finance health care is to pay directly out-of-pocket for health care services. These financial systems dominate developing countries. An alternative to this model is the concept of the user fee. This refers to cost sharing, cost recovery, or copayment, and it has been widely used since the Bamako Initiative in 1987.

The Bamako Initiative was an attempt to decentralize health care to the district level, create an essential drug policy, and provide these drugs to communities.[62] The financing mechanism behind the Bamako Initiative was supposed to be a combination of central government, regional governments, local governments, and individual patients. In theory, user fees were created to aid the development of health services and not to replace government funding. The hope was that there would be a combination of different financing mechanisms, including social insurance, fee for service, and out-of-pocket payment, for drugs, which would lead to a sustainable structure. However, from the Bamako Initiative, governments focused mostly on fee-for-service payment schemes.

In the early 1980s, the World Bank was a major proponent of user fees for health services. They saw it as a major mechanism to finance health care. A significant concern with the implementation of user fees is that they disproportionately affect the poor, who are often reluctant to use health care services until they are extremely sick. Yet there is significant concern that the abolishment of user fees may adversely affect primary health care services, by taking away much needed basic financing for these services.

A 2004 World Bank publication reversed the position on user fees.[63] In contrast, it focused on three major ideas: protecting the economic abilities of the poor, building sustainable health care services, and allocating resources more efficiently.

Community Insurance

Finance systems may lead to some collective attempts to pool resources to decrease individual risk. Community insurance is a prepayment scheme that focuses at the community level. Community health insurance may be a village or a group of villages or an employee group that negotiates with suppliers of health care services for discounted health services. In most community health insurance services, primary care is integrated, whereas secondary and tertiary services are separated.

The advantage of community financing is that in negotiating with health care suppliers, there is a higher incentive for doctors to attend regularly and provide higher quality service. Furthermore, it bypasses the concern of government regulation and corruption in other prepayment schemes. Community financing raises money at the local level, and in turn, the community has clear control of the movement of funds.

Community health care services in many developing countries are composed of a basic primary health care service provision and contracts with secondary and tertiary institutions for catastrophic health events. There is compulsory membership by all members in the community. A portion of funds are often reinvested in income-generating activities (microfinance) to further encourage investment within the community.

A major disadvantage of community financing is that it requires significant community buy-in, or adverse selection will occur. Furthermore, there are concerns over moral hazard. The financing is also extremely tenuous, especially during financial downturns, when many rural farmers lose their main sources of income. Hence there needs to be strong community ties and agreements to sustain community health insurance.

Social Insurance

Social insurance is an extension of community health insurance. Social insurance refers to prospectively collecting funds in advance to purchase health care in the future. The first social health insurance program, an amalgamation of many community health insurance schemes, began in 1883 in Germany. Today, the two most common ways to raise funds is either through employers or through the government.

There are three main properties of social insurance. First, insurance must be compulsory. Otherwise adverse selection will play a role and only the sickest will buy insurance. Second, social insurance requires a social compact. There are expectations that individuals will pay and the funds will be used fairly by those within the social insurance scheme. Third, funds are raised and targeted specifically to finance the social health insurance system. In some countries such as

France, social insurance is compulsory for all citizens; in other countries, social insurance is provided only for people in the formal work sector.

Social health insurance funds often have their own health care networks. Often a network of providers negotiates with a social health insurance organization and draws up a specified list of health care provisions that will be provided.

Countries that have adopted social insurance programs include countries in Europe (France, Netherlands, and Hungary), Latin America (Mexico, Argentina, and Brazil), and East Asia (South Korea, Taiwan, and the Philippines).

Social health insurance schemes increase the pool of resources and funds. This, in turn, because of its negotiation power, leads to a more responsive system. Second, social health insurance systems are easily implemented if formal sector workers can be identified.

There are a number of disadvantages to the social health insurance system. First, it helps finance only those enrolled in the social health insurance system, which are usually formal worker employees. It does not make provisions for the poor and the most vulnerable groups. Second, the cost of social insurance is shifted from employer to employee in the form of lower wages.[64] Third, if there are competing social health insurance systems, they compete to get the healthiest individuals. Fourth, there needs to be an ability to collect the tax revenues and to administrate the financial and health care systems.

General Taxation

In many countries, general taxes may support health care. In general, as countries become wealthier and the government is more able to collect taxes, an increasing amount of health spending is financed through general taxes. Various types of taxes may pay for health care, including income taxes, sales and value-added taxes, import taxes, and corporate taxes. Usually revenues for health increase if the economy grows. However, at the same time, health care suffers if there is sudden economic downturn.

The major advantage of general taxation is that there is a strong source of steady revenue. Furthermore, general taxation is politically controllable, and it requires a large degree of financial accountability. Depending on the type of taxation used, it may be progressive and improve equity, and it can pool health risks across an entire population. Certain services, such as immunization and public health surveillance, are almost always best covered by general taxation.

Health care faces competition for general tax revenue from other sources of interest, including defense, infrastructure development, industry, and education. A major concern with general taxation is that it requires a strong administrative infrastructure and transparency, especially to collect taxes. There is always some concern of favoritism toward certain groups; for example, spending may favor larger urban centers over rural areas.

Private Insurance

Private insurance refers to purchasing insurance on a voluntary basis from individual competitive sellers. A key difference is that the premiums charged are based on a purchaser's risk rather than their ability to pay. One of the clear advantages of private insurance is that it clearly defines the preferences for different levels of services at different income levels. Therefore, private insurance acts as a spur to medical technological advancement. There is also an argument that private insurance empowers individuals to act in their best health interests.

Private insurance is becoming increasingly prevalent in wealthier countries without strong generalized taxation schemes. One of the ways corporations build loyalty in these countries is by providing health insurance as an additional perk for employees. Therefore, companies purchase insurance on behalf of their employees.

Historically, private health insurance is often characterized by the culprit of adverse selection. Insurers prefer to take people who are healthiest, and those that tend to be sickest prefer to get the best insurance possible. A second problem is the poor and the sick tend to find it very difficult to purchase health insurance. The third issue is that there are often high administrative and marketing costs that add to the cost of the health care insurance.

The best example of a private health insurance market is the United States, which has the highest cost of care in the world and almost 45 million uninsured individuals.

SUMMARY

- Health and wealth flow bidirectionally. More wealth can buy better health care services and goods that can improve health. Conversely, better health can lead to more wealth through four key mechanisms: productivity, education, investment in physical capital, and impacts on the demographic dividend.
- Both low-income levels and high income disparities can adversely affect overall population health.
- Health care spending is a large part of government spending.
- Four key prioritization methods exist in determining how to finance health care: financial resources,

stage of economic development, the ability to administrate financial services, and the political will and structure.

- Key basic concepts in financing health care include risk pooling, risk aversion, adverse selection, and moral hazard.
- Five financing systems include direct purchaser payment, community insurance, social insurance, general taxation, and private insurance.

STUDY QUESTIONS

1. You are a minister of health in a developing country. You would like to improve the health care status of people in your country. What financing system exists now? What type of financing system would you like? Justify why you think this financing system would improve your health care. What criticism could you receive from the finance minister and other members of the cabinet?

2. You are the minister of health in China. Explain how avian influenza may affect your economic systems and what impacts it could have on overall development.

3. "Money, money, money" are the three things needed for better health. Do you agree with this statement? Why or why not?

ACKNOWLEDGMENTS

I would like to acknowledge the constructive comments of David Bloom, Rosemary Marotta, and Larry Rosenberg.

REFERENCES

1. Preston SA. Causes and consequences of mortality decline in less developed countries during the twentieth century. In: Easterlin RA, ed. *Population and Economic Change in Developing Countries*. Chicago: University of Chicago Press, 1980:289–360.

2. Fuchs VR. Time preference and health: an exploratory study. In: Fuchs VR, ed. *Economic Aspects of Health*. Chicago: University of Chicago Press, 1982:93–120.

3. Fogel RW. Economic growth, population theory and physiology. *Am Econ Rev* 1994;84(3):369–395.

4. Wagstaff A. Poverty and health. Commission on Macroeconomics and Health Working Paper Series. Paper No. WG1: 5. March 2001. www2.cid.harvard.edu/cidcmh/wg1_paper5.pdf.

5. Pritchett L, Summers LH. Wealthier is healthier. *J Hum Resources* 1996;31(4):841–868.

6. Case A. Does money protect health status? Evidence from South African pensions. Princeton University and the NBER, 2001:1–30.

7. Wilkinson RG, ed. *Class and Health: Research and Longitudinal Data*. New York: Tavistock, 1986.

8. Marmot MG, Theorell T. Social class and cardiovascular disease: The contribution of work. *Int J Health Serv* 1988;18(4): 659–674.

9. Marmot MG, Smith GD, Stansfeld S, et al. Health inequalities among British civil servants: the Whitehall II study. *Lancet* 1991;337:1387–1393.

10. Wilkinson RG. Income distribution and mortality—a natural experiment. *Health Illness* 1990;12:391–412.

11. Deaton A. Inequalities in income and inequalities in health. National Bureau of Economic Research Working Paper Series No. 7141, 1999:1–37.

12. Deaton A, Paxson C. Mortality, education, income and inequality among American cohorts. National Bureau of Economic Research Working Paper No. 7140, 1999:1–49.

13. World Bank. *World Development Report 1993: Investing in Health.* Oxford: Oxford University Press, 1993.

14. Bloom DE, Canning D. The health and wealth of nations. *Science* 2000;287(5456):1207–1209.

15. Schultz TP. *Productive benefits of improving health: evidence from low-income countries.* New Haven, CT: Yale University, 2001. http://www.econ.yale.edu/~pschultz/productivebenefits

16. Strauss J. Does better nutrition raise farm productivity? *J Political Econ* 1986;94(2):297–320.

17. Deolalikar A. Nutrition and labor productivity in agriculture. *Rev Econ Stat* 1988;70(3):406–413.

18. Sahn DE, Alderman H. The effect of human capital on wages, on the determinants of labor supply in a developing country. *J Develop Econ* 1988;29(2):157–183.

19. Foster AD, Rosenweig M. A test for moral hazard in the labor market: effort, health and calorie consumption. *Rev Econ Stat* 1994;76(2):213–227.

20. Strauss J, Thomas D. Human resources: empirical modeling of household and family decisions. In: Behrman JR and Srinivasan TN, eds. *Handbook of Development Economics.* Vol IIIA, Chapter 34. Amsterdam: North-Holland, 1995.

21. Thomas D, Strauss J. The micro-foundations of the links between health, nutrition and development. *J Econ Lit* 1998; 36:766–817.

22. Bloom DE, Canning D, Sevilla J. The effect of health on economic growth: a production function approach. *World Dev* 2004;32(1):1–13.

23. Bhargava A, Jamison DR, Lau LJ, Murray CJL. Modelling the effects of health on economic growth. Geneva: World Health Organization, Global Programme on Evidence Discussion Paper, 2000.

24. Schultz TP. Investments in the schooling and health of women and men: quantities and return. *J Hum Resources* 1993;28(4): 694–734.

25. Schultz TP. Health and schooling in Africa. *J Econ Perspect* 1999;13(3):67–88.

26. Bleakley H. Disease and development: evidence from the American South. *J Eur Econ Assoc* 2003;1(2–3):376–386.

27. Barro R, Lee JW. Sources of economic growth. *Carnegie-Rochester Conference Series on Public Policy* 1994;40:1–46.

28. Bloom DE, Williamson JG. Demographic transitions and economic miracles in emerging Asia. *World Bank Econ Rev* 1998; 12(3):419–455.

29. Jamison DT, Lau LJ, Wang J. Health's contribution to economic growth, 1965–1990. In: *Health, Health Policy and Economic Outcomes.* Final report of the Health and Development Satellite WHO Director. Geneva: World Health Organization, 1998.

30. Barker DJ. Fetal and infant origins of adult disease. *Br Med J* 1990;301(6761): 1111.

31. Fogel RW. Catching up with the economy. *Am Econ Rev* 1999; 89(1):1–21.

32. Leslie J, Jamison DT. Health and nutrition considerations in education planning: educational consequences of health problems among school-age children. *Food Nutr Bull* 1990;12:204–214.

33. Mincer J. *Schooling, Earning and Experience.* New York: Columbia University Press, 1974.

34. Bloom DE, Canning D, Chan KJ. *Higher Education and Economic Growth in Africa.* Washington, DC: World Bank, 2006.

35. Nur E. The impact of malaria on labour use and efficiency in the Sudan. *Soc Sci Med* 1993;37:1115–1119.

36. Conference Board of Canada. The economic impact of SARS. May 2003. Ottawa: Conference Board of Canada: 1–3.

37. Bloom DE, Canning D. Contraception and the Celtic tiger. *Econ Soc Rev* 2003;34:229–247.

38. World Health Organization. *World Malaria Report.* Geneva: WHO, 2012. www.who.int/malaria/publications/world_malaria_report_2012/en/index.html.

39. Breman JG, Mills A, Snow RW, et al. Conquering malaria. In: *Disease Control Priorities Project.* 2nd ed. files.dcp2.org/pdf/DCP/DCP21.pdf.

40. Gallup Jl, Sachs JD. The economic burden of malaria. CID Working Paper No. 52. Cambridge, MA: Centre for International Development, Harvard University, 2000.

41. Filmer D. Fever and its treatment in the more and less poor in sub-Saharan Africa. Development Research Group. Washington, DC: World Bank, 2000.

42. Chima RI, Mills A. Estimating the economic impact of malaria in sub-Saharan Africa: A review of the empirical evidence. 1998. Unpublished manuscript.

43. Malaney P. Benefits of malaria control. Cambridge: Harvard Institute for International Development, 1998.

44. World Health Organization. *Global Tuberculosis Report, Executive Summary.* Geneva: WHO, 2012. www.who.int/tb/publications/global_report/gtbr12_executivesummary.pdf.

45. Dye C, Floyd K. Tuberculosis. In: Jamison DT, Breman JG, Measham AR, eds. *Disease Control Priorities.* 2nd ed. Washington, DC: World Bank, 2006.

46. Murray CJL. Epidemiology and demography of tuberculosis. In: Timaeus IM, Chackiel J, Ruzieka L, eds. *Adult Mortality in Latin America.* Oxford: Clarendon Press, 1996.

47. World Health Organization. *The Economic Impacts of Tuberculosis.* Geneva: WHO, 2000.

48. World Health Organization. Report from a consultation on the socioeconomic impacts of HIV/AIDS on households. UNAIDS/97.3. Geneva: WHO, 1997.

49. Croft RA, Croft RP. Expenditure and loss of income incurred by tuberculosis patients before reaching effective treatment in Bangladesh. *Int J Tuberculosis Lung Dis* 1998;2(3): 252–254.

50. World Health Organization. Global health observatory, HIV/AIDS. Geneva: WHO, 2013. www.who.int/gho/hiv/en/.

51. Haacker M. The economic consequences of HIV/AIDS in southern Africa. IMF Working Paper WP/02/38. 1–41.

52. Ainsworth M, Over M. AIDS and African development. *World Bank Research Observer* 1994;9(2):203–240.

53. Bloom DE, Bloom LR, Steven D, Weston H. *Business and HIV/AIDS: Who Me?* Geneva: World Economic Forum, 2003:1–9.

54. Aventin L, Huard P. The cost of AIDS to three manufacturing firms in Côte d'Ivoire. *J Afr Econ* 2000;9(2):161–188.

55. Arndt C, Lewis JD. The macro implications of HIV/AIDS in South Africa: a preliminary assessment. *South Afr J Econ* 2000;68(5):856–887.

56. Arndt C, Lewis JD. The HIV/AIDS pandemic in South Africa: sectoral impacts and unemployment. *J Int Dev* 2001;13:427–449.

57. Bonnel R. *HIV/AIDS: Does It Increase or Decrease Growth?* Washington DC: World Bank, 2000.

58. ING Barings. *Economic Impact of AIDS in South Africa: A Dark Cloud on the Horizon.* Johannesburg: ING Barings, 2000.

59. World Health Organization. *World Health Report 2000.* Geneva: WHO, 2000.

60. National Coalition on Health Care. Health insurance cost. www.nchc.org/facts/cost.shtml.

61. Hsiao W. Financing. In: *Getting Health Reform Right.* Oxford: Oxford University Press, 2004.

62. Camara YB, El Abassi A, Knippenberg R, et al. *State-Civil Society Partnership Improves Health Services Delivery for the Poorest in West Africa.* Washington, DC: World Bank, 2003.

63. World Bank. *World Development Report 2004: Making Services Work for Poor People.* Washington, DC: World Bank, 2004.

64. Atkinson A, Stiglitz J. *Lectures in Public Economics.* New York: McGraw-Hill, 1980.

65. World Bank. *World Development Indicators 2006.* Washington DC: World Bank, 2006.

Health Systems, Management, and Organization in Global Health

20

David Zakus, Onil Bhattacharyya, and Xiaolin Wei

LEARNING OBJECTIVES

- *Explore the most current issues of health services management in low- and middle-income countries*
- *Understand the structure of health systems*
- *Understand the concept and dimensions of health system performance*
- *Explore national, organizational, provider, and patient interventions to improve the performance of health systems*

INTRODUCTION TO HEALTH SYSTEMS

Have you ever wondered why, in light of great scientific advances, modern communications, and the availability of many cures, treatments, and preventive measures for most diseases commonly found in low- and middle- income countries (LMICs), those diseases still persist and often with great prevalence and incidence? This is the conundrum that we hope to explore in this chapter, especially as it relates to the organization, management, and delivery of services to reach those in need of prevention or treatment of the many diseases, both chronic and infectious, found in LMICs.

To begin, it is important to understand how services that maintain, improve, and restore health are provided to individuals and populations in both urban and rural areas, in light of growing disparities in privilege.[1,2]

The perspective that is most often used in understanding the delivery of health and medical services is that of a "system," which is a set of components and their interrelationships, attributes, and properties. From systems theory we understand a system as the continuum of inputs, processes, and outputs. Therefore, within our understanding of the need for health services, the health system is:

- The totality of the required resources, including human, mechanical, material, and financial
- The formal and informal organization interactions and conversions of these resources in the provision of services to individuals and populations to help them maintain good or acceptable health status and improve on it when it is perceived in need, either from disease, physical disability, trauma, or even when perceived as suboptimal[3]
- The final product of health, which can vary in definition but is commonly understood as the state of complete physical, mental, and social (and even spiritual) well-being or the ability to live one's life in a manner compatible with achieving one's social and personal goals, achieving dignity and human rights.

The last theoretical component of systems, for now, is that they are either "closed" or "open." Closed systems are completely self-contained, are not influenced by external events, and eventually must die because nothing is self-sustainable on its own. Open systems, in contrast, interact with their external environments by exchanging materials, energies, or information, and they are influenced by or can influence this environment; they must adjust to the environment to survive over time. The environment can generally be classified as political, economic, social, and technological, as well as physical (the space available and the way system components relate physically to each other). Thinking of natural disasters and climate and population change, the environment always has an ecological perspective, too.

Health systems are open and must be approached from this perspective. They are open to their local and national environments, and now, ever increasingly, to international and global influences. All the world's national health ministries are members of the World Health Organization (WHO), are often accountable to more local government, and at times to the people they serve.

Health systems are one of several determinants of health, and high-performing health systems can improve the health of populations.[4] Although there is no perfect health system, an understanding of the system in its current form allows us to gain a comprehensive picture of how it and its constituent parts contribute to maintaining health. This, then, helps in understanding the interactions required of its various components. There is an important need for ethical considerations and promotion of equity.

Theoretically, components within a system can be deterministic; that is, the components function according to a completely predictable or definable relationship, as in most mechanical systems; or they can be probabilistic, where the relationships cannot be perfectly predicted, as in most human or human-machine systems, like health care. The WHO suggests that health system boundaries should encompass all actors whose primary intent is to improve and protect health, and to make it fair and responsive to all, especially those who are worst off and most vulnerable to disease and illness.[4]

What then makes a health system good? What makes it equitable? And how does one evaluate a health system or components of it? The WHO report entitled "Health Systems: Improving Performance"[4] provides a detailed presentation and analysis of why health systems matter, how well they are performing, organizational failings, resources needed, financing, and governance. In summary, it defines four key functions of a health system: "providing services; generating the human and physical resources that make service delivery possible; raising and pooling the resources used to pay for health care; and, most critically, the function of stewardship."[4]

The then director general, Dr. Gro Bruntland, stated, "Whatever standard we apply, it is evident that health systems in some countries perform well, while others perform poorly. This is not due just to differences in income or expenditure: we know that performance can vary markedly, even in countries with very similar levels of health spending. The way health systems are designed, managed, and financed affects people's lives and livelihoods. The difference between a well-performing health system and one that is failing can be measured in death, disability, impoverishment, humiliation and despair."[4]

The report concluded that:

- The ultimate responsibility for the performance of a country's health system lies with government.
- Dollar for dollar spent on health, many countries are falling short of their performance potential. The result is a large number of preventable deaths and lives stunted by disability. The impact of this failure is borne disproportionately by the poor.
- Health systems are not just concerned with improving people's health, but with protection from the financial costs of illness.
- Within governments, many health ministries focus on the public sector, often disregarding the (frequently much larger) privately financed provision of care.

Health systems have not always existed; nor have they existed for long in their present form. Early attempts to provide organized national and international access to health services have gone through various stages of evolution throughout the last century and will continue to evolve in this century. Early attempts to found national health systems were common throughout Western Europe, starting with the protection of workers, and are now being followed by most countries around the world, in some attempt to provide health care for all their citizens. The first attempt was in Russia following the Bolshevik revolution in 1917, but it took many more years and a Second World War for most governments to catch on. New Zealand, though, introduced a national health service in 1938; in Britain it was in 1948 with the National Health Service; and in Canada, which is widely known for its national and provincial Medicare health system, it was only in 1971. The United States remains the only Organization for Economic Co-operation and Development country without a national health delivery system (although there have been recent attempts in moving toward one), and Cuba remains a model of what a public system can achieve with limited financial resources.[5]

Today, most countries' health systems have evolved along two lines: the employee/employer payment scheme or the tax-based model, whereby all tax payers contribute all or part of the required financial input. Both involve a mix, to widely varying degrees, of public versus private service provision. Comparing health systems is an often useful exercise, especially for learning new ideas.

The WHO came into being in 1946, and its efforts to promote viable and effective health services culminated with the Declaration of Alma Ata in 1978, which advocated the concept and strategy of primary health care[6] as a means to achieve health for all. Although much debate has persisted concerning the value and utility of primary health care, it remains a viable and recently renewed approach for providing an acceptable level of health services in countries at all levels of economic and social development.[7–9] Debate now centers on how best to deliver services through public or private providers, and the appropriate mix of financing mechanisms: government expenditure, out-of-pocket, or various other types of insurance.

Moving toward universal access and insurance coverage is now considered mandatory,[10] and the world is moving toward achieving universal health coverage, aimed at giving everyone in a country the health services they need without financial barrier.[11] Most developed countries have already achieved this momentum except the United States, where the movement is still under political debate. Canada presents one of the best examples of universal health coverage in rich countries. The five principles of the Canadian Medicare scheme (comprehensiveness, universality, accessibility, portability and public administration) have sufficiently ensured that every Canadian is entitled to the health care they need across the country without financial burdens. Many LMICs such as Mexico, Thailand, Philippines, Vietnam, and Ghana are moving in this direction. Large developing countries such as China and India have made significant progress in insurance coverage in the last decades.[3] Since 2002, the New Cooperative Medical Scheme (NCMS), a form of rural health insurance, together with various other urban health insurance plans, have achieved over 90% health insurance coverage of the total population in China.[12] Recent studies have identified that NCMS was associated with increased use at the primary care level and reduction in out-of-pocket spending in township hospitals and village clinics.[13] India, today, is implementing various state level universal access policies. This unprecedented revolution of health reform will change how health care is financed and paid, relieve the health need of the poor, and contribute to more equitable human development in general. At the health system level, universal coverage will reshape the organization of health delivery and health financing. New perspectives of health financing, including tax-based and employer-based insurance, as well as public private partnerships, have been explored in different countries.[14] Universal coverage, together with a primary care–based health delivery system, will contribute to advancing the Millennium Development Goals related to more equitable health rights and better accessibility to health services.[15]

Health systems matter in the achievement of health, especially for those at the lower end of the socioeconomic spectrum, but also for the wealthy. Although health systems are complex,[16] proper health system stewardship and management offers the potential for coordination of multi- and intersectoral services,[17] and accessibility of these services for those who need them according to their needs. Health service providers may be from the public and/or private sectors, and how they interact and are coordinated are all issues of great concern within the health system perspective. A systems perspective on health also helps us get out of our "health" box, in thinking that only medical services and technologies are important; rather, through a systems perspective we come to understand that addressing inequalities in income and housing,[18] seatbelt laws, safe roads, antismoking legislation, firearm registries, dietary recommendations, workplace safety, and weather predictions all help to maintain good health and longevity. In 2008, the WHO published the final report of a special commission mandated to investigate the social determinants of health. In their report *Closing the Gap in a Generation: Health Equity Through Action on the Social Determinants of Health*, they demonstrate very clearly the importance of many social factors, previously not considered central and yet having a direct impact on health status. They conclude that "Social injustice is killing people on a grand scale."[19]

THE PERFORMANCE OF HEALTH SYSTEMS

We have already argued that health systems are important to people's health and that some systems seem to achieve more than others; but to assess this critically, we must measure it against the objectives and intended outcomes of a health system. Health system assessment is essential and practical.[20] The *World Health Report 2000* defines three objectives for health systems: improving the health of the populations they serve; responding to people's expectations; and providing financial protection against the costs of ill health.[4] Furthermore, it attempts to assess the average level of attainment of a given objective and its distribution across the population. This follows a growing interest in equity, making it an essential element of performance.[21] These objectives and measures are discussed here in a general sense, without specifically referring to those from the WHO report. The first, the health status of a population, would be measured by an average, such as life expectancy, maternal mortality, or infant mortality as well as the range of life expectancy across subgroups within a population. It is always important to disaggregate average measures to get a fuller understanding of the actual situation. Today, for instance, we are now learning how to save 1.2 million stillborn babies per year.[22]

Health systems that systematically neglect certain subgroups while having a good overall average would have a worse performance than one with the same average but more even distribution across subgroups. These subgroups are generally defined by social characteristics such as wealth, education, occupation, ethnicity, sex, rural or urban residency, or religion.[23] These groups are chosen because these characteristics should not affect people's health (although they often do), and health systems should attempt to mitigate these effects where possible by providing targeted access to appropriate services. The difference in health status between these groups—for example, maternal mortality in rural versus urban areas—would be minimized in a high-performing health system. This reflects the degree of distributive justice within a system, which is also a measure of overall effectiveness.

Responsiveness of a health system is also an objective due to interest in governance and a concern for patient preferences, and not only their epidemiologically defined health needs. This is important because patient preference has an impact on health service utilization, as shown by the widespread use of private health services in LMICs, even among the poor and even when free public services are available.[24] Fair financing is an important objective because health care costs are unpredictable and may be catastrophic. For example, in China family bankruptcies due to medical expenditures accounted for a third of rural poverty in 2004.[25] Universal coverage may not necessarily reduce financial burden on patients because many barriers of health insurance plans such as co-payment, user fees, thresholds and ceilings may prevent patients using them. The rapid expansion of health insurance coverage in China was associated with a 2.5 times increase of hospitalization rate between 2003 and 2011; the proportion of families bankrupted because of hospitalization increased 20%.[26] Health insurance plans should be scrutinized using the effective coverage rate, that is, the actual coverage of health insurance plans after, including all patient-related out-of-pocket costs. Thus health systems have a responsibility to reduce the financial impact of health care costs and make payments more progressive, such that they are related to ability to pay rather than likelihood of becoming ill. As part of health performance, health systems research is gaining emphasis. It is important for informing policy,[27] including universal health coverage.[28,29]

Functions of the Health System

The formal health care system may not be the only or even the main provider of care to a population, but it nevertheless has several functions that promote the objectives of the system (see Figure 20-1). These functions are stewardship, the creation of resources, delivery

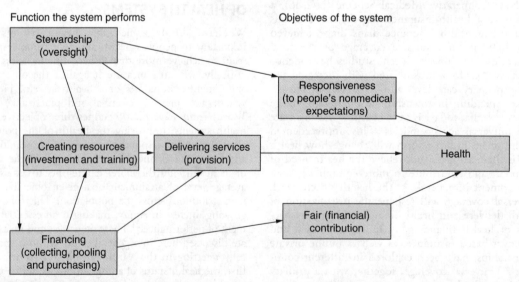

Figure 20-1. Functions of a health system. (*Reproduced, with permission, from World Health Organization. The World Health Report 2000. Health Systems: Improving Performance. Geneva: WHO, 2000.* http://www.who.int/whr2001/2001/archives/2000/en.)

of services, and financing.[4] *Stewardship* is oversight of the components and functions of the health system, and it is the one function that is undeniably best done by national governments. However, national governments have tended to neglect this function because of a lack of budget, managerial capacity, data, and the unorganized nature of many LMIC health systems, which make this a considerable challenge. The focus of many national health systems has been on service delivery, with most of a health system's budget being taken up by recurrent costs of curative care, particularly staff salaries and large (capital) city services. Effective oversight would allow governments to assess the performance of the system with respect to the other functions and allow it to target certain areas for reform and monitor the impact of health care reforms.

Creating resources refers to investment in health care infrastructure and training of health professionals. This function is commonly undertaken by the public sector, although some middle-income countries have large private sectors that include medical schools and high-technology facilities with private financing (e.g., in Nepal there are 18 medical schools only 2 of which are public).[30] *Service provision* has traditionally been the main role of health systems, but this is increasingly being questioned because of difficulties with public management in many LMICs. These difficulties have included poor incentives for public providers leading to poor quality and quantity of care (particularly with regard to responsiveness) and widespread use of private sector providers.[24] As a result, some authors have suggested that the government's role should be to purchase services and monitor the quality, as part of the financing function.

Revenue to fund health systems may come from income taxes, like in the United Kingdom and Canada, employment insurance schemes, as in most of Latin America, the purchase of private insurance, or out-of-pocket payments by patients at the point of care, as in India. Because the health expenditure of individuals is unpredictable, prepayment systems with significant coverage protect patients from impoverishment due to health care expenditures. The financial impact of illness also varies according to how risk of illness (and therefore expense) is pooled. Prepayment systems where insurance premiums are based on ability to pay (rather than propensity for illness) allow for cross-subsidy from the rich to the poor and from the healthy to sick. In a sufficiently large risk pool, the costs from year to year will be more predictable and with an appropriate mix of young, old, rich, poor, healthy, and sick, the costs will be affordable for all. Health systems that are financed by income tax provide the greatest potential for pooling risk, whereas those financed primarily by out-of-pocket payments have the worst impact on fair financing. This is because the poor pay a higher proportion of their income than the rich when costs are fixed, and the unpredictable nature of out-of-pocket costs is greater for those with no financial cushion or with limited access to credit.

THE STRUCTURE OF HEALTH SYSTEMS

Health systems in industrialized countries are highly structured and were developed in a context of economic stability, with a moderate pace of social change, rule of law, efficient systems for taxation, strong regulatory frameworks, and sufficient numbers of skilled personnel to run these institutions. These conditions are still not found in most LMICs.[31] In the second half of the 20th century, many developing countries established national health systems ostensibly designed to provide comprehensive services for the whole population, much like the United Kingdom's National Health Service, which served as an international model. However, many countries did not fund or staff these services sufficiently to achieve their stated goals, either due to financial crises or a lack of commitment to population health and universality. Most LMIC governments' incapacity to provide comprehensive health services for the whole population has led to the emergence of other service providers to meet growing patient demand. In these mixed health systems, the distinctions between public and private are sometimes blurred. The more important distinction is between the organized sector, which is subject to some measure of government oversight, and the unorganized or informal sector, which operates according to locally negotiated rules and is largely independent of the state and its regulatory oversight.[31]

Table 20-1 shows the types of providers and institutions that support the basic functions of a health system, namely public health, consultation and treatment, provision of drugs, physical support for the infirm, and management of intertemporal expenditure (i.e., unpredictable and potentially costly health expenses).[32] The providers and institutions are divided into the organized and the unorganized health sectors. The former includes public services run by the government and licensed private providers; the latter includes market-based services, such as those given by unlicensed private providers, and the nonmarket-based services provided by household members, neighbors, and community members. The importance of the various sectors varies tremendously according to the history and relative capacity of each health system. Health policy recommendations should not be transferred from one context to the next without understanding

Table 20-1. Pluralistic health systems

Health-related function	Unorganized health sector		Organized health sector
	Nonmarketized	**Marketized**	
Public health	Household/community environmental hygiene		Government public health service and regulations Public or private supply of water and other health-related goods
Skilled consultation and treatment	Use of health-related knowledge by household members	Some specialized services such as traditional midwifery provided outside market Traditional healers Unlicensed and/or unregulated health workers and facilities Covert private practice by public health staff	Public health services Licensed for-profit health workers and facilities Licensed/regulated Nongovernmental organizations (NGOs), faith-based organizations, etc.
Medical-related goods	Household/community production of traditional medicines	Sellers of traditional and western drugs	Government pharmacies Licensed private pharmacies
Physical support of acutely ill, chronically ill, and disabled	Household care of sick and disabled Community support for AIDS patients and people with chronic illnesses and disabilities	Domestic servants Unlicensed nursing homes	Government hospitals Licensed or regulated hospitals and nursing homes
Management of intertemporal expenditure	Interhousehold/intercommunity reciprocal arrangements to cope with health shocks	Money lending Funeral societies/informal credit systems Local health insurance schemes	Organized systems of health finance: Government budgets Compulsory insurance Private insurance Bank loans Microcredit

(*Reproduced, with permission, from Standing H, Bloom G. Beyond Public and Private? Unorganised Markets in Health Care Delivery. Background paper for the World Development Report [WDR] 2003/4. Oxford: Presented at Making Services Work for Poor People workshop, November 2002.*)

their comparability. For example, in Niger 16% of deliveries are attended by trained birth attendants, so the vast majority of obstetric services are provided by family members in the home (in the nonmarketized sector) or by a traditional midwife charging fees (in the local marketized sector).[30] In Sri Lanka, 97% of births are attended by trained personnel, so initiatives to reduce perinatal mortality in these two countries would target very different segments of the health system to achieve similar goals.[30]

For each of the key functions of the health system, it is important to understand in which sector the service is being provided for rational planning of the health system. For example, India expanded

the number of primary health centers between 1961 and 1988, in an effort to increase access to care.[33] Government health planners did not take into account the existing capacity of private health providers (which were widely used); nor did they attempt to provide a service that was considered complementary or competitive by patients, who continued to frequent the private sector. As a result, they invested in public service facilities that remained underfunded, understaffed, underutilized, and uncompetitive with preexisting private and informal providers. For the government to provide adequate stewardship of health reforms, policies should take the existing structure and utilization of the health system into account.

APPROACHES TO IMPROVING THE PERFORMANCE OF HEALTH SYSTEMS

Now that we have broadly defined the goals, functions, and the general criteria for assessing the performance of health systems, we review a series of approaches to improving performance. Does more health care mean better health?[34] We have subdivided these approaches according to the perspective they take or the level of the health system on which they act. There is the *national or regional perspective*, which refers to policy measures relating to the locus of decision making within the system, the structure of the health system, and the degree of integration of its component parts. The *local or organizational level* refers to the management of institutions that provide care. Below this is the *provider level*, the management of health service providers, and the *individual perspective*, which relates to the engagement or modification of the behavior of health system users.

National Perspectives

The organizational structure and management of national health systems are areas that have profound impact on outcomes. Health system organization can be defined as "the systematic arrangement of various resources, with designated responsibilities and special channels of communication and authority, intended to attain certain objectives. The ultimate objective of organizations in a health care system is to promote and/or protect people's health, but this ultimate goal is approached through the intermediary role of many agencies with more focused objectives. These agencies may be involved with financing, planning, administration, regulation, provision, or any other health-related function."[35]

Loosely, we can include in these agencies:

- Ministries of health and other ministries (e.g., agriculture, finance, labor, housing, transportation, sanitation, education) either nationally or regionally
- Insurance organizations
- Public enterprises
- Private sector players
- Professional groups and unions
- Voluntary organizations
- Health education institutions
- Public participation
- International actors (e.g., WHO, other UN, World Bank, bilateral donor agencies, nongovernmental organizations [NGOs], foundations, some public-private partnerships, etc.)

REGULATION OF HEALTH MATTERS

Regulation is a core function of government that cannot be delegated to other system actors. Regulatory laws are generally designed to protect the public interest, but new laws can also be highly contentious.[36]

BOX 20-1. HEALTH SYSTEM CHALLENGES FOR THE POOR: MEDICAL POVERTY TRAP

One of the goals of a health system is to minimize the financial impact of ill health on the population. In countries with limited insurance coverage, the cost of health services is a common cause of impoverishment.[6] The descent into poverty is the result of a sequence of events that are largely preventable.[24] A breadwinner becomes ill; he or she is no longer able to work, with resultant loss of income. Either the person goes without treatment, or the costs of treatment lead to the sale of assets and debt for the family. Food becomes scarce; children become malnourished and may be taken out of school and put to work to support the family. The poor family has been further impoverished, often irrevocably. The adult who has fallen ill may die, increasing the proportion of dependents to providers, and if the adult remains disabled, he or she is a further burden on the family's resources.

Many factors predispose to the sequence of events. The first is untreated morbidity because poor patients may not consult health providers for financial reasons and may not be hospitalized when it is recommended because they cannot afford it. For example, in China, a quarter of patients were not hospitalized despite medical recommendations, and of these the majority were for financial reasons.[25] Access to all forms of care may be reduced because user fees are common in many LMIC health systems. Formal and informal user fees are high compared with salaries of the poor, and lack of insurance means that they do not have any financial protection for catastrophic health costs, which often lead to long-term impoverishment. Lastly, the care the poor access is often of low quality, with irrational use of drugs that may be wasteful and potentially harmful. The widespread and unnecessary use of intramuscular and intravenous treatments for conditions such as viral infections is an example of this.[4]

Moving beyond policy toward a justly governed regulatory system is the stipulation and enforcement of various standards and is often regarded as government surveillance.[37] This surveillance can focus on a wide variety of health system components, such as:

- Health professions, including licensing, registration, salary, training and supply
- Technical specifications and standards, including the quantity and assessment of high-technology equipment and waiting times for patients to access them
- Pharmaceuticals, including safety and approval for sale, supply lists, pricing, and grossly fraudulent production and sales
- Movement from primary to tertiary, health center to hospital and rural to urban, including governance, accreditation, budgets, physical structures, and local guidelines. Procedures may involve wait lists, records management, use of eHealth and eLearning, enhancing access to services and overall quality control
- Insurance plans and sickness funds

Although governments are the best positioned to regulate health systems, in practice their ability to generate and implement appropriate policies is highly variable. This is generally due to political market imperfections, policy contradictions, lack of oversight, problems with collective action (e.g., no effective representation of patients), and moral hazard (e.g., public officials suffer no consequences for inappropriate action or inaction).[38]

Decentralization

The role of the public sector is in the development, financing, and implementation of policies to guide service delivery, including public health and health promotion. One of the more common policies has long been decentralization or the delegating of decision-making power from central to local levels of government, including forms of community participation.[39] The three key elements of decentralization include the amount of choice or options that are transferred from central institutions to institutions at the periphery, including the most important component of financial resources; what choices local officials make with their increased discretion; and what effect these choices have on the performance of the health system.[40] Decentralization can therefore take various forms.[35]

- *Deconcentration* involves passing some administrative authority from central government offices to the local offices of central government ministries.
- *Devolution* involves passing responsibility and a degree of independence to regional or local government, with or without financial responsibility (i.e., the ability to raise and spend revenues).

- *Delegation* involves passing responsibilities to local offices or organizations outside the structure of the central government such as quasi-public (nongovernmental, voluntary) organizations, but with central government retaining indirect control (as in many national Global Fund funded activities).
- *Privatization* involves the transfer of ownership and government functions from public to private bodies, which may consist of voluntary organizations and for-profit and not-for-profit organizations, with varying degrees of government regulation.

Over the past decades, bilateral and multilateral financial and development agencies have been encouraging decentralization as an important strategy in achieving better health outcomes by facilitating greater efficiency, effectiveness, equity, participation, and multisectoral collaboration. In theory, it sounds good to decentralize and get decision making closer to where the decisions need to be made and where they can have the greatest impact. But, as some analysts have concluded, it is also important to understand the political and economic contexts of any decentralization activity. Birn, Zimmerman, and Garfield[41] looked at Nicaragua in the 1990s when decentralization was implemented alongside International Monetary Fund (IMF) structural adjustment policies that favored budget cuts to social services, including primary health care, promotion of user fees, and privatization. They concluded that decentralization brought few benefits to Nicaragua, particularly in the areas of health policy development, priority setting, and programming; and that it is not sufficient to analyze decentralization as a sector-specific reform that can be understood through solely technocratic modifications. The political context must also be taken into account, which is consistent with a systems perspective.

Decentralization can be at the health delivery level, for example extending specific health services from the city center to rural areas so the service can be closer to patients. This process needs systematic planning, training of health staff, and establishing quality assurance to ensure that the service at the lower level has good quality and can be sustainable. For example, a tuberculosis decentralization program into the rural townships in Guangxi China has resulted in better treatment outcomes and lower medical out-of-pocket costs.[42]

In some occasions, decentralization may be used as an excuse to shift government involvement. The case in Indonesia showed that decentralization reform was associated with less transparency of health service at local levels, and public health centers were turned into profit-seeking organizations due to the lack of government investment.[43]

Privatization

Most countries have health systems in which both the public and private sectors play a role. The degree to which each is allowed to flourish is usually controlled by the government, although the private sector and multilateral finance and development agencies may also play major roles. The debate regarding whether the public or private sector should be promoted has raged since the 1990s and continues today. There is agreement on a strong government role in building effective health systems through regulation, compensating for market failures (particularly in the area of health insurance), addressing inequalities in access to care, and building a strong primary health care system. However, whether government should be primarily involved in care provision or should contract it out to the private sector and regulate quality also remains an area of varying opinions. Most economically successful countries have high involvement of government in health care expenditures. Many LMICs simply do not invest enough of their wealth in health and education. China is an exception with extensive postsecondary training programs and national health care reform.

Health markets are fragmented, not only in terms of their structure as noted in Table 20-1, but also in terms of their clientele. The rich tend to use the highest quality private services and the best government referral hospitals, whereas the poor use low-end government services and informal sector private providers.[44] The rich and powerful push for the development of high-end private facilities and public tertiary care in urban areas, which reduces funds available for the provision of public health measures and basic care for the poor in rural areas. In this way, the health system reproduces the inequalities found in society at large.

Private/Public Partnerships

Because many LMIC governments do not prioritize health care and are not in a position to implement a health system that meets the needs of their more wealthy citizens, they may enter into partnerships with the private sector for the delivery of a variety of medical interventions. Although historically most health service delivery was done privately (often by churches), the number of private health system actors, both in the not-for-profit and for-profit sectors, has grown substantially. Many private businesses, especially in the pharmaceutical and health technology sectors, have substantial roles to play, and they are now being courted by governments to join with them in the delivery of services. However, it is in the voluntary sector or NGOs and private voluntary organizations where the greatest growth has been seen in recent years.

Large international NGOs like Oxfam, World Vision, Caritas, CARE, PLAN, SAVE, MSF, and so on, have been increasingly vocal about their role within the health care system because they are able to deploy large sums of money and large numbers of personnel quite effectively. Add to these the growing number of private philanthropic organizations, like the Rockefeller Foundation, Ford Foundation, and now the colossal Bill and Melinda Gates Foundation. This part of the private sector is now highly competitive with the usual forms of bilateral (national aid agencies) and multilateral (UN agencies and World Bank) aid in the health sector.

With the WHO's emphasis on improving health systems, it became a staunch advocate of partnering with the private sector in dealing with worldwide health problems, including the infectious diseases of public health importance. This partnership led to the creation in 2001 of the Global Fund for HIV/AIDS, Tuberculosis, and Malaria as the lead financial agency. The Global Fund is a partnership between governments, civil society, the private sector, and affected communities, and it acts primarily as an agent to review and finance projects. Drug and vaccine development, too, has increasingly adopted this type of organizational structure. "A large variety of public-private partnerships, combining the skills of a wide range of collaborators, have arisen for product development [and] disease control through product donation and distribution, or the general strengthening or coordination of health services. Administratively, such partnerships may either involve affiliation with international organizations (i.e., they are essentially public-sector programs with private-sector participation), or they may be legally independent not-for-profit bodies."[45] Such partnerships show promise but are not a panacea, and they should be regarded as social experiments, perhaps especially so with the current alignment of Coca-Cola with the GAVI Alliance for vaccine delivery.

Research has to be conducted in a way that contributes to health service delivery. Operational and now implementation research play a key role in bridging knowledge and disease control programs,[46] that largely strengthen the health delivery system and benefit communities in developing countries. This is called research into practice. There are many specific examples of tuberculosis and cardiovascular programs where research priorities are informed by the field and can then be developed to improve health delivery and subsequently generate new evidence.[47,48] Operational research has been a theme in health system studies, and international programs such as the Global Fund against HIV, Tuberculosis, and Malaria, which has a specific budget and goals dedicated to operational research. A set of questions, such as how to initiate the research topic, conduct the research, and disseminate the results have to be carefully considered to meet needs at the operational and health policy levels.[49]

Professional bodies, such as medical councils and disease associations, are important types of partners, and they influence health service delivery in different ways. For example, medical councils regulate how health professionals are credited and quality ensured. In many developing countries, the professional body may provide service directly in its own hospitals. Professional bodies may disseminate and review medical algorithms and guidelines that directly affect health delivery.

The partnership among public organizations is also crucial in achieving health system goals. Hospitals are the major health care provider in most countries, whereas specific disease control programs are often managed outside of hospitals, such as so-called vertical programs that operate directly under the management of the Ministry of Health. Hospitals may not comply with national guidelines in treating patients with tuberculosis. This may cause treatment delays, failures, and an increase in drug-resistant tuberculosis. For example, China's tuberculosis case detection rates were as low as 30% before 2005, substantially lower than the 70% WHO target. This was largely due to the lack of case referral from public hospitals to tuberculosis dispensaries. After the outbreak of severe acute respiratory syndrome (SARS), all hospitals were required to report tuberculosis suspects and cases online within 24 hours.[50] In addition, guidelines improving the collaboration between hospitals and tuberculosis dispensaries were published by the Ministry of Health.[51] These efforts, plus government commitment and the strengthened public health system after SARS, resulted in substantial improvement of case detection in China to 70% by 2005.[52] Recent development of the new model of integrating hospital and tuberculosis services has also improved patient outcomes and reduced their financial costs.[53]

Contracting

Health managers easily recognize that they often cannot control all the necessary inputs for ensuring good health and good services to their patients and other clientele. From the open systems perspective they realize there are many patient-based services that might be more efficiently delivered by organizations outside of their own or in cooperation with them. This has led to the contracting out of certain services. Services can be described by the degree to which their quality can be measured and the contestability or level of competition for provision of that service. It is best to contract out services whose quality can be easily assessed and for which there are a number of providers competing to provide that service. Examples of these services are laundry, laboratory, food production, and maintenance. Services whose quality is harder to assess include ambulatory care (for which there is ample competition) and health policy (for which there is much less). The difficulty in contracting out these types of services is that providers may reduce quality while keeping costs constant to increase profit, and the contracting agent may not realize it.

Accreditation

Human resources to carry out daily activities are a key component of any health system. Although the medical profession continues to dominate health services, it has lost some ground to other players (such as nurses and allied health professionals) in recent years. Hospitals continue to be at the center of most health systems, although there has been an appropriately increasing emphasis on ambulatory and primary care in many countries. But whether it is a doctor, a nurse, or a community health agent, it is only through the development and implementation of competency based criteria that patients and communities can be assured that they are getting good health service providers. These criteria are put together into a system of accreditation, which also includes forms of membership, compliance, and enforcement. Appropriate accreditation procedures are often lacking in most LMICs, and companies like JCI (United States) and Accreditation Canada International market such services overseas.

Accreditation is common for health professionals and also for major health facilities in the more wealthy countries, but it is sorely lacking in countries with fewer resources. Although professional peer-regulated associations provide some control over the training, work, and standards of a particular group of providers (e.g., doctors and nurses), they have varying degrees of credibility in the sense of what they can enforce. A problem, particularly in LMICs, is how to integrate and accommodate traditional healers within the broader health system.[54,55] Large proportions of such populations seek help from traditional practitioners for a wide range of problems. Whether it is an herbalist, bone setter, or spiritualist, these practitioners often constitute the first line of health-seeking behavior. They present a particular challenge to the coordination of health services, but also to any attempts at accreditation and standardization.

Worldwide, there are an increasing number of complementary health services and products being purchased and used. The most legitimate ones are being slowly integrated into the more conventional (or Western) services. This is especially so in China where its traditional Chinese medicine has been systematized for centuries and is widely practiced and integrated with more modern services, both at large urban hospitals and local community health centers.

APPLICATION OF THEORIES OF MANAGEMENT AND ORGANIZATIONAL BEHAVIOR

In the management of any organization, much is left to the discretion of the managers. This discretion is informed by knowledge, experience, and intuition. Although experience and intuition are personal and acquired over time in a somewhat haphazard way, the knowledge component is one that can be actively addressed in a systematic manner, either through formal education, including continuing education, or informal reading. The validity of such knowledge, then, comes into question, especially when its source is the popular press, a common source of information for managers. However, much can be done to ensure validity of this knowledge through good research.

Health systems, policy, and management research, as a discipline, is now about 40 years old, and it continues to grow. Research specific to international health and development is scarce, and most research addresses private sector companies, usually those with many employees. However, there is much happening today to promote health system and policy research, especially in the multilateral sector, which has recently seen the birth of the Alliance for Health Systems and Policy Research, and within universities, where more and more young researchers are interested in applying their skills to international health. Many universities are starting global health programs. Popular Global Health Systems Research Symposia were held in Switzerland in 2010 and China in 2012. A Centre for Health Systems Studies has opened at the Bangladesh Rural Advanced Committee (BRAC) University, and a Canadian group has made an inventory of all the international health systems researchers in their country.[56]

The theoretical perspectives of resource dependency,[57] population ecology, institutionalization, and theories of evaluation can all provide more information on how to make health systems and interventions more effective, efficient, and equitable. Concerning equity, the People's Health Movement is at the forefront (www. phmovement.org).

Organizational culture is a theory particularly relevant to management. By learning from aspects of national cultures, and focusing on issues like values and beliefs, rites and rituals, symbols and heroes, myths and cultural networks, managers who apply them in their workplace can make significant changes to achieve better outcomes in many aspects of organizational life.[58]

Whether a manager is working in a private or public environment, he or she can gain valuable insight by reading the literature on health management,[59] which contains many years of research insight regarding the behavior of organizations and the people that work in them. There is also now much literature on leadership and teamwork, both very important, although often lacking components of any well-functioning health system.

PERFORMANCE OF NGOs, GOVERNMENT INSTITUTIONS, AND PRIVATE COMPANIES

The dominant actors in governance, diplomacy, and implementation of health services worldwide continue to change.[60] For much of the period around Alma Ata and into the 1980s, the WHO held a leading role. Then several of the multilaterals, especially the World Bank, began to occupy a more central role as they created new divisions with a health mandate and increased spending in this area. All the while, NGOs were becoming increasingly prevalent and gaining in number and importance, especially those with large international profiles or strong roots in communities. However, there is some action now on the part of large bilateral donors to take greater control of the development agenda and underfund NGOs who are seen as more independent but innovative. Private donor agencies are also growing in importance in global health. These trends result in the medium to small NGOs and community-based organizations having more of a struggle to stay alive and do their work, even though this work is often recognized as being more effective due to the close proximity to communities and families.

Evaluation of the impact of all levels of organizational involvement in overseas development requires further attention. It was only after much damage was done that the World Bank and IMF began to understand the devastating impact to health and other social services resulting directly from their structural adjustment programs.[61] In 2012, the leadership of the World Bank was passed to a global health expert. Governments in high-income countries, with their large bilateral aid agencies, also struggle to understand their effectiveness. NGOs and community-based organizations, although much closer to the people who have the opportunity to directly see the impact of their work, are still in need of good monitoring and evaluation. This evaluation can be done through participatory methodologies that can provide information on outcomes while building capacity. Overall, there is a great need for enhanced accountability in all forms of international cooperation.[62]

Provider Perspective

Addressing health system issues from the perspective of providers is important because they do the work of the health care system. Whether they belong to formal professional associations or are unlicensed individuals working in isolation, they collectively make decisions that have a large impact on health resource utilization and, to a lesser extent, population health outcomes. Who are the providers? The broadest definition includes health service providers and health management and support workers.[30] Health service providers are those who directly provide services to patients, whereas health management and support workers set up and run the infrastructure needed to provide health services. This section only discusses the former because there is more on this group, although future work may study a broader range of health human resources.

Numerous challenges face the health workforce, including its size, distribution, skill mix, and working conditions. The WHO estimates that there is a global shortage of approximately 4 million health service providers, although not every region has a shortage.[30] The global distribution of health workers is imbalanced; the largest numbers of health service providers are in the regions with the healthiest populations. For example, the WHO region of the Americas has 10% of the global burden of disease, but 37% of the world's health workers and 50% of the resources for health. In contrast, Africa bears 24% of the global burden of disease with only 3% of the world's health workers and less than 1% of the global expenditure on health.[30]

The distribution within countries is similarly skewed, with most providers located in cities, where health outcomes tend to be better than in rural areas. Such a dire situation has changed little in decades for much of the world's population.

The skill mix of nurses, doctors, midwives, and public health workers should vary according to the needs of the population, but this rarely occurs because these needs are not taken into account in basic training programs. The working conditions of providers are not always conducive to high performance, and low pay in the health sector often leads providers to seek informal payments or work in different fields altogether.

The key health human resource issues for creating a high performance place to work are:

1. Managing the entry into the workforce
2. Enhancing the performance of existing workers
3. Limiting rates of attrition
4. Continuing education
5. Competency regulation

Getting the right mix of skills and diversity (racial, gender, and regional) in the health workforce is a key issue for educational institutions. This is being addressed through reforms in medical and nursing curricula, the opening of schools of public health (particularly in Asia), and the use of quotas for disadvantaged minorities. The latter is common in India, where a significant number of university spots are reserved for lower caste and ethnic minority students.[30] In North America, some medical schools have spaces reserved for indigenous native students (e.g., Washington and Alberta).

Improving the performance of existing workers is a strategy that may have the greatest short- and medium-term effect, given the time required to train a new generation of health care providers. The key elements for improvement are:

- Availability (to meet demand)
- Competence (to inspire demand by improving capabilities)
- Responsiveness (to improve efficiency)
- Productivity (to improve efficiency)

The strategies to achieve these include:

- Matching skills to tasks
- Appropriate supervision
- Financial incentives and sufficient remuneration
- Ensuring organization commitment
- Promoting lifelong learning
- Promoting responsibility with accountability[30]

There is extensive literature on improving the appropriateness of care in developed countries but very little from developing countries. There is no consensus on which methods are most effective for bringing the current practice of health providers in line with "best practice" theory (based on the best available evidence).[63] Furthermore, approaches that have worked in developed countries may not be as effective in developing countries given the differences in practice environments. Retaining the health workforce is another challenge because wealthier countries often draw health professionals away from poorer countries (with greater need) or people leave the profession because of low pay or other poor working conditions.[64]

Individual/Patient Perspective

One of the goals of a health system is *responsiveness*, a term that means the system provides services that reflect the needs and preferences of its users.[4] This is one of the keys to ensuring that the system is appropriate, promotes the dignity of patients, and optimizes patient satisfaction. In general, a patient-focused or -centered approach is an important and key strategy in all direct service and related health care organizations. One of the most systematic attempts to understand the perspective and experience of the lower socioeconomic stratum of health system users was conducted by the World Bank and compiled in a report called "Voices of the Poor."[65] It concludes that the poor generally felt state health and education services to be ineffective, inaccessible, and disempowering. Preferential treatment is given to those who were well dressed, or have money or influence, whereas the poor complain of callous, rushed, or ineffective consultations. Many state institutions reproduce the social inequalities that are present elsewhere in society.

Patients generally consult private or informal services for minor acute problems and government facilities for more severe problems. The experience varies in different countries, but generally government health agencies are not used because they may be difficult to access, may lack medicines, and their staff may be unsympathetic. The barriers to consultation for the poor include:

- Distance
- Transportation
- Time for travel
- Shortage of medicine
- Costs
- Discrimination or disdain by staff
- Staff absenteeism
- Ineffective treatment

Health services are very expensive for the poor when one includes cost of consultation, travel, informal payments, medicine, and lost income. Furthermore, the cost of informal payments in so-called free government services is unpredictable and is regressive, meaning that costs are a much higher proportion of income for the poor than the rich.

Using the Patient Perspective to Improve Health System Performance: The Demand Side in Health Service Delivery

Although the national, organizational, and provider perspectives mentioned previously are key factors in health system performance, ultimately it is the patients who choose which type of health service to seek under which circumstances and which provider instructions to follow and which to ignore. In countries where out-of-pocket expenditure is one of the main sources of health care finance (as in India or China), patients' purchasing power can be harnessed to improve access or quality. Approaches that go through health system users to enhance performance usually refer to the demand side in health services (as opposed to the supply side as discussed in the previous sections).

The demand side in health care has several meanings.[66] It includes leveraging inputs, from communities to health facilities, such as contribution of land, labor, and time (local representation), as well as the private purchase of health goods like oral rehydration salts or insecticide-treated nets to prevent malaria. It also refers to understanding and changing demand side behaviors, such as those to seek and promote health.

The demand side can also be stimulated to provoke changes in provider behavior through consultative processes or involvement in planning, designing, managing, and monitoring health services. The most direct form of intervention in this area is demand-side financing, which channels resources directly to users who then purchase health services. An example of this is giving vouchers for treatment of sexually transmitted disease to commercial sex workers.[24] These patients then use the voucher to obtain treatment from approved health care providers, who then present the vouchers to a financing agent who reimburses them for their services. Enhancing patient's purchasing power in this way can create a market for services to a group that is either too poor or marginalized to be considered viable customers by existing providers.

Ideally, empowered citizens/consumers use their collective voice and any local press to hold providers and policymakers accountable for fulfilling their contract to deliver competent, responsive services. The more direct form of accountability is between service providers and users, involving the poor in monitoring and providing services and making provider income dependent on accountability to users, as in Guatemala.[46] The indirect form of accountability is between government and citizens, where broader political change allows citizens to use democratic means to have input into the reform of health systems.[67]

Internationally, too, there exist vast and huge disparities of wealth and health outcomes among and within countries around the world.[68] But global studies suggest the need to combat disease and unhealthy lifestyles among both poor and rich.[69]

DETERMINANTS OF HEALTH SERVICE PROVIDER BEHAVIOR

In the previous section, we discussed the various levels at which one can intervene to improve the performance of health systems. Ultimately, health systems should provide the right service to the right patient at the right time in the most cost-effective setting (a focus on effectiveness and efficiency). As one might imagine, this is not often the case in either high-income countries or LMICs. However, the degree to which appropriate management of patients' conditions is practiced in the health system depends on a series of factors relating to the national and organizational context, and the providers and patients themselves. Figure 20-2 is inspired by a model of the determinants of the behavior of private providers by Brugha and Zwi,[70] although it could be applied to all health service providers.

The national context includes the structure of the health system and the degree of interaction between the public and private sector. It also refers to the bureaucratic and regulatory environment, the influence of pharmaceutical companies, and the availability of health-related technologies and treatments (which may or may not be effectively regulated by the government). The practice and social environments include incentive structures for providers to compensate for ownership (e.g., market exposure for private practitioners with recurrent expenses), provider pay

mechanisms, supervision, and the expectations of the community or patients. The next level is the providers, their level of training, opportunities for continuing education, the degree to which their knowledge and practice is influenced by the drug industry, their ability to access timely information on evidence-based practice in the form of guidelines[71] and systematic reviews,[72] and their general overall sense of responsibility as potentially highly esteemed community members. Lastly, the interaction between providers and patients is affected by a provider's caseload; the number of patients seen in a day; the provider's ability to choose the correct management and consult good information sources; and the availability, acceptability, and affordability of this approach. All these factors contribute to the either good or poor provider relationship with patients and management of their health conditions.

Case Study: Private Providers in India

The following case study examines the determinants of the behavior of health care providers in one country (India) in more depth.

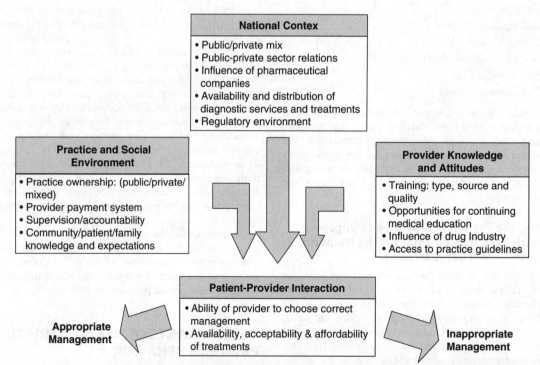

Figure 20-2. Determinants of health service provider behavior. (*Reproduced, with permission, from Brugha R, Zwi A. Improving the quality of private sector delivery of public health services: challenges and strategies. Health Policy Plan 1998;13:107–120.*)

National Context

India has a population of 1.15 billion and a gross domestic product (GDP) per capita of $2,460 at purchasing power parity (PPP). Life expectancy is 63, infant mortality is 57/1,000, and maternal mortality is 450/100,000.[73] The total expenditure on health care is 4.9% of GDP, which comes to approximately $109 per capita (PPP). Public spending accounts for 20% of all health expenditure. Private expenditure accounts for the rest, 97% of which is out-of-pocket at point of service. This indicates a very low level of insurance coverage,[73] although there are some plans for state-level universal coverage.

After independence, the Indian government set up a health care system modeled on the United Kingdom's National Health Service, with comprehensive, free services for all. However, government mostly invested in infrastructure, creating a vast network of facilities that were chronically underfunded.[74] Increasing, unmet demand for services, along with decreasing government investment in health, left a gap in which the private sector could flourish. The National Health Policy was to promote the private sector starting in 1982,[75] although the government did little to assess its capacity or monitor its behavior, and did not include it in planning strategies.[76] Private expenditure on health has been growing rapidly since 1960 and was expected to double between 2004 and 2012.[77] There are 645,000 registered providers, of whom 75% are in private practice.[73] A detailed survey of private and public providers found that 72% of qualified paramedical staff members work in the private sector, primarily in rural areas. In this study, there were six times more 'less than fully qualified' staff personnel than doctors, again mostly working in rural areas.[78] It is estimated that 93% of all hospitals and 64% of hospital beds are in the private sector. A total of 91% of private facilities are owned and managed by one person, and 86% are small outpatient clinics with one or two beds. The private sector provides 81% of all outpatient care and 46% of inpatient care.[77]

Policy Context

The government has made several attempts at regulating the behavior of private providers. The first approach was through the use of professional bodies, by establishing the Medical Council of India, which regulates medical education and registers physicians through its branches at the state level. Early studies showed that there is no systematic database of its members[79] and few private providers are aware of or follow its recommendations.[80] Furthermore, there are allegations that the council exists more to protect the interests of its members than to protect the public.

This claim is supported by the fact that few state councils have ever suspended any members, despite numerous complaints.[81]

There has been very little legislation specific to private medical facilities. Only Delhi and the state of Maharashtra have passed a Nursing Home Act, which requires small private hospitals (fewer than 25 beds) and dispensaries to register with local authorities. An early study in Delhi found that only 130 of approximately 1200 eligible nursing homes were registered under this act.[79] Official inspection of nursing homes and cancellation is rare, although an independent study from Mumbai showed that 63% of hospitals were on residential premises, 12.5% were in sheds with inadequate roofing, and 50% were in poorly maintained buildings. The lack of oversight may be due to staff shortages and the ability of these organizations to influence local authorities.[82]

SUMMARY

The health system perspective is very useful in working toward the improvement of individual and population health by helping to identify and respond to important management and organizational issues. Issues of coordination, integration, effectiveness, efficiency, reliability, accessibility, equity, public-private involvement, primary versus tertiary care, and community participation are all important to consider in the delivery of health services.[39,57] Added to these various national concerns are now those of globalization.[83] Diseases are crossing borders with high speed and volume, health professionals are migrating to greener fields, populations are growing rapidly, technology is becoming more widely available, finances are available, advocacy is on the increase, and we are all communicating more with each other. How these things can be brought to improve our global health and not denigrate it is, especially at this time of dire ecological consequence, is the ongoing emerging question of the day. Understanding these phenomena and making use of them toward sustainable development[84] in a highly connected and evolving world,[10] and in the management and organization of health services to meet the growing and changing needs of all is the challenge we leave with you.

STUDY QUESTIONS

1. List the functions of a health system, how they interact, and explain the level of priority given to each function in your country.

2. What are some advantages and disadvantages to nations in decentralization, public finance and ownership, privatization, public-private partnerships,

contracting in the health sector, and community engagement for social justice?

3. Using the case study of private providers in India as an example, look at the determinants of health service provider behavior in another country. Include the national context, provider knowledge and attitudes, patient-provider interactions, and the practice and social environments.

REFERENCES

1. Diez Roux A. *Conceptual Approaches to the Study of Health Disparities.* Ann Arbor, MI: Center for Social Epidemiology Health, Department of Epidemiology, University of Michigan, 2012: 41–58.

2. Bleich S, Jarlenski M, Bell C, LaVeist T. *Health Inequalities: Trends, Progress, and Policy.* Baltimore, MD: Department of Health Policy and Management and Hopkins Center for Health Disparities Solutions, Johns Hopkins Bloomberg School of Public Health, 2012: 7–40.

3. World Health Organization. *Changing mindsets: WHO Strategy on Health Policy and Systems Research.* Geneva: WHO, 2012.

4. World Health Organization. *The World Health Report 2000. Health Systems: Improving Performance.* Geneva: WHO, 2000. http://www.who.int/whr2001/2001/archives/2000/en.

5. Spiegel J, Yassi A. Lessons from the margins of globalization: appreciating the Cuban health paradox. *J Public Health Policy* 2004;25(1):85–110.

6. Zakus D, Cortinois A. Primary health care and community participation: its origins, implementation and future. In: Fried B, Gaydos L, eds. *World Health Systems: Challenges and Perspectives.* Chicago: Health Administration Press, 2002.

7. World Health Organization. *Primary healthcare-now more than ever.* Geneva: WHO, 2008.

8. Starfield B, Shi L, et al. Contribution of primary care to health systems and health. *Milbank Q* 2005;83(3):457–502.

9. Walley J, Lawn J, et al. Primary health care: making Alma-Ata a reality. *Lancet* 2008;372(9642):1001–1007.

10. Best A, Greenhalgh T, Lewis S, Saul J, et al. Large-system transformation in health care: a realist review. *Milbank Q* 2012;90(3):421–456.

11. Sachs J. Achieving universal health coverage in low-income settings. *Lancet* 2012;380(9845):944–947.

12. Barber L, Yao L. Development and status of health insurance systems in China. *Int J Health Plan Manage* 2011;26(4): 339–356.

13. Babiarz K, Miller G, et al. New evidence on the impact of China's New Rural Cooperative Medical Scheme and its implications for rural primary healthcare: multivariate difference-in-difference analysis. *BMJ* 2010;341:c5617.

14. Lagomarsino G, Garabrant A, et al. Moving towards universal health coverage: health insurance reforms in nine developing countries in Africa and Asia. *Lancet* 2012;380(9845):933–943.

15. United Nations. *The Millennium Development Goals Report 2011.* New York: UN, 2011.

16. Glouberman S, Zimmerman B. *Complicated and complex systems: what would successful reform of Medicare look like?* Discussion Paper No. 8 from the Commission on the Future of Health Care in Canada, July 2002. http://c.ymcdn.com/sites/ www.plexusinstitute.org/resource/collection/6528ED29-9907-4BC7-8D00-8DC907679FED/ComplicatedAndComplexSystems-ZimmermanReport_Medicare_reform.pdf.

17. Health Systems 20/20. 2012. *The Health System Assessment Approach: A How-to Manual*, v.2.0. www.healthsystemassessment. org.

18. Zheng H. Do people die from income inequality of a decade ago? *Soc Sci Med* 2012;75(1):36–45.

19. World Health Organization. *Closing the Gap in a Generation: Health Equity Through Action on the Social Determinants of Health.* Geneva: WHO, 2008.

20. Norton A, Rogerson A. *Inclusive and sustainable development: challenges, opportunities, policies and partnerships.* Ministry of Foreign Affairs of Denmark, September 2012. http://www.odi.org.uk/ sites/odi.org.uk/files/odi-assets/publications-opinion-files/7809. pdf.

21. Gwatkin D. The need for equity-oriented health sector reforms. *Int J Epidemiol* 2001;30(4):720–723.

22. The enormous, invisible toll of stillbirths in low-income and middle-income countries. *NewsRx Health & Science*, May 1, 2011. http://www.verticalnews.com/premium_newsletters/NewsRx-Health-and-Science/2011-05-01/246NHS.html.

23. Braveman P, Starfield B, Geiger HJ. World Health Report 2000: how it removes equity from the agenda for public health monitoring and policy. *BMJ* 2001;323(7314):678–681.

24. Mills A, Brugha R, Hanson K, et al. What can be done about the private health sector in low-income countries? *Bull World Health Organ* 2002;80(4):325–330.

25. Liu Y, Rao K. Providing health insurance in rural China: from research to policy. *J Health Polit Policy Law* 2006;31(1):71–92.

26. Meng Q, Xu L, et al. Trends in access to health services and financial protection in China between 2003 and 2011: a cross-sectional study. *Lancet* 2012;379(9818):805–814.

27. Luft H. *From Small Area Variations to Accountable Care Organizations: How Health Services Research Can Inform Policy.* Palo Alto, CA: Department of Health Policy Research, Palo Alto Medical Foundation Research Institute, 2012: 377–392.

28. Rodin J, de Ferranti D. Universal health coverage: the third global health transition? *Lancet* 2012;380(9845):861–862.

29. The struggle for universal health coverage [editorial]. *Lancet* 2012; 380(9845):859.

30. World Health Organization. *World Health Report 2006: Working Together for Health.* Geneva: WHO, 2006.

31. Bloom G. *Private Provision in Its Institutional Context: Lessons from Health.* London: DFID Health Systems Resource Centre, 2004.

32. Standing H, Bloom G. *Beyond public and private? Unorganised markets in health care delivery.* Background paper for the World Development Report (WDR) 2003/4. Oxford: Presented at Making Services Work for Poor People workshop, November 2002.

33. Berman P. Rethinking health care systems: Private health care provision in India. *World Dev* 1998;26:1463–1479.

34. Brown R. *More Health Care Doesn't Mean Better Health.* EvidenceNetwork.ca with the Canadian Institute of Actuaries, September 5, 2012. http://umanitoba.ca/outreach/evidencenetwork/archives/7695.

35. World Health Organization. *Health Care Systems in Transition: Production Template and Questionnaire.* Copenhagen: WHO Regional Office for Europe, 1996.

36. White H, Waddington H. *Why Do We Care About Evidence Synthesis? An Introduction to the Special Issue on Systematic Reviews.* New York: Routledge, 2012.

37. Ellen M, Shamian J. How We Move Beyond a Policy Prescription to Action. *Healthcare Papers* 2011;11(1):76–83.

38. Wild L, Chambers V, King M, Harris D. Common constraints and incentive problems in service delivery. London: Overseas Development Institute, Working Paper 351, August 2012. http://www.odi.org.uk/publications/6767-service-delivery-accountability-international-development-aid-contraints-incentives.

39. Zakus D, Lysack C. Revisiting community participation. *Health Policy Plan* 1998;13(1):1–12.

40. Bossert T. Analyzing the decentralization of health systems in developing countries: decision space, innovation, and performance. *Soc Sci Med* 1998;47(10):1513–1527.

41. Birn A, Zimmerman S, Garfield R. To decentralize or not to decentralize, is that the question? Nicaraguan health policy under structural adjustment in the 1990s. *Intl J Health Serv* 2000;30(1):110–128.

42. Wei X, Liang X, et al. Decentralizing tuberculosis services from county tuberculosis dispensaries to township hospitals in China: an intervention study. *Int J Tuberculosis Lung Dis* 2008;12(5):538–547.

43. Kristiansen S, Santoso P. Surviving decentralization? Impacts of regional autonomy on health service provision in Indonesia. *Health Policy* 2006;77(3):247–259.

44. Bloom G. *Private Provision in Its Institutional Context: Lessons from Health.* London: DFID Health Systems Resource Centre, 2004: 12–17.

45. Widdus R. Public-private partnerships for health: their main targets, their diversity, and their future directions. *Bull WHO* 2001;79(8):159–173.

46. Flores W, Zakus D. Engaging country actors and communities in Implementation Research for adoption and scale up: a participatory approach. In: Kengeya-Kayondo J, Gonzalez-Block M, Bochorishvili I, eds. *Implementation Research for the Control of Infectious Diseases of Poverty.* Geneva: Tropical Disease Research, WHO, November 2010.

47. Walley J, Graham K, et al. Getting research into practice: primary care management of noncommunicable diseases in low- and middle-income countries. *Bull World Health Organ* 2012;90(6):402.

48. Walley J, Khan A, et al. How to get research into practice—first get research into research: lessons learned from TB partnerships in Pakistan and China. *Bull World Health Organ* 2007;85(6):1–2.

49. Zachariah R, Ford N, et al. Is operational research delivering the goods? The journey to success in low-income countries. *Lancet Infect Dis* 2012;12(5):415–421.

50. Ministry of Health. *Notice About Further Strengthening of TB Report and Patient Management.* Beijing: Disease Control Department, 2004.

51. Wang L, Cheng S, et al. Model collaboration between hospitals and public health system to improve tuberculosis control in China. *Int J Tuberculosis Lung Dis* 2009;13(12):1486–1492.

52. Wang L, Liu J, et al. Progress in tuberculosis control and the evolving public-health system in China. *Lancet* 2007;369:691–696.

53. Zou G, Wei X, et al. Factors influencing integration of TB services in general hospitals in two regions of China: a qualitative study. *BMC Health Serv Res* 2012;12:21.

54. Weeks J. Major trends in the integration of complementary and alternative medicine. In: Fasss N, ed. *Integrating Complementary Medicine into Health Systems.* New York: Aspen, 2001: 12–21.

55. Bannerman R. The role of traditional medicine in primary health care. In: World Health Organization, *Traditional Medicine and Health Care Coverage: A Reader for Health Administrators and Practitioners.* Geneva: WHO, 1983: 318–327.

56. Haddad S, Zakus D, Mohindra, et al. *Promoting Canadian Involvement and Capacity Building in Global Health Policy and Systems Research (GHPSR): Perspectives and Recommendations.* Ottawa: Université de Montréal & University of Toronto, Canadian Institutes of Health Research, May 2002.

57. Zakus D. Resource dependency and community participation in primary health care. *Soc Sci Med* 1998;46(4–5):475–494.

58. Denison D, Haaland S, Goelzer P. Corporate culture and organizational effectiveness: is Asia different from the rest of the world? *Organizational Dynamics* 2004;33(1):98–109.

59. Shortell S, Kaluzny A. *Health Care Management: Organization Design and Behaviour.* 5th ed. Clifton Park, NY: Thomas Delmar Learning, 2005.

60. Kickbusch I, Berger C. Global Health Diplomacy. In: Sommer M and Parker R, eds. *The Routledge International Handbook of Global Public Health.* New York: Routledge, 2010.

61. Abbasi K. The World Bank on world health: under fire. *BMJ* 1999;318:1003–1006.

62. Kirsch D. *Improving Results and Reducing Costs Through Greater Accountability.* Ottawa: Presented at the Canadian Conference on Global Health, October 22, 2012.

63. Grimshaw J. Is evidence-based implementation of evidence-based care possible? *Med J Australia* 2004;180:50–51.

64. Labonte R, Packer C, Klassen N, Kazanjian A, et al. *The Brain Drain of Health Professionals from Sub-Saharan Africa to Canada.* African Migration and Development Series No, 2, Southern Africa Migration Project. Cape Town, SA: IDASA, 2006.

65. Narayan D, Patel R, Schafft K, et al. *Voices of the Poor: Can Anyone Hear Us?* New York: Oxford University Press, 2000.

66. Standing H. *Understanding the "Demand Side" in Service Delivery: Definitions, Frameworks and Tools from the Health Sector.* London: DFID Health Systems Resource Centre, 2004.

67. World Bank. *World Development Report 2004: Making Services Work for Poor People.* Washington, DC: World Bank, 2004.

68. Kumanyika S. *Health Disparities Research in Global Perspective: New Insights and New Directions.* Philadelphia: Department of Biostatistics and Epidemiology, Perelman School of Medicine, University of Pennsylvania, 2012: 1–6.

69. Global Study Suggests Need for Strategies to Combat Unhealthy Lifestyles among the Poor and the Rich. *Science Daily*, August 26, 2012. http://www.sciencedaily.com/releases/2012/08/120826142847.htm.

70. Brugha R, Zwi A. Improving the quality of private sector delivery of public health services: challenges and strategies. *Health Policy Plan* 1998;13:107–120.

71. Zheng ZH, Cui SQ, Lu XQ, et al. Analysis of the status of Chinese Clinical Practice Guidelines development. *BMC Health Serv Res* 2012;12:218.

72. Tran M. Human rights are the best weapon to combat hunger. *The Guardian*, September 26, 2012. http://www.guardian.co.uk/global-development/2012/sep/26/human-rights-combat-hunger-report.

73. World Health Organization, Country indicators, 2010. http://www.who.int/gho/countries/en/.

74. World Bank. *India: Raising the Sights: A Better Health System for India's Poor*. Washington, DC: Health Nutrition and Population Sector Unit, South Asia Region. World Bank, November 3, 2001.

75. Baru R. *Private Health Care in India: Social Characteristics and Trends*. New Delhi, India: Sage, 1998.

76. Berman P. Rethinking health care systems: private health care provision in India. *World Dev* 1998;26:1463–1479.

77. Rao K, Nundy M, Dua A. *Financing and Delivery of Health Care Services in India, Section II: Delivery of health services in the private sector*. New Delhi: National Commission on Macroeconomics and Health Report, Ministry of Health and Family Welfare, 2005.

78. De Costa A, Diwan V. Where is the public health sector? Public and private sector healthcare provision in Madhya Pradesh, India. *Health Policy* 2007;84:269–276.

79. Bhat R. Regulation of the private sector in India. *Int J Health Plan Manage* 1996;11:253–274.

80. Bhat R. Characteristics of private medical practice in India: a provider perspective. *Health Policy Plan* 1999;14:26–37.

81. Thaver I, Harpham T. Private practitioners in the slums of Karachi: professional development and innovative approaches for improving practice. In: Bennett S, McPake B, Mills A, eds. *Private Health Providers in Developing Countries: Serving the Public Interest?* London: Zed Books, 1997.

82. Yesudian C. Behaviour of the private sector in the health market of Bombay. *Health Policy Plan* 1994;9:72–80.

83. Waters W. Globalization, socioeconomic restructuring, and community health. *J Comm Health* 2001;26(2):79–92.

84. Neufeld B, ed. *Health Diplomacy Monitor*. Ottawa: The Centre for Trade Policy & Law, September 2012;3(5).

Global Health Ethics

21

Anvar Velji and John H. Bryant

LEARNING OBJECTIVES

- *Define the emerging discipline of global health ethics and its components*
- *Expand the dialogue on global health ethics and its relationship to human rights; culture, including race, gender, ethnicity, and religion; poverty; and ill health*
- *Discuss the concept of the "global being" or the "global person" in the milieu of equity, equality, justice, and benchmarks of fairness*

DEFINING GLOBAL HEALTH AND GLOBAL HEALTH ETHICS

The world is changing, and one product of this change is the rapid emergence of a new discipline: *global health ethics, the theory and practice of ethics in a holistic manner informed by multiple disciplines.* These disciplines include public and population health and health systems; biotechnology and other scientific research; philosophy, including ethics; and other fields, such as anthropology, psychology, sociology, economics, religion, and law. Practitioners of global ethics thus include not only health care workers and researchers but also practitioners of international biolaw, philosophers, bioethicists, moral and civic leaders, human rights advocates, environmentalists, experts in religion, social and biologic scientists, governmental officials, and nongovernmental organizations. Once considered independent of (and often competing with) one another, this diverse group has converged to achieve a common overarching goal: the well-being and thriving of the *global being (person)* within the worldwide community. This collective entity is embodied in each person and transcends differences between groups of people regardless of whether these differences are based on race, ethnicity, political affiliation, economics, culture, education, language, gender, age, or religion.

Whereas the traditional concept of *international* health focused on bilateral interactions between well-to-do and poor countries, the concept of *global* health reaches beyond the rich-poor dichotomy and geographic borders to the forces that separate the powerful, free, privileged population from the population that is powerless, unfree, and marginalized. In its acceptance of human diversity, global health is an expression of support for human rights. And with human rights as a key value, global health ethics thus provides moral guidance for world health systems and governance. It is critical that a very comprehensive World Health Organization (WHO) definition of health be used in our discussion, that is, *health as a state of physical, social, mental, and spiritual well-being that extends beyond the absence of physical disease or infirmity.*

For the purpose of our discussion, two definitions highlight different aspects of global health but to a certain extent are complementary: Velji and Bryant's understanding and definition of global health "with a human face" emphasizes shared ideas, ideals, and values: global health is a new paradigmatic vision and action that rests on human ideas, ideals, and values of providing high quality of health for all globally. It has at its core equity, compassion, altruism, sharing, sensitivity, dignity, respect, philanthropy, and professionalism. It is bound by a global ethical code of conduct and governance that transcends borders, socioeconomic standing, ethnicity, caste, and religions. It enshrines the notion of the "global good." Global health as a collective entity and enterprise is beyond the component disciplines, philosophies, and sciences but is informed by them. As a new mindset, global health is mindful of individual liberties and societal good. It enshrines the principles of equity, solidarity, beneficence, avoidance of malfeasance, promotion of fairness, and autonomy with responsibility. Global health is mindful of the privileged connections that exist between all human beings. It is science and evidence based and informed by the socially sensitive input of all parties involved.[1]

Koplan et al define global health in more practical terms with an emphasis on study, research, and practice: "Global health is an area for study, research, and practice that places a priority on improving health and achieving equity in health for all people worldwide. Global health emphasizes transnational health issues, determinants, and solutions; involves many disciplines within and beyond the health sciences and promotes interdisciplinary collaboration; and is a synthesis of population-based prevention with individual-level clinical care."[2]

In recent decades, the development of global health was greatly influenced by the 1978 International Conference on Primary Health Care, convened by the WHO and UNICEF in Alma-Ata (Kazakhstan, USSR).[3] At that landmark conference, primary health care was established as a fundamental component of health care, with equity and the right to health care as core features. The conference responded to ongoing global changes, particularly with regard to their ethical dimensions.

Because it encompasses clinical/medical ethics, public health ethics, population health ethics, and bioethics, the study and practice of global health ethics are potent tools for alleviating human suffering, poverty, disease, and environmental degradation, both locally and globally. For instance, in the field of research, global health ethics challenges its practitioners not only to identify promising research subjects but also to assure respect for their equity, dignity, and human rights when interacting with them and their communities. Furthermore, global health researchers continue to be challenged by the extensive imbalance in research support available to well-to-do countries compared with resources available to poor countries: ninety percent of all medical research funds are expended by and for the wealthiest countries to address 10%—their share—of the worldwide disease burden.

Today, global health practitioners and policymakers recognize that individual health security—an essential component of personal well-being—is a human right that every civil society is obliged (and therefore must be empowered) to protect. This obligation is emphasized in the United Nations (UN) Millennium Development Goals, which insist that major obstacles to human social, economic, and health development be addressed. In partnership with global health ethicists, these goals recognize that ethical reform in national and global governance is a necessity in the 21st century amid the threats and spread of global violence, erosion of health gains accumulated during the past two centuries, and emergence of novel health challenges.

PUBLIC HEALTH ETHICS, CLINICAL ETHICS, AND BIOMEDICAL ETHICS

Public health ethics focuses on the general public good of the population (instead of the individual). The "macro-ethics" of public health transcend both the "micro-ethics" of medicine (with its provider-patient relationship) and "meso-ethics," which operate at institutional levels. Public health concerns envelop health and safety issues at the city, state, and country level. The principles and practice of public health may be at odds with the "micro-ethics" of individual rights and autonomy. A case in point is the classical ethical conundrum of mandating quarantine for a patient with a communicable disease such as tuberculosis or severe acute respiratory syndrome (SARS).

Clinical ethics (also called *clinical medical ethics*) is a burgeoning field that focuses on improving the quality of patient care by identifying, analyzing, and attempting to address the ethical problems that arise in clinical practice. Clinical ethics is acknowledged to be an inherently inseparable part of good clinical medicine and includes concerns of the patient's family.[4] Clinical ethics as a discipline consists of research, teaching, committee work, and consultation activities.[4] The primary emphasis of clinical ethicists is the quality of end-of-life care and conflict resolution within the framework of clinical ethics committees. To date, clinical ethics as a distinct discipline has been primarily a phenomenon of developed countries and is based on secular premises: "Clinical ethics is not founded in philosophy, law or theology but instead on the subdiscipline of medicine, centering upon the doctor patient relationships."[4] In many institutions, committees that meet to discuss issues of clinical ethics are called "bioethics committees" or "biomedical ethics committees." As an academic discipline, clinical ethics addresses questions at the clinical level, such as informed consent, autonomy, and death and dying.

Often called "bioethics," *biomedical ethics* is an academic discipline limited to learned societies and academicians; it is the purview of departments of philosophy. At the national level, bioethical forums discuss institutional and national policies and issues such as health care rationing and access. Bioethics relates to the ethical questions and dilemmas that arise at the interfaces between medicine, biology, cybernetics, politics, law, theology, philosophy, technological research, and the ethics of morality, duty, and obligations. In the global context, newly emerging issues related to human genomic research and other major developments of biotechnology, such as cloning, xenotransplantation, and stem cell research, have become focuses of bioethics.

The post–World War II emergence of bioethics in the United States evolved around the Protestant values that predominated in US culture. This concept was elegantly encapsulated by Jonsen, who stated, "US medicine had in the immediate postwar years begun to build a wall around itself and within that wall a complex edifice. Three streams of bioethical concerns highlighted that reality. The therapeutic stream, which brought new treatments, found that it had to exclude persons from them, as the 'God Committees' chose some to live, others to die. The experimental stream, on the other hand, seemed to capture some, entrusting them into treatment they did not want or need, and repelling others from treatment they needed. The scientific stream was perhaps the most ominous, suggesting in the power the remaking of humans in an engineer's image."[5] In the early 1960s, vigorous debate in the "God Committees" centered on the first genuinely life-supporting, lifesaving technology: chronic hemodialysis.[5]

The second bioethical model is that of "Euro-Ethics." This model also has limited value because it lacks diversity and the notion of plurality. The focus of Euro-Ethics is the philosophy of medicine and epistemology; this focus contrasts with the American model of bioethics, which is more closely aligned with applied and practical ethics.[5]

Nominally and conceptually, the modern discipline of bioethics is seen as an offspring of a Western, predominantly US, model characterized by scientific voluntarism or the technological imperative and libertarian or secular morals. This focus demonstrates radical change of the tradition of "*bios* (life) and *ethike* (ethos) through manipulation of life."[6] The discipline of bioethics as viewed by the developing world is "conceptually a synthesis of the advances of science and the mandates of conscience."[6] The Roman Catholic perspective, expressed predominantly in Latin America, is succinctly described as containing bioethical premises based on the principle of holiness of life and on the imperatives of natural law as supported by the moral theology of the Catholic church.[6]

Can the rules, laws, and principles of secularism be separated from religious rationales and the sanctions of God's reward and punishment? Secularists and religious fundamentalists are at odds on several issues of current relevance in the new millennium. One danger of the Western (and particularly the American) form of biomedical ethics is the "unleashing of absolute individualism and moral atomism of a socially destructive kind."[7] This powerful, incessant drive operates in issues such as euthanasia, assisted suicide, abortion, purchase of organs for transplantation, all

forms of reproductive technology and surrogate parenthood, preservation of confidentiality, and the use of public health funding for research.[7]

FROM "INTERNATIONAL HEALTH" TO "GLOBAL HEALTH": EXPANDING OUR LANGUAGE AND PERCEPTIONS

Traditionally, medical practitioners have focused on personal health from a limited perspective (prevention, diagnosis, and treatment) and were bound by ethics and covenants traceable to ancient civilizations (India, Persia, Egypt, China, Greece), whereas the new discipline of global health requires a vocabulary that defines health as a state of physical, social, mental, and spiritual well-being that extends beyond the absence of physical disease or infirmity. The new dialogue on global health has already outgrown the limitations of current terminology (e.g., "international health"), and no consistent vocabulary yet exists that adequately describes the conceptual framework and operationalization of global health ethics. Language is needed to fully convey the global cultural contexts for such terms as individual and public good, equity, inequality, rights, solidarity, beneficence, autonomy, justice, fairness, dignity, virtue, and responsibility. Indeed, with the onset of globalization—a set of new economic realities amid disappearing political boundaries—the world's thinking must be reoriented to achieve health in this new millennium.

This reorientation is being guided by leaders in the emerging field of global health who contribute their experience and ideas regarding major health-related concerns of social science (e.g., societal discrimination and inequality, health care rights, population displacement, poverty, ethics of environmental practices and technology transfer, access to primary health care services, health care financing, education, global networking) and of natural science (e.g., diagnosis and treatment of diarrheal, respiratory, tropical, and infectious diseases; malnutrition; and global disease burden), summarized in two seminal volumes edited by Velji.[8,9]

Two volumes on global health, *Global Health Education* and *Infectious Disease in the New Millennium*, extended this dialogue further by engaging more global health thought leaders to focus on the 21st-century challenges and solutions.[10,11]

As an example of steps taken to address human rights and social determinants of health, both locally and globally, through education, service, and research, a consortium—originally named International Health Medical Education, subsequently renamed Global Health Education Consortium and now a merged entity, Consortium of Universities for Global Health,[12] was founded in 1991, to address new challenges of global health, global health development, and education.[13] The cofounders of this consortium stated their intent to impart a systemic networking approach to global health education by focusing on marginalized populations around the world. This intent was subsequently articulated also in the historic 1997 WHO policy statement, which stated that "Health for All in the 21st century . . . [must be] built on the genuine expressions of moral obligations to protect the vulnerable and to mitigate inequities . . . with . . . science-based and socially sensitive methods."[14]

Accordingly, a director general of WHO articulated its changing role as the world's health conscience: "The role of WHO . . . must include ethical standard setting to meet today's and tomorrow's needs in such areas as cloning, reproductive health, and access to triple-drug treatment for persons with HIV infection, or the use of interferon for hepatitis C carriers. Many issues relating to fair access to preventive, therapeutic and rehabilitative technologies should be considered, and ethical guidelines should be prepared."[15]

HEALTH-RELATED ETHICS OF GLOBALIZATION

From the perspective of the developing nations, globalization is manifested as an onslaught of ethico-religious, cultural, technological, economic, and informational changes that disrupt established societies. These globalization-related changes result in the marginalization of vulnerable populations, whose health is further affected negatively by additional phenomena present throughout the world: unethical organ donor policies, militarization, privatization, unfair trade practices, and economic sanctions.[16–18] All these phenomena cause continuous and sporadic societal paradigm shifts that transcend national boundaries and affect the politics, ecology, economics, education, and health of entire societies. Without a commitment to ethical principles—human rights and freedom, justice, fairness, equity—the weak, disadvantaged global citizen is denied access to education, housing, jobs, and food and is placed in a lopsided struggle against the privileged citizen within a neoliberal, highly individualistic environment. Lack of ethical intervention will continue to erode health care not only in the developing countries but also in the developed nations.

EQUITY AS A CORE ELEMENT OF GLOBAL HEALTH ETHICS

The enormous size of these challenges calls for ethical policies that benefit the vulnerable and have equity at the core. This essential element was affirmed in

the WHO Declaration of Alma Ata[3] and was a centerpiece of renewing the WHO *Health for All* call.[19] Health equity involves more than equality and is not a "vague but politically popular desire for social justice."[20] Instead, health equity is "a feasible and tangible process" in which health benefits are received according to measurable need, not on the basis of economic or political status.[20]

Surveillance of equity status is a practical management tool that makes the moral imperatives of social justice feasible.[21] Inequities in health care—and especially in health outcomes—imply presence of a subset of measurable inequalities that are both unfair and avoidable. Equitable distribution of health care is not necessarily sufficient to overcome health inequities; health equity is measured also by the extent to which disadvantaged populations can exercise their human right to justice and fairness in the context of achieving well-being.

EQUALITY AS A CORE ELEMENT OF GLOBAL HEALTH ETHICS

The 19th-century British epidemiologist William Farr is credited with having initiated the scientific study of health inequalities,[22] a central feature of the European tradition, especially in the United Kingdom. Unlike the normative concept of health equity, health inequality is a primarily empirical concept that emphasizes the disparity between rich and poor populations and thereby avoids focusing on the health of the poor.[23] The most daunting challenge of the third millennium is to understand the causes of health inequity and how health care is distributed within and between countries. Central to this concern is the need to create health systems on the basis of fairness, distributive justice, human rights, democracy, and peace-building—a suggestion echoed by a Rockefeller Foundation report,[24] which presents diverse dimensions of health equity in 13 countries. The report explores fundamental issues, such as ethics and its measurement as well as causal analysis related to underlying social determinants (e.g., gender, globalization) and argues explicitly that specific fairness-related values are involved in distributing health care and facilitating positive health outcomes. The report discusses remediable health inequalities, including unequal access to resources—financial assistance, education, job security, clean air and water, sanitation, health care—and gender inequality. Within any society, health inequity is both a proxy and a barometer for marginalization, for deficiencies in social justice and human rights, and for lack of democracy.[24]

To be accurate, any ethics-based measurement of inequalities in health care requires a sophisticated technique. Ideally, this measurement technique would consider the distribution of ill health across the full socioeconomic gradient and not only within a selected segment of the population.

The classical health status indicators used for monitoring global health achievement includes rate of infant mortality, overall mortality and morbidity, and combined rates of mortality and morbidity (described by indicators such as quality-adjusted life years, disability-adjusted life years [DALYs], and health life years). (See Chapter 2 for more information on these measures.) However, these indicators fall short of monitoring equity in health care. The Council of International Organizations for Medical Sciences (CIOMS) working group suggested monitoring of other health services indicators, including accessibility, affordability, utilization, and coverage of health care along with its appropriateness and procedural fairness. Moreover, processes of decision making must be visible, and caregivers must be accountable.[25]

The sea-change in the ethical search for cost-effective and equitable care has focused on one vexing philosophical, theological question: How should life be valued? This question subsumes others: should life be valued in terms of economic and social productivity or in terms of a given duration of life, with its intrinsic value and variation by age, economic productivity, and social status? How do we measure the value of future life versus that of the present? As Morrow and Bryant state,[26] measuring and valuing human life contribute importantly to understanding the disease burdens in populations and to guiding thinking about the most appropriate ways to address those burdens with health care intervention. Such interventions are mindful of ethical dimensions of health and human development.[26] Are DALYs considered to be an ethical measure that is also sensitive—both quantitatively and qualitatively? How do these concepts fit into the ethics of public, global health decision making versus the traditional, doctor-patient–based ethics?[26,27]

The 1993 World Bank Report *Investing in Health*[28] focused on quantifying and comparing the disease burden borne by diverse populations. The metric created for this purpose was the DALY.[29,30] Subsequently, the concept of the benchmarks of fairness, initially introduced by Daniels et al,[31] queried various equity-related dimensions of health care reform, including provision of universal access to services, comprehensiveness of services, uniformity of benefits, equitable financing as determined by ability to pay value for money (clinical financial efficiency), public accountability, and degree of choice.[32-34] Thailand, Pakistan, Mexico, and Colombia have modified and refined some of these matrices. In Pakistan, for instance, the following benchmarks were introduced: intersectoral public health; financial- and gender-related barriers to access;

comprehensiveness and tiering of benefits; equitable financing; effectiveness, efficiency, and quality of health care; administrative efficiency; democratic accountability; and patient-provider autonomy.[33]

In the setting of low-income and insufficient data, unique thinking and creation of novel benchmarking tools are needed for building greater capacity to monitor and analyze policies from an equity-ethical perspective. In postapartheid South Africa, another tool—the *equity gauge*—was invented to enable legislators at both the national and subnational levels to monitor the impact of government policy on health systems.[34]

HEALTH-RELATED ETHICS OF GLOBAL POVERTY, DISTRIBUTIVE JUSTICE, AND THE POOR–RICH DIVIDE

One cannot discuss global health ethics without addressing poverty, inequity, and injustice. This section examines some examples of these issues and how they affect the health of people around the world.

Orphans and Other Vulnerable Children of the Urban Slums of Africa

Of the 350 million children under 17 years of age who currently live in sub-Saharan Africa, 43 million (12.3%) are orphans.[35] In addition to these children, however, a very large number of nonorphaned children in sub-Saharan Africa are nonetheless highly vulnerable for other reasons; therefore, focusing concern on orphans exclusively would be unfair and unjust. The orphans and other vulnerable children of Africa are the most disadvantaged of any in the world. The dimensions of such disadvantage reach far beyond what usually comes to mind in considering the lives of such children, whether these factors are physical, economic, social, cultural, educational, ethical, or rights based.

The practical realities of vulnerable children include a broad range of deeply troubling circumstances, including the circumstance of being orphaned, abandoned, or physically handicapped; forced to become a child soldier; being displaced by war or exposed to hazardous work; becoming a victim of human trafficking and other forms of abuse and neglect; living in extremely poor conditions; being homeless, living on the streets; or a combination of these circumstances. To these threats to health and well-being must be added the further burdens imposed by the HIV/AIDS pandemic: of the 43 million orphans living in sub-Saharan Africa, 28% were orphaned as a result of HIV/AIDS.[35] (See Chapters 4 and Chapter 5 for more on this subject.)

These vulnerable children can thus be defined as those whose safety, well-being, and development are threatened. Of the many factors contributing to these children's vulnerability, the most important are lack of care and affection, adequate shelter, education, nutrition, or psychological support, and, of course, frequent discrimination.

Recent research has identified two fundamental qualities that determine the caregiver's ability to provide effective care: *sensitivity* and *responsiveness to the child*. These skills enable the caregiver to detect the child's signals and to respond appropriately, in synchrony, to meet the child's needs and promote the development of a child who is physically, intellectually, and socially healthy and more resilient to the damaging effects of poverty and violence.[36] A useful approach might be to reach beyond the generalizations relating to these children to focus on the extremely vulnerable population of children living in Africa's urban slums. Of people living in the large urban slums of Nairobi—70% of that city's population—79% live in one-room homes without running water or sanitation and usually without electricity. One can only begin to imagine the extreme difficulties of families trying to build constructive lives under such circumstances; not surprising, therefore, is the exceedingly high mortality rate for children under 5 years of age. In some areas, this rate reaches 25% of children. More than half of these childhood deaths are associated with malnutrition.[37]

To address the needs of those living in the slums, UN Habitat has committed its members to the Millennium Development Goal of improving the well-being of 100 million people dwelling in the urban slums of Africa, simultaneously expressing concern for the orphans and other vulnerable children in those slums.[38]

Given the immense burden on the health and well-being of those children, one can easily understand the existence of multiple approaches to alleviating these children's problems. Indeed, no fixed set of answers exists, and accessible resources fall far short of need for them. Multiple approaches are thus needed and used, and a great challenge is to create coherent interaction among those responses.[39]

One distinct pattern of need is relatively new and underappreciated. There have been recent advances in the science of early childhood development that are exceedingly important. The National Academy of Science USA[40] and the WHO[41] report that early caregiver-child interactions, beginning in the early days of life, are strong foundational determinants of social, psychological, physical, emotional, and cognitive capacities of the young child; a strongly nurturing, loving, protective, stimulating caregiver-child interaction is essential for the child's early development. In contrast, a negligent, unprotective, non-loving interaction can be disruptive, damaging, and produce lifelong negative effects. The nature of these caregiver-child interactions or attachments has been further defined as representing *secure attachment* (which is supportive, nurturing, and loving) or *insecure attachment* (which is negligent and disruptive). Considerable research has been focused on the nature of these attachments and their positive and negative consequences.

Applying these concepts to the circumstances of the lives of vulnerable children in slum settings adds insight not only into the risks to these children's well-being but also into the nature of equity. Let us consider for a moment the place of equity in caring for these children. Equity in child care calls not for equal distribution of care but for delivery of care according to need. Health care programs for vulnerable children in the urban slums are challenged by the extreme scarcity of resources and active community participation. The aim of these programs is therefore to identify those children most in need and to respond accordingly.

A disturbing equity-related issue is the widespread underappreciation of the importance of early caregiver-child attachments for the foundational development of the child. For example, little local concern is expressed for orphans and other vulnerable children sitting in the trash and mud of an African slum community; the response to this situation is often, "They are poor to be sure, and perhaps hungry, but they are not being harmed." In addition to the potential damage of malnutrition and exposure to infectious disease, the lack of sufficient, positive caregiver-child interactions early in these children's lives does indeed cause them harm. The development of life skills—in particular, the ability to cope with the complex difficulties of their corner of the world—is seriously diminished in these children. Thus this emerging example illuminates the unseen inequities affecting a large number of children in Africa.

That these children lack opportunity to have a good life is a violation of their human rights, and this deprivation also must not be neglected. Working with UN Habitat in the slums of Nairobi, Bryant and colleagues have developed a project focused on the health care and social support of orphans and vulnerable children under 5 years of age in three slum communities of Nairobi, Kenya. One of the purposes is to develop a methodology that could be extended to other African communities. A prime focal point is to demonstrate the feasibility of achieving assessment of caregiver-child attachment by community health workers (CHWs) as a routine component of community-based primary health care (PHC). Given the effectiveness of such assessment, further community-based actions are to be taken, in support of secure attachment or corrective actions relating to insecure attachment.[36]

Thus an important component of the project is the selection and training of CHWs, eight in each of the three communities. There are now 2,400 community households in the three communities, each containing one or more children under 5, and the CHWs arrange to visit each of those households once every 1, 2, or 3 months, depending on the needs of the children. There are two major components of the work of the CHWs. One is to extend PHC to those children, including growth monitoring, immunizations, and use of insecticide-treated bed nets, handwashing with soap to prevent diarrhea, oral rehydration therapy, nutritional supplementation, and general child well-being. The second component includes assessment and monitoring of caregiver-child attachments. A methodology for assessing caregiver-child attachment was developed through an iterative process, building on other validated assessment tools.

Of the 2,560 children assessed from July to December 2010, 2,391 (90.2%) were assessed as having a secure attachment with a parent or other caregiver; 259 (9.8%) were assessed as having an insecure attachment. Children with a secure attachment were more likely to have a normal weight-for-age compared with children assessed as insecure, and they were less likely to have diarrhea or malaria at the initial CHW visit. Following workshops focusing on methods to strengthen caregiving relationships, follow-up assessments showed that among the 259 children initially assessed as insecure, 215 (83%) were assessed as having a secure attachment.

Thus it is apparent that assessment of caregiver-child attachment in the setting of routine home visits by CHWs in a PHC context is feasible and may yield valuable insights into household-level risks and responsive actions. This reaches beyond a goal of child survival to important gains in early child development.

Further, we see here the affirmation of a methodology for encouraging and supporting secure caregiver-child attachments that can be community based and equitably distributed, accessible to all of sub-Saharan Africa. We do appreciate the complexities of building collaborative relationships supportive of such processes, but we see the potential benefits as exceedingly attractive to African communities.[36] Special attention should be given to the five key strategies (see Table 21-1) discussed in "Framework for the Protection, Care, and Support of Orphans and Vulnerable Children living in a World with HIV and AIDS," which appeared in Children on the Brink 2004.[35]

Inequity and Poverty in the Global Health Equation

Inequity is deeply rooted in the soil of poverty, and the oft-expressed question, "Am I poor because I am

Table 21-1. Key strategies for improving the health and development of orphans and other vulnerable children in poor communities worldwide.

- By prolonging the lives of parents and by providing economic, psychosocial, and other support, strengthen the ability of families to protect and care for orphans and other vulnerable children.
- Mobilize and support community-based responses to provide both immediate and long-term assistance to vulnerable households.
- Ensure that orphans and other vulnerable children have access to essential services, such as education, health care, and birth registration.
- Ensure that governments protect the most vulnerable children by improving policies and legislation and by directing resources to communities.
- To create a supportive environment for children affected by HIV/AIDS, raise awareness at all levels through advocacy and social mobilization.

sick, or am I sick because I am poor?" points to the inter-penetrating relation between poverty and global health. Accordingly, global opinion is now focused on the health of the poor along with the ethical notion of inequality in health care. Poverty-oriented economics has thus gained recognition on the world stage.[42] (See Chapter 19 for more information on this topic.) Nonetheless, societal discrimination at various levels and predatory unethical practices—prevalent globally, regionally, and locally—still prey on the vulnerable. After a long study of AIDS, Mann stated, "The central insight from a decade of hard work against AIDS is that societal discrimination is at the root of individual and community vulnerability to AIDS and other major health problems of the modern world."[43]

Table 21-2 outlines a three-step process focused on ethics, which has been proposed for addressing the societal risk factors operating worldwide.[43] Central to this three-step process is a concept applicable to a wide variety of global health problems, "A careful analysis of the major causes of preventable illness, disability, and premature death—including cancer, heart disease, injuries and violence and infectious disease—shows that they, like AIDS, are linked to societal discrimination and lack of respect for fundamental human rights and dignity."[43]

In the 21st century, the primary cause of ill health is poverty. Recent climatologic and geologic catastrophes in the first few years of the present millennium—the Indian Ocean tsunami; Hurricane Katrina in the United States; and earthquakes in Turkey, Iran, Pakistan, and Haiti—garnered global attention to the

Table 21-2. Proposed three-step ethics-based process for addressing societal risk factors operating worldwide.

- Identification of the basic forms of discrimination within one community or nation
- Identification of societal discrimination that leads to risk of HIV exposure and diminished access to health care
- Identification of processes that can reduce this societal discrimination

Table 21-3. Sustainable development goals contained within the Millennium Development Goals endorsed by 189 countries in December 2000 at the Millennium Summit in New York.

- Eradicate extreme poverty and hunger. By the year 2015, halve the proportion of people in extreme poverty and the proportion of people who suffer from hunger.
- Achieve universal primary education. By 2015, ensure that all children can complete a full course of primary schooling.
- Promote gender equality and empower women to eliminate gender disparity in primary and secondary education by 2005 and in all levels of education by 2015.
- By the year 2015, reduce child mortality by two thirds.
- By 2015, improve maternal health by reducing the maternal mortality rate by 75 percent.
- By 2015, combat HIV/AIDS, malaria, and other diseases and begin to reverse their spread.
- Ensure environmental sustainability. By 2015, halve the proportion of people without sustainable access to safe drinking water.
- Develop a global partnership for development. Develop further rule-based, predictable, nondiscriminatory trading and financial systems and address the special needs of the least-developed countries.

susceptibility of vulnerable populations, especially the poor, to natural disasters, and massive amounts of aid were offered to help disaster victims. However mind-numbing "daily tsunamis" never register on the radar of the same donor communities in the same proportion. For instance, the HIV/AIDS pandemic costs the African subcontinent 1% of its gross domestic product each year. Malaria alone kills 2,800 Africans a day,[44] and 314 million Africans—nearly twice as many as in 1981—live on less than $1 a day. Moreover, Africa is home to the world's 48 poorest countries, including 24 of the 32 countries ranked lowest in human development.[44] Every week, 10,000 women in the developing world die during childbirth and 200,000 children under the age of 5 years die from disease. Each day, more than 8,000 people die from AIDS-related conditions. In 2005 alone, 2 million people died from AIDS. Another hallmark of this impoverishment is the observation that an estimated 115 million children in developing countries have no schooling.[44] And even Europe has not been spared: the Roma population for instance—a people once known as gypsies—is the largest, poorest, and fastest growing minority worldwide.[44]

In 2000, in response to the challenges of poverty and discrimination, 189 countries became signatories to the Millennium Development Goals (MDG) project, which clearly outlined targets for reducing poverty and other sources of human deprivation as well as promoting eight sustainable development goals (SDGs)[44–46] (see Table 21-3).

Private philanthropic foundations have also had a major ethical and practical role in addressing the problems of global health. The long-standing philanthropic efforts of the Rockefeller Foundation, the Aga Khan Foundation, the Aga Khan Health Services, and other key players[47–49] have now been boosted by more recent contributors, such as Ted Turner, the Bill and Melinda Gates Foundation, and Warren Buffett.

In 1999, the Bill and Melinda Gates Foundation assumed a major leadership role in the global fight against HIV/AIDS, malaria, tuberculosis, and other underfunded diseases endemic in the developing world. A total of US$6 billion had been pledged by the foundation until June 2006, when Warren Buffett announced his contribution of some US$38 billion to the foundation for its global efforts. The Global Fund to Fight AIDS, Tuberculosis, and Malaria promised $4.8 billion to 128 countries, and the [US] President's Emergency Plan for HIV/AIDS Relief (PEPFAR) pledged US$15 billion to help "selected countries." The Global Alliance for Vaccines and Immunization (GAVI) has been involved in 72 countries, using a budget half of which was contributed by the Bill and Melinda Gates Foundation.[50]

In 2009, President Obama's complex Global Health Initiative proposed a 6-year $63 billion effort to develop a comprehensive US response to global health challenges,[51] but it is currently facing opposition due to US policymakers' efforts to rein in runaway budget deficits. In addition to the budget impasse, the global financial crisis, and the economic stagnation in donor countries, the annualized rate of growth in development assistance for health has slowed from prior years, which will result in the inability to meet the goals of the MDGs by 2015.[52] However, a bigger challenge will be in selecting, launching, and funding the post-2015 SDGs.

Aside from these financial challenges, ethical questions abound as to appropriate priorities in distributing health services and funds for these and related services and measuring their impact. A recent focus on global health is the complicated, confusing interrelationships between 30 stakeholders—Tanzania, for example, where the HIV/AIDS epidemic highlights ethical dilemmas.[50,53] Aid to intended recipients is often blocked by the "architectural indigestion" that can result from the differing political agendas of multiple donors combined with their often inadequate attention to health ethics.

In response to the mounting evidence and research on social determinants of health inequalities, the WHO Commission on Social Determinants of Health was launched to focus on the world's most vulnerable populations.[54] The commission seeks to ensure that public policy is based on a vision of the world where people matter most and where social justice is therefore paramount.

The G8 countries—the United States, Canada, Great Britain, France, Germany, Japan, Italy, and (nominally) Russia—account for roughly halve the world's economic activity and dominate the decision-making processes of both the World Bank and the International Monetary Fund (IMF).[55] Support from the G8 is therefore critical for improving the key social determinants of health, which include education, housing, sanitation, nutrition, and safe, clean food and water. Intervention by the G8 is pivotal also for reversing the severe debt crises of developing nations (especially those in sub-Saharan Africa), where fragile, destabilized economies are susceptible to internal strife and further crises, health crises foremost among them. The roots of these debt crises are sociopolitical, historical, and economic; for example, postcolonial African nations experimented with Marxism and socialism, which furthered both the extension of debt and loss of infrastructure. Famine, drought, and wars added more burdens. A recognized effect of deep national debt in the developing countries is the *debt-death link*: The higher the interest payment owing on a nation's debt, the lower the mean life expectancy of that nation's citizens. This link is now well accepted internationally as a necessary focus of debt relief,[56] especially given that the heavily indebted developing countries spend far more money for arms than for reducing debt. By 1990, for example, sub-Saharan Africa was receiving US$11 billion annually for military weaponry; and developing countries, including those south of the Sahara, sent to the developed countries a staggering US$220 billion more than these developing countries received in aid.[56] Under this scenario, the 1994 World Bank report predicted that the sub-Saharan black states will require

40 years to reach the level of wealth that existed there 20 years previously.[57] For the world's poorest countries, debt burden is thus the "new slavery."[58] Jubilee 2000, a coalition of more than 90 organizations, including Oxfam, Christian Aid, and the British Medical Association, have spotlighted this relation between the creditor nations, the IMF and World Bank.[58]

These health-related issues become more critical each year as the poor-rich divide increases—so much so that the UN secretary general has called for urgent action to raise the living standards of the world's poor.[59] At the ceremony where he was awarded the Nobel Peace Prize, former US president Jimmy Carter stated that the greatest challenge facing the world is the universal, growing chasm between the richest and the poorest people on earth and that this disparity causes most of the world's unsolved problems, including starvation, illiteracy, environmental degradation, violent conflicts, and unnecessary illnesses from guinea worm to HIV/AIDS.[60]

This enormous, growing disparity is illustrated by many statistics. Of the world's total consumption, the richest fifth of the world's people consume 86% of all goods and services, whereas the poorest fifth consumes only 1.3%; and the three richest people in the world have assets that exceed the combined gross domestic product of the 48 least-developed countries.[59,61,62] The world's 225 richest individuals (of whom 60 are American) have a combined wealth of more than $1 trillion—equal to the annual income of the poorest 47% of the world's population.[59,61,62] The amount of money spent each year by Americans and Europeans on pet food alone—US$17 billion a year—is $4 billion more than the estimated annual amount needed to provide basic health and nutrition for everyone in the world.[59,61,62] The rising economic tide expected to flow from market economics is said to be a force that will "lift all boats," but "the poor have no boat and are drowning in this tsunami of corporate profit."[63]

Health Care Inequity and Its Worldwide Association with Culture, Race, Ethnicity, and Gender

Global inequities of socioeconomic position and health are disproportionately distributed along racial lines. Disadvantaged groups and countries identifiable by race sustain higher burdens of disease and deprivation than their advantaged cohorts identifiable by race. This inequity exists despite current genomic research, which shows that 99.9% of DNA is shared by all human beings, regardless of the anatomic and physiologic aspects of "race"[64] and that genetic variation within socially recognized human populations exceeds the genetic variation between population groups. Race is therefore meaningful only socially, not biologically,[64] and the rational taxonomy traditionally used by anthropologists, epidemiologists, researchers, and nations around the world is clearly outdated.

During the past century 26 different schemes, most of them motivated by politics of isolation and marginalization, have sought to categorize racial differences in the US population.[65] Over time, several of these schemes have been replaced by others. For instance, Jews were defined as nonwhite along with certain other groups but were "deracialized" later in the century. Similarly, persons of South Asian origin were at first classified as "Hindus"[64] but were later classified as whites regardless of skin tone. In South Africa, the apartheid classified Japanese and Chinese persons—along with other Asians and even Jews—as "colored." Subsequently, with the rising force of the Japanese economy, Japanese persons were classified as "whites" under the apartheid system.

Ethnicity, in comparison, emphasizes the cultural, socioeconomic, religious, and political characteristics of human groups; these characteristics include language, dress, customs, kinship, and historical identification with territory.[66] *Culture* denotes fundamental beliefs, art, language, literature, customs, ideals, and laws in general[7] and provides an inextricable link to morals and ethics of the human species. To violate a person's cultural beliefs and practices is therefore tantamount to assaulting that person's humanity,[7] and imposition of beliefs and practices on an individual or a society is also a violation and is immoral.[7] A cardinal principle of global health ethics is to respect others and uphold their inviolable dignity.

Of course, health disparities based on a person's "race" and skin "color" are prevalent in many countries other than the United States. In Brazil, for instance, the mortality rate among children under 12 months of age is 62.3 for black and brown children as compared with 7.3 for white children.[64] Similarly, in Australia, the life expectancy at birth for nonindigenous males is 75.2 years and 81.1 years for females, whereas the lifespans of indigenous people are considerably shorter: 56.9 years for males, and 61.7 years for females. In the United States, where most studies on "racial disparities" are conducted, the diabetes-related mortality rate among Native Americans is 27.8 per 100,000—380% higher than that of whites (7.3 per 100,000). Black women in the United States have a three-fold higher rate of childbirth-related mortality than their white female cohorts, and the rate among Hispanic women is 23% higher. Across social lines, similar differences in health outcomes have been shown for asthma, hypertension, heart disease, cancer, diabetes, HIV/AIDS, and end-stage renal disease.

Examples of factors that create barriers to health care—and therefore, inequity—for these disadvantaged populations include lack of economic access to health care, institutional barriers encountered by health care providers, discriminatory health care policies and practices, and lack of language and cultural competency among health care practitioners and policymakers.[64] The Kaiser Permanente National Diversity Council within the Kaiser Permanente Medical Care Program (a large nonprofit managed care organization headquartered in California) has issued several publications and provider handbooks about techniques for rendering culturally competent care for various populations, including African American, Latino, Southeast Asian, Pacific Islander, gay, bisexual, and transgender patients as well as those with medical disabilities. Nonetheless, except for the United Kingdom where researchers have substantially documented barriers to health care, data are as yet insufficient to describe these barriers as they exist across Europe and in developing nations, where many "nonwhite" members of society have undergone health care–related discrimination in connection with their ethnicity and culture. Such data are needed to address disparities in health care and in health outcomes; however, they are also susceptible to the hazards inherent in planning delivery of health care on the basis of specified ethnic populations notwithstanding any scientific basis for such "racialization" of disease.

For example, the frequency of the BRCA-1 genetic mutation (present in women with breast cancer) in the general US population is 1 in 1,666, whereas the frequency is 1 in 107 among Ashkenazi Jewish women of Eastern European origin.[64] Identifying female patients with this heritage might therefore facilitate testing that would allow some women to obtain appropriate medical care earlier than would be possible without such testing. However, such targeted testing based on advances in genomic technology can easily lead to both stigmatization and discrimination and raises legitimate ethical questions: Are our genes being singled out as "mutant"? Should the specified female population receive breast screening and "prophylactic" mastectomy?

Specified genetic traits, such as that for sickle cell disease (the first "racialized" disease), might be used inappropriately as a surrogate marker of race. Screening the African American population for sickle cell trait and screening persons of Mediterranean and Southeast Asian ancestry for thalassemia are thus additional examples of issues that raise ethical concerns.

Gender is another factor influencing worldwide disparities in the quality and availability of health care, and a perspective of shared values, equity, and human rights used to transform the health of the global person must challenge historical cultural norms and notions that value males over females. Current measures of aggregate health fail to adequately quantify household assets by gender—a demographic survey marker that has great potential to improve equity in women's and children's health. A seminal paper[67] invoked human rights as well as economic considerations in valuing women's worth.

The burden of disease is carried from one life period to another—from girlhood to motherhood and throughout daughterhood—as multiple male-dominated, paternalistic institutions (political, social, legal, and religious) view the woman's role as that of procreator over whom males are granted the life-and-death power of decision making. In most nations and societies, the law favors males through male-operated and supported agencies and in the name of religion and morality. Until 1969, for example, Canadian law prohibited distribution of information and materials for contraception, which was regarded as a "crime against morality."[68] In societies where these paternalistic forces operate, women lack power to assert their own priorities and aspirations in making reproductive choices and other health-related decisions. Ownership rights to pregnancy and its termination are vested in the males of these societies; the husband owns proprietary and matrimonial rights, including the legal right of control over the fetus.[68]

Gender-based health disparities are evident also in rates of infant mortality. In Bangladesh, India, Pakistan, and China, more male infants survive to the age of 2 years than do female infants; more than 1 million girls die each year as a result of being born female.[69] Each year, more than 95% of an estimated 20 million unsafe abortions—considered by many as a product of moralistic laws and social injustice—occur in developing countries as a result of repressive colonial laws,[68,70] "religious morality," culture, and misguided ideas about family "nobility."

Disparity—and denial—of reproductive rights around the world and throughout history is evident also in various involuntary sterilization practices. The Nazi practice of "ethnic cleansing" and involuntary sterilization to create an uncontaminated "master race" was one such practice that horrified the civilized world. Similarly appalling is the long history of abusive nonconsensual sterilization of persons designated as "intellectually subnormal" or classified by other unprofessional, sometimes racist criteria. For many of these vulnerable members of society, reproduction was controlled by the state, which considered their reproduction to be a social menace.[68]

Ethical Case Study 1: Rights of Mother over the Zygote (Embryo)

The debate over gender-based health care is related to questions of reproductive rights and other issues, such as the sanctity of unborn human life and the relative value of the zygote and mother. In North America,

Europe, and certain other countries, viable fetuses are protected in utero as "legal persons," entities who are protected by law and who possess legal rights. Some ethical issues in this area are illustrated by the following case:

> *A court of law orders a pregnant woman with placenta previa to have the fetus delivered by cesarean delivery. The woman insists on vaginal delivery and refuses elective cesarean delivery on grounds of religious belief. The obstetrician and the hospital fear that litigation against them will ensue if the fetus dies. A court injunction to perform a cesarean delivery without the mother's consent is granted. Fortunately, the woman has a successful vaginal delivery.[68]*

What are the rights of the fetus, and should they override the mother's rights? In handing down the injunction, did the court violate the rights and autonomy of the mother? Were the caregivers justified in basing their actions on the fear of litigation?

A case such as this was documented along with its negative outcome: a mother and her fetus both died after the mother received a court-ordered involuntary cesarean delivery requested by her physicians and the hospital.[68]

This new millennium brings with it great hopes of improving women's rights, health, and educational opportunities. "Just as health care and medical education are critical beacons in the struggle of a community to achieve its highest potential, the status of women and the professions they serve are decisive criteria,"[71] and these criteria are intrinsically related inasmuch as elevated health status is an outcome of elevated societal status.

THE FOUR PRINCIPLES OF ETHICS IN GLOBAL HEALTH AND CULTURE

In the past four decades, both the dialogue of global health ethics and that of clinical bioethics have benefited from the articulation of the four principles of ethics: autonomy, beneficence, nonmaleficence, and justice. These principles have undergone several challenges, especially within the developing countries milieu,[72-74] but nonetheless they provide a common moral language for use as an analytic framework for ethics-related dialogue.

Autonomy (from the Greek *autos,* "self" and *nomos,* "rule") designates a norm of respecting the decision-making capacities of autonomous persons.[74] The proper priority to be given this principle has formed the basis of much debate. In modern dialogue, the original sense of autonomy as self-rule (applied to the independent Greek states) has been extended to diverse meanings including self-governance, liberty rights, privacy, individual choice, freedom of the will, causing one's own behavior, and being one's own person.

Nonmaleficence is a term used to designate a norm of avoiding causation of harm.[74] Throughout the centuries the concepts and practice of nonmaleficence and beneficence have played a central role in medical ethics in all recorded cultures and civilizations. In the setting of global health, the moral objective of providing beneficence (doing good deeds) and avoiding harm assumes production of net benefit to one individual or to society. The maxim "Above all, do no harm" has thus been a foundational part of medical ethics teaching. This concept did not originate within the Hippocratic traditions of medical ethics despite the Hippocratic Oath itself, which states, "I will use treatment to help the sick according to my ability and judgment, but I will never use it to injure or wrong them."[74]

Beneficence—the flip side of nonmaleficence—describes a group of norms for providing benefit and for balancing benefit against risk and cost.[74] Accordingly, acts of mercy, kindness, and charity—colored by altruism, love, humanity, and a sense of obligation—drive global health work and its associated philanthropy.

Justice describes a group of norms for fairly distributing benefit, risk, and cost.[74] Justice is commonly understood as law or lawfulness; in the context of global health, the meaning of "justice" is closer to fairness and is considered a virtue. The concepts of legal justice, criminal justice, distributive justice, social justice, and the fair and equitable allocation of resources and benefits further refine the notion of justice. Philosophical theories and approaches to justice include egalitarianism, communitarianism, libertarianism, and utilitarianism. For constructive reflection on global health policies, various approaches with different emphases should be considered; the diverse problems in global delivery of health care are only partially addressed by any particular theory. Current emphasis on distributive justice focuses on equality, equity, and fairness, especially in allocating benefits and resources.

Aristotle's principle of formal justice or equality—that equals must be treated equally and that unequals must be treated unequally—is found in several theories of justice.[74] Many countries use one or several principles of distributive justice, such as "to each person an equal share," "to each person according to need," "to each person according to effort," "to each person according to contribution," "to each person according to merit," or "to each person according to free market exchanges."[74] In a related line of thinking, also used in constructing benchmarks of fairness, the Rawls-Daniel theories of fair and equal opportunity in health care

have gained currency in global health ethics. *Virtue* is a moral quality, which, like character, addresses the ethics of the agent (whether human being, society, or nation). This moral quality is inherent in the human psyche and as such contrasts to the *active* quality of the four ethical principles (autonomy, beneficence, nonmaleficence, and justice), which refer to the ethics of action. Moral virtues and character are expressed in different measures. In contemplating virtue and human character, the ancient Greek philosophers—Socrates, Plato, and Aristotle—identified five character types ranging from the great-souled human being to the moral monster.[75] According to Plato, the cardinal virtues included courage, temperance, wisdom, and justice; and to these cardinal virtues Thomas Aquinas in the 13th century added the Christian values of faith, hope, and charity.[75] However, Aristotle believed that a stupid person could have no true virtue; like other ancient Greek philosophers, Aristotle emphasized perfectionistic ideals and ethics that could not accommodate the equality of democracy.[75]

Many virtues—including compassion, discernment, trustworthiness, integrity, and conscientiousness—are central to health professionals[74] and equally admirable and desirable at many levels of global health care practice. Within the global binding matrix of values and ethics, these virtues have been made explicit by oaths whose recorded historical roots extend back to the great physician-surgeon Susruta of ancient India.[76] The idealistic, distinct professional ethics and morals incumbent on practitioners were further refined over centuries. Similarly, the Oath of Hippocrates, the Oath of the Muslim Physicians, and the Oath of Maimonides transcended cultures and boundaries.

The famed physician, alchemist, and Taoist Sun Szu-Miao (AD 581–682) wrote perhaps the oldest ethical text in China, *On the Absolute Sincerity of Great Physicians*. This treatise emphasized compassion, humaneness, self-discipline, education, and rigorous conscientiousness.[77] Value-based ethics clearly dominated and continues to dominate in most non-North American cultures.

THE ROLE OF RELIGION IN GLOBAL HEALTH ETHICS: CHRISTIANITY, ISLAM, AND JUDAISM

Ethics are grounded in sociocultural, philosophical, or religious convictions as well as in conventions deeply ingrained in the social fiber and culture of societies around the world. Health care choices and options are thus immensely influenced by religion. By their very nature, religions possess prescriptive moral ground rules for ethical judgment and fairness. As the cradle of 11 faiths, including the three major monotheistic faiths (Judaism, Christianity, and Islam) as well as Hinduism, Buddhism, Jainism, Confucianism, Shintoism, Baha'i, Taoism, and Zoroastrianism, Asia has a rich recorded tradition of values, ethics, and humanism. Ideals such as love, harmony, tolerance, respect, and reverence were often expressed in theological principles and as a way of life, whereas Western societies emphasized autonomy, justice, and rights—values that may be considered more measurable and practical. All these religions, as well as secularism, have influenced health ethics.

In many societies, religion and culture influence greatly how health care services are perceived, developed, accessed, and built upon. In many cultures around the world, beliefs regarding causation of health and recovery from illness were significantly affected by belief in the power of the "evil eye" as well as other concepts, such as karma, kismet, magic, spells, incantations, possessions by ghosts or spirits (evil and good), jinn, devil, witches, voodoo, departed ancestors, bad humors, and gods. Charismatic and revivalist Christian churches share with others a powerful belief that sin is a cause of disease.

Ecological wisdom and sacredness of the universe (especially earth) is enshrined in many of the major religions along with the unique stature and nobility of the human being. Even now, the quality of life, the environment, consumption, and the ecological crisis are at the center of expanded religious dialogue and response.[78]

HUMAN RIGHTS IN RELATION TO GLOBAL HEALTH ETHICS

The visionary WHO constitution, adopted in 1946, emphasizes the central tenet of the "right to health": "The enjoyment of the highest attainable standard of health is one of the fundamental rights of every human being without distinction of race, religion, political belief, economic, or social condition."[79]

The right to health was further strengthened by the Universal Declaration of Human Rights (UDHR), which was signed on December 10, 1948,[80] and enshrined the universal principles of freedom, dignity, and rights of individuals embedded in "reason and conscience." Article 25 of the UDHR is visionary in its broad outlook on the health of the "global individual" and states that "everyone has the right to a standard of living adequate for the health and well-being of himself [sic], and his [sic] family, including food, clothing, housing, medical care and necessary social services."[80]

Several other declarations and treaties strongly advocated elimination of discrimination against women; bolstered the rights of children; emphasized elimination of all forms of discrimination, torture, and other inhuman or degrading treatment as well as punishment, intolerance, and discrimination based on religion and belief.[81] Ample evidence exists to demonstrate that a violation of any of these rights leads to ill health.

The 1978 WHO Declaration of Alma Ata identified equity, human rights, and social justice as essential elements for achieving health for all.[82] The 1993 World Bank Report *Investing in Health*[28] further supported and connected rights-based principles to global health development in alleviating poverty and ill health and granting empowerment through education.

The powerful language and concepts expressed in human rights declarations of global health ethics—including equity, fairness, and justice—have been harnessed by groups of health care providers and lawyers devoted to empowering people globally in issues relating to their health. Groups such as the International Physicians for Prevention of Nuclear War, Physicians for Social Responsibility, Physicians for Human Rights, Médecins Sans Frontières, Médecins du Monde, Global Lawyers and Physicians, the Consortium for Health and Human Rights, Amnesty International, and the [US] National Academy of Sciences Committee on Human Rights have developed effective strategies for promoting health and for preventing and treating diseases and destruction of ecology.[82]

In the 21st century, the language and action of human rights pervades global politics, law, morality, and health and is expanding rapidly—as it should in its role as a premier global health ethics principle. Dialogue on human rights is central for global health governance.

THE ROLE OF SCIENTIFIC RESEARCH IN THE ADVANCEMENT OF GLOBAL HEALTH AND THE GLOBALIZATION OF RESEARCH ETHICS

Scientific research and innovation continue to be recognized as the key drivers for delivering health, equity and development beyond aid to low- and middle-income countries (LMICs).[83] The concept of "Beyond aid is about development that builds and consolidates countries' capacity to address their challenges themselves and to generate the necessary resources".[83] Whereas in 1990 the focus was on closing the "10/90 gap" for health research for development by transferring more resources to LMICs from high income countries,[84] today it is a reality that thriving economies and democracies, rule of law, human rights, and poverty reduction are the key drivers of good global health, development, and research.[83] As much as research is a quintessential tool for advancing global health, yet societies and nations worldwide have made uneven progress in the basic sciences, clinical sciences, and epidemiology. And like the research itself, ethical frameworks of research often suffer from lack of political will, poor economics, low levels of education, inadequate human resources, political corruption, and unexercised rights to information and justice. To secure a safer and more secure future, a 2011 editorial addressed the transformation of global health, global health education, infectious disease, and chronic conditions in the 21st century.[85]

However, as this scientific, educational, and research transformation accelerates, it must be recalled that global public health interventions, vaccines, and drug trials (whether randomized, controlled, clustered, or operational) are frequently done without clearly having the good of subjects as an end point. Ethical research controls used in developed countries are easily abandoned when studies are done in resource-poor settings. The primary good inheres to the academicians and to the large pharmaceutical companies and global consortia that fund these studies. The intent of intervention is often not to promote sustainability and ongoing involvement in the community but to prove a scientific point and then move on. The process of *globalization of research ethics* commenced with Article 25 of the Universal Declaration of Human Rights, a pivotal document that emphasizes that the benefits of scientific research must be accessible and of benefit to all humankind equally, so as to address the injustice prevalent in earlier decades.[80] Designed by European physicians as a professional guideline, this physicians' code of ethics was subsequently adopted by the World Medical Assembly at the 1964 Helsinki Meeting. Since then, the "Declaration of Helsinki" has undergone several revisions.[86]

The 1993 World Human Rights conference, held in Vienna, adopted the following template for global cooperation on ethical research:

> Everyone has the right to enjoy benefits of scientific progress and its applications ... and notes that advances, notably in the biomedical and life sciences as well as information technology may have potentially adverse consequences for the integrity, dignity, and human rights, of the individual and calls for international cooperation to ensure that human rights and dignity are fully respected in this area of universal concern.[87]

The UNESCO (IBC) document titled *Universal Declaration on Human Genome and Human Rights* succinctly affirms this statement and adds the language of nondiscrimination based on genetic characteristics.[88]

The CIOMS/WHO Guidelines reflect a paramount concern for protecting the rights and welfare of research subjects and of vulnerable individuals or groups. These guidelines are equally applicable in developed and developing countries. For instance, guideline 8 states that the research should be responsive to the health of the community and insists on familiarity with community customs, traditions, and priorities.[89] Guideline 15 states that the committees in both the sponsoring and hosting countries are responsible for conducting both scientific and ethical review. Equitable selection of subjects, privacy, and consent also are emphasized.[89–91]

GLOBAL HEALTH ETHICS: PRACTICAL ISSUES AND APPLICATIONS

To understand the practical issues and applications of global health ethics, various historical and ongoing ethical failures should be studied along with the remedial actions taken in response.

The "Doctors' Trial" at Nuremberg (1946–1947) led to the indictment of 16 of 23 Nazi German doctors, seven of whom were later executed by hanging, and nine of whom were imprisoned.[92] In this first-of-its-kind international trial, the physicians were convicted of murder and torture in the conduct of medical experiments on concentration camp inmates.[92] The central facts at issue in the trial related to physiologic research experiments, such as high-altitude, hypothermia, and seawater experiments, which were ordered by the state to benefit German pilots and soldiers.[92]

The defense pointed out that ethics were "similarly compromised" during the Statesville Penitentiary experiments on malaria (conducted in Illinois, USA, on more than 800 prisoners) and that no written consent had been given by its subjects (prisoners), although they were supposedly informed and had supposedly consented.[92] With its 10 standards, the Nuremberg ethical code was the first to establish the concepts of consent and full disclosure, including risks, benefits, safety, and the right to choose participation, protection of human subjects, avoidance of harm, use of initial animal studies, and a focus on useful research. This code merged Hippocratic ethics—with its maxim *primum non nocere* ("first, do no harm")—and human rights into a single code, thus widening the scope of research ethics. For the first time, consideration focused on the human subject, not the interests of either the researcher or the state.

Ethics violations committed in the United States early in the 20th century have included the use of prisoners as human subjects of research, a subject that has been reviewed extensively.[92] During the Nuremberg trials, the Nazi doctors drew attention to several instances of rights violations by American researchers; from the 1906 cholera experiments on inmates of the Bilibid Prison in Manila (where fatalities resulted from accidental bubonic plague serum injections) to pellagra studies in Mississippi.[92]

Other ethical violations captured the attention of the American public: testicular implants in San Quentin State Prison, tuberculosis experiments at Denver's National Jewish Hospital, and several post–World War II experiments with plasmapheresis, chemical warfare agents, pain threshold, and hepatitis.[92]

Violations of ethics and human rights have occurred in many countries (including the former communist countries of Europe) and continue today. Many of these violations have been documented and publicized in published literature.

Strict legislation came into effect in 1976, only after further unethical violations occurred. Examples of such violations included the thalidomide trials, the use of 22 senile patients for live cancer cell studies (at the Jewish Chronic Disease Hospital in New York City), and the Tuskegee syphilis experiments. Despite the Nuremberg pronouncements, researchers—including those working at major pharmaceutical and chemical companies—seemed unable to resist the wealth of test material contained within prisons.[92]

Ethics of Racial Profiling

Case Study 2: Racial Profiling of Blood Donors

Large inequalities exist globally in the distribution of safe blood: 80% of the world's population has access to only 20% of the world's blood supply.[93] Moreover, fewer than 30% of countries have nationwide blood transfusion services. Family members and paid donors are recognized sources of unsafe blood in approximately 50% of blood donations.[94] Each year, an estimated 80,000 to 160,000 people are infected with HIV as a result of receiving a blood transfusion.[95] The worldwide supply of safe transfusion products is thus inadequate, and tainted transfusion products are highly dangerous. Strategies are urgently needed for obtaining safe transfusion products effectively and efficiently. Epidemiologic data showing differences among some donor groups in rates of infection has led to instances of racial profiling in selection of blood donors.

Blood donation is thus an area of medical practice that has raised issues of global health ethics. In the context of national and global health, "racial profiling" and the use of "race" and ethnicity for making medical decisions have been the subjects of debate in both national and global health contexts. At present, race is at best an imperfect surrogate associated with many other variables, including language, health beliefs, culture, and socioeconomic status.[65]

In South Africa, a policy of profiling by race, gender, and donor came to light in 2004 after the public learned that South African president Mbeke's blood donation had been discarded as a result of the policy.[96] This revelation raised several ethical questions. One such question was whether profiling by race (or gender) can be a fair and just (ethical) process for ensuring the safety of health care practitioners as well as the safety of persons who receive transfusion products. The urgency of this question was evident in 1999 when antenatal HIV seroprevalence was higher than 20%. HIV prevalence in the blood donor pool reached 0.26%, and an estimated 26 HIV-infected units had entered the blood supply. Since that time, the procedure for processing blood donations was changed so that the new costs added $15 per unit. This new procedure avoids racial profiling, but how many nations can afford this added expense? Should it be a national budget priority?

This issue affects all nations regardless of their relative prosperity. In the United States in the early 1980s, for example, Haitian immigrants were identified by the US Centers for Disease Control and Prevention (CDC) as one of four major groups at risk for HIV/AIDS. In 1990, the US Food and Drug Administration refused to accept blood from Haitian donors.[97]

Ethics of Selection for Medical Treatment

The issue of selecting 3 million "lucky" persons globally to receive AIDS treatment by 2005 created an urgent problem for the WHO. The process should ensure transparency, fairness, and equality.[98] In this case, what constitutes distributive fairness? Should patients who have been "accidentally" infected by transfusions, health care workers at high risk, teachers, or tribal leaders have priority in receiving treatment over women and children? How was the transparency and fairness ensured?

Ethics of Research

Case Study 3: A Short-Term AIDS Clinical Trial in a Developing Country

A pharmaceutical company has a new AIDS drug. The focus of the initial clinical trials is a Latin American country. Participants are selected by "lottery" for a year-long study to be carried out at a local clinic. The protocol requires other components for the multidrug "cocktail."

At the end of the year, the enrolled patients gain weight and can work, earn a living, and look after their household. Their CD4 counts have improved dramatically, and the viral loads are "undetectable." The company stops the trial.[99]

Who benefited from this study? Were the patients appropriately notified that they were participating in a study for 1 year only and that, after completion of the study, they would be released without drugs and that progress of their AIDS would consequently accelerate?

Was the developing country chosen because of lax ethical guidelines? Would the trial become ethically appropriate if local researchers participated? Were the company and investigators obligated to ensure drug subsidies or free drugs for study participants for a reasonable number of years, considering that drugs are required for lifelong suppression of HIV?

Case Study 4: A Placebo-Controlled Study in a Developing Country

A study protocol showed that zidovudine (AZT) reduced perinatal transmission of HIV by 65%. Use of AZT was therefore considered highly efficacious therapy and rapidly became the standard of care in the United States. The National Institutes of Health (NIH) and CDC subsequently sponsored randomized placebo-controlled trials of alternative, less costly protocols of AZT.

Is the use of a placebo-control study protocol ethical in countries or communities where the standard of care is no drug or no other active intervention? Is the use of a placebo-control protocol in this case an example of scientific and imperialistic colonialism? Are the researchers in this case "mosquito scientists," that is, researchers who enter a country to extract blood samples and take them out of the country, releasing the results only at publication of the study?[100,101] Did the researchers consider the culture and health beliefs of the participants outside the United States?

The study rationale was that administering a placebo is justified when effective treatment exists because placebo-controlled trials are the quickest way to validate drug efficacy. Is this argument valid?

Case Study 5: The Tuskegee Syphilis Study

The historic Tuskegee study of untreated syphilis was sponsored by the US Public Health Service and lasted for 40 years, beginning in 1932 and ending in 1973.[102–105] A total of 412 impoverished African American men with untreated syphilis were monitored and compared with 204 disease-free men to determine the natural history of syphilis. The research continued despite the availability of penicillin and despite the known fact that penicillin cures syphilis.

No informed consent was signed by any of the 412 study participants.

Multiple serious ethical violations were committed in this study and were documented. Did the researchers have a valid argument when they stated that "these poor African American males probably would not have been treated anyway" and that the investigators were therefore "merely observing what would happen"?[102–105]

Case Study 6: Race and Study Design

In 1997, a total of 16 randomized trials were conducted in several African nations as well as the Dominican Republic and Thailand to evaluate use effectiveness of a less costly method of preventing perinatal transmission of HIV. A total of 17,000 pregnant women participated in the trials. In all except one trial, a placebo was used as the control. Subsequently, the study participants gave birth to more than 1,000 babies who were infected with HIV. None of the 16 trials was funded by either the CDC or the NIH.[106]

Did the fact that all participants were nonwhite represent an ethically questionable study design? Was this series of trials an example of exploitation because no benefits accrued to the study population beyond the study period?

Case Study 7: Clinical Trials in Children

A trial of a new antibiotic, trovafloxacin, was conducted during a meningitis epidemic in Kano, Nigeria,[107] an impoverished city already devastated by concomitant outbreaks of cholera and measles. In a 2-week period, six physicians employed by a large American pharmaceutical company conducted the trial in children by using an oral formulation of Trovan along with a reduced dose of the comparison drug, ceftriaxone. The study perpetrated several ethical breaches, including deviation from protocol, lack of informed consent, inaccurate record keeping, inadequate follow-up, and failure to offer subjects a choice of alternative treatment. In addition, no previous research was conducted to study the pharmacokinetics in children. The study thus violated Nigerian law as well as the Helsinki Declaration of Human Rights and the UN Convention on the Rights of Children. In its defense, the pharmaceutical company claimed that the study was "a philanthropic act."

Was this trial an example of opportunistic research that unscrupulously exploited the needs of a vulnerable population?

Case Study 8: Clinical Trials and the Standard of Care

A placebo-controlled arm was included in a Ugandan clinical trial of various regimens of prophylaxis against tuberculosis in HIV-infected adults, most of whom had positive results of tuberculin skin tests.[108] Meanwhile, in the United States, the standard of care for HIV-infected persons with positive tuberculin skin test results called for prophylaxis against tuberculosis.

Should future studies in developing and developed countries include a placebo arm if a standard of care exists for other populations?[109,110]

Defining the Ethical Parameters of Global Health Research

Bhutta's discussion of ethics in global health research from the perspective of the developing world is valuable not only because it points out examples of poorly designed studies, but also because it illustrates studies done properly.[111] Important lessons are also learned from other studies, including the groundbreaking Gambian studies on hepatitis B and *Haemophilus influenzae* type b vaccine,[112] the Gadchiorli neonatal study of suspected sepsis in India,[113] and the randomized controlled trial of the effect of handwashing on child health.[114]

Another admired effort in epidemiology, the International Clinical Epidemiology Network, has successfully developed a sustainable network of clinical epidemiology units in the developing world with technical assistance from European and North American universities.[27,115] Focusing on health research needs in developing countries, where data are meager and often unreliable and where new health research needs and tools are prioritized in the national context, Morrow and Lansang[27] based their equity-oriented approach on the needs of people in developing countries. In the developing world, limited resources, expertise, and capacity for research, as well as poor infrastructure, competing national agendas, and loss of human resources (in the form of internal and external "brain drain") pose tremendous challenges. Implementation of ethical principles and creation of equitable, sustainable, mutually beneficial partnerships focusing on equity and societal needs require innovative solutions. The CIOMS[91]and the Swiss Commission Guidelines[116] clearly enunciated important principles and parameters for culturally sensitive, appropriate research. Central points included in the Swiss guidelines[116] include: collective formulation of objectives; building mutual trust; sharing information, responsibility, and responses; developing networks; creating transparency; monitoring and evaluating the collaboration; disseminating and applying results equitably; increasing the research capacity; and building on past achievements.

A casebook with a collection of 64 case studies, each raising important and difficult ethical issues connected with not only the planning but conducting health-related research was published by the WHO.

This valuable tool is suitable to train scientists and research ethics committee members or for use in developing certificate courses.[117]

Ethics of Responsibility

Western technologic, scientific, and informational civilization has created a massive gap in the moral-ethical arena, especially with ecological concerns, including eradication of the rainforest; depletion of earth's atmospheric ozone layer; global warming; degradation of air, water, and soil quality; loss of biodiversity; species extinction; misuse of animals; disappearance of wetlands and open lands; and need for wilderness preservation and animal biotechnological interventions.[118]

Geologic deposits of sewage, garbage, and toxic waste provoked the comment, "Surely no creature other than the human being has ever managed to foul its nest in such short order."[119] Powerful industrial and commercial forces have unleashed tremendous hurt onto our biosystems and have shifted the naturally self-rejuvenating balance of the ecosystem—a balance that is closely interwoven with human health. Global health and eco-health are hurt by nations as well as by large corporations operating with unlimited ecological autonomy despite a local and global obligation to act as stewards of the earth and its resources. The WHO report *Ecosystems and Human Well-Being: Health Synthesis* highlights the complex links between preservation of health and biodiversity, natural ecosystems, and human health and concludes, "Over the past 50 years, humans have changed natural ecosystems more rapidly and extensively than in any comparable period in human history."[120]

Case Study 9: Conflict of Interest

In 2000, a group of 30,000 indigenous persons and peasants filed a lawsuit against an oil company operating in Ecuador, accusing the oil company of inflicting irreparable damage to the Amazon rainforest. The lawsuit was dismissed by a US court.[121] Negative consequences of oil exploitation have occurred also in Bolivia, Colombia, Peru, and other Latin American, African, and Asian countries.

In evaluating the merits of this case, consider the following two statements:

- "Oil is a major source of income for Ecuador and since the 1970s has been the 'engine' of the nation's economy, which averages 7% growth annually. Per capita income rose from US$290 in 1972 to US$1,200 in 2000, and oil makes up 40% of the national budget. Petroecuador, the government-owned company, is responsible for 55% of the total oil production."[121]

- Morbidity and mortality rates in oil-producing areas are higher than in communities without this involvement.

What should be the ethical response of the government? What should be the response and responsibility of all oil companies? Does the WHO or the UN have a role in this situation? Is this case an example of a human rights violation?

Case Study 10: Conflicts of Interest Concerning Pandemics

In 1918, a total of 20 to 50 million people perished from the "Spanish flu," a strain of influenza that seems to have been a variant of the avian flu virus.[122] The HIV epidemic has caused more than 13 million children to become orphaned. The late-20th-century limited outbreak of SARS and subsequent threat of pandemic avian influenza refocused global energy on planning and on ethical and legal issues such as equity, access, fair process, vulnerability, civic engagement, and allocation of existing resources globally and locally.[122] Regulation, intellectual property, market incentives, and liability issues have further added more complex ramifications.

In ethical planning regarding higher attack rates in younger, healthy populations and regarding availability of scarce resources, does an altruistic, equity-based process take precedence over a selection process favoring intergenerational group priority (e.g., for the elderly, the frail, the chronically ill, infants, and pregnant females)?[122] How should such consideration be applied in sub-Saharan nations? The SARS outbreak in Toronto raised further questions, such as risks to providers and their families. Key ethical issues and underlying values such as individual liberty, protection of the public from harm, proportionality, reciprocity, transparency, privacy, protection of communities from undue stigmatization, duty to provide care, equity, and solidarity have been highlighted.[123]

Therapeutic and Reproductive Cloning and Stem Cell Research: Ethical Challenges

Now that mapping and sequencing of the human genome have enabled human beings to look into the mirror of self cloning, current debate focuses on the science of cloning (especially reproductive cloning), cloning technologies, stem cell research applications, and moral consequences of these activities. This novel encounter with the basic elements of life, prospects of self regeneration, and the ability to choose future progeny has led all religions to ban cloning of an entire human being.

Cloning Californians? The Report of the California Advisory Committee on Human Cloning[124] summarized notes for members of the California State Legislature on the ethics of human cloning and stem cell research and addressed some complex aspects of the debates. Limited stem cell research is currently occurring globally after successful cloning of sheep (despite adverse consequences to the test animals).

At the beginning of the new millennium, a global consensus across nations and faiths states that reproductive cloning should not be allowed. The most robust opposition to all forms of cloning has been declared by the Roman Catholic Church, which is spread across several countries. Differences of opinion between Arab states and other Muslim nations have been expressed. Some of these Muslim countries have conducted highly advanced genomic research, whereas some Arab states are considering a regionwide ban on human cloning. Participants at the November 2003 session of the UN General Assembly reached no consensus on the issue of cloning.[125]

Ethical debate on cloning remains within the matrix of religious beliefs, values, and norms of societies and within the progress of science. Increasingly, however, therapeutic cloning is gaining favor because its central concepts and objectives relate to curing disease as well as improving health and quality of life for all humanity. Nonetheless, as of this writing, regenerative cloning has been banned globally by all major religions. Limited research on human cloning for harvesting stem cells is occurring in the United Kingdom, Japan, and the United States. Current thorny, fundamental debate centers on the concept of life itself. Is the embryo a "human being" after the second week of gestation (when differentiation of the sensory system begins), after the third week (when early signs of heartbeat can be detected), when fetal movement occurs as noted by ultrasound (at the tenth week of gestation), or when the fetal movements are first noticed by the mother (at 16 weeks of gestation)?[125]

In Islam, three stages of inception have been defined: the fusion of the "spermed" ovum (zygote stage), implantation, and "ensoulment" at 120 days of inception. Some believe that the latter occurs at the 40th day.[125] Today, consensus in Islam maintains that any debate on cloning need not rest on scientific merit alone and that advances in science should not be regarded as a threat to religious belief as long as human dignity, values, and cultures are honored. However, very conservative Muslims, like their conservative Christian counterparts, tend to draw a line in the sand and are totally opposed to any form of cloning. Recent controversies revolve around the legality, morality, and social responsibility of somatic cell nuclear transfer and commercialization of cloning technology and its various applications from cloning pets and endangered animal species to therapeutic cloning to produce stem cells for the treatment of several chronic diseases such as diabetes, Parkinson's, and Alzheimer's.[126–128] Thus science and commercial interests will henceforth continue to be the driving force, and our expectations are that the societal moral forces will continue to be the guiding modifiers to prevent excesses and abusive practices.

TOWARD A BRAVE NEW VISION OF GLOBAL HEALTH ETHICS IN THE NEW MILLENNIUM

The ethical values and principles enshrined in the covenants and oaths of the global physician are increasingly being challenged by a new world order that emphasizes consumerism and greed at the expense of health. Historically, like the medical profession's central dictum—that disease and illness transcend boundaries and borders—"cybernations" also transport knowledge and cures across borders and across castes, creeds, religions, and cultures. Certain universal guiding principles and values bind all physicians and health care providers, and even more so the global health physician, in unremitting pursuit of health for all. Taylor[76] outlined such ethical principles for the "international physician" in a "free version of the Hippocratic Oath" (see Table 21-4), which still relates well to the global health physician.

Table 21–4. Taylor's "Free Version of the Hippocratic Oath"[a]

- I will share the science and art by precept, by demonstration, and by every mode of teaching with other physicians regardless of their national origin.
- I will try to help secure for the physicians in each country the esteem of their own people, and through collaborative work see that they get full credit.
- I will strive to eliminate sources of disease everywhere in the world and not merely set up barriers to the spread of disease to my own people.
- I will work for understanding of the diverse causes of diseases, including social, economic, and environmental.
- I will promote the well-being of mankind in all its aspects, not merely the bodily, with sympathy and consideration for a people's culture and beliefs.
- I will strive to prevent painful and untimely death, and also help parents to achieve a family size conforming to their desires and to their ability to care for their children. In my concern with whole communities I will never forget the needs of its individual members.

---

[a]Taylor CE. Ethics for an international health profession. Science 1966 Aug 12;153(3737):716–720. (Reproduced with permission.)

Kofi Annan's poignant and pragmatic reminder of the "Butterfly effect" is indeed the new ethical world order: "Today's real borders are not between nations, but between powerful and powerless, free and fettered, privileged and humiliated. Today, no walls can separate humanitarian or human rights crises in one part of the world from national security crises in another."[129]

The global human being must be the focus of global health ethics as proclaimed by the WHO charter[129] and by the UN Charter. If the 19th century was the century of public health action and the 20th century, that of international health and the beginning of global health, then the 21st century will certainly be defined by a new and more profound awareness of health ethics, rights, equity, fairness, justice, and solidarity, each concept centered on the dignity of the global human being. We entered the new millennium through a "gate of fire," the tragedy and horror of September 11, 2001, which was masterminded by one global human being. Similarly, genocide and ethnic "cleansing" begins with the killing of one global human being, not for what was done but because of who that individual is.[120] "What begins with failure to uphold the dignity of one life, all too often ends with calamity for entire nations."[129]

Accordingly, the UN has outlined three key priorities for the new millennium: eradicating poverty, preventing conflict, and promoting democracy. These priorities are also key elements in ensuring health advancement. They are of paramount importance if the 21st century is to show improvement over the 20th century, which saw numerous and extensive wars, violence, hatred, poverty, exploitation, ethnic cleansing, and other human violations that caused millions of people to lose their lives or become permanently injured or displaced.

Worldwide application of global health ethics requires the competent cooperation of all the world's governments. Currently, however, global public health governance is justifiably perceived as antiquated and structurally weak.[130,131] Ethical reform processes are needed to address national and global governance in this 21st century amid threatened and spreading global violence, novel health challenges, and loss of many health gains acquired during the past two centuries. Transforming the words of treaties, declarations, and understandings into practical reality cannot take place in a vacuum of autonomy claimed by powerful nations, dictators, or global corporations; indeed, insular self-interests as well as relevant, limited aspects of state sovereignty have recently been relinquished to address transnational health threats such as SARS, avian influenza, and the Global Framework on Tobacco Control.[132,133]

To accelerate the agenda to reshape global governance for health, reduce inequalities, improve transparency, define national and international roles and responsibilities in a post-MDG world, the Joint Action and Learning Initiative on National and Global Responsibilities for health has formed an international campaign to advocate for a Framework Convention on Global Health. This initiative has received endorsement from the UN Secretary General.[134]

Global Health Training and Ethics

There has been considerable activity to ensure that we construct bridges and partnerships based on mutual respect, trust, beneficence, and solidarity within the framework of a new world order, amid increasing global vulnerability, safety, and security concerns. The building blocks of these efforts include shared knowledge, generation and application of new knowledge, a shared global workforce, resources, including natural resources, peace, and effective, fair, and representative governance. Shared safety and security have many components, such as basic rights to food, clean water, shelter, jobs, education, and freedom of worship.[135]

With a tremendous recent welcome emphasis on global health education and training and the proliferation of global health institutes and centers of excellence, a number of authors have developed valuable ethical principles and guidance, some with working case examples, in how to structure ethical, mutually beneficial, transparent, sustainable training, service, and research partnerships.[136–142]

In a collective partnership nurtured by ethics and harmony, civil societies must be reenergized and empowered to protect individual health and rights because these rights—primarily health security and well-being—are intimately tied to societal obligations. To achieve these goals, ethical concepts operating for the good of all human beings—the global person— have been described by a vocabulary first recorded many centuries ago. Ancient Asian concepts of harmony, tolerance, values, and love can serve as bridges to more concrete, practical, and secular Western concepts of ethics.[143]

STUDY QUESTIONS

See each case study for study questions on various global health ethical issues.

ACKNOWLEDGMENTS

Bibliographic assistance was provided by Yvonne Sargent and Carolyn Fishel for this chapter in both this edition and the first edition of this text. Editorial assistance was provided by the staff of the Medical Editing Service of the Permanente Medical Group Physician Education and Development Department: Lila Schwartz, David W. Brown, Janet H. Startt, and Juan Domingo, for the first edition.

REFERENCES

1. Velji A, Bryant J. Global health: evolving meanings. *Infect Dis Clin North Am* 2011;25(2):299–309.
2. Koplan J, Bond T, Merson M, et al. Towards a common definition of global health. *Lancet* 2009;373(9679): 1993–1995.
3. Declaration of Alma-Ata. International Conference on Primary Health Care, Alma-Ata, USSR, September 6–12, 1978. http://www.who.int/publications/almaata_declaration_en.pdf.
4. Singer P, Pellegrino E, Siegler M. Clinical ethics revisited. *BMC Med Ethics* 2001;2:E1.
5. Jonsen A. The origins of bioethics in the United States of America. In: Bankowski Z, Bryant J, eds. *Poverty, Vulnerability, the Value of Human Life, and the Emergence of Bioethics: Highlights and Papers of the XXVIIIth CIOMS Conference, Ixtapa, Guerrero State, Mexico, 17–20 April 1994.* Geneva: CIOMS, 1994:38–40.
6. Mainetti J. Academic and mundane bioethics in Argentina. In: Pellegrino E, Mazzarella P, Corsi P, eds. *Transcultural Dimensions in Medical Ethics.* Frederick, MD: University Publishing Group, 1992: 43–55.
7. Pellegrino E. Prologue: intersections of Western biomedical ethics and world culture. In: Pellegrino E, Mazzarella P, Corsi P, eds. *Transcultural Dimensions in Medical Ethics.* Frederick, MD: University Publishing Group, 1992: 13–19.
8. Velji A, ed. International health. *Infect Dis Clin North Am* 1991;5(two-theme issue):183–435.
9. Velji A, ed. International health. Beyond the year 2000. *Infect Dis Clin North Am* 1995;(two-theme issue):223–461.
10. Velji A, ed. Global health, global health education, and infectious disease: the new millennium, part I. *Infect Dis Clin North Am* 2011;25(2):xiii–xxi.
11. Velji A, ed. Global health, global health education, and infectious disease: the new millennium, part II. *Infect Dis Clin North Am* 2011;25(3):xiii–xxii.
12. Stuck C, Bickley L, Wallace N, et al. International health medical education consortium. Its history, philosophy, and role in medical education and health development. *Infect Dis Clin North Am* 1995;9(2):419–423.
13. Velji A. Global health education consortium: 20 years of leadership in global health and global health education. *Infect Dis Clin North Am* 2011;25(2):323–335.
14. Bryant J. [opening of the conference]. In: Bankowski Z, Bryant J, Gallagher J, eds. *Ethics, Equity and the Renewal of WHO's Health-for-All Strategy: Proceedings of the XXIXth CIOMS Conference, Geneva, Switzerland, 12–14 March 1997.* Geneva: CIOMS, 1997: 1–3.
15. Nakajima H. [opening of the conference]. In: Bankowski Z, Bryant J, Gallagher J, eds. *Ethics, Equity and the Renewal of WHO's Health-for-All Strategy: Proceedings of the XXIXth CIOMS Conference, Geneva, Switzerland, 12–14 March 1997.* Geneva: CIOMS, 1997: 4–6.
16. Delamothe T. Embargoes that endanger health [editorial]. *BMJ* 1997;315(7120):1393–1394.

17. Fort M, Mercer M, Gish O, eds. *Sickness and Wealth: The Corporate Assault on Global Health.* Cambridge, MA: South End Press, 2004.

18. Kim J, Millen J, eds. *Dying for Growth: Global Inequality and the Health of the Poor.* Monroe, ME: Common Courage Press, 2000.

19. Bankowski Z, Bryant J, Gallagher J, eds. *Ethics, Equity and the Renewal of WHO's Health-for-All Strategy: Proceedings of the XXIXth CIOMS Conference, Geneva, Switzerland, 12–14 March 1997.* Geneva: CIOMS, 1997.

20. Taylor C. Ethical issues influencing health for all beyond the year 2000. *Infect Dis Clin North Am* 1995;9(2):223–233.

21. Taylor C. Surveillance for equity in primary health care: policy implications from international experience. *Int J Epidemiol* 1992;21(6):1043–1049.

22. Whitehead M. William Farr's legacy to the study of inequalities in health. *Bull World Health Organ* 2000;78(1):86–87.

23. Gwatkin D. Health inequalities and the health of the poor: what do we know? What can we do? *Bull World Health Organ* 2000;78(1):3–18.

24. Evans T, Whitehead M, Diderichsen F, et al., eds. *Challenging Inequities in Health Care: From Ethics to Action.* New York, NY: Oxford University Press, 2001.

25. Brock D. Working Group III. Measurement/surveillance for equity: health status and health systems functions. In: Bankowski Z, Bryant J, Gallagher J, eds. *Ethics, Equity and the Renewal of WHO's Health-for-All Strategy: Proceedings of the XXIXth CIOMS Conference, Geneva, Switzerland, 12–14 March 1997.* Geneva: CIOMS, 1997: 171–173.

26. Morrow R, Bryant J. Measuring and valuing human life: cost-effectiveness, equity and other ethics-based issues. In: Bankowski Z, Bryant J, eds. *Poverty, Vulnerability, the Value of human life, and the Emergence of Bioethics: Highlights and Papers of the XXVIIIth CIOMS Conference, Ixtapa, Guerrero State, Mexico, 17–20 April 1994.* Geneva: CIOMS, 1994:53–56.

27. Morrow R, Lansang M. The role of clinical epidemiology in establishing essential national health research capabilities in developing countries. *Infect Dis Clin North Am* 1991;5(2):235–246.

28. World development report 1993: Investing in Health. The World Bank Web site. http://econ.worldbank.org/external/default/main?pagePK=64165259&theSitePK=469382&piPK=64165421&menuPK=64166093&entityID=000009265_3970716142319.

29. Murray C. Quantifying the burden of disease: the technical basis for disability-adjusted life years. *Bull World Health Organ*1994;72(3):429–445.

30. Murray C, Acharya A. Understanding DALYs (disability-adjusted life years). *J Health Econ* 1997;16(6):703–730.

31. Caplan R, Light D, Daniels N. Benchmarks of fairness: a moral framework for assessing equity. *Int J Health Serv* 1999;29(4):853–869.

32. Daniels N, Bryant J, Castano RA, et al. Benchmarks of fairness for healthcare reform: a policy tool for developing countries. *Bull World Health Organ* 2000;78(6):740–750.

33. Daniels N, Flores W, Pannarunothai S, et al. An evidence-based approach to benchmarking the fairness of health-sector reform in developing countries. *Bull World Health Organ* 2005;83(7):534–540.

34. Ntuli A, Khosa S, McCoy D. The equity gauge. Health Systems Trust Web site. http://www.healthlink.org.za/publications/104 Published 1999.

35. Joint United Nations Program on HIV/AIDS, United Nations Children's Fund, and United States Agency for International Development. Children on the brink 2004: a joint report of new orphan estimates and a framework for action. United Nations Children's Fund Web site. http://www.unicef.org/publications/files/cob_layout6-013.pdf. Published 2004.

36. Bryant J, Bryant N, Williams S, Ndambuki R, Erwin P. Addressing social determinants of health by integrating assessment of caregiver-child attachment into community-based primary health care in urban Kenya. *Int J Environ Res Public Health* 2012;9:3588–3598.

37. Population and health dynamics in Nairobi's informal settlements: report of the Nairobi Cross-Sectional Slums Survey (NCSS) 2000. African Population and Health Research Center Web site. http://www.aphrc.org/images/Downloads/ncss%20report.pdf. Published 2002.

38. The challenge of slums: global report on human settlements 2003. United Nations Human Settlements Programme Web site. http://www.unhabitat.org/pmss/listItemDetails.aspx?publicationID=1156

39. Subbarao K, Coury D. Reaching out to Africa's orphans: a framework for public action. The World Bank Web site. http://siteresources.worldbank.org/INTHIVAIDS/Resources/375798-1103037153392/ReachingOuttoAfricasOrphans.pdf Published 2004.

40. Committee on Integrating the Science of Early Childhood Development, Shonkoff JP, Phillips DA, eds. From neurons to neighborhoods: the science of early childhood development. National Academies Press Web site. http://www.nap.edu/books/0309069882/html/. Published 2000.

41. The importance of caregiver-child interactions for the survival and healthy development of young children: a review. World Health Organization Web site. http://www.who.int/maternal_child_adolescent/documents/924159134X/en/index.html. Published 2004.

42. Feachem R. Poverty and inequity: a proper focus for the new century. *Bull World Health Organ* 2000;78(1):1–2.

43. Mann J, Tarantola D. The global AIDS pandemic: toward a new vision of health. *Infect Dis Clin North Am* 1995;9(2):275–285.

44. Annual Report 2005. The World Bank Web site. http://web.worldbank.org/WBSITE/EXTERNAL/EXTABOUTUS/EXTANNREP/EXTANNREP2K5/0,,menuPK:1397361~pagePK:64168427~piPK:64168435~theSitePK:1397343,00.html Published 2005.

45. Millennium Development goals. The World Bank Web site. http://www.mdgawards.org/webroot/index.php?option=com_content&view=article&id=50&Itemid=56 Published 2004.

46. Sachs J, McArthur J. The Millennium Project: a plan for meeting the Millennium Development Goals. *Lancet* 2005; 365(9456):347–353.

47. Velji A. International health. Beyond the year 2000. *Infect Dis Clin North Am* 1991;5(2):417–428.

48. Umhau T, Umhau J, Morgan R. National and international health agencies. Profile of key players. *Infect Dis Clin North Am* 1991;5(2):197–220.

49. Howard L. Public and private donor financing for health in developing countries. *Infect Dis Clin North Am* 1991;5(2):221–234.

50. Cohen J. Global health. The new world of global health. *Science* 2006;311(5758):162–167.

51. US Global Health Policy. *US Funding for the Global Health Initiative (GHI): the President's FY 2013 Budget Request Fact Sheet.* Menlo Park, CA: Henry Kaiser Family Foundation, February 2012. http://www.kff.org/globalhealth/upload/8160-02.pdf.

52. Leach-Kemon K, Chou D, Schneider A, et al. The global financial crisis has led to a slowdown in growth of funding to improve health in many countries. *Health Affairs* 2012;31(1):1–8. http://www.healthmetricsandevaluation.org/sites/default/files/publication_summary/2011/Global_Financial_Crisis_Led_Slowdown_Health_Affairs_Dec_2011_IHME.pdf.

53. Bissell R. International health: beyond the year 2000. Project selection. Many needs, few resources. *Infect Dis Clin North Am* 1995;9(2):377–389.

54. Marmot M. Social determinants of health inequalities. *Lancet* 2005;365(9464):1099–1104.

55. Labonte R, Schrecker T, Grupta AS. A global health equity agenda for the G8 summit. *BMJ* 2005;330(7490):533–536.

56. Osuntokun B. A developing-country perspective on the emergence of bioethics. In: Bankowski Z, Bryant J, eds. *Poverty, Vulnerability, the Value of Human Life, and the Emergence of Bioethics: Highlights and Papers of the XXVIIIth CIOMS Conference, Ixtapa, Guerrero State, Mexico, 17–20 April 1994.* Geneva: CIOMS, 1994: 42–46.

57. World development report 1994. The World Bank Web site. http://econ.worldbank.org/external/default/main?pagePK=64165259&theSitePK=469382&piPK=64165421&menuPK=64166322&entityID=000011823_20071010172019.

58. Abbasi K. Free the slaves [editorial]. *BMJ* 1999;318(7198):1568–1569.

59. Crossette B. Kofi Annan's astonishing facts! *New York Times,* September 27, 1998. http://www.nytimes.com/1998/09/27/weekinreview/kofi-annan-s-astonishing-facts.html.

60. Carter J. The Nobel lecture, December 10, 2002, Oslo, Norway. The Nobel Peace Prize Web site. http://nobelpeaceprize.org/en_GB/laureates/laureates-2002/carter-lecture/.

61. Human Development Report 2000: human rights and human development. United Nations Development Programme Web site. http://hdr.undp.org/reports/global/2000/en/. Published 2000.

62. Handful hog most of the wealth. *Business Times* (Johannesburg, South Africa), September 13, 1998. http://webcache.googleusercontent.com/search?q=cache:TXIZAYchXE8J:http://www.btimes.co.za/98/0913/world/world04.htm%2BHandful+hog+most+of+the+wealth&hl=en&gbv=2&prmd=ivns&strip=1.

63. Mukherjee J. Global injustice. In: Fort M, Mercer MA, Gish O, eds. *Sickness and Wealth: The Corporate Assault on Global Health.* Cambridge, MA: South End Press, 2004: xiii.

64. Lee S, Mountain J, Koenig B. The meanings of "race" in the new genomics: implications for health disparities research. *Yale J Health Policy Law Ethics* 2001;1:33–75.

65. American Anthropological Association response to OMB Directive 15: race and ethnic standards for federal statistics and administrative reporting. American Anthropological Association Web site. http://www.aaanet.org/gvt/ombdraft.htm Published September 1997.

66. Barth F. Introduction. In: Barth F, ed. *Ethnic Groups and Boundaries: The Social Organization of Cultural Differences.* Boston: Little, Brown, 1969: 9–38.

67. Curlin P, Tinker A. Women's health. *Infect Dis Clin North Am* 1995;9(2):335–351.

68. Cook R, Dickens B, Fathalla M. *Reproductive Health and Human Rights: Integrating Medicine, Ethics, and Law.* Oxford: Clarendon Press, 2003.

69. Grant G. *The State of the World's Children 1992.* New York: Oxford University Press, 1992.

70. Safe abortion: technical and policy guidance for health systems. World Health Organization Web site. http://extranet.who.int/iris/bitstream/10665/70914/1/9789241548434_eng.pdf Published 2003.

71. Velji A. Preface. *Infect Dis Clin North Am* 1991;5(2):xii–xv.

72. Gillon R. Medical ethics: four principles plus attention to scope. *BMJ* 1994; 309(6948):184–188.

73. Gillon R. Ethics needs principles—four can encompass the rest—;and respect for autonomy should be "first among equals." *J Med Ethics* 2003;29(5):307–312.

74. Beauchamp T, Childress J. *Principles of Biomedical Ethics,* 5th ed. New York: Oxford University Press, 2001.

75. Pence G. Virtue theory. In: Singer P, ed. *A Companion to Ethics.* Oxford: Blackwell, 1991: 249–258.

76. Taylor C. Ethics for an international health profession. *Science* 1966;153(3737):716–720.

77. Tsai D. Ancient Chinese medical ethics and the four principles of biomedical ethics. *J Med Ethics* 1999;25(4):315–321.

78. Tucker M, Grim J. Series forward: the nature of the environmental crisis. Center for the Study of World Religions Web site. http://www.hds.harvard.edu/cswr/research/ecology/foreword.html Published 2005.

79. Constitution of the World Health Organization. World Health Organization Web site. http://www.searo.who.int/LinkFiles/About_Searo_const.pdf.

80. Universal declaration of human rights. United Nations Web site. http://www.un.org/Overview/rights.html.

81. Mann J, Gostin L, Gruskin S, et al. Health and human rights. *Health Hum Rights* 1994;1(1):6–23.

82. Annas G. Human rights and health—the Universal Declaration of Human Rights at 50. *N Engl J Med* 1998;339(24):1778–1781.

83. COHRED, The Ministry of Science and Technology, The Ministry of Health. *Beyond AID: Research and Innovation as Key Drivers for Health, Equity and Development.* Final Report to Forum 2012: Cape Town, SA, 2012 http://www.forum2012.org/2012/10/final-report-to-forum-2012-on-beyond-aid-research-and-innovation-as-key-drivers-for-health-equity-and-development/.

84. Commission on Health Research for Development. *Health Research: Essential Link to Equity Development.* New York: Oxford University Press, 1990.

85. Velji A. Transforming global health, global health education, infectious disease, and chronic conditions in the 21st century. *Infect Dis Clin N Am* 2011;25:485–498.

86. Declaration of Helsinki. World Medical Association Web site. http://www.wma.net/en/30publications/10policies/b3/17c.pdf Published 2003.

87. Report of the World Conference on Human Rights. United Nations Web site. http://www.unhchr.ch/Huridocda/Huridoca.nsf/TestFrame/76a62cb583c2a55c802567c9004c62ea?Opendocument.

88. Mayor F. Message from Federico Mayor, Director-General, UNESCO. In: Bankowski Z, Bryant JH, Gallagher J, eds. *Ethics, Equity and the Renewal of WHO's Health-for-All*

strategy: Proceedings of the XXIXth CIOMS Conference, Geneva, Switzerland, 12–14 March 1997. Geneva: CIOMS, 1997: 7.

89. Bankowski Z, Levine R. A decade of the CIOMS programme: health policy, ethics and human values: an international dialogue. In: Bankowski Z, Bryant J, eds. *Poverty, Vulnerability, the Value of Human Life, and the Emergence of Bioethics: Highlights and Papers of the XXVIIIth CIOMS Conference, Ixtapa, Guerrero State, Mexico, 17–20 April 1994.* Geneva: CIOMS, 1994: 13–25.

90. Bankowski Z, Bryant J, Last J, eds. *Ethics and Epidemiology: International Guidelines: Proceedings of the XXVth CIOMS Conference, Geneva, Switzerland, 7–9 November 1990: cosponsored by the World Health Organization.* Geneva: CIOMS, 1991.

91. International ethical guidelines for biomedical research involving human subjects. Council for International Organizations of Medical Sciences (CIOMS) Web site. http://www.cioms.ch/publications/guidelines/guidelines_nov_2002_blurb.htm.

92. Hornblum A. They were cheap and available: prisoners as research subjects in twentieth century America. *BMJ* 1997;315(7120):1437–1441.

93. WHO: protect the public from contaminated blood: 55th session of the WHO Regional Committee. World Health Organization Regional Office for the Western Pacific Web site. http://www2.wpro.who.int/rcm/en/archives/rc55/press_releases/pr_20040916_3.htm. Published 2004.

94. Fact sheets: blood safety and voluntary donations. World Health Organization Regional Office for the Western Pacific Web site. http://www.wpro.who.int/mediacentre/factsheets/fs_20040610/en/index.html. Published 2004.

95. Blood supply and demand [editorial]. *Lancet* 2005;365(9478):2151.

96. Global challenges: South African blood service to stop calculating donors' risk of HIV infection based on race. Henry Kaiser Family Foundation Web site. http://www.kaiserhealthnews.org/Daily-Reports/2004/December/07/dr00027102.aspx?p= 1 Published December 7, 2006.

97. Donor exclusion policy under review. *FDA Consumer*1990; 24(6):6.

98. Daniels N. Fair process in patient selection for antiretroviral treatment in WHO's goal of 3 by 5. *Lancet* 2005;366(9480): 169–171.

99. Edejer T. North-South research partnerships: the ethics of carrying out research in developing countries. *BMJ* 1999;319(7207):438–441.

100. Angell M. The ethics of clinical research in the Third World. *N Engl J Med* 1997;337(12):847–849.

101. Lansang M, Olveda R. Institutional linkages: strategic bridges for research capacity strengthening. *Acta Trop* 1994; 57(2–3):139–145.

102. Caplan A. Twenty years after. The legacy of the Tuskegee Syphilis Study. When evil intrudes. *Hastings Cent Rep* 1992; 22(6):29–32.

103. Edgar H. Twenty years after. The legacy of the Tuskegee Syphilis Study. Outside the community. *Hastings Cent Rep* 1992; 22(6):32–35.

104. King P. Twenty years after. The legacy of the Tuskegee Syphilis Study. The dangers of difference. *Hastings Cent Rep* 1992;22(6):35–38.

105. Jones J. The Tuskegee legacy. AIDS and the black community. *Hastings Cent Rep* 1992;22(6):38–40.

106. Randall V. Race, health care and the law: regulating racial discrimination in health care. United Nations Research Institute for Social Development Web site. http://www.unrisd.org/80256B3C005BCCF9/(httpPublications)/603AC6BDD4C6AF8F80256B6D005788BD?OpenDocument. Published 2001.

107. Stephens J. As drug testing spreads, profits and lives hang in balance. *Washington Post,* December 17, 2001: A01. http://www.washingtonpost.com/ac2/wp-dyn/A11939-2000Dec15?language=printer.

108. Whalen C, Johnson J, Okwera A, et al. A trial of three regimens to prevent tuberculosis in Ugandan adults infected with the human immunodeficiency virus. Uganda-Case Western Reserve University Research Collaboration. *N Engl J Med* 1997;337(12):801–808.

109. Angell M. Ethical imperialism? Ethics in international collaborative clinical research. *N Engl J Med* 1988;319(16): 1081–1083.

110. Angell M. The Nazi hypothermia experiments and unethical research today. *N Engl J Med* 1990;322(20):1462–1464.

111. Bhutta Z. Ethics in international health research: a perspective from the developing world. *Bull World Health Organ* 2002;80(2):114–120.

112. Mulholland E, Hilton S, Adegbola R, et al. Randomized trial of *Haemophilus influenzae* type-b tetanus protein conjugate vaccine [corrected] for prevention of pneumonia and meningitis in Gambian infants. *Lancet* 1997;349(9060): 1191–1197.

113. Bang A, Bang R, Baitule S, et al. Effect of home-based neonatal care and management of sepsis on neonatal mortality: field trial in rural India. *Lancet* 1999;354(9194):1955–1961.

114. Luby S, Agboatwalla M, Feikin D, et al. Effect of handwashing on child health: a randomized controlled trial. *Lancet* 2005; 366(9481):225–233.

115. Neufeld V, Alger E. Network is a verb. The experience of the network of community-oriented educational institutions for health sciences. *Infect Dis Clin North Am* 1995;9(2):407–418.

116. Guidelines for research in partnership with developing countries; 11 principles. Commission for Research Partnerships with Developing Countries Web site. http://www.kfpe.ch/download/Guidelines_e.pdf. Published 1998.

117. Cash R, Wikler D, Saxena A, et al, eds. *Case Book on Ethical Issues in International Health Research* [online monograph]. Geneva: World Health Organization, 2009. http://whqlibdoc.who.int/publications/2009/9789241547727_eng.pdf.

118. Donnelley S. Humans within nature. Hans Jonas and the imperative of responsibility. *Infect Dis Clin North Am* 1995; 9(2):235–244.

119. White L. The historical roots of our ecologic crisis. *Science* 1967;155(3767):1203–1207.

120. Human health under threat from ecosystem degradation: threats particularly acute in poorer countries. World Health Organization Web site. http://www.who.int/mediacentre/news/releases/2005/pr67/en/index.html.

121. San Sebastian M, Hurtig A. Oil exploitation in the Amazon basin of Ecuador: a public health emergency. *Rev Panam Salud Publica* 2004;15(3):205–211.

122. Gostin L. Medical countermeasures for pandemic influenza: ethics and the law. *JAMA* 2006;295(5):554–556.

123. Singer P, Benatar S, Bernstein M, et al. Ethics and SARS: lessons from Toronto. *BMJ* 2003;327(7427):1342–1344.

124. Summary notes for members of the California State Legislature on the ethics of human cloning and stem cell research: a report from "California cloning: a dialogue on state regulation" held at Santa Clara University, October 12, 2001. Markkula Center for Applied Ethics Web site. http://www.scu.edu/ethics/publications/cloning.html.

125. Development of a regional position on human cloning. World Health Organization Regional Committee for the Eastern Mediterranean Web site. http://applications.emro.who.int/docs/EM_RC51_infDoc11_en.pdf.

126. Noogle S, et al. Human oocytes reprogram somatic cells to a pluripotent state. *Nature* 2011;478:70–75.

127. Williams B, Cavico F, Mujtaba B. Integrating modern business values and cloning. The legality, morality, and social responsibility of somatic cell nuclear transfer. *Adv Manage App Econ* 2011;1:53–92.

128. Global Legal Research Center. *Bioethics Legislation in selected Countries. Bioethics in International Law.* Washington, DC: The Law Library of Congress, October 2012. http://www.loc.gov/law/help/bioethics_2012-008118FINAL.pdf.

129. Annan K. Nobel lecture, December 10, 2001, Oslo, Norway. Nobel Peace Prize Web site. http://nobelprize.org/peace/laureates/2001/annan-lecture.html.

130. Gostin L. International infectious disease law: revision of the World Health Organization's International Health Regulations. *JAMA* 2004;291(21):2623–2627.

131. Smolinksi M, Hamburg M, Lederberg J, eds. Committee on Emerging Microbial Threats to Health in the 21st Century, Board on Global Health. Microbial threats to health: emergence, detection, and response [monograph on the Internet]. National Academies Press. http://www.nap.edu/openbook.php?isbn=030908864X Published 2003.

132. Taylor A, Bettcher D. WHO Framework Convention on Tobacco Control: a global "good" for public health. *Bull World Health Organ* 2000;78(7):920–928. http://www.who.int/bulletin/archives/78(7)920.pdf.

133. Novotny T, Carlin D. Ethical and legal aspects of global tobacco control. *Tobacco Control* 2005;14(Suppl II):ii26–ii30. http://tobaccocontrol.bmj.com/content/14/suppl_2/ii26.full.

134. Gostin, L. A framework convention on global health: health for all, justice for all. *JAMA* 2012;307(19):2087–2092.

135. Velji A. Transforming global health, global health education, infectious disease, and chronic conditions in the 21st century [editorial]. *Infect Dis Clin North Am* 2011;25(3):485–498.

136. Barnard D, Bui T, Chase J, Jones E, et al. Ethical issues in global health education. In: Chase J, Evert J., eds. *Global Health Training in Graduate Medical Education: A Guidebook.* 2nd ed. San Francisco: Global Health Education Consortium, 2011:30–52.

137. Evert J, Huish R, Heit G, et al. Global health ethics. In: Illes J, Sahkian J, eds. *Oxford Handbook of Neuroethics.* New York: Oxford University Press, 2011:835–856.

138. Pinto A, Upshur R. Global health ethics for students. *Dev World Bioeth* 2009;9(1):1–10.

139. Crump J, Sugarman J; Working Group on Ethics Guidelines for Global Health Training (WEIGHT). Ethics and best practice guidelines for training experiences in global health. *Am J Trop Med Hyg* 2010;83(6):1178–1182.

140. Student handbook for global engagement. University of Michigan Web site. http://open.umich.edu/education/sph/resources/student-handbook-global-engagement/2011 Published 2011.

141. Dharamsi S, et al. *Global Praxis: Exploring the Ethics of Engagement Abroad.* Vancouver, BC: Ethics of International Engagement and Service Learning Project, 2011. http://ethicsofisl.ubc.ca/downloads/_2011-EIESL-kit-loRes.pdf.

142. White M, Evert J. Developing ethical awareness in global health: four cases for medical educators. *Dev World Bioethics* 2012. doi:10.1111/devb.12000 http://www.ncbi.nlm.nih.gov/pubmed/23025791.

143. Macer D. Bioethics in and from Asia [editorial]. *J Med Ethics* 1999;25(4):293–295.

Education and Careers in Global Health

22

Jessica Evert and Scott Loeliger

LEARNING OBJECTIVES

- *Appreciate the landscape of global health education for health science and other trainees*
- *Describe global health workforce challenges and opportunities*
- *Define competencies of global health education and structural models for educational programs*

OVERVIEW

The multifaceted, interdisciplinary nature of global health makes for a field that has many career and educational paths leading into and stemming from it. In the last decade many health disciplines and programs have embraced global health education. This embrace has come in the forms of global health content and pathways, educational competencies, and consensus of the globalization of health science education. Despite the increasing popularity of global health education and careers, there are still many hurdles to fully actualizing this globalization. Central challenges include ensuring that global engagement occurs in an ethical fashion and garnering sustainable institutional support. Increasingly there is recognition of the necessity for interdisciplinary approaches to global health issues, which contrasts with the traditional discipline-specific silos in academic settings. There has been an emergence of organizations and schools dedicated to cutting across these silos and increasing academic institutions' relevance in the area of global health engagement, specifically in the areas of education, research, service, and advocacy.[1]

There are a variety of global health program structures, content, and focus within health science and public health schools. Many Westerners who discuss global health education are referring to training students from the global north about health and health determinants in the global south. The *north* is the collective term for economically developed, industrialized countries, whereas the *south* refers to low- and middle-income countries.[2] Many of these educational approaches are based on empirical evidence or impact on trainees, without attention to impact on the low-resource community hosts. There is a need for research and program development in the areas of true interdisciplinary educational engagement, program sustainability, impact on host communities, as well as cost effectiveness. Furthermore, the best use of Western professionals in global health circles is still not clear. Although some education programs encourage Westerners to be direct care providers, others see the roles as advocates and empowerment agents as more appropriate and sustainable. Lastly, there is considerable development of global health education that is occurring with south-south collaborations and within countries that show promise of developing a sustainable global health workforce.

INCREASED SOCIAL ACCOUNTABILITY AND THE TRANSFORMATION OF HEALTH EDUCATION

Two pivotal reports provide impetus for and evidence of the momentum in global health education. The Lancet commission, *Education for Health Professionals for the 21st Century*, produced a 2010 report to examine the state of health education worldwide and propose needed actions to address the "collective failure to share the dramatic health advances equitably."[3] The commission shared this vision:

> All health professionals in all countries should be educated to mobilize knowledge and to engage in critical reasoning and ethical conduct so that they are competent to participate in patient and population-centered health systems as members of locally responsive and globally connected teams. The ultimate purpose is to assure universal coverage of the high-quality comprehensive services that are essential to advance opportunity for health equity within and between countries.

The report provides a diagnosis of current ills of the health and education systems, elaborates on their intersections, and their mutual influences. Interdependent reforms are espoused as necessary next steps. The Lancet commission included stewardship mechanisms, one of which is socially accountable accreditation of educational institutions.

A parallel effort on behalf of 65 delegates from medical education and accreditation is reflected in the Global Consensus on Social Accountability of Medical Schools (GCSA). The GCSA defined 10 areas for schools to address to achieve social accountability. Examples of these areas include anticipating society's health needs and adapting to the evolving role of doctors and other health professionals. Importantly, the GCSA suggests that communities where the medical school is embedded provide feedback as to the social accountability of the institution. The Consensus suggests this community assessment be used in addition to national standards for accreditation. This focus on local responsiveness and partnership is a cornerstone of the GCSA framework.[4] The Training for Health Equity Network (THEnet), a consortium of community-based health education institutions that are committed to health equity, published a subsequent framework for evaluating socially accountable health professional education.[5] THEnet's efforts to increase the visibility of community-based medical schools (most of which are in the global south) that train local individuals to address local health challenges are unique. The nature of THEnet's efforts is in contrast to many schools in the global north that train predominantly outsiders to address global health challenges in communities geographically removed from the medical school itself.

Efforts to move in the direction of more socially accountable educational institutions to affect health systems and disparities are at the heart of the global health education movement. Students have a growing interest in global health issues, health equity, and international practice.[6] In response to this interest and the resultant education reform movements, a variety of global health education programs have emerged and existing programs have been strengthened. Educational programs are diverse and reflect the many facets of global health. Likewise these programs are evidence of the efforts to globalize educational systems and the health care workforce.

Workforce Needs

In thinking about the global workforce for health and medical care. it is important to carefully define what part of the health workforce is being described. In addition to physicians, this term also includes administrators, pharmacists, radiologists, phlebotomists, nurse midwives, physician assistants, and many other workers in health systems. We must include in the discussion the segment of the workforce that contributes to behavior change, public health, and the environment because clinical health care contributes to only about 10% of the determinants of health.[7] We must not only talk about global health workers coming from Europe and North America in academic or aid projects. We should also focus on the massive shortage of many categories of skilled professionals that represents one of the greatest barriers to improved health in all countries around the globe (Figure 22-1). An all-inclusive discussion should rightly include elements of equity of salary and careful attention to true academic and intellectual exchange programs. Finally we should address not only the needs or benefits of our learners and faculty, but also the processes that promote, guide, and give local professionals in under-resourced countries the ability to gain knowledge, be retained, and have access to continuing medical education.

The Global Health Workforce Alliance (GHWA) was created in 2006 to address the crisis of chronic shortage of health care workers, approximately 4.2 million worldwide and 1.5 million in Africa alone. This new alliance represents a global partnership of national governments, civil society, international agencies, finance institutions, researchers, educators, and professional associations. Its membership now includes over 300 organizations around the world such as Johns Hopkins University, BP Korala Institute of Health Sciences in Nepal, Family Health International, Fiji School of Medicine, and the GAVI Alliance (formerly the Global Alliance for Vaccines and Immunisation).[8] At the First Global Forum on Human Resources for Health in Kampala, Uganda, in 2008, GHWA issued a declaration about an agenda for global action to address the health workforce crisis. It calls for coordinated action from governments, multilateral and bilateral, academic institutions, civil society, the private sector, and health workers' professional associations and unions.[9]

Achievement of Millennium Development Goals 4, 5, 6, and 8 (child mortality, maternal health,

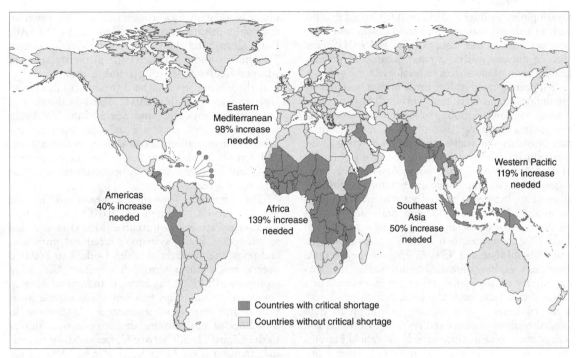

Figure 22-1. Countries with a critical shortage of health care workers.

infectious diseases, and global partnerships) hinges on a rapid increase in health care workers. For physicians, addressing these goals is an important opportunity to work with other professional groups to understand how to distribute energy and dollars toward programs that support other health workers who are needed in a functional local and national health care system.

The current definition of global health properly includes the underserved and impoverished areas of all nations, developed and developing. Many have struggled with how to provide a description that allows for a common ground for discussions, proposals, and actions. Koplan and others offered that:

> Global health is an area for study, research, and practice that places a priority on improving health and achieving equity in health for all people worldwide. Global health emphasizes transnational health issues, determinants, and solutions, involves many disciplines within and beyond the health sciences and promotes interdisciplinary collaboration. It is a synthesis of population-based prevention with individual-level clinical care.[10]

There is a recognized contradiction when health care personnel from high-resource countries get on planes that fly over their own urban slums and poor rural communities in an effort to address impoverished communities across the globe. The issue of persistent local health disparities, particularly in the United States, must be considered. It is fairly recognized that successful health systems require a primary health care workforce and infrastructure to be sustainable, cost effective, and culturally competent. Among physicians from developed countries there is an emerging tension about the focus of work that is needed to support improved health care. Traditionally, medical missions often consisted of surgeons, obstetrician/gynecologists, and infectious disease specialists that focused on specific diseases that could be addressed by one-time medications, treatments, and procedures. This specialist view is often supported by academic institutions in the less developed countries, which have been modeled on specialist-oriented sister institutions in North America and Europe. The emergence of primary care and primary health care as central foci of health care services and human resources in health in both the developed and developing world has created an increased demand for family physicians, primary care internists, pediatricians, obstetricians, nurse practitioners, physician assistants, and nurse midwives, both as providers and educators. Dr. Margaret Chan, in an address to the International Conference on Health for

Development in Buenos Aires in 2007, noted that the path to reduced maternal and child deaths and more coverage for malaria, tuberculosis, HIV/AIDS, and chronic diseases will be a rapid buildup of primary health care staff more than technology.[11]

Supporting rapid scaling up of primary health care capabilities in the developing world will be difficult to achieve without a retooling of medical education and postgraduate training that produces more primary care providers and health care workers inherent in the new primary care model. For the struggling countries of Asia, Africa, and Central/South America, this enormous task seems impossible unless efforts to help are adapted to increasing the relevant human resources for health. The impact of brain drain and conflict on shortages of physicians continues to worsen. As of early 2008, countries such as Kenya, Ghana, Angola, and Mozambique had 43% to 75% of their trained physicians working abroad.[12] South Sudan, the newest country on the planet, offers a stark example of a country that lacks both the basic workforce to staff a central hospital or a training institution to train needed medical students and residents. Conflicts and lack of basic infrastructure outside the capital prevents the establishment of even the most rudimentary primary care outposts.

The huge workforce focus on vertical programs, such as HIV/AIDS, tuberculosis, and malaria, exposed more than ever the inequities and inadequacies of human resources in developing countries. This realization has driven the most recent, and somewhat controversial, effort to scale up the physician workforce to address the inequities in the developing world. The Institute of Medicine (IOM), as requested by the Office of the US Global AIDS Coordinator, began to study options for placing US health care professionals in 15 focus countries. The IOM proposed a Peace Corps–style recruitment and mobilization effort. The report stated, "Nothing less than a Peace-Corps scale contingent of health care professionals and other experts should be mobilized to plan, carry out, and sustain a campaign against the disease."[13]

The proposed Global Health Service, circa 2005, envisioned six programs:

1. Global Health Service Corps
2. Health Workforce Needs Assessment
3. Fellowship Program
4. Loan Repayment Program
5. Twinning Program
6. Clearinghouse

The Global Health Service Corps is now a reality with the July 2012 launch of the Global Health Service Partnership. The workforce goal is to offset shortages in human resources and to promote direct work with local communities. This program is a public-private partnership between the PEPFAR, Peace Corps, and the Global Health Service Corps. The nurses and physicians will primarily serve as adjunct faculty in existing training programs. The first three countries will be Tanzania, Malawi, and Uganda starting in July 2013. These positions will use licensed physicians and nurses, but, like Peace Corps volunteers, they will only get monthly stipends, transportation, medical care, vacation time, and a readjustment allowance. The initial commitment will be 1 year with an opportunity to extend for a second year.[14]

The "twinning" program, mentioned in the original proposal, started in 2010. The Medical Education Partnership Initiative (MEPI) is intended to strengthen health systems, educational programs, and boost the numbers of health workers to 140,000 over a much longer term.[15] This effort, also using repurposed PEPFAR funds, is an attempt to develop "twinned" relationships between US academic institutions and severely under-resourced institutions in a number of sub-Saharan African countries. Similar to the Global Health Service Corps, much of the initial attention is on Africa because it has 24% of the global burden of disease, but only 3% of the global health workforce and only 1% of the world's health expenditure.[16] MEPI has a $130 million budget and uses the resources of Health and Human Services, PEPFAR, the Fogarty International Center of the National Institutes of Health (NIH), and more than 15 major American universities working with multiple educational institutions in over 10 sub-Saharan African countries. This project, in part, was an effort to address the redirecting of funds from AIDS programs. Many experts felt these programs overlooked the needs of many countries to have more trained health care workers and to pay more attention to the basic health issues of water, sanitation, nutrition, and chronic diseases.[17]

These recent efforts to focus more on the training and support of health systems development should stimulate debate and discussion about ethical issues to avoid harm and to be thoughtful about future outcomes of current actions or assistance. This is especially important for students, trainees, and residents who are contemplating going abroad either as individuals or part of a larger academic or nongovernmental organization. Although the phrase *primum non nocere* "first do no harm," generally applies to the care and treatment of individual patients, it should also apply to communities and governmental agencies in the countries being supported. Much like the traditional "vertical" programs that diverted health care workforce and resources from preexisting nutritional, public health, and chronic disease programs in many countries, a new dependence on a Peace Corps model of short-term medical volunteers may retard longer term more sustainable solutions in developing countries.

A public debate on the *New York Times* editorial page in 2008 underscored this dilemma. Two former volunteers, one a US senator and the other a former recruiter and country director, offered their opinions about either doubling the number of volunteers (the senator) or being more circumspect in sending short-term volunteers that are not requested and may not be needed.[18] Older programs, such as the Foundation for the Advancement of International Medical Education and Research, were focused on improving capacity and capability of faculty in medical/nursing training institutions abroad to innovate and develop appropriate models for trainees. This type of indirect aid, not medications or workforce, has the potential to keep foreign physicians in place and, simultaneously, develop professional and equitable relationships with medical educators around the world.[19]

One model of low-budget cooperative efforts, called the Friends of Family Medicine Uganda (FFMU), under the aegis of an international advisory committee, stresses the collaborative development of family medicine curricula, residency programs, and family medicine faculties in that country. Rather than spend weeks or months struggling to treat diseases and place bandages on broken delivery systems, participating FFMU faculty from Europe, Canada, and the United States work with their African counterparts electronically and in periodic visits/conferences.

Another larger project, funded by the European ACP-Eu-Edulink, works from a similar framework in a collection of sub-Saharan countries. Known as Primafamed, faculties from Europe and the United States supported meetings and the development of an online primary health care and family medicine journal established in 2009.[20] The Primafamed network currently provides a platform for those African educational institutions concerned with issues of primary health care and family medicine. It helps to provide training to increase the necessary capacity in countries such as South Africa, Sudan, Uganda, Nigeria, Ghana, the Democratic Republic of the Congo (DRC), Rwanda, Tanzania, and Kenya.[21]

Moreover, the VLIR ZEIN 2009 program, funded by the Belgian government and the Flemish Interuniversity Council, has established a "South African family medicine twinning project." The departments of family medicine in South Africa twin with those training complexes that have been or will be set up in Namibia, Zambia, Mozambique, Malawi, Lesotho, Swaziland, the DRC, and Botswana. Primafamed gives support in terms of capacity building, content development, and the monitoring of

postgraduate training in family medicine. This network is fostering the principle of south-south cooperation, by encouraging the sharing of unique knowledge and wisdom among different African institutions, as well as by creating an institutional network.[22]

Of particular concern to global health is the increasing emigration of health care workers in response to market forces.[23] With the movement of physicians, nurses, and pharmacists out of economically disadvantaged environments to developed countries, there looms a crisis of care in developing countries. For example, Africa bears 25% of the world's disease burden but has only 0.6% of the world's health care professionals. More than a third of South African medical school graduates immigrate to the developed world each year. In Zimbabwe, where pharmacists provide substantial primary care, only 40 are trained each year, and in 2001, 60 migrated abroad. Ethical solutions to these labor flows are needed; these may include educational and institutional incentives that link academic institutions in developed countries to partner institutions in developing countries. In 2011, approximately 2,700 non-US international medical graduates matched for residency training in the United States.[24] This represents over 10% of all first-year residents and represents a significant loss of physician workforce for countries that can least afford it. It also shows how the United States (and likely Europe) is simultaneously taking talent from less resourced countries while preparing a legion of their own physicians to go there through the new global health service corps.

Certainly, models for the contribution of health manpower from better resourced environments to high-need areas exist. Cuba has been contributing physicians to developing countries for decades as a community service requirement for its new graduates; in fact, it has extended its concern for underserved areas by training US medical students to treat poor urban Americans. Thousands of medical students from other less developed countries are trained in Cuba to return home to serve local needs.[25]

Other Models for Cooperation and Partnership

As discussed in the section about research activities, health research partnerships have considerable benefits that enhance the quality of research, the exchange of knowledge between counterparts, and the development of focused research capacity in global health. A recent product of just such a focus, conducted by the Canadian Coalition for Global Health Research and supported by the International Development Research Centre, was the development of a "Partnership Assessment Toolkit."[26] A central goal of the toolkit is to break down the tension that exists in many research and assistance initiatives from developed countries and the lack of true empowerment and ownership created by top-down neocolonial models.

Recently an important report by the Global Commission on Education of Health Professionals for the 21st Century in *Lancet* attempted to point the way toward closing gaps in health equity and workforce within and between countries.[3] The primary focus of the report was transforming education to strengthen health systems. This systems centered approach has clear implications for the health care workforce and for North American and European students, postgraduates, and residents. A commentary by several European students from Austria and the Netherlands endorses this new approach:

> *We encourage the proposed team-based education to breakdown professional silos. Working in health care means working within multidisciplinary and interdisciplinary teams. As teamwork is a soft skill which can be learned, its development should be fostered by the proposed inter-professional courses starting at an early age. In the past seven years, international health-care students recognized the importance of inter-professional education, and launched an international forum which brings together students of medicine, nursing, pharmacy, and allied health professions.[27]*

FRAMEWORKS FOR GLOBAL HEALTH EDUCATION

Global health education occurs at all levels of medical education: premedical undergraduate, undergraduate medical education (medical school), graduate medical education (residency), and postgraduate medical education (i.e., residencies and fellowships). It also occurs in allied health, public health, nursing, and other health education schools. In addition, global health and similar themes are studied in most non-health disciplines, with particular attention in geography, women's studies, anthropology, and other social sciences. Because determinants of health are so broad, especially in the developing world, global health education is the subject of business, engineering, political science, and many other disciplines. Even when not conceived as explicitly global health education, the concepts, principles, and interventions of most disciplines when applied in a globalized fashion are integrated into global health in its most inclusive form.

Within health-specific and health-related disciplines, explicit global health education takes many forms:

- Undergraduate programs (nonprofessional schools) in international relations, public health, anthropology, etc.

- Certificate programs, applying to both visiting scholars and professional school students who concentrate on global health.

- Global health tracks for students in medicine, pharmacy, nursing, dentistry, and veterinary medicine.

- A global health elective or required coursework during undergraduate medical, nursing, or allied health education.

- Master's degrees in global health sciences or clinical research focusing on global health topics.

- Areas of concentration for doctoral students in basic sciences, nursing, or other fields to support research projects in global health.

- Clinical scholar programs for residents who wish to expand their clinical training to include research, service, or program work abroad.

- Participation in student-run local, national, and international organizations (i.e., IFMSA, GlobeMed, Unite for Sight, Global Brigades) as well as participation in professional groups (i.e., AAFP's Global Health Workshop, ACS Operation Giving Back, AAP Section on International Child Health), consortiums (i.e., CUGH, WONCA), and other national/international organizations (i.e., Doctors for Global Health, Physicians for Social Responsibility).

- Participation in international rotations or study abroad programs through academic institutions or nongovernmental organizations (i.e., Child Family Health International, Cross Cultural Solutions, others).

There is no agreed upon or universal structure to global health education.[28] Bozorgmehr and colleagues presented key characteristics of global health education that emphasizes important concepts such as inter-professionalism, focus on social justice, and critical thinking (Table 22-1).[29] However each program is a reflection of its own institutional strengths, faculty capabilities, global health agenda, unique philosophy, and underlying ethical approach.[30]

Many from the global north refer to global health education programs as those at global north institutions that teach global health concepts to a predominantly Western trainee population. However there are also those that focus on training individuals from the global south to serve their own communities. This occurs through grassroots capacity building activities, formal educational institutions, and twinning programs. Grassroots capacity building usually occurs at the community or provincial level. These activities include training of community health workers, existing health care professionals, and others. Although this process occurs internally, the literature predominantly reflects education programs and capacity building that involves facilitators from the global north.[31–33]

Table 22-1. Key characteristics of "global health" education

Category	Characteristics	Implication	Rationale
Object	Focuses on social, economic, political and cultural forces which influence health across the world	Learning opportunities in "global health" focus on the underlying structural determinants of health	To ensure that educational interventions cover the social, economic, political and cultural etiology of ill health, and not merely its disease-oriented symptoms on a global level
	Concerned with the needs of developing countries; with health issues that transcend national boundaries; and with the impact of globalization	Learning opportunities in "global health" link territorial up to supraterritorial dimensions of underlying structural determinants of health	To ensure that educational interventions clarify the links between territorial health situations (either domestic ones and/or situations in other countries) and their underlying transborder and global determinants
Orientation	Toward "health for all"	Learning opportunities in "global health" should adopt and impart the ethical and practical aspects of achieving 'health for all'	To ensure that educational interventions are relevant to people's needs on community, local, national, international and global level
	Toward health equity	Learning opportunities in "global health" should emphasize issues of health equity (or health inequity) within and across countries	To ensure that educational interventions orientate on the challenge of achieving health equity worldwide
Outcome	Identification of actions	Learning opportunities in "global health" facilitate the identification of actions (by the student), undertaken to resolve problems either top-down or - more important- bottom-up	To ensure that educational interventions foster critical thinking and present options for professional engagement on different dimensions towards "health for all" and health equity
Methodology	Cross-disciplinarity	Learning opportunities in "global health" involve educators and/or students from various disciplines and professions	To ensure that educational interventions lead to an understanding of influences on health beyond the biomedical paradigm and respect the importance of sectors other than the health sector in improving health
	Bottom-up learning and problem-orientation	Learning-opportunities in "global health" require unconventional methods for teaching and learning	To ensure that educational interventions clarify the relevance for the health workforce to deal with transborder and/or global determinants of health

Adapted from: Bozorgmehr K, Saint V, Tinnemann P. Global Health Education Framework: A Conceptional Guide for Monitoring, Evaluation and Practice. *Globalization and Health* 2011; 7: 8.(29)

Formal educational institutions that train local student populations exist throughout the world. There has been a growth and collaboration of such institutions dedicated to educating local individuals to be physicians, midlevel providers, nurses, and pharmacists who are dedicated to caring for the underserved in their own countries and regions. THEnet is a consortium of 11 medical schools around the world committed to training health care providers who are embedded in the community, responsive to its needs, and dedicated to a social justice agenda. This is in contrast to the traditional ivory tower view of medical schools. Traditional ivory tower academic institutions are perceived as out of touch with the communities where they are located, concerned with technological advancement at the expense of equitable dissemination of existing resources, and generally not exemplifying priorities consistent with health equity.[34-37]

Although there is still a dearth of training institutions, particularly in sub-Saharan Africa, the support of institutions training local populations to address their own health needs and engage in global health from the southern perspective is crucial for sustainable impacts. There is an increasing role for south-south partnerships for education and health services, in addition to north-south partnerships aiming to improve education and retention.[38-40]

Competencies and Global Health Education

In addition to multiple frameworks that exist for global health education programs and partnership structures, there are also many lenses through which to view the competencies and goals of such an education.

The utilization of competencies as predefined outcomes of medical, health science, and other fields of education has surged in recent years. Known as Competency-Based Medical Education (CBME) in the medical field, this approach is defined as "an outcomes-based approach to the design, implementation, assessment, and evaluation of medical education programs, using an organized framework of competencies." Frank et al identified four overarching themes that guide CBME: focus on outcomes, emphasis on abilities rather than solely knowledge, de-emphasis on time-based training, and promoting greater learner centeredness.[41]

The global health education community has called for increased reliance on competencies and standardization of curriculum.[42,43] A nominal group process at the Bellagio Conference, convened at the Rockefeller Center in 2008, found that cultural humility was the most important global health education competency. Several sets of competencies have been developed for global health education. However, there still is no consensus or standardization of competencies, and many programs are developed without even the guidance of learning objectives.[44]

Competencies in global health can be categorized into essential core competencies and specialized competencies. Core competencies are those necessary for all medical students regardless of interest in global health. Specialized competencies are relevant for trainees seeking expanded global health training, usually through tracks, distinction, certificates, fellowships, or the like. Four domains of competencies have been suggested as core for all medical students: global burden of disease, traveler's medicine, immigrant health, and cultural awareness.[45,46] These domains were expanded

by the Joint US/Canadian Committee on Global Health Essential Core Competencies (Table 22-2). In addition to identifying knowledge domains and competencies, the committee went a step further to discuss how students can demonstrate each competency.

Peluso and colleagues divided competencies into general and local competencies (Table 22-3). General competencies are applicable to all sites around the world regardless of national origin of the trainee when the trainee is working in a novel cultural setting. Local global health competencies are site specific and location dependent.[44]

The Accreditation Council for Graduate Medical Education's (ACGME) general competencies for medical residents are patient care, medical knowledge, practice-based learning and improvement, interpersonal skills, professionalism, and systems-based practice.[47] The American Academy of Pediatrics Section on International Child Health has created curriculum guidelines that underscore how global health exposure and topics can help fulfill requirements from the ACGME.[48] The American Academy of Family Physicians has delineated a recommended curriculum in global health for residents that includes competencies, attitudes, knowledge, and skills domains.[49] Anspacher and colleagues propose objectives for each ACGME competency as they relate to global health, as well as to specific population considerations.[50]

Although ACGME competencies drive graduate medical education in the United States, CanMEDS is a framework developed by the Royal College of Physicians and Surgeons of Canada to improve patient care by organizing training and practice competencies around seven themes. These themes are also roles required by physicians: medical expert, communicator, collaborator, manager, health advocate, scholar, and professional.[51] These competency themes were built on by the Ontario Global Health Family Medicine Curriculum Working Group to develop an evidence-informed shared curricular framework.[52] This group defined eight components of a Global Health Education Framework:

1. Definition of global health
2. Mission of global health
3. Principles and values
4. Global health competencies
5. Curriculum delivery
6. Mentorship
7. Service learning and practice settings
8. Evaluation

This framework guides the development of programs and is graphically depicted in Figure 22-2.

Table 22-2. Joint Us/Canadian Core Competencies In Global Health

Knowledge Domains	Competencies
Global Burden of Disease	• Knowledge of the major global causes of morbidity and mortality and how health risks vary by gender and income across regions. • Be able to knowledgeably discuss priority setting, health care rationing and funding for health and health-related research.
Health Implications of Travel, Migration, and Displacement	• Understand health risks associated with travel, with emphasis on potential risks and appropriate management, including referrals. • Understand the health risks related to migration, with emphasis on the potential risks and appropriate resources. • Understand how travel and trade contribute to the spread of communicable diseases.
Social and Economic Determinants of Health	• Understand the relationship between health and social determinants of health, and how social determinants vary across world regions.
Populations, Resources, and the Environment	• Understand the impact of rapid population growth and of unsustainable and inequitable resource consumption on important resources essential to human health, including water, sanitation and food supply and know how these resources vary across world regions. • Describe the relationship between access to clean water, sanitation, and nutrition on individual and population health. • Describe the relationship between environmental degradation, pollution and health.
Globalization of Health and Health Care	• Understand how global trends in health care practice, commerce and culture contribute to health and the quality and availability of healthcare locally and internationally • Be familiar with major multinational efforts to improve health globally. • Understand and describe general trends and influences in the global availability and movement of health care workers.
Health Care in Low Resource Settings	• Identify barriers to health and health care in low-resource settings locally and internationally. • Demonstrate an understanding of health care delivery strategies in low-resource settings, especially the role of community-based healthcare and primary care models. • Demonstrate an understanding of cultural and ethical issues in working with underserved populations. • Demonstrate the ability to adapt clinical skills and practice in a resource-constrained setting. • For students who participate in electives in low-resource settings outside their home situations, demonstrate that they have participated in training to prepare for this elective.
Human Rights in Global Health	• Demonstrate a basic understanding of the relationship between health and human rights.

Each program must customize its content to reflect its local context, resources, available experts, and focus.[48]

International Placements and Global Health Education

It has been argued that the only settings that will challenge medical trainees' attitudes and prompt the transformative development necessary for successful global health education are those outside the student's reference culture, geographic location, and perhaps language.[44] There is evidence that, in graduate medical education, international placements may be the crux of a resident's global health exposure,

often existing without a wider curricular context.[53] Although many assume this to be outside the student's country of origin, others argue this change in student thinking and understanding can be catalyzed by an experience in a domestic low resource or culturally novel community.[54] Regardless of whether global health related placements occur in under-resourced, culturally novel settings at home or abroad, the components of such experiences should be similar. Recently, a key component of these placements, predeparture training (PDT), was made mandatory for LCME accreditation of the medical schools in Canada. This affirms the important role PDT plays in global health programs. This requirement, like many

Table 22-3. General and local core competencies for global health.

General global health core competencies
   Individual competencies
      Cross-culture competence
      Communication and linguistic skills
      Understanding the geographic burden of disease
      Problem solving with limited resources
      Identifying social and environmental determinants of health
      Recognizing health inequities and their effect on individual health
      Teamwork and collaborative problem solving
      Professionalism and ethical behavior
      Awareness of requirements for global health workers
   Community competencies
      Conducting a limited, population or community-based study
      Applying knowledge of preventive care
      Understanding the impact of migration and marginalization on health
      Understanding key global health "players"
Local global health core competencies
      Knowledge of local history, culture, social structure, politics
      Understanding local health care service structure
      Knowledge of local medical terminology

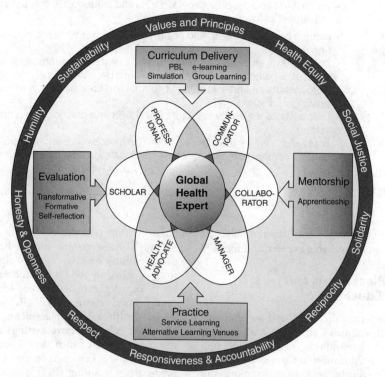

Figure 22-2. A global health education framework. (*Reproduced from Redwood-Campbell L, Pakes B, Rouleau, et al. Developing a curriculum framework for global health in family medicine: emerging principles, competencies, and educational approaches. BMC Med Educ. 2011 Jul 22;11:46. doi: 10.1186/1472-6920-11-46. http://www.biomedcentral. com/1472-6920/11/46*)

efforts to expand and improve medical school global health training, has been student led, in this case by the Canadian Medical Student Association and its Quebec counterpart, FEMC.[55] PDT curricular components aim to prepare students for entering into a new community, to help students cope with the stress of resource-limited settings, and to provide a way to process the experience. Although many institutions have not integrated compulsory global health curriculum, students have turned in large numbers to international rotations and other placements abroad to pursue global health interests.[56] In 2011, 30.5% of graduating US medical students reported going abroad during their training.[57] Although there is evidence for the benefit of such experiences,[58–60] there is concern about the local impact, ethical issues, sustainability, and potential risks to patients and students posed by these experiences.[61–63] To mitigate these risks, a curricular continuum before, during, and after the international placement is ideal.

Preparing Trainees for Global Health Placements: Predeparture Training

PDT can be defined as "any preparation that students complete before taking part in a global health elective that has as its goal to build trainee competence in the skills necessary to maximize learning while also minimizing harm to themselves and the communities in which they study."[64] Five areas of PDT have been suggested:

- Personal health
- Travel safety
- Cultural awareness
- Language competencies
- Ethical considerations[65]

Cheung and colleagues suggest this useful outline for PDT that integrates several sources.[66]

Recommended PDT for International Trainee Placements

1. **Personal health**
   This includes a discussion of:
   - Basic health precautions
   - Immunizations
   - Health insurance
   - Personal protective equipment
   - Postexposure prophylaxis
   - How and where to access medical care while on elective

2. **Travel safety**
   This includes gaining prior knowledge of:
   - Local contacts
   - Transportation options and housing arrangements

- Packing requirements
- Registration with the embassy of the learner's home country
- Local laws and customs
- Awareness of the most current travel advisory warnings and how to access this information
- Emergency preparedness and evacuation plans

3. **Cultural competency**
   Learners should have an understanding of:
   - The concept of culture
   - Acting with humility
   - The specifics of the culture of communities within their placement
   - Intercultural relationships
   - Historical trends in the region and community
   - Religion
   - Role of traditional healers
   - Gender norms
   - Appropriate dress
   - The meaning of purchasing and consuming alcohol in the host community
   - Norms of professionalism of the sending and hosting institutions
   - Standards of practice of the sending and hosting institutions
   - Valuing the knowledge and experience of collaborators (both individuals and institutions)
   - Appropriate conflict resolution and communication skills (in the context of the culture)

4. **Language competencies**
   Learners should have an understanding of:
   - The language requirements of the International Medical Experience (IME) and the host institution's expectations for level of language competency
   - At minimum, language basics (learners should gain experience working with interpreters, if applicable)

5. **Ethical considerations**
   If not previously addressed during other global health training, as discussed previously, PDT is an opportunity for students to reflect on the ethical challenges they may encounter on their elective. Discussions should include:
   - Personal motivations for going on an IME
   - An ethical framework to approach various problems
   - An expected professional code of conduct
   - Patient confidentiality (e.g., in light of blogs)
   - Establishing goals, objectives, level of training, and limitations early on with supervisors

- Ensuring appropriate and effective supervision and mentorship of IME learners and associated costs to local learners and care provision
- Appropriate licensing and privileges for clinical work during the IME
- Research-specific considerations
  - Focus on interest, priorities, needs, and relevance to host
  - Follow research procedures of host and sending institution
  - Obtain ethics committee approval before initiation of research
  - Receive appropriate training in research ethics
  - Follow international standards for authorship of publications
  - Discuss issues and plans for presentations early in collaborations

Outcomes and Evaluation of Global Health Education

International travel and experiential learning have traditionally been a component of liberal arts education. Outcome assessments of such learning have until recently been quite scarce, but the value of study abroad has been linked to needs arising from globalization.[67] Evidence-based outcomes reflect personal growth, improved clinical and patient care skills, and effects on career choice. Results of one outcome study show that students who studied abroad generally showed improvement in intercultural communication skills compared with those who did not study abroad. However, the study abroad experience alone was not the only determinant of cultural competency; prior experiences and training also likely have effects on ultimate outcomes, suggesting that a longer term integrated learning program may be important to optimize

---

BOX 22-1. MYTHS AND FACTS FOR TRAINEES

- *Myth: The demand for global health professionals outweighs the supply.*
- **Fact:** Although there are health labor shortages, there are not enough paid positions in organizations to provide solid career tracks for most interested professionals. Instead, one must take a strategic approach to career development that can assure a useful outcome of this interest. This would include appropriate clinical training, extra degrees, and of course, experiential learning.
- *Myth: Working in global health is a good way to find one's self.*
- **Fact:** This outcome may result from working in global health, but such work is not a cure for career uncertainty or personal crisis. Global health is public service, not therapy.
- *Myth: You will be able to treat patients.*
- **Fact:** It is difficult to combine clinical work (licensing abroad is only one issue) with programmatic work. Ethical concerns about our learners practicing on the community members they come in contact with have grown with the increased numbers going abroad. Global health is by its nature *public* health, with nonclinical interventions the most effective. However, volunteer health professionals still find their place in relief work and occasional clinical service opportunities (e.g., Doctors Without Borders (MSF) and faith-based organizations).
- *Myth: You must be a doctor or nurse to work in global health.*

- **Fact:** This is clearly not the case; technical knowledge, community-based interventions, sanitation, and public health education do not require clinical degrees. Newer workforce initiatives are focusing on total workforce needs and co-training of health care workers based on each locale's needs and resources. Physicians, however, still provide certain leadership potential and medical management vital to successful improvements in health status.
- *Myth: Volunteering overseas will expand your technical skills.*
- **Fact:** It can certainly expand one's creativity and perhaps inform one better as to appropriate technology, but it will not improve technical acumen in most cases. It may also teach the learner how to adopt approaches that utilize appropriate technology and the limits of local resources to achieve the best possible health outcomes.
- *Myth: More health care is the best solution to health problems in the developing world.*
- **Fact:** Health care access is usually a good idea, but again, much of the solution to global health problems lies with public health approaches and not individual health care. The current focus of programs such as MEPI and Global Health for Social Change are based on support and training for in-country personnel, along with improvements in basic standards of living and equitable access to care for all people in the community. Even unlimited funding does not necessarily create sustainable results.

outcomes of short- and medium-term experiential learning. Longitudinal studies would be very important in evaluating career implications and lasting communication skills resulting from experiential learning.[68]

A 2003 literature review to identify the outcomes of cross-cultural experiences for nursing and medical students reported qualitative and some quantitative data showing positive outcomes for professional development, including cultural competence, personal development, clinical learning, and host population benefits.[69] A broadened perspective about the world (and presumably global health) was the most frequently cited outcome of such experiences. However, the review pointed out the dearth of evidence regarding clearly defined outcomes for medical students or for host populations. Another literature review[70] of outcome studies, including 522 medical students and 166 house staff suggested that international health electives may be associated with choosing careers in primary care and focusing careers on underserved populations. Many of the studies reviewed noted positive effects on clinical skills as well as a greater appreciation of the importance of public health, culture, and health care systems. In addition, the review suggested that participants in experiential learning may be more competent in tropical medicine, potentially supporting better care for both immigrants and travelers. Other reports have confirmed the positive effects of experiential learning on competence with multicultural communities.[71]

Studies from non-US institutions show similar results. A Dutch survey of undergraduate medical students reported meaningful learning outcomes for international experiences in medical knowledge, skills, health care organization, society and culture, and personal growth.[72] The International Health and Medical Education Centre at University College London developed Student Selected Modules and International Health electives, combining experience abroad with appropriate didactic training (see the following section). A preliminary evaluation of this integrated program suggested that the value of experiential learning is enhanced by the integration of such learning with a comprehensive program of teaching about global health.[73]

A randomized control trial of such programs would be essentially impossible, but better long-term follow-up studies on participants versus nonparticipants using validated instruments are needed. One long-term follow-up of an integrated didactic/experiential program at Drew University of Medicine and Science reported that of 52 alumni who completed the course as medical students, two thirds joined national or international relief organizations, and 80% returned to the elective site for additional work or cultural experience.[74]

An association between international health experience and practicing primary care, public health, or working in underserved communities seems consistent across studies. Although these findings are probably influenced by the selection of service-minded future physicians for global health experiences during residency (thus "selection bias"), they may also reflect an important outcome of global health exposure on career choice.

Not unlike other educational subject matter, there are multiple ways to approach assessment and evaluation in global health education. It is important to both assess the outcomes for learners and the overall impact and quality of global health education programs. Utilizing one method of assessment or evaluation may not be sufficient to understand the multifaceted impact of global health education.[75] Commonly used mechanisms for participant assessment include self-reflection, scholarly projects, standardized testing, competency-based, and multisource or 360 evaluations. Self-reflection and critical reflection are increasingly used in medical education arenas, including global health. Critical reflection advances self-reflection to create action-oriented planning and objective assessment of transformations. There is evidence that students can increase their perception of compassionate care using reflection.[76–79]

Regardless of the methods used for assessment and evaluation, these are important components of any global health education program. Basing evaluation on competencies and learning objectives helps to establish desired outcomes. When possible, evaluation of program impact and achievements of trainees should solicit input from a variety of perspectives, including host communities, faculty, peers, and self.

Research Opportunities and Responsibilities

Research activities in the developing world are complicated by the relatively short time that Western academics, students, and volunteer health care workers actually spend in the countries getting assistance from abroad. It is well recognized that high-quality research efforts and results can inform quality approaches to health care, infectious and chronic diseases, and the development of health systems that truly improve health indices. There are many biomedical research efforts focused on disease etiology, the distribution and effectiveness of treatments, and the impact of improved health system measures, such as access to maternity care that reduces both infant and maternal mortality. This newer focus seeks to broaden the research efforts performed globally through American academic institutions or private entities. Paired with concerns about the ethics of foreign involvement in workforce matters are additional concerns about which components of global health should be studied. Many of the foundation studies performed in developing countries involve research about diseases, effectiveness of drugs and medical treatments, and descriptive research about public health matters. However, the heart of effective and efficient health care in all countries, rich and poor, is a strong primary health care system. Years of research by Barbara Starfield and others have shown that primary health care improves both access and equity and predicts a better health status.[80–82] As Starfield pointed out in one editorial, primary care research informs more equitable care and changes the focus to "what sort of patient has a disease" rather than "what sort of disease a patient has."[83]

Investments in personnel, vaccines, and medicines have generally been the principal foci of global health assistance. It seems realistic—and appropriate—that similar increases in investment promoting basic research, research networks, and evidence-based activities now follow those massive efforts. There is already some effort to reformat global health HIV/vertical program funding into support for cooperative multi-institutional programs to improve the academic training capacity in various sub-Saharan countries as previously described in the workforce section.

The enormously changed landscape of philanthropy and investment in global health has further complicated so-called brain drain impacts in developing countries.[84] Shortages of trained personnel stymie the best intentions of foundations, bilateral donors, the World Bank, and other multinational organizations to bring new resources to the problems of AIDS, tuberculosis, and malaria, as well as to vaccine-preventable diseases. Deteriorating or transitional health systems do not adequately support dissemination of effective pharmaceuticals and vaccines. Traditionally inadequate attention to research on diseases of the poor has ignored development of new drugs, vaccines, diagnostics, and other appropriate technology for underserved global populations. One of the main ethical responsibilities of any health research enterprise is to ensure an equitable response to problems that contribute to the main causes of the global burden of disease and to the vicious cycle of ill health and poverty. (See Chapter 21 for more on this topic.) An ethical code for conducting research parallels elements of the NGO Code of Conduct for Health Systems Strengthening.[85] This health systems strengthening code is intended specifically to address international NGOs and their roles in training, securing, and deploying human resources in the countries where they work. There are six areas where NGOs can improve: (1) hiring policies, (2) compensation schemes, (3) training and support, (4) minimizing the management burden on governments due to multiple NGO projects in their countries, (5) helping governments connect communities to the formal health system, and (6) providing better support to government systems through policy advocacy. This code offers sustainable practices in each of these areas

of concern. Likewise, concerns about the selection of research topics, the use of the results, and the dissemination of the results to local academic institutions and communities are increasing. One research group, the Canadian Coalition for Global Health Research, has proposed using a partnership assessment toolkit to enhance the quality of research, improve the exchange of knowledge between counterparts, and further develop research capacity on a global scale.[86]

The imbalance in research investment has been known as the 10/90 Gap in health research wherein 90% of global health research funding is focused on only 10% of the global population.[87] This gap has narrowed in recent years due to increased investment in global health research.

Three main causes for this gap have been identified:

1. Failure of the public sector in high-income countries to allocate funding on the basis of global health priorities
2. Limited capacity for research in many low- and middle-income countries as a result of limited funding, labor, and progressive policies
3. Limited research by the private sector on neglected diseases and determinants resulting from insufficient commercial incentives, although this is changing

Again, Barbara Starfield led the push for primary care research and its essential role in global health systems and the charge to improve equity in health services for the world's poorest and least healthy people.[88] Through the first decade of the 21st century, there were multiple calls for primary care research in global health settings that included the recognition that research should be not only about but also within primary health care.

Included in this primary care emphasis should be community-based participatory research (CBPR). CBPR is a research orientation that equitably involves all partners in the process and recognizes the unique strengths that each partner brings. It has been said that such collaboration is often lacking in many global health research efforts. The advantages of CBPR include:

- Joining partners with diverse expertise to address complex public health problems.
- Improving intervention design and implementation by facilitating participant recruitment and retention.
- Increasing the quality and validity of research.
- Enhancing the relevance and use of data.
- Increasing trust and bridging cultural gaps between partners.
- Providing resources for the communities involved.
- Benefiting the community and researchers alike through the knowledge gained and actions taken.

- The potential to translate research findings to guide the development of further interventions and policy change.[89]

Another refocusing of aid and assistance that supports health care training institutions and infrastructure is found within a Gates Foundation program called "Grand Challenges." This program seeks to fund research that is both community-based and supports the research capabilities and capacity of in-country organizations.

Grand Challenges in Global Health is modeled after the grand challenges ideals formulated more than 100 years ago by mathematician David Hilbert. His list of important unsolved problems has encouraged innovation in mathematics research ever since. Grand Challenges in Global Health will focus on 16 major global health challenges with the aim of engaging creative minds across scientific disciplines—including those who have not traditionally taken part in health research—to work on solutions that could lead to breakthrough advances for those in the developing world.

Since 2003, grants have totaled $458 million for research in 33 countries. It birthed a subsequent program in 2008 from the Bill and Melinda Gates Foundation called Grand Challenges Explorations. This is an agile, accelerated grant initiative with two-page applications and no preliminary data requirement, meant to encourage anyone with a bold idea. To date, 700 Grand Challenge Explorations have been awarded in 45 countries.[90]

RESOURCES, CONTACTS, AND AGENCIES FOR STUDENTS/RESIDENTS

There are many organizations available to those interested in career development in global health. The American Public Health Association, the Global Health Council, the Global Health Education Consortium, the Consortium of Universities for Global Health, the American Society for Tropical Medicine and Hygiene, and nearly all the professional organizations (in pediatrics, family practice, surgery, obstetrics/gynecology, etc.) have global health sections that support student interests as well as professional development in global health.

The classic way that a practicing or newly certified health professional entered a career in global health was through volunteerism. This is less likely to be a successful and rewarding pathway in the 21st century because even the voluntary organizations now prefer people with appropriate experience. For example, MSF will only accept initial volunteers who can provide at least 6 months of service, who have specified clinical training, and who have significant international experience. Experiential learning in professional school may be the best option to gain this experience. With this in hand, voluntary groups will be more confident in the professional's cultural orientation, flexibility, and dedication. Language training cannot be overemphasized, and training acquired in the context of a medical experience would be the best preparation.

Various agencies are actively seeking individuals trained in global health. In the next section some of these groups are considered in detail.

Department of Health and Human Services

Even though the US Department of Health and Human Services (DHHS) is a domestic agency, it has an increasingly important role in global health, with numerous opportunities for career development. Health professionals from across disciplines may serve as Public Health Service (PHS) officers or civilian employees. A partial list of these opportunities includes:

- **The Epidemic Intelligence Service.** This 2-year fellowship in applied epidemiology is conducted by the Centers for Disease Control and Prevention (CDC). It is the main workforce for investigation and program application in public health for DHHS and many US public health leaders are alumni of this program. There is substantial training in basic epidemiology, scientific

---

BOX 22-2. OTHER OPPORTUNITIES IN GLOBAL HEALTH RESEARCH

HIVCorps Internships in Zambia
The American Society of Tropical Medicine Fellowships
Robert E. Shope International Fellowship in Infectious Disease
Burroughs Wellcome Fund/American Society of Tropical Medicine and Hygiene Postdoctoral Fellowship in Tropical Infectious Diseases
Sarnoff Cardiovascular Research Foundation
CDC Epidemiology Elective
Fulbright Program for US Students
The Erasmus Summer Programme
NIH-Duke Training Program in Clinical Research
CDC Foundation
IHCAI Foundation Scholarships and Fellowships Fund
Child Family Health International
Lambarene Schweitzer Fellows Program
The Global Health Fellows Program (GHFP)
TDR Clinical Research & Development Fellowships
American Society for Microbiology Fellowships[91]

Source: Fogarty International Center Website, http://www.fic.nih.gov/

writing, epidemiologic investigation, analysis, and program evaluation. Substantial international opportunities within the training involve outbreak investigation, HIV/AIDS, malaria, emerging infections, surveillance, immunizations, and other subjects. Although this program is directed to US citizens, international applicants may qualify for a fellowship that essentially duplicates the experience.[92]

- **Fogarty International Center, NIH.** This is the international component of the NIH; it addresses global health challenges through innovative and collaborative research and training programs and supports and advances the NIH mission through international partnerships. It supports research grants (with collaboration from other NIH institutes), international training programs, regional exchanges of information, and supports specific projects such as the Disease Control Priorities Project (DCPP) and the Multilateral Malaria Initiative, as well as the Fogarty-Ellison International Fellowship.[93]

- **US Public Health Service.** As one of the seven Uniformed Services of the United States, the Corps is a specialized career system designed to attract, develop, and retain health professionals who may be assigned to federal, state, or local agencies or international organizations. Headed by the surgeon general, it is a personnel system that integrates within DHHS and other federal agencies (such as the Coast Guard, National Oceanographic and Aeronautic Administration, CDC, NIH, Indian Health Service, Food and Drug Administration, and Health Resources and Services Administration). PHS officers are often deployed in response to emergencies and crises abroad; they may serve as EIS officers in the CDC. As in the military, this is a 20-year career for retirement purposes (less service does not count toward retirement), with good training, benefits, and support for career development.

- **Office of Global Health Affairs (Formerly Office of International and Refugee Health).** This staff office to the secretary of DHHS represents the department to other governments, other federal departments and agencies, international organizations, and the private sector on international and refugee health issues. It develops US policy and strategy positions related to health issues and facilitates collaborative involvement of the US PHS in support of these positions and organizations. Nearly all agencies within DHHS have international offices or key officials focusing on global health—coordinated by this office; thus within specific agencies there are global health opportunities serving departmental interests. (www. globalhealth.gov).[94]

- **Global Health Service Corps.** As discussed in an earlier section, this previously planned entity is an NGO that will be working with the Peace Corps office to place experienced physicians and nurses in academic institutions for the purpose of training a local provider work force. The first three countries will be staffed in July 2013.

USAID/Department of State/Peace Corps

The US Agency for International Development (USAID) is an independent federal government agency that receives overall foreign policy guidance from the secretary of state. Its work intends to support long-term and equitable economic growth by advancing US foreign policy objectives for economic growth, agriculture, and trade; global health; and democracy, conflict prevention, and humanitarian assistance. The Bureau of Global Health within USAID provides leadership to improve the quality, availability, and use of essential health services. It focuses on HIV/AIDS, other infectious diseases (such as tuberculosis and malaria), maternal and child health, family planning, environmental health, and nutrition. Much of this work is done through competitively awarded contracts to NGOs and some US government agencies such as the CDC and USPHS. For example, PHS officers serve in the Office of Foreign Disaster Assistance at USAID, coordinating across agencies for support to disaster and postconflict situations. Career opportunities may be direct or through contractors and DHHS agencies.[95]

USAID is gradually becoming more closely integrated with the US Department of State (DOS), the foreign policy arm of the US government. Within this agency, there are rare opportunities for global health careers, but there are clinical opportunities for physicians, nurses, and midlevel practitioners within DOS international facilities, primarily serving DOS employees and programs abroad.[96]

The Peace Corps, a branch of the DOS, has an Office of Medical Services in Washington, DC, serving the public health and clinical needs of volunteers. This is supplemented by midlevel health providers stationed abroad as Peace Corps Medical Officers. In addition, the Peace Corps now has an integrated Masters International (MI) Program with several schools of public health, wherein a prospective student will apply simultaneously to both the Peace Corps and the participating graduate school. After being accepted by both, candidates will complete 1 to 2 years of graduate coursework at the respective university while continuing to prepare for work overseas. Each MI Program has its own requirements and will award credit for Peace Corps service accordingly. This is an extraordinary opportunity to acquire a MPH degree (probably not for MD students, but ideal for nursing or midlevel health professionals) while gaining unsurpassed field experience.[97]

Military

Military service may provide numerous opportunities for global health service, research, and training. For example, the US Army Research Laboratories (ARL) include scientists, engineers, administrators, and support staff, all of whom make valuable contributions both to the ARL's mission and to global health. Often, such laboratories and other military services provide crisis response to natural disasters, first-line response to emerging epidemics (e.g., avian influenza), and laboratory support for identification and research on potential bio-pathogens or emerging infections. Postdoctoral research programs are available in military facilities.[98]

Nongovernmental Organizations

NGOs perhaps provide the most extensive opportunities for variety in service, research, and practice. These range from direct clinical service providers to specific program contractors and consultants to bilateral and multilateral organizations. Most require substantial training and experience for employment, and most do not have long-term "hard money" career tracks. The Global Health Council (www.globalhealth.org) was an association of healthcare professionals and organizations that included NGOs, foundations, corporations, government agencies, and academic institutions that work in global health. It is currently being reconstituted after closing its doors in 2012.

Private Voluntary Groups/Faith-Based Organizations

Volunteerism has been the mainstay for short-term, and sometimes career, involvement in global health. This can take many forms including, faith-based or missionary-associated commitments, but also short-term response to emergencies and crises as well as specific clinical specialty needs such as in ophthalmology, maxillofacial surgery, orthopedic and reconstructive surgery, and cardiac surgery. MSF is perhaps the quintessential private voluntary relief group, having won the Nobel Peace Prize in 1999 as well as many other international awards. Its focus—like that of the International Rescue Committee, Oxfam, and Save the Children—is generally on crisis and humanitarian urgencies with some longer term programs meant to improve the standards of health in a variety of impoverished countries.

Contractors

Private, for profit, or not-for-profit groups may act as contractors for donor organizations, multilateral organizations, and governments to carry out specific projects in global health. The headquarters for many of these organizations may be found close to Washington, DC, or near UN agency headquarters in New York and elsewhere. Some, such as Family Health International, are large organizations that focus on a particular area (reproductive health); others specialize in government-funded projects, often blurring the boundaries between government agencies and the private sector. Many were members of the Global Health Council. Employment is largely task specific, and consortia of universities, individuals, or other companies may be formed in response to task orders to respond to specific needs of the funding agencies. One may obtain a flavor of the range, quantity, and complexity of USAID contractors by accessing the USAID Yellowbook, a compendium of awarded contracts in a given year.[99]

Multinational Organizations

Multinational organizations are those composed of member states (countries), either under the United Nations auspices, or through some other basis of affiliation such as defense or economic cooperation. Career opportunities are difficult to obtain within these organizations, but many have "Young Professional" entry programs, internship opportunities, and opportunities for secondments from government or other agencies through interagency personnel agreements. In many cases, consultants are brought into the agencies as a result of valuable contributions through contractual relationships.

UN Organizations

The United Nations is the world's largest international employer. Over 60,000 staff members come from all over the world, including about 4,500 from the United States. Among them are health professionals such as sanitarians, physicians, sociologists, nurses, health economists, and health system managers. UN staffing levels are determined by member state contributions and nonbudgetary support as well as cultural integration. The United Nations is a complex array of organizations, commissions, and councils, many with a health focus.

The World Health Organization (WHO) (www.who.int), the United Nations Children's Fund (UNICEF), the United Nations Development Programme (UNDP), and other health-related multinational agencies are separate autonomous organizations related to the United Nations by special agreements. They have their own membership, legislative and executive bodies, secretariats, and budgets, but they work with the UN and with each other through the Economic and Social Council. Although UN staff are found in nearly every country, the majority work in New York at UN headquarters, and in regional or agency headquarters' offices in Bangkok, Cairo, Copenhagen, Geneva (WHO), Harare, Manila, Montreal, Nairobi, New Delhi, Paris, Rome, Vienna, and Washington (Pan-American Health Organization [PAHO]). There are official and unofficial quotas for Americans in these organizations, owing in part to the influence of the world's largest economy on almost all decision making. There is a conscious effort by the secretariats of these groups to involve Part II countries (developing economies) rather than be influenced predominantly by Part I countries (developed economies).

One of the most important components of the WHO is the GHWA. The alliance was created in 2006 as a common platform for action to address the health crisis. The alliance is a partnership of national governments, civil society, international agencies, finance institutions, researchers, educators, and professional associations dedicated to identifying, implementing, and advocating for solutions.

Most professional positions require an advanced degree, competency in at least two official UN languages (Arabic, Chinese, English, French, Russian, and Spanish), and several years of specialized professional experience, much of it gained from service in a particular country or region. Types of employment in UN organizations are usually divided into (1) professional positions and (2) experts and consultants. The experts and consultants are hired for a short term to provide technical advice on specific projects in developing countries. The United Nations and many of its organizations have their own standard application form, although most now accept individual résumés or CVs, and many applications can be filled out online (www.jobs.un.org). Some assistance may be provided to US citizens through the DOS (http://www.state.gov/p/io/empl/).

World Bank

The World Bank, headquartered in Washington, DC, with 7,000 employees, focuses on poverty alleviation, and with it, health and human development (www.worldbank.org). It works closely with UN agencies and health ministries of member states. Founded as the International Bank for Reconstruction and Development in the wake of World War II, and governed by a board of directors with voting power based on gross domestic product, it has assumed the dominant global role in health development financing since the early 1990s. This role grew from the 1993 World Development Report, an annual Bank report that focused for the first time on how health and economic development were inextricably linked. With a loan portfolio of more than $20 billion, and at least $2.5 billion devoted to health-related projects, the World Bank influences health policy and works with

other partners to support key health interventions. Many of these interventions center around health systems development, but public health projects, including infectious diseases, tobacco control, injuries, and mental health have all received investment. The Bank has health professional staff as part of the Human Development Network, with both central office resources and country team professionals who develop health projects.

Research is an extensive Bank activity, especially in health economics, macroeconomics and health, and evidence-based health interventions. The Bank has a Young Professionals program that occasionally admits physicians but requires substantial economics training for these applicants. Consultants have an important role in both project development and implementation. These consultants may be NGO employees, university faculty, for-profit companies, or simply individuals with personal contacts within the Bank.[100]

Others

Economic multinational organizations such as the Organization for Economic Co-operation and Development (OECD), with 30 member countries, are committed to the global market economy. Their interests cover economic and social issues from macroeconomics, to trade, education, development, and science and innovation. Health and economics are invariably intertwined, with development dependent on health, and with health expenses and values increasingly of concern to both developed and developing countries. Health economists play a key role in the analyses and publications produced by such organizations, and these publications may drive global health policy and financing. Jeffry Sachs, a key promoter of the Millennium Development Goals, is an economist and uses these theories to push for rapid correction of global health inequities.

Another example is the Asia-Pacific Economic Cooperation (APEC), which has a Health Task Force dedicated to sharing information and responding to emerging health issues that directly affect trade, movement of people, tourism, and economic development. Severe acute respiratory syndrome (SARS) and avian flu are of particular interest, and health consultants have been mobilized to help address these regional global health problems.

The World Trade Organization (WTO) is the global international organization dealing with rules of trade between nations. The WTO agreements are negotiated and signed by the bulk of the world's trading nations and ratified in their parliaments. The goal is to help producers of goods and services, exporters, and importers conduct their business. Often, rules on intellectual property rights, especially regarding essential health drugs, may play an important part in health. Although there is no significant representation by health officials in the WTO, there is considerable input by health ministries and health organizations concerned with emergency responses to health crises and health inequity due to lack of availability of essential medicines.

The Network: Towards Unity for Health (TUFH) is an academic-oriented NGO in an official relationship with the WHO. Started over 30 years ago during the era of primary health care, TUFH has a primary goal of fostering community-oriented innovations that lead to curriculum reforms in health and medical institutions around the globe. TUFH has over 200 member institutions, organizations and individuals—many from developing countries.[101]

Academia

Research, training, and consultation are all important career tracks for academic health professionals. The range of subjects is limitless, and often academic health professionals may combine occasional work abroad with an active clinical practice. However, international health research in the 21st century may require more specific training in health diplomacy, cultural understanding, health economics, and area studies to prepare researchers and trainers for appropriately collaborative research. Training opportunities in tropical medicine, laboratory diagnostics, vector control, and public health practice are especially important to potential global health research professionals, and these subjects have not been adequately addressed by existing institutions. Thus some have proposed the establishment of a new academic institution that would provide interdisciplinary training for the next generation of global health scientists.[97]

The Global Health Education Consortium (GHEC) has served as an important clearinghouse and networking site for all things global health. Established in 1991, it has offered guidebooks, teaching modules, annual conferences, and a place for programs to announce activities related to global health work and learning (http://www.ghec.org). GHEC has now been folded into the Consortium of Universities for Global Health (CUGH), but the Website still offers tremendous resources for students, residents, and faculty. CUGH continues to hold an annual conference and aims to:

- Define the field and discipline of global health
- Standardize required curricula and competencies for global health
- Define criteria and conditions for student and faculty field placements in host institutions
- Provide coordination of projects and initiatives among and between resource-rich universities and less-developed nations and their institutions

CUGH is dedicated to creating balance in resources and in the exchange of students and faculty between institutions in rich and poor countries. It recognizes the importance of equal partnership between the academic institutions in developing nations and their resource-rich counterparts in the planning, implementation, management, and impact evaluation of joint projects.[102]

Given the new philanthropy in global health research and practice, the interests of students, residents, research scientists, and faculty in service and global health equity, and the demands of a globalized economy, academic careers will increasingly focus on global health, and academia must respond with appropriate curriculum, administrative support, and opportunities. The careers on the near and distant horizon in academic global health are exciting, without bounds, and within reach to those who seek them out. We hope this chapter has whetted the appetite of today's students who will be tomorrow's global health leaders.

STUDY QUESTIONS

- Why is there an increasing focus on making global health education programs and initiatives interdisciplinary? What hurdles to this collaboration exist in our current educational institutions and practice models?
- The competencies necessary for a global health expert go well beyond the traditional biomedical knowledge emphasized in medical school curricula. What are some of the important competencies and professional domains for a global health expert?
- Global health workforce migration occurs in two directions—from poorer to richer countries and vice versa. Contrast the motivations behind these two types of migration.
- What is the 10/90 gap, and why does it exist?
- The Global Health Workforce Alliance was begun in 2006 to address workforce needs around the globe. If you could create an organization that would address the global health workforce challenge, what would your organization be called, what would be its mission, and how would it achieve this mission?

ACKNOWLEDGEMENT

Dr. Thomas Novotny authored this chapter in the previous edition of this text. Some content from the earlier version has been used in this updated version of the chapter, and we would like to acknowledge Dr. Novotny's valuable contributions.

REFERENCES

1. Merson M, Page K. *The Dramatic Expansion of University Engagement in Global Health: Implications for US Policy.* Washington, DC: Center for Strategic and International Studies, 2006. Consortium of Universities for Global Health, http://www.cugh.org/.

2. Patrick W. The Asia Pacific Academic Consortium for Global Public Health and Medicine: stabilizing south-south collaboration. *Infect Dis Clin N Am* 2011;25:537–554.

3. Frenk J, Chen L, Bhutta Z, et al. Health professionals for a new century: transforming education to strengthen health systems in an interdependent world. *Lancet* 2010;376:1923–1958.

4. Global Consensus for the Social Accountability of Medical Schools. December, 2010. http://healthsocialaccountability.sites.olt.ubc.ca/files/2011/06/11-06-07-GCSA-English-pdf-style.pdf.

5. The Training for Health Equity Network. *THEnet's Social Accountability Evaluation Framework Version 1. Monograph I.* Baisy-Thy, Belgium: The Training for Health Equity Network, 2011.

6. Panosian C, Coates T. The new medical "missionaries"—grooming the next generation of global health workers. *N Engl J Med* 2006;354(17):1771–1773.

7. Schroeder S. We can do better—improving the health of the American people. *N Engl J Med* 2007;357:1221–1228.

8. The Global Health Workforce Alliance, 2012, WHO. http://www.who.int/workforcealliance/about/en.

9. The Global Workforce Alliance and the Kampala Declaration, 2010, WHO. http://www.who.int/workforcealliance/knowledge/resources/kampala_declaration/en/.

10. Koplan J, Bond C, et al. Towards a common definition of global health. *Lancet* 2009;373:1993–1995.

11. Chen M. The contribution of primary health care to the Millennium Development Goals. Buenos Aires: World Health Organization, 2007. http://www.who.int/dg/speeches/2007/20070816_argentina/en/index.html.

12. Africa 'being drained of doctors.' BBC News, 2008. http://newsvote.bbc.co.uk/mpapps/pagetools/print/news.bbc.co.uk/2/hi/health/7178978.stm.

13. Institute of Medicine of the National Academies. *Healers Abroad: Americans Responding to the Human Resource Crisis in HIV/AIDS report brief.* Washington, DC: National Academies Press, 2005.

14. Peace Corps. The Peace Corps now accepting applications for Global Health Service Partnership Positions. 2012. http://www.peacecorps.gov/resources/media/press/2092/.

15. Mullan F, et al. The Medical Education Partnership Initiative: PEPFAR's effort to boost health worker education to strengthen health systems. *Health Affairs* 2012;31(7):1561–1572.

16. Global Health Service Corps. Building Capacity through Health Service. Boston, 2012. http://globalhealthservicecorps.org/need-by-the-numbers.

17. McNeil D. *Africa: $130 million from United States to train doctors in a dozen countries.* New York Times, 2010. http://www.nytimes.com/2010/10/12/health/12global.html.

18. Strauss R. *Too many innocents abroad.* New York Times, 2008. http://www.nytimes.com/2008/01/09/opinion/09strauss.html.

19. Education Commission for Foreign Medical Graduates (ECFMG), 2012. www.ecfmg.org.

20. African Journal of Primary Health Care and Family Medicine (PHCFM) http://www.phcfm.org.

21. Primafamed Africa Network. http://www.primafamed.ugent.be.

22. De Maesseneer J. Primary health care in Africa: now more than ever! *Afr J Prm Health Care Fam Med* 2009;1(1): Article112.

23. Davies A. Health care worker migration: Why should we care? *Migration,* March 2006:15–18. http://publications.iom.int/bookstore/index.php?main_page=product_info&cPath=40&products_id=465.

24. ECFMG-Fact Card Summary Data, 2012. http://www.ecfmg.org/forms/factcard.pdf.

25. Connor G. Cuba's Latin American Medical School: can socially-accountable medical education make a difference? *MEDICC Rev* 2012;14(3):5–11.

26. Canadian Coalition for Global Health Research (CCGHR). www.ccghr.ca.

27. Stigler F, et al. Health professionals for the 21st century: a student's view. *Lancet* 2010;376:1877–1878.

28. Peluso M, et al. Guiding principles for the development of global health education curricula in undergraduate medical education. *Med Teach* 2012;34(8):653–658.

29. Bozorgmehr K, Saint V, Tinnemann P. The 'global health' education framework: a conceptional guide for monitoring, evaluation and practice. *Global Health* 2011;7:8.

30. Evert J, Chase J, eds. *Graduate Medical Education in Global Health: A Guidebook.* 2nd ed. Global Health Education Consortium, 2011.

31. Lewin SA, et al. Lay health workers in primary and community health care. Cochrane Database Syst Rev 2005: CD004015.

32. Brown A, Cometto G, Cumbi A, et al. Mid-level health providers: a promising resource. *Rev Peru Med Exp Salud Publica* 2011;28(2):308–315.

33. Petroze R, et al. Collaboration in surgical capacity development: a report of the inaugural meeting of the Strengthening Rwanda Surgery Initiative. *World J Surg.* In press.

34. Glasper A. Escaping the ivory tower: emancipation of the modern clinical academic. *Br J Nurs* 2012;21(8):496–497.

35. Kolars J. Taking down 'the ivory tower': leveraging academia for better health outcomes in Uganda. *BMC Int Health Hum Rights* 2011;11(Suppl 1): S1.

36. Gugushe T. Beyond the ivory tower: service learning for community engagement. *SADJ* 2010;65(3):138, 140.

37. Schur C, Berk M, Silver L, et al. Connecting the ivory tower to main street: setting research priorities for real-world impact. *Health Aff (Millwood)* 2009;28(5):w886–w899.

38. Eichbaum Q, Nyarango P, Bowa K, et al. Global networks, alliances and consortia in global health education—the case for south-south partnerships. *J Acquir Immune Defic Syndr* 2012; 61(3):263–264.

39. Chen C, Buch E, Wassermann T, et al. A survey of Sub-Saharan African medical schools. *Hum Resour Health* 2012;10:4.

40. Kasper J, Bajunirwe F. Brain drain in sub-Saharan Africa: contributing factors, potential remedies, and the role of academic medical centres. *Arch Dis Child* 2012;97(11):973–979.

41. Frank J, Snell L, Cate O, et al. Competency based medical education: theory to practice. *Med Teach* 2010;32(8):638–645.

42. Brewer T, Saba N, Clair V. From boutique to basic: a call for standardized medical education in global health. *Med Educ* 2009;43(10):930–933.

43. Battat R, Seidman G, Chadi N, et al. Global health competencies and approaches in medical education: a literature review. *BMC Med Educ* 2010;10:94.

44. Peluso M, et al. Guiding principles for the development of global health education curricula in undergraduate medical education. *Med Teach* 2012;34(8):653–658.

45. Houpt E, Pearson R, Hall T. Three domains of competency in global health education: recommendations for all medical students. *Acad Med* 2007;82(3):222–225.

46. Association of Faculties of Medicine of Canada Resource Group on Global Health. Creating Global Health Curricula for Canadian Medical Students. Report of the AFMC Resource Group on Global Health, 2007. http://www.afmc.ca/pdf/pdf_2007_global_health_report.pdf.

47. University of Maryland. Graduate Medical Education: ACGME Competencies. Baltimore, MD: University of Maryland, 2008. http://www.umm.edu/gme/core_comp.htm.

48. Evert J, Stewart C, Chan K, Rosenberg M, Hall T. *Developing Residency Training in Global Health: A Guidebook*. San Francisco: Global Health Education Consortium, 2008.

49. American Academy of Family Physicians (AAFP). *Recommended Curriculum Guidelines for Family Medicine Residents, Global Health*. American Academy of Family Physicians, Reprint 287, 2011. http://www.aafp.org/online/etc/medialib/aafp_org/documents/about/rap/curriculum/globalhealth.Par.0001.File.tmp/Reprint287.pdf.

50. Anspacher M, Hall T, Herlihy J, et al. Competency-based global health education. In: Chase J, Evert J, eds. *Global Health Training in Graduate Medical Education: A Guidebook*. 2nd ed. San Francisco: Global Health Education Consortium, 2011.

51. Royal College of Physicians and Surgeons of Canada. The CanMeds Framework. http://www.collaborativecurriculum.ca/en/modules/CanMEDS/CanMEDS-intro-background-01.jsp.

52. Redwood-Campbell L, Pakes B, Rouleau K, et al. Developing a curriculum framework for global health in family medicine: emerging principles, competencies, and educational approaches. *BMC Med Educ* 2011;11(1):46.

53. Castillo J, Castillo H, Dewitt TG. Opportunities in global health education: a survey of the virtual landscape. *J Grad Med Educ* 2011;3(3):429–432.

54. Anderson K, Slatnik M, Pereira I, et al. Are we there yet? Preparing Canadian medical students for global health electives. *Acad Med* 2012;87(2):206–209.

55. Canadian Federation of Medical Students. Pre-Departure Training, 2012. http://www.cfms.org/index.php/global-health/projects/pre-departure-training.html.

56. Izadnegahdar R, Correia S, Ohata B, et al. Global health in Canadian medical education: current practices and opportunities. *Acad Med* 2008;83(2):192–198.

57. AAMC. Medical School Graduation Questionnaire. AAMC, 2012. https://www.aamc.org/download/300448/data/2012gqallschoolssummaryreport.pdf.

58. Godkin M, Savageau J. The effect of medical students' international experiences on attitudes toward serving underserved multicultural populations. *Fam Med* 2003;35(4):273–278.

59. Mutchnick I, Moyer C, Stern D. Expanding the boundaries of medical education: evidence for cross-cultural exchanges. *Acad Med* 2003;78(10 Suppl):S1–S5.

60. Thompson M, Huntington M, Hunt D, Pinsky L, Brodie J. Educational effects of international health electives on U.S. and Canadian medical students and residents: a literature review. *Acad Med* 2003;78(3):342–347.

61. Hanson L, Harms S, Plamondon K. Undergraduate international medical electives: some ethical and pedagogical considerations. *J Studies Int Educ* 2011;15:171–185.

62. Pinto A, Upshur R. Global health ethics for students. *Dev World Bioeth* 2009;9(1):1–10.

63. Crump J, Sugarman J. Ethics and best practice guidelines for training experiences in global health. *Am J Trop Med Hyg* 2010;83(6):1178–1182.

64. Anderson K, Slatnik M, Pereira I, Cheung E, Xu K, Brewer T. Are we there yet? Preparing Canadian medical students for global health electives. *Acad Med* 2012;87(2):206–209.

65. Anderson K, Bocking N. Preparing medial students for electives in low-resource settings: a template for national guidelines for pre-departure training. AFMC Global Health Resource Group and CFMS Global Health Program, 2008. http://www.cfms.org/downloads/Pre-Departure%20Guidelines%20Final.pdf.

66. Cheung E, Abelson J, Matthews D. Going global: approaching international medical electives as an institution. In: Evert J, Drain P, Hall T, eds. *Developing Global Health Programming for Medical and Other Professional Schools*. San Francisco, CA: CFHI. In press.

67. Marcum J. What direction for study abroad? Eliminate the roadblocks. *Chron Higher Educ* 2001;47(36):B7–B8.

68. Williams T. Exploring the impact of study abroad on students' intercultural communication skills: adaptability and sensitivity. *J Studies Int Educ* 2005;9(4):356–371.

69. Mutchnick I, Moyer C, Stern D. Expanding the boundaries of medical education: evidence for cross-cultural exchanges. *Acad Med* 2003;78(10Suppl):S1–S5.

70. Thompson M, Huntington M, Hunt D, et al. Educational effects of international health electives on US and Canadian medical students and residents: a literature review. *Acad Med* 2003;78(3):342–347.

71. Godkin M, Savageau J. The effect of medical students' international experiences on attitudes toward serving under-served multicultural populations. *Fam Med* 2003;35:273–278.

72. Niemanstsverdriet S, Majoor G, van der Vleuten C, et al. "I found myself to be a down to earth Dutch girl": a qualitative study into learning outcomes from international traineeships. *Med Educ* 2004;38:749–757.

73. Miranda J, Yudkin J, Willott C. International health electives: four years of experience. *Travel Med Infect Dis* 2005;3(3):133–141.

74. Esfandiari A, Gill G. An international health/tropical medicine elective. *Acad Med* 2001;76(5):516.

75. Epstein R. Assessment in medical education. *N Engl J Med* 2007;356(4):387–396.

76. Jones E. Students going abroad for service-learning experiences: questions considered. *The Advisor,* June 2009: 25–29.

77. Kalish R, Dawiskiba M, Sung Y-C, Blanco M. Raising medical student awareness of compassionate care through reflection of annotated videotapes of clinical encounters. *Educ Health (Abingdon)* 2011;24(3):490.

78. Aronson L. Twelve tips for teaching reflection at all levels of medical education. *Med Teach* 2011;33(3):200–205.

79. Belani H, Dempsey K, Stone G, et al. Competencies and assessment. In: Evert J, Drain P, Hall T, eds. *Developing Global Health Programming for Medical and Other Professional Schools*. San Francisco, CA: CFHI. In press.

80. Starfield, B, Leiyu S, Macinko J, et al. Contribution of primary care to health systems and health. *Milbrook Q* 2005;83(3):457–502.

81. Starfield B. Toward international primary care reform. *CMAJ* 2009;180(11):1091–1092.

82. Starfield B. The hidden inequity in health care. *Int J Equity Health* 2011;10:15.

83. Osler W. Remarks on specialism. *Boston Med Surg J* 1892;126: 457–459.

84. Cohen J. The new world of global health. *Science* 2006;311: 162–167.

85. NGO Code of Conduct for Health Systems Strengthening. Seattle, WA: Health Alliance International, 2007. http://ngocodeofconduct.org.

86. Afsana K, Habte D, Hatfield J, et al. *Partnership Assessment Method*. Ottawa, ON: Canadian Coalition for Global Health Research, 2009. http://www.ccghr.ca/Resources/Documents/Resources/PAT_Interactive_e.pdf.

87. Global Forum for Health Research. *Strategic Orientations 2003–2005*. Geneva: World Health Organization, 2003.

88. Beasley J, Starfield B, et al. Global health and primary care research. *J Am Board Fam Med* 2007;20(6):518–526.

89. Office of Behavioral and Social Sciences Research. Community Based Participatory Research (CBPR). Washington, DC: 2012. http://obssr.od.nih.gov/scientific_areas/methodology/community_based_participatory_research/index.aspx.

90. Grand Challenges Explorations. Grand Challenges in Global Health, 2012. http://www.grandchallenges.org/about/Pages/Overview.aspx.

91. Fogarty International Clinical Research Scholars and Fellows Support Center (FICRS-F). Nashville, TN: 2012. https://fogartyscholars.org/resources/global-health.

92. Centers for Disease Control and Prevention. Epidemic Intelligence Service. Atlanta, GA. http://www.cdc.gov/eis/index.html.

93. National Institutes of Health. Fogarty International Center. Bethesda, MD. http://www.fic.nih.gov/.

94. US Department of Health and Human Services. Office of Global Health Affairs. http://www.globalhealth.gov.

95. USAID. Global Health, 2012. http://www.usaid.gov/what-we-do/global-health.

96. Foreign Service Careers. http://www.foreignservicecareers.com/specialist/self_evals/med_jobs.html.

97. Peace Corps. Master's International, 2012. http://www.peacecorps.gov/index.cfm?shell=learn.whyvol.eduben.Mastersint.

98. US Army. US Army Research Laboratory (ARL), 2012. http://www.arl.army.mil/main/Main/default.cfm?Action=3.

99. Contractors: USAID Yellowbook, 2001. http://gemini.info.usaid.gov/yellowbook/.

100. The World Bank. Jobs, 2012 http://web.worldbank.org/WBSITE/EXTERNAL/EXTJOBSNEW/0,,contentMDK:23122244~menuPK:8680050~pagePK:8454306~piPK:7345678~theSitePK:8453353,00.html.

101. The Network: Towards Unity for Health (TUFH), 2011. http://www.the-networktufh.org.

102. Consortium of Universities for Global Health (CUGH), 2012. http://cugh.org/about-us.

Index

interventions, disaster-related, 343–348

key interventions, 343–348

milestones in, 1–2

overview, 1

priorities and humanitarian aid, 339

priorities of medical and, 339

public private partnerships (PPPs), 321

public relations, 413

public service announcements (PSAs), 410

publication bias, 63

public/private partnerships, 453–454

pulmonary tuberculosis, 240

purified protein derivative (PPD) test, 240

PYLL (potential years of life lost), 33

pyrazinamide, 241

Q

QALYs (quality-adjusted life years), 30–31, 35

quantitative buffy coat, 226

quantitative risk assessment, 38

quarantine, 67

quinine, 228

quinupristin-dalfopristin resistant isolates, 293

R

R_0 (basic reproductive rate of infectious diseases), 66

race

and health care inequity, 471–473

and study design, 478

racial profiling, 477

radiological threats, 348–350

radionuclides, 154

radios, 420

radon, 154

rainwater, 144, 153

randomization, 50, 51, 60, 62

rapid impact package (RIP), 281

rapid malnutrition assessment, 172–173

RBM (Rollback Malaria Program), 231

ready-to-use therapeutic foods (RUTFs), 183

real-time evaluations and humanitarian aid, 343

recall bias, 50, 51

recreational water exposure, 151

Red Cross and Red Crescent Societies (IFRC), 330, 428

re-emerging diseases, 287–290

reflective equipment, 303

Refugee Law, 337

Refugee Nutrition Information System (RNIS), 172

refugees, 17–18, 331. *See also* humanitarian work

regional perspective, 451

regulations

antimicrobial use, 297–298

health system, 451–455

relationship information tracking system (RITS), 429

relative risk (RR), 59

relevance of health communications programs, 410

reliability, 69

religion in ethics, 474–475

religious fundamentalists, 465

religious minorities, 352–353

renal dialysis-dependent patients, 355

reproducibility, 69

reproductive and urogenital disorders, 127

reproductive cancer, 101–103

reproductive choice, 79

reproductive cloning, 480–481

reproductive health, 94, 95

reproductive rate, basic, of infectious diseases (R_0), 66

reproductive rights, 473

research

and emergency aid, 343

of emerging diseases, 290

ethics of, 477–478

and global health education, 499–501

scientific, and ethics, 475–476

and social marketing, 416–421

reservoirs, infectious disease, 64–65

resources, financial, 438

resources, human, 200–202

respeto, 411

respiratory disease, 378

responsibility, ethics of, 479–480

retrospective cohort studies, 59

revenue to fund health systems, 449

rickets, 169, 170

rifampicin, 245

rights, 473, 475

Rights of the Child and its two Optional Protocols (2000), 353

ring treatment, 67

ring vaccinate, 345

RIP (rapid impact package), 281

risk aversion, of financing systems, 439

risk factors, 373

and burden of disease, 35–40

for noncommunicable disease, 38, 378–379

risk pooling, of financing systems, 439

RITS (relationship information tracking system), 429

RNIS (Refugee Nutrition Information System), 172

"road to health" chart, 173

road traffic injuries, 15–16, 34, 302–303

Rockefeller Foundation, 148, 453, 466, 470

Rollback Malaria Program (RBM), 231

Roman Catholicism, 465

Ross, J. A., 79

Rotary International, 7

RR (relative risk), 59

RTS, S/AS01 vaccine, 234

rural-to-urban migration, 367, 371–372

RUTFs (ready-to-use therapeutic foods), 184

Rwanda-Canada paradigm, 322

S

Sachs, J. D., 436

Salmonella, 142, 153, 291, 292

Salmonella typhi, 142

salt iodization, 167

Salter scales, 173

SAM (severe acute malnutrition), 180

sanatoria movement, 243

sand filtration, 147, 150

sanitation, 148–151

SARS (severe acute respiratory syndrome), 5, 67, 285–286, 480

SARS CoV (Severe Acute Respiratory Syndrome coronavirus), 285

scald burns, 304